Intravenous Infusion Therapy for Nurses:

PRINCIPLES & PRACTICE

SECOND EDITION

Dianne L. Josephson, RN, MSN

Infusion Therapy Consultant, El Paso, Texas
Nursing Education Consultant Services, El Paso, Texas

(915)-855-6299

THOMSON

DELMAR LEARNING

Australia   Canada   Mexico   Singapore   Spain   United Kingdom   United States

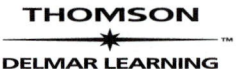

THOMSON

DELMAR LEARNING

Intravenous Infusion Therapy for Nurses: Principles & Practice, Second Edition
by Dianne L. Josephson

Vice President, Health Care Business Unit:
William Brottmiller

Editorial Director:
Cathy L. Esperti

Acquisitions Editor:
Matthew Kane

Developmental Editor:
Darcy M. Scelsi

Editorial Assistant:
Erin Silk

Marketing Director:
Jennifer McAvey

Channel Manager:
Tamara Caruso

Project Editor:
Bryan Viggiani

Production Coordinator:
Kenneth McGrath

Art and Design Coordinator:
Jay Purcell

For permission to use material from this text or product, contact us by
Tel   (800) 730-2214
Fax   (800) 730-2215
www.thomsonrights.com

Library of Congress Cataloging-in-Publication Data

Josephson, Dianne L.
  Intravenous infusion therapy for nurses : principles & practice /
Dianne L. Josephson.-- 2nd ed.
    p. ; cm.
  Includes bibliographical references and index.
    ISBN 1-4018-0935-9 (alk. paper)
  1. Infusion therapy. 2. Nursing.
    [DNLM: 1. Infusions, Intravenous--methods--Nurses' Instruction.   WB 354 J83i 2004] I. Title.
    RM170.J68 2004
    615'.6--dc21
                                              2003013664

NOTICE TO THE READER

Publisher does not warrant or guarantee any of the products described herein or perform any independent analysis in connection with any of the product information contained herein. Publisher does not assume, and expressly disclaims, any obligation to obtain and include information other than that provided to it by the manufacturer.

The reader is expressly warned to consider and adopt all safety precautions that might be indicated by the activities described herein and to avoid all potential hazards. By following the instructions contained herein, the reader willingly assumes all risks in connection with such instructions.

The publisher makes no representation or warranties of any kind, including but not limited to, the warranties of fitness for particular purpose or merchantability, nor are any such representations implied with respect to the material set forth herein, and the publisher takes no responsibility with respect to such material. The publisher shall not be liable for any special, consequential, or exemplary damages resulting, in whole or part, from the readers' use of, or reliance upon, this material.

Contents

UNIT 1

Foundations of Intravenous Infusion Therapy Practice

UNIT ■■■

Intravenous Infusion Needs of the Pediatric and Gerontologic Populations

APPENDICES

IV THERAPY SKILLS

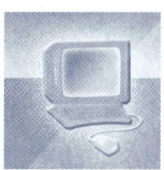 This icon is found next to each skill in the book. It indicates that the skill can also be found on our *IV Therapy Skills* product. Additional skills covered on *IV Therapy Skills* that are not covered in the book are:

Secondary Infusion Setup

Administering Local Anesthesia

Performing Venipuncture for Blood Sampling

Assisting with Insertion of a Central Venous Catheter

CVC Damage and Repair

BOXED FEATURES

Critical Thinking

Nursing Alerts

Nursing Checklists

Case Study/Care Plan

DEDICATION

I dedicate this second edition of Intravenous Infusion Therapy for Nurses: Principles & Practice in memory of my parents, Judy and Jim Diaz, and to all my nursing colleagues who generously dedicate themselves to the care and well-being of others and to all nursing students who will benefit from the material contained herein.

ACKNOWLEDGMENTS

I wish to express my sincere appreciation to those individuals who contributed to the preparation, development, and production of this second edition of *Intravenous Infusion Therapy for Nurses: Principles & Practice*. A special word of thanks is imparted to my loving husband, Rick; my children Jennifer, Jeffrey, and Bethany. To my devoted friends, Charlotte Rowe and Nancy Mattinson, who are always there to share and listen, I am forever grateful. I want to thank, posthumously, my dear friend and colleague, Joan Bury McCollister, who entrusted to me the task of developing the infusion therapy continuing education curriculum, among other courses, at El Paso Community College. It was a joy to work for a person of such integrity and competence and, more significantly, an honor to have our professional relationship evolve into a true and lasting friendship. Special thanks goes to Martha Yee-Nevarez and Cerena Henderson Suarez, the contributing authors for Chapter 15 and 16 of this book, for imparting their knowledge and expertise in the areas of pediatric and gerontologic nursing.

Appreciation goes to the personnel at Thomson Delmar Learning, especially Darcy Scelsi, Developmental Editor, who has been extremely helpful, kind, and patient, and Matthew Kane, Acquisitions Editor, as well as Bryan Viggiani, Project Editor, Cathy Ciardullo, Production Coordinator, and Jay Purcell, Art and Design Coordinator.

The author and publisher would like to thank the following reviewers for their useful observations and notes that were of benefit in bringing this second edition up to date:

Patricia Richter Sipe, BSN, EdM
Howard Community College
Columbia, MD

Catherine Lazo-Miller, MS, RN
Prairie State College
Chicago Heights, IL

Tracy Lynn Collins, RN, BSN
St. Anthony Hospital
Denver, CO

Marty Bachman, BSN, MSN, PhD
Front Range Community College
Fort Collins, CO

Patricia Lavin, BA, RN
St. Anthony Central Hospital
Denver, CO

Appreciation is given to the following companies who provided clinical data, product information, and useful illustrations:

Abbott Laboratoties Hospital Products Division, Abbott Park, IL

AstraZeneca, Wilmington, DE

BARD Access Systems, Salt Lake City, UT

Baxter International, Inc., Round Lake, IL

BD Medical Systems, Sandy, UT

Block Medical, Carlsbad, CA

Braun Medical, Inc., Bethlehem, PA

Clintec Nutrition Company, Deerfield, IL

CONMED Corporation, Utica, NY

Delta Medical Specialties, Division of ARROW International, El Paso, TX

GESCO International, Norcross, GA

HDC® Corporation, San Jose, CA

Infusaid Corporation, Norwood, MA

IMED Corporation, San Diego, CA

Johnson & Johnson Endosurgery

McGaw, Inc., Irvine, CA

Menlo Care, Inc. Menlo Park, CA

Pall Biomedical Products Company, East Hill, NY

SIGMA International, Medina, NY

Deltec, St. Paul, MN

Smith and Nephew United, Inc., Largo, FL

SoloPak®, Boca Raton, FL

Strato/Infusaid, Inc., Norwood, MA

3 M Health Care, St. Paul, MN

United Ad Label, Inc., Brea, CA

Venetec

Venoscope, LLC, Lafayette, LA

VYGON Corporation, East Rutherford, NJ

Preface

Approximately 90% of the patients in acute care settings receive some form of intravenous infusion therapy, and up to 75% of home-bound patients undergo continuous or intermittent IV treatment. The nurse practicing today is accountable for the safety and welfare of a diverse population of patients, most of whom require such treatment. Nursing care, which is based on the nursing process, must incorporate the biologic, physiologic, and physical sciences while approaching the patient from a bio-psycho-social-cultural standpoint. The nurse must adhere to state nurse practice acts and the mandates and guidelines set forth by governmental and institutional groups, maintain strict standards of infection control, and sustain expertise in using new and sophisticated equipment, all while working efficiently under the constraints of time and cost-containment. The nurse is accountable to the profession by adhering to the Infusion Nurses Society Standards of Practice, which define the criteria for nursing accountability in the practice of IV infusion therapy in all health care settings and provide a framework to evaluate the outcomes of nursing care. *Intravenous Infusion Therapy for Nurses: Principles & Practice,* Second Edition, addresses all of these concepts for nurses who deal with patients requiring IV care.

Intravenous Infusion Therapy for Nurses: Principles & Practice, Second Edition, provides the reader with a complete guide to venipuncture and intravenous therapy. While its contents are germane to a broad health care constituency, its format is such that it targets two primary audiences and their purposes. First, it serves baccalaureate and associate degree nursing students (and faculty) by providing a text that is a learning tool with material that is an adjunct to clinical, laboratory, and other course work. It ties together and reinforces the principles and concepts presented in other phases of the curriculum, while introducing all the theories and practical applications of IV therapy in a step-by-step, easy-to-comprehend format with accompanying illustrations and tables. For the second audience, registered professional nurses, it provides a comprehensive reference source and valuable, all-in-one, on-the-job review tool. The concepts presented in this text are relevant to multiple health care fields: hospitals (all areas and services), extended care facilities, freestanding surgery centers, endoscopy and other outpatient care departments, nursing consultant and education groups, medical-dental offices, and the home health environment. It is an excellent reference for nurses in colleges and universities who develop nursing board-approved intravenous courses. It is a versatile reference in that it saves time and effort in looking for intravenous therapy-related information in several different sources.

Intravenous Infusion Therapy for Nurses: Principles & Practice, Second Edition, discusses all aspects of venipuncture and intravenous therapy. Because the text is written for both nursing students and practicing nurses, it gives background information on the process of communication, patient and family education, and the nursing process, and it includes a thorough review of fluid and electrolyte balance. While this may be conventional information for most nursing students, it is often far-removed from many practicing nurses, who may have been away from the academic setting for varying time spans and may be less familiar with some of these concepts. It is also needed because (due to restructuring of the health care delivery system and industry downsizing, as well as nursing shortages in some geographic areas) practical-vocational nurses are becoming involved in intravenous infusion therapy and taking on more and more responsibilities that were formerly carried out only by registered nurses and physicians.

Intravenous Infusion Therapy for Nurses: Principles & Practice, Second Edition, is composed of 16 chapters contained in three units. Unit I outlines the foundations for practice that underlie the intravenous infusion therapy process. Unit II covers all of the actual practice issues associated with IV nursing. Unit III discusses two specialty areas of IV therapy: pediatrics and gerontology.

Each chapter is introduced with a list of measurable learning competencies. Key terms are highlighted throughout the text and are defined in the glossary. A set of key concepts with thought-provoking questions and learning activities, formulated to stimulate critical thinking, conclude each chapter. The appendices provide essential information that often requires extra time and effort to locate.

Chapter 4 is devoted exclusively to infection control guidelines, encompassing the latest recommendations set forth by the Department of Health and Human Services Centers for Disease Control and Prevention, the Occupational Safety and Health Administration, and the Association for Practitioners in Infection Control. With this data, the reader has all the current information necessary to implement IV therapy correctly and in a safe manner.

This book gives complete information regarding intravenous infusion therapy from initiation of treatment through maintenance and discontinuation. It incorporates the legal and ethical implications facing today's practitioner. Categories of fluid and medication administration as well as the delivery of blood and blood products are included. State-of-the-art equipment and instructions for use, with accompanying illustrations, are included. All procedures include the underlying scientific principles and rationales needed to successfully monitor patient care.

While the book deals mainly with the average adult population, two chapters address the pediatric and gerontology populations, since there are increasing numbers of patients being served from these groups. The text, as a whole, provides guidelines of safety for the nurse, the patient, and all members of the health care team. Principles of patient-family teaching and accurate documentation are stressed throughout all portions of the book. The Infusion Nurses Society Standards of Practice are cited as they apply to the specific content areas.

The patient is viewed as a unique, holistic individual, with the family and significant others fully incorporated into the regimen of care. To enhance this view, nursing care plans, utilizing the steps of the nursing process, and case studies are presented along with strategically located Critical Thinking, Nursing Tips, and Nursing Alert displays. Thought-provoking questions stimulate critical thinking and encourage problem-solving on the part of the reader. There are numerous checklists as well as detailed step-by-step procedures and illustrations included for every component of venipuncture and intravenous therapy.

Appendix E, Study Questions for Further Review, is a valuable tool for nursing students preparing for the NCLEX as well as registered nurses who are preparing to take the CRNI certification examination.

It is usually necessary to explore several references to find all of the information needed to answer questions regarding venipuncture or various phases of intravenous therapy.

Intravenous Infusion Therapy for Nurses: Principles & Practice, Second Edition, provides a complete source of information in one book.

NEW TO THIS EDITION

- Reflects the most current INS Standards
- Incorporates the latest CDC infection control standards, including guidelines for hand hygiene and intravenous line antisepsis
- All intravenous skills are highlighted in a step-by-step form, and include rationales for comprehension
- Skill checklists have been incorporated to allow feedback on clinical aspects of care
- New color design enhances visibility
- Most current approved antineoplastic and chemotherapeutic agents

Delmar Learning provides a complete solution to all your intravenous learning needs! Check out these related products:

IV Therapy Skills

Now that you have begun your quest to learn IV Therapy by using *Intravenous Therapy for Nurses: Principles & Practice,* Second Edition, hone your skills further with *IV Therapy Skills*. This unique media product allows the user to practice IV skills in an interactive environment. Walk through each step of the skills in a fully interactive lab with 3D models and animations. Review the nursing process, watch video demonstrations of the skills with real nurses and clients, then proceed to the lab where you can rehearse the skill on a 3D client. You can train in "Learning Mode," which prompts you as you go, or you can train in "Testing Mode," in which you are provided with a case study that simulates real-world experiences.

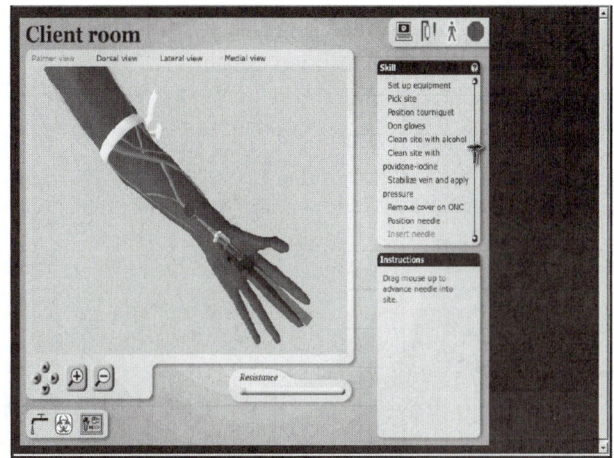

The organization of this program allows the user to comprehend, observe, and take action in IV therapy.

READ IT—An overview of each skill is provided based upon the steps of the nursing process. Animations, photographs, and tables help illustrate concepts. Common Nursing Errors, Nursing Alerts, and Changes of Age are related to further enhance your understanding of the skill.

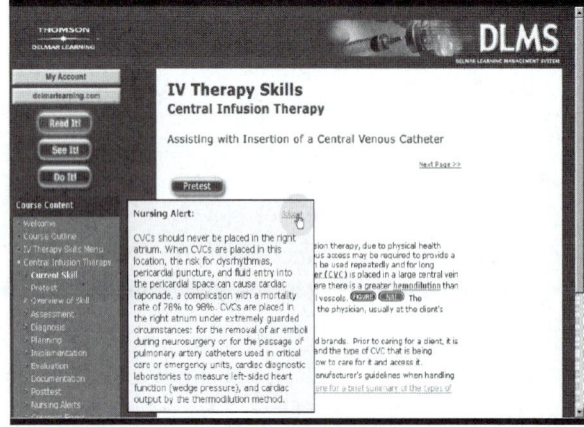

SEE IT—View a video of the skill being performed by a real nurse on a patient. Each step will be reviewed as you see it demonstrated in the video.

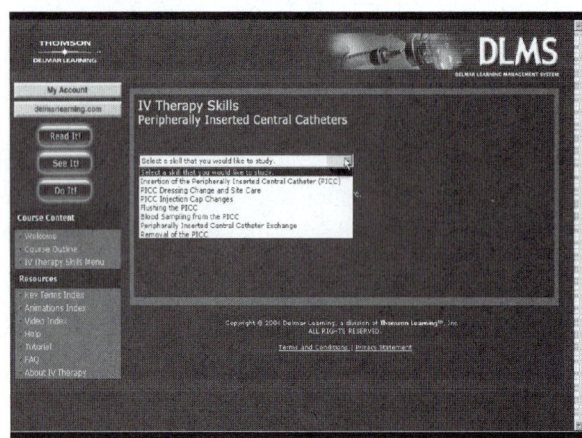

DO IT—An interactive learning lab allows you to perform the skill on a three-dimensional client.

To see a demonstration of *IV Therapy Skills,* go to www.delmarhealthcare.com.

Individual Version (CD-Rom): 0-7668-4010-7
Individual Version (online): 1-4018-5765-5

Institutional Version (CD-Rom): 0-7668-4011-5
Institutional Version (online): 1-4018-5766-3

The Venatech IV Trainer

Still not ready to practice on a real person? Here is the next best thing. The Venatech IV Trainer is a patented IV training device that is so economical you can purchase your own to practice venipuncture skills. No need to waste precious class time waiting your turn. This IV trainer is easily attached to a person's arm so the user can perform venipuncture techniques on a live person, including proper positioning on an actual human arm all without the risk associated with puncturing live tissue. The human interaction allows the user to practice essential communication skills while working with the IV trainer.

The Venatech IV Trainer includes the three main veins used in phlebotomy—cephalic, basilica, and median cubital—all in correct anatomical position. An arterial vessel is present on the trainer for arterial blood gas simulation, and can also be used as a tool for showing how to correct the puncture through a vein into an artery. Go to www.delmarhealthcare.com to see a demonstration of the product.

Light pigmentation trainer ISBN: 1-4018-1580-4
Dark pigmentation trainer ISBN: 1-4018-1582-0
Clear trainer ISBN: 1-4018-1830-7

With Delmar Learning, IV Therapy is as easy as one, two three:

ONE—Read *Intravenous Infusion Therapy for Nurses: Principles & Practice, 2e*

TWO—Practice and explore the interactive IV Therapy Skills CD

THREE—Perform on a real person with the Venatech IV Trainer

HOW TO USE THIS TEXT

The content within *Intravenous Infusion Therapy for Nurses,* Second Edition, has been supplemented with key nursing information designed to structure the learning process and maximize your understanding of the subject matter. The following tools will encourage you to set priorities, analyze clinical situations, apply knowledge, and master procedures.

Case Study

Exemplars from actual practice bring you into the clinical setting and demand nursing action. Each **Case Study** will describe a realistic scenario that requires your knowledge of IV therapy to provide effective nursing care.

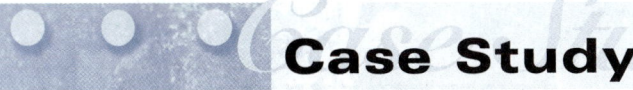

Case Study

COMPOUNDING MEDICATION PROBLEMS IN THE ELDERLY

Case Presentation

A 68-year-old woman in an acute care hospital was experiencing severe pain. She was treated with intravenous morphine sulfate. During her treatment, she complained of nausea, a common side effect of morphine. She was treated with intravenous metoclopramide. She later complained of

itching, another common side effect of narcotics, and received small doses of intravenous diphenhydramine. Urinary retention was also a problem, and she was treated with Urecholine and intermittent urinary catheterization. After several hours, the patient became progressively more confused, agitated, and unable to communicate with family members.

Nursing Diagnosis

Risk for Injury Related to Acute Confusion as Evidenced by Disorientiation and Agitation

Competencies

"What do I need to know?" This common question is answered on the opening page of each chapter. **Competencies** set the goals and expectations for the user upon reading the content that will follow.

C O M P E T E N C I E S

Upon completion of this chapter, the reader should be able to:

✸ Evaluate the dual importance of psychological and physical preparation for the patient in need of infusion therapy.

Critical Thinking

Nursing is a challenging profession because it requires knowledge, physical skills, and the exercise of proper judgment in potentially life-threatening situations. **Critical Thinking** will call upon you to examine your thoughts and actions in light of the responsibilities surrounding IV therapy.

C R I T I C A L   T H I N K I N G

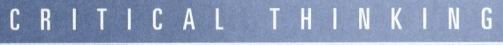

Maintaining Priorities

You are preparing to set up an IV infusion that is ordered stat. The only IV pole on your unit was just used by another patient and is contaminated with splatters of blood. What would you do in this situation?

Key Concepts

Summarizing critical items reinforces one's comprehension level. **Key Concepts** serve as a reminder of the most important material in a given chapter and as a guide for you to re-read any content that may not have been understood.

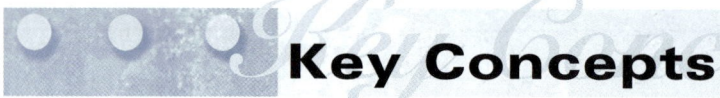

Key Concepts

✳ Physical and psychological preparation go hand-in-hand when administering infusion therapy to a patient.

✳ By using simulation mannequins and training devices, the nurse develops the confidence and dexterity necessary to successfully perform venous cannulation on patients.

Nursing Alert

Because mistakes in calculation and administration often lead to injury or even death, **Nursing Alerts** call attention to the hazards of practicing intravenous infusion therapy.

N U R S I N G   A L E R T

Checking for a Needle in the Patient's Bedding

Do not leave the needle or stylet in the patient's bed. Check before completing the procedure.

Nursing Checklist

The responsibilities of the nurse can seem overwhelming. The **Nursing Checklist** has been created to serve as a reminder of the "must-do" and "must-know" information surrounding the specific topic areas of IV therapy.

N U R S I N G 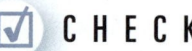 C H E C K L I S T

The Three Checks of Medication Administration

☑ Check the medication as it is removed from its location.

☑ Check the medication with the MAR.

☑ Check the medication before administering it to the patient.

Nursing Tip

Applying a helpful hint received from an experienced nurse can enhance the effectiveness of nursing care. **Nursing Tips** include clinical suggestions, guiding principles, and even key statistics to foster safety and professionalism.

N U R S I N G   T I P

Latex Balloons

Remember, latex balloons, which are often brought to patients in the home or hospital setting, are a source of latex allergy exposure. Mylar balloons should be used instead of latex to protect latex-sensitive individuals.

Introduction

The practice of infusion therapy has become such a considerable component of nursing practice that in 1981 the U.S. Congress proclaimed January 25th as National IV Nurses Day. The majority of all patients receive some form of IV therapy, making it absolutely imperative that the nursing student be introduced to, and become fully acquainted with, all of the major concepts and components of infusion therapy throughout the academic curriculum. The registered professional nurse who is engaged in active practice needs to be thoroughly familiar with all aspects of infusion therapy, and develop competence and maintain expertise in its application. With the plethora of facts and skills the nurse must possess and apply in this discipline, it is imperative not only to have the knowedge but to know where to find the information that is relevant to safe IV practice. With this in mind, *Intravenous Infusion Therapy for Nurses: Principles & Practice,* Second Edition, was written.

The book is sequenced in such a way that it incorporates a review of previously learned concepts with state-of-the-art information that provides the nurse with the material needed for the practice of infusion therapy. The term *patient* (rather than client) refers to the individual in need of nursing care as well as the individual's family and significant others. To avoid any gender bias, the reader will note that use of *he* for patient and *she* for nurse, and vice versa, is interchanged in alternate chapters. The care settings in which the nurse practices infusion therapy are the acute care setting (hospital and free-standing surgical centers), long term care facility (extended care nursing or convalescent home), subacute care unit (intermediate, or step-down from acute care), outpatient department, medical-dental office, home, or the community. The material presented in this text is apropos to any of these domains.

Intravenous Infusion Therapy for Nurses: Principles & Practice, Second Edition, presents accurate information from a holistic perspective regarding the essentials of IV nursing practice all in one source. Special features make the text user-friendly, for both the novice and the practicing nurse. These are conveyed via true-to-life case studies, nursing care plans, problem-solving exercises, and thought-provoking questions. All of the material the reader needs for the safe, effective delivery of infusion therapy is presented in this all-inclusive text, so the time that might otherwise be used to look for information from several sources can be better spent practicing the art and science of nursing.

ABOUT THE AUTHORS

Author

Dianne L. Josephson, RN, MSN

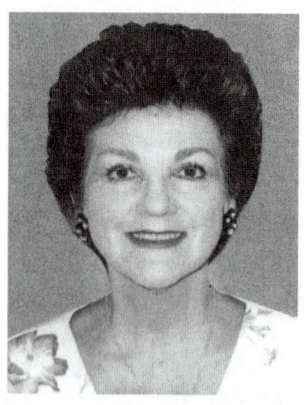

Dianne Josephson is a nurse educator and author, with clinical experience in medical-surgical nursing, infusion therapy, pharmacology, end of life care, and bereavement support. She is currently self-employed as a nursing education consultant and legal consulting expert. Her past employment experience includes Hotel Dieu Hospital in El Paso, Texas, where she worked as a nurse manager, supervisor, and patient/staff educator and the El Paso Community College where she served as a nursing faculty member and clinical mentor in the Health Occupations Division and was employed in the areas of curriculum development and instruction in the Division of Continuing Education for Health and Public Service. She developed and taught an extensive refresher course for inactive registered nurses and provided numerous infusion therapy courses for registered and licensed vocational nurses. Ms. Josephson has also worked as a Clinical Specialist at the University of Texas at El Paso College of Nursing and Health Sciences and has developed and presented numerous nursing education and training courses for hospitals and nursing agencies in the El Paso area. She is a faculty member at Tepeyac Institute, the international Roman Catholic formation center in the Diocese of El Paso, Texas where she presents programs on anticipatory grief and bereavement support. She has advanced training as a bereavement facilitator through the American Academy of Bereavement and is an active member of the Texas Partnership for End of Life Care.

Ms. Josephson is a graduate of Barry University in Miami, Florida where she received her B.S.N. She earned her M.S.N. from the University of Texas at El Paso College of Nursing and Health Sciences. She was selected as a participant in the Master Teacher Project at the El Paso Community College where she also received the Part-Time Faculty Award for Teaching Excellence. She is a member and past officer of the Delta Kappa Chapter of Sigma Theta Tau International Nursing Honor Society, the Intravenous Nurses Association, and is listed in *Who's Who in American Nursing*, *Notable Women of Texas*, *The National Dean's List*, and *The Society of Nursing Professionals*. She has been listed as a Sigma Theta Tau International Media Guide Expert in the areas of infusion therapy, pharmacology, and bereavement support since 1998.

Ms. Josephson is a published author and has been a textbook reviewer for Delmar Learning since 1991, has written articles for nursing journals, reviewed for a variety of publishing companies, and recently developed an interactive multimedia learning program on IV Therapy skills for Delmar Learning. Ms Josephson is currently co-authoring a nursing pharmacology textbook.

Contributing Authors

Martha Yee-Nevárez, RN, MSN, C

Martha Yee-Nevárez is a Pediatric Critical Care Nurse Practitioner in El Paso, Texas. She is a graduate of the University of Texas at El Paso where she received her BSN and her MSN. She received her post-graduate certificate as a pediatric critical care nurse practitioner at the University of Pennsylvania in Philadelphia, PA. Ms. Yee-Nevárez has dedicated her career to critically ill children and has served as speaker for pediatric conferences at an international level. Ms. Yee-Nevárez would like to extend her gratitude to her parents, Martin and Emma Yee, her brother, sisters, nephews, niece, and her husband, M. Bernardo Nevárez for being an inspiration throughout her life.

Cerena Henderson Suarez, RN, MSN, FNP

Cerena Henderson Suarez is a Family Nurse Practitioner in El Paso, Texas. She is a graduate of West Texas State University in Canyon, Texas where she received her B.S.N. She earned her M.S.N. from the University of Texas at El Paso College of Nursing and Health Sciences. Ms. Henderson Suarez is a member of Sigma Theta Tau International, Delta Kappa Chapter. She is a published writer for various nursing journals and has presented nursing workshops and been a speaker for nursing seminars.

Foundations of Intravenous Infusion Therapy Practice

Chapter 1

Introduction to Intravenous Infusion Therapy

COMPETENCIES

Upon completion of this chapter, the reader should be able to:

- ✳ Define nursing accountability as it applies to intravenous infusion therapy.
- ✳ List the five steps of the nursing process.
- ✳ Differentiate between objective data and subjective data.
- ✳ Discuss the components of writing nursing diagnoses.
- ✳ Outline the nursing responsibilities for each step of the nursing process.
- ✳ Explain therapeutic communication as a mechanism of nursing accountability.
- ✳ Describe the teaching-learning process as a mechanism of accountability.
- ✳ Identify the role of the nurse in intravenous infusion therapy.
- ✳ List three indications for venipuncture and intravenous infusion therapy.
- ✳ State three advantages of intravenous infusion therapy.
- ✳ State three disadvantages of intravenous infusion therapy.

KEY TERMS

accountability	label	related factors
assessment	learning	risk factors
communication	long-term goal	short-term goal
database	nursing diagnosis	sign
defining characteristics	nursing process	subjective data
definition	objective data	symptom
evaluation	phlebotomy	teaching
implementation	planning	therapeutic communication

The nurse practicing in today's world is faced with a myriad of duties and responsibilities involving specialized skills and techniques. She is answerable for all decisions and performances associated with the delivery of a safe level of care. It is expected that the nurse function within legal parameters and employer guidelines while utilizing the steps of the nursing process, therapeutic communication skills, and the principles of teaching-learning. For her to practice safely, she must understand the concepts of health and disease as they relate to the total person as a bio-psycho-social being.

Infusion therapy is one of the major responsibilities the nurse faces in her day-to-day practice of nursing and is an area that is continually expanding. "Infusion nursing should be defined as the utilization of the nursing process as it relates to the following: technology and clinical application, fluid and electrolyte balance, pharmacology, infection control, pediatrics, transfusion therapy, antineoplastic therapy, parenteral nutrition, (and) quality assurance/performance improvement" (INS, 2000, Standard 5, S15). The nurse is expected to understand all aspects of such therapy—the indications, expected consequences for the patient, any anticipated side effects or adverse reactions, and all interventions needed to maintain the patient's safety and well-being.

ACCOUNTABILITY AND INFUSION THERAPY

Accountability is the act of being professionally responsible and answerable for one's actions, inactions, decisions, and judgments. The nurse is accountable to herself, her profession, her employer, and to the members of society she serves in the practice of nursing. The patient and his family have the right to expect the highest level of care provided by a qualified individual. The nurse is accountable for doing for the patient what he would do for himself, were he able to do so. In order to do this she must utilize her educational training and background and her professional learning experiences, while keeping up with the ongoing changes in health care through continued learning. The nursing process must serve as the underlying concept for all that she does in the course of her work.

In dealing with intravenous infusions the nurse is accountable for knowing what is ordered, why it is indicated, its intended impact on the patient, and any possible side effects or adverse reactions that may occur. She is expected to prepare the patient physically and psychologically, to administer the infusion correctly, to maintain it, to monitor the patient and support him emotionally, and to discontinue it properly. All documentation and reporting associated with the infusion therapy is her responsibility.

CRITICAL THINKING

Know Your State RN Practice Act Regulations

What does the Registered Nurse Practice Act in your state dictate regarding intravenous infusion therapy by registered nurses? What does your employer's policy and procedure manual state?

The Registered Nurse (RN)

The registered nurse, based on the dictates of her employer and the state in which she practices, is expected to know and understand all necessary policies and procedures needed to safely manage the patients in her charge. In addition, she must often delegate certain nursing tasks to other licensed and unlicensed individuals. These people assist the RN in her duties, but do not act as her substitute. Whenever the nurse delegates nursing tasks, she is still responsible for their safe outcome. When depending on others to carry out certain duties, she must evaluate their competency, instruct them, or verify that they are properly trained. She then must supervise their performance, be available to them for any consultation or assistance, and monitor the patients in their care. "The RN remains accountable and responsible for all delegated tasks and must have clear knowledge of the nursing scope of practice relative to assessment, planning, implementation, and evaluation of infusion therapy, as well as legal responsibilities associated with delegating nursing care activities" (INS, 2000, S8).

The RN also delegates tasks, for the purpose of learning, to nursing students who are unlicensed. This can be done only if the students are enrolled in accredited nursing programs and have had the appropriate course background in the tasks they are to carry out. When performing any invasive procedures, such as intravenous infusion therapy, students should always be supervised by an RN. Even though nursing students and their instructors are present, the RN is still responsible for the patients to whom they are assigned.

CRITICAL THINKING

Know Your State PN/VN Practice Act Regulations

What does the Practical or Vocational Nurse Practice Act in your state dictate regarding venipuncture and intravenous infusion therapy? What does your employer's policy and procedure manual state?

The Licensed Practical Nurse (LPN) or Licensed Vocational Nurse (LVN)

In some states, the practical, or vocational, nurse (LVN) performs duties that are usually only relegated to the registered nurse. Because of downsizing, restructuring, and the nursing shortage in some areas of the country, the tasks of intravenous infusion therapy may be carried out by the LVN. While such duties may be delegated, the responsibility still remains with the RN to whom the LVN reports. When performing these tasks, the practical or vocational nurse must have the necessary preparation and experience, and she must be authorized by her employer and the state where

she works to perform these procedures. Such a nurse may not perform, or attempt to perform, any procedures without the proper training, experience, and the supervision of an RN. Once assignments are accepted and tasks are executed by the LVN, she is accountable for the outcome of her actions or inactions.

The Nursing Process

The nurse demonstrates accountability by using the **nursing process**—the organized and systematized approach to managing nursing care that is composed of five distinct, but interrelated, steps: assessment, nursing diagnosis, planning, implementation, and evaluation (Table 1-1). This tool enables the nurse to administer comprehensive care in a safe, efficient, and thorough manner. The nurse is expected

Table 1-1 | The Nursing Process

STEP	COMPONENTS
Assess	Collect data Take nursing history Perform nursing physical assessment Review records, reports, literature Validatie data Review database
Nursing diagnosis	Analyze data Organize data Formulate nursing diagnosis Validate nursing diagnosis
Plan	Collaborate Prioritize Establish short-term goals Establish long-term goals Write nursing care plan (NCP) Plan for discharge
Implement	Utilize Nursing Interventions Classification (NIC) System Utilize Nursing Outcomes Classification (NOC) System Carry out nursing care plan (NCP) Review NCP Revise NCP Teach patient Explain discharge instructions Document Report
Evaluate	Evaluate goal achievement Reassess Revise NCP (if appropriate) Analyze outcomes Terminate; goals achieved

to understand and utilize the nursing process, then integrate it into everything she does.

Prior to administering care to patients, the nurse needs to be educated regarding the theoretical and clinical components of the nursing process. Such information can be derived from nursing process course work, independent study, or both. While this chapter provides a basic overview, the reader should already have a good working knowledge of the nursing process. The only way such information can be fully understood and internalized is by using it on a regular basis.

Assessment

Assessment is the first step of the nursing process, in which the nurse gathers information about the patient acquired from the nursing interview and history, and the nurse's physical examination (in which the tools of inspection, palpation, auscultation, and percussion are used). This is a thorough investigation in which objective and subjective data are reviewed, sorted out, and organized.

Objective data is information the nurse detects by means of sensory input. A **sign** is the objective evidence of disease. This may include what the nurse sees, the patient's appearance, color and demeanor, and the general condition of his body. It also includes what she externally hears when listening to the patient and what she internally auscultates with a stethoscope. Sensations of warmth, cold, pressure, hardness, and so forth, that are felt or palpated, and any odors emitted from the body or its secretions, are all objective assessment data. Also included in objective data are reports that can be read, such as laboratory and diagnostic studies, progress reports, and the physician's history. Objective data is always measurable.

Subjective data comprises any information the nurse obtains from the patient—any verbalizations regarding his condition. It also includes what his family says. A **symptom** is subjective evidence of disease. It includes opinions, feelings, and beliefs that are communicated.

Once all the information about a patient is gathered, the nurse must review and validate it to be sure that it is accurate. She then can organize and categorize the data to determine any actual or potential problems or health alterations that exist in the patient. Any information that needs to be reported to other members of the health care team to expedite the delivery of care is communicated as soon as possible. All recorded information that the nurse gathers during her assessment makes up the patient's database.

Nursing Diagnosis

Once the assessment is complete and the database for a patient is established, there is a smooth transition into the second phase of the nursing process, where the analysis and synthesis of the collected data begins. During this component, the patient's strengths, weaknesses, and problems are identified and analyzed and a nursing diagnosis is made so that a plan of care can be established. The **nursing diagnosis** is a clinical judgement regarding an actual or a potential health problem or life process that the nurse, by virtue of her background, education, and experience, is legally able to identify and treat. As the professional organization for nursing in the United States, the American Nurses Association has defined the nature and scope of nursing. In 1980 the ANA defined nursing as "the diagnosis and treatment of human responses to actual or potential health problems."

For a nursing diagnosis to be made, the nurse must have an understanding of basic human needs, normal anatomy, physiology, psychology, the social sciences, and the concepts of growth and development. She must be able to identify the deviations from normal processes that result in illness and disease and fine-tune her therapeutic communication skills and observation competencies. The ability to formulate an appropriate nursing diagnosis is dependent on clinical and experiential expertise. The medical diagnosis labels a pathologic state or disease process that the physician treats, whereas the nursing diagnosis describes a human response to a health impairment that the nurse can treat. Whereas a medical diagnosis, once made, is infrequently changed, the nursing diagnosis changes with the patient's day-to-day situation.

When formulating the nursing diagnosis, the nurse takes into consideration all of the signs and symptoms presented by the patient. The North American Nursing Diagnosis Association (NANDA), a group responsible for developing and updating diagnostic categories, has formulated an extensive list of nursing diagnoses that should be used by every nurse in her practice of nursing. Each NANDA category is made up of five necessary components: a label, a definition, defining characteristics, risk factors, and related factors. The **label** or title concisely names the diagnosis so that it corresponds to a pattern of related indicators. The **definition** provides a clear, accurate description that explains its meaning and distinguishes it from comparable diagnoses. The **defining characteristics**, or observable cues, are assumptions that when grouped together present signs of an actual or wellness nursing diagnosis. The **risk factors** are those elements (physiologic, psychologic, or genetic) or environmental considerations that increase the individual, family, or communal potential for an unhealthful situation. The **related factors** are patterned components that connect to the nursing diagnosis in terms of being antecedent to, associated with, related to, or abetting it.

When writing a diagnostic statement (P-E-S), a format that is often used consists of the patient problem (P) (title or label), the etiology (E), and the signs/symptoms (S). The problem statement (nursing diagnosis) is joined to the etiology statement by the phrase *related to* (R-T), which is then joined to the signs/symptoms statement by the phrase *as evidenced by* (A-E-B). An example of a diagnostic statement is, "fluid volume deficit R-T diarrhea A-E-B dry skin and mucous membranes."

Once the assessment data are properly collected, organized, and validated, the nursing diagnosis can be formulated. If the nurse takes the time to do this correctly, the groundwork is laid for the smooth transition to the planning and implementing of care.

Planning

During the **planning** phase of the nursing process, the actual goal-directed nursing care plan is formulated and recorded. This component consists of all the measurable actions that will actually progress the patient toward the desired goal, because his unique individual needs are addressed. It is the link that unites all members of the nursing team (and ancillary care providers) by giving them the specific directions needed to solve patient problems.

Since no two patients are alike, neither are their problems alike; therefore, no two care plans are the same. Each patient's plan of care must be individualized and organized, and have specific, realistic goals that he can meet. In addition, priorities need to be set so that what needs to be done gets done (simultaneously or in order of importance).

In setting priorities appropriately, several lesser problems are usually solved as an indirect result of handling the most important ones first. There are several methods of prioritizing, based on established models or theories. Abraham Maslow's hierarchy of human needs and Erik Erikson's growth and development patterns are models frequently used. Nursing education programs often make care planning policies parallel the philosophy of their program, which may be founded on one of the established nursing theory models. The method used may vary as long as patient goals are realistic and accomplish the desired outcome.

When writing goals, the focus is on what the patient will accomplish, not what the nurse will do. Goals are written so that interventions can be directed toward resolving the problem identified in the diagnostic statement. They must be realistic, specific, and measurable and should be accomplished within a reasonable time frame. Goal statements should include who (subject; patient) is to perform the action, what the action (verb) is, the circumstances under which it will occur, how it is to be performed, and when it should be done. For example, "Mr. Rose will ambulate with his walker around the block, three times a day after meals for the next two weeks."

A short-term goal is one that can be achieved in a relatively short period of time (usually hours or days), such as "will drink 50 cc of water every hour while awake for the next 48 hr." **A long-term goal** is reached over a longer period of time (weeks or months) or is ongoing on a daily or weekly basis. An example would be "will lose 20 lb by June 5" or, "will lose 2 lb/week between March 27 and June 5."

The types of care plans available vary from one facility to another. Standardized care plans that are documented according to protocols are used in many agencies. The Joint Commission on Accreditation of Healthcare Organizations (JCAHO) requires that care plans become a permanent part of the medical record, but it does not dictate the format to be used.

Implementation

The **implementation** phase of the nursing process is closely bound to the planning phase because the nurse now intervenes to carry out the written plan of care for the patient. It is now that she links appropriate actions with the previously stated nursing diagnosis to carry out a treatment strategy. In delivering care, the nurse has to make decisions and prioritize what needs to be done, always allowing for unpredictable changes that may occur.

Just as the nursing diagnosis is a universal means used to describe patient problems, the Nursing Interventions Classification (NIC) provides a care planning tool that describes what the nurse actually *does* to carry out the plan of care. Each NIC is a concise title, or label, that defines the needed intervention for resolution of the problem defined by the nursing diagnosis. The Nursing Outcomes Classifications (NOC) is a comprehensive listing of defined patient outcomes that assist in the evaluation of nursing interventions. An outcome is a quantifiable behavior that is measurable in terms of its response to nursing interventions.

The implementation phase is unique because, in the process of carrying out the care plan, the nurse uses all steps of the nursing process simultaneously. She is continually assessing, reassessing, and evaluating the patient and his situation to determine what is being resolved. She is identifying and diagnosing new or different health alterations, and updating and revising the original written plan of care. During this step of the process, the nurse calls upon her experience, training, and expertise to carry out interventions needed by the patient. She identifies learning needs, carries out necessary patient and family teaching, and participates in discharge planning. She documents in the medical record, collaborates with other members of the health care team, and verbally reports significant data via the appropriate channels of communication. It is here that she validates that the care provided effectively solved the identified patient problem.

Evaluation

The final step of the nursing process is **evaluation**, when the nurse determines whether or not the patient's goals were achieved, and records the outcome. Although this step is stated as a distinct entity, it is actually an ongoing process that begins with the first meeting with the patient. It involves the continuous assessment and reassessment of any variables that influence the patient's progress and goal achievement. It is a dynamic process when the nurse can look at the whole picture and decide whether the plan is correct to begin with, if it needs to be modified, or, if the goals are attained, to terminate the plan. It is the tool that decides whether nursing care is effective and to what degree it is operative.

Communication

Another component that supports the nurse's accountability is her ability and willingness to communicate effectively with her patients and other members of the health care team. The nursing process depends on her skill in communicating verbally, nonverbally, and in writing so that the appropriate interactions and outcomes occur, and she acts as the patient's advocate when he is experiencing health impairments. Every nurse should base her practice on formally learned and practiced communication skills and should periodically update her knowledge and take a self-inventory to determine that she is using such skills to their fullest extent.

Communication is the dynamic interchange of self-expression, emotions, beliefs, information, and knowledge between individuals. All behavior in the presence of another person constitutes communication, whether it is intentional or not. Communication occurs when a message is sent by one individual, received by another, and feedback is then imparted. The mode by which the message is transmitted can be verbal or nonverbal, using various symbols, signals, and vocabulary. The brain receives and interprets the input, then either stores the information for later use or immediately initiates a response (feedback). If any of these components (sender, message, mode of transmission, signals, receiver, and feedback) are missing or deficient, communication is distorted (Table 1-2).

The nurse must always remember that all of her behaviors, whether intentional or not, constitute communication. She must never forget that communication is a potpourri of sensory input and reception and that there is a constant interplay of such factors in each individual's personality that affects communication.

Therapeutic Communication

In all settings there are stumbling blocks to communication, but in the health care setting, any deterrent can be magni-

Table 1-2	Communication Components	
SENDER	**NURSE OR PATIENT**
Message	Explanations
	Inquiries
	Instructions
	Questions
	Teaching
Receiver	Patient or nurse
Mode	Spoken word
	Touch
	Visuals
	Written word
Signals	Distance
	Facial expression
	Gestures
	Odors
	Personal appearance
	Posture
	State of health
	Tone of voice
	Touch
	Vocabulary
Feedback	Demonstration
	Discussion
	Drawing
	Illustration
	Listing

fied. Illness and disease, the presence of unfamiliar people and a strange environment, and various foreign terms and unusual procedures can distort communication tremendously. This is why it is so important for the nurse, or anyone dealing in health care, to use the best communication skills possible, so that a therapeutic goal can be reached. When the nurse uses effective communication skills, she is conveying to the patient a sense of compassion and empathy and offering him the highest degree of respect. **Therapeutic communication** is the planned and goal-directed interchange between individuals that results in a desired and mutually agreed-upon outcome. Communication can also be social in nature, serving to foster the nurse-patient relationship and enhance interaction. What the nurse must always remember, however, is that all of her verbalizations, gestures, expressions, and postures, even if unplanned and unintended, are being communicated with each patient contact.

Fostering Therapeutic Communication

One of the most important assets the nurse has in maintaining therapeutic communication is self-awareness and self-acceptance, that is, the ability to understand her own feelings, to be able to laugh at herself, to know how to take care of herself, and to like herself. Without this, the nurse may seem to be just doing her job, rather than conveying a genuine respect and sensitivity for people she associates with in the practice of nursing.

Empathy is probably one of the most important features that contributes to therapeutic communication. Sympathy is the ability to feel sorry for someone else, whereas empathy is the capacity to mentally project oneself into another's state of being so as to understand and feel what he is experiencing at a particular time, for example, his emotional state, his pain, joy, and so forth. The late Fulton J. Sheen once said, "To work with the sick, one must have two things—a sense of humor and an incision." This is something to think about. Even though the nurse may have never been in a patient's situation, her knowledge of human behavior and health and disease processes, as well as her level of comfort with herself, all enable her to be empathetic.

As mentioned earlier, the nurse needs to understand and use techniques that promote good communication. She must periodically take a self-inventory to evaluate her use of the skills that foster a therapeutic relationship between herself and the patient, and others in her work. She needs to look at her attitudes and beliefs and avoid judgmental, closed-minded behaviors.

Whenever the nurse and the patient are not on the same wavelength, communication can be distorted. The nurse needs to use language the patient understands and to elicit feedback to be sure he is clear on what she is saying and doing. Cultural, social, and religious beliefs must be taken into consideration and respected. Being forceful, authoritarian, and judgmental can hinder communication between the nurse and patient. The nurse must respect the patient by taking care not to talk down to him or his family, thus causing them to feel inferior to her.

Therapeutic Communication and Infusion Therapy

With intravenous infusion therapy, therapeutic communication must exist between the patient and all members of the medical and nursing team so that the patient's safety, comfort, and well-being are not jeopardized. It is the duty of the physician to write clear and understandable infusion orders that are appropriate for the patient. The nurse must have a good working knowledge of infusion therapy and every patient in her charge so that she can verify that the medical orders are correct and appropriate for the patient and that they are carried out properly. She must communicate to all other members of the nursing staff so that everyone is carrying out the orders correctly. It is important to explain and reinforce medical directives for the patient so that he knows what is going to be done and why. She needs to communicate to him his part in complying with the therapy, so he can

report anything unusual. It is necessary to prepare and support him physically and emotionally throughout all aspects of infusion therapy, to document correctly, and to report any untoward reactions using correct communication channels.

The Teaching and Learning Processes

Another important aspect of accountability is the nurse's capability to understand and use the principles of teaching and learning in her work. This is a concept that must be utilized in order to implement the nursing process. **Teaching** is the verbal, nonverbal, visual, or written act of transferring information from one person to another in order to impart knowledge and effect a desired change in behavior. **Learning** is the taking in and processing of information with a resultant change in behavior. While the nurse, herself, must continue to learn in order to be effective, she must also impart to her patient any information that will support the achievement of desired goals and support the plan of care.

Before teaching and learning can begin, the nurse must first assess the situation and evaluate all of the variables that dictate whether the timing is right and what methodology will be used. The patient's developmental and chronological ages, educational history, and life experiences are considered. Until a person sees the importance of and need for any learning, and is physically and emotionally ready, there is no point in teaching, as learning will probably not occur.

After the nurse determines that a patient is ready to learn, she selects the teaching strategy that is most appropriate for him. She investigates what he already knows and by what method he best learns. She then proceeds in a manner that will fit his needs. It is also important for her to determine if the patient has learned the material before and just needs to review it, or if he needs to learn it again, thus trying to break previous habits associated with it. Learning objectives that are measurable can then be developed. As with any outcome, the situation must be evaluated to see if the objectives of learning are met. Therefore, the goals must be written in terms that allow for specific measurement of the results.

Patient Rights and Nursing Accountability

When a person experiences health impairment and enters the health care setting, he may be faced with numerous physical and emotional obstacles. If he is unable to meet his own needs, he has the right to expect that they will be met by the nurse and other members of the health care team. When others act on his behalf, it does not mean that his rights as a unique, autonomous human being are altered.

During illness and disease, when medical and nursing interventions are required, the nurse acts as the patient's

Right to Refuse Treatment

Having fully explained the procedure you are about to perform, you approach your patient with the injection the physician has ordered. As you are about to administer the medication, the patient says, "I don't want the shot." What would you do?

Remember, the adult patient who is mentally competent has the right to refuse treatment. Although it is wise to investigate and find out why he doesn't want this medication, then document and report his response to the physician, you may not force anything on a patient against his will (or it may be deemed assault/battery).

advocate to support him throughout such processes. She is responsible for honestly explaining all procedures to him and monitoring his safety. Even though he may have given previous permission for any care and procedures, he always has the right to change his mind and rescind his authorization for treatment. The nurse must respect this choice whether or not she agrees with it. Under all circumstances she is expected to maintain the patient's dignity through the provision of privacy and by maintaining confidentiality. She imparts a sense of caring and consideration by respecting his cultural and religious beliefs and fostering his independence.

INTRAVENOUS INFUSION THERAPY

As technology rapidly advances, it affects all aspects of the health care industry. One area that has been greatly impacted involves the pharmacologic development of life-preserving fluids and medications, many of which are administered intravenously. Such products are ordered by the physician, but the responsibility for delivering them to patients rests mainly with the nurse. She initiates infusion therapy, maintains it, monitors the patient, and is responsible for discontinuing it.

Indications for Venipuncture and Intravenous Therapy

Although there are numerous risks associated with accessing the venous system, removing blood, or administering any

product directly into the circulating blood, the intravenous route is often the best, or only, route of choice. It is indicated for situations when oral or other parenteral routes are not appropriate. The purpose of venipuncture is to access the venous circulation in order to draw blood for laboratory screens and diagnostic tests or to administer fluids, electrolytes, medications, blood, blood products, and nutritional supplements (Table 1-3).

Fluid Volume Maintenance

Fluid volume maintenance aims to preserve circulatory equilibrium by supplying the body's daily need for water, electrolytes, nutrients, vitamins, and minerals. In many situations the patient's fluid volume is monitored and an infusion line kept in place to maintain the correct circulatory volume if needed. This is often the situation when a patient may have nothing by mouth (NPO) for a short period of time, such as during minor surgical and dental procedures or when undergoing certain diagnostic tests and procedures.

Fluid Volume Replacement

Whenever there is a loss of blood, body water, electrolytes, and nutrients, infusion therapy is indicated as a replacement regimen. Replacement is a critical factor during the life-threatening situations associated with shock, hemorrhage, and severe burns, where there is a drastic loss of fluid volume.

In cases of prolonged nausea, vomiting, and diarrhea, the replacement of both lost fluids and electrolytes is necessary. When there is any type of inflammatory bowel disease, infection, gastrointestinal obstruction, or stasis, intravenous fluid replacement is needed. It is also necessary for malabsorption

Table 1-3 | Intravenous Infusion Access and Therapy

Blood sampling for diagnostic tests
Donor phlebotomy for transfusion
Fluid volume maintenance
Fluid volume replacement
Medication administration
Blood or blood product administration
Nutritional supplementation
To keep a vein open for emergency or special use
Hemodynamic monitoring

syndromes or for people who have gastric or enteral tubes in place for decompression. Two of the most common situations in the hospital associated with fluid loss occur during strenuous labor and delivery and with major surgical procedures.

Medication Administration

Many medications cannot be given orally or by other routes without losing their potency or becoming denatured. These need to be administered directly into the vein over a short period of time or diluted in other infusates and given over several hours. Because of the health status of some patients who might have inconsistent absorption from the gastrointestinal system, medications are given intravenously to achieve consistent blood levels of the drug. Some medications are administered intermittently through a temporary port connected to a venous access device. Many chemotherapeutic agents are delivered by vein because they would be toxic, irritating, or rendered ineffective by other routes. For patients whose muscle mass is reduced because of disease or damaged from repeated injections, drugs that are normally given intramuscularly must be administered intravenously.

Blood and Blood Product Donation and Administration

Phlebotomy is the venipuncture and withdrawal of blood for the purpose of autotransfusion at a later time or for donation and transfusion to others. Although whole blood is rarely given anymore, blood and any one of its components must be administered directly into the circulatory system by special intravenous techniques (see Chapter 14).

Nutritional Support

When a state of negative nitrogen balance exists for any reason and the body is unable to assimilate oral nutrients, nutrition is supplied intravenously. This occurs with anorexia, burns, tumor growth, some malabsorption syndromes, and gastrointestinal disease, among others. High concentrations of dextrose or proteins, fats, electrolytes, vitamins, and minerals are given directly into one of the large veins of the body (see Chapter 13).

Advantages of Intravenous Infusion Therapy

The main advantage of intravenous infusions is to provide an access route for medications, fluids, and anesthetics in emergency situations. It is also ideal for delivering a rapid, even supply of an infusate that can exert a systemic effect in a short period of time. Once a vein is accessed, an indwelling device can be inserted and the vein can be used

numerous times. This alleviates the need for multiple punctures, which are uncomfortable and are a route for infections to develop as a result of breaks in the skin.

For persons who are unconscious or unable to take anything by mouth for long periods of time, the intravenous route is often used, especially when gastrointestinal intubation is contraindicated. It is the route of choice for any products that are irritating to body tissues or are not absorbed orally or by the other parenteral pathways.

Because of new and improved equipment, the intravenous route provides a safe and efficient delivery system. It is convenient and a time-saver for the nurse, especially with the availability of electronic infusion devices (Table 1-4).

Disadvantages of Intravenous Infusion Therapy

While the advantages far outweigh the disadvantages, there are several hazards associated with intravenous infusion therapy (Table 1-5). In some patients, it is difficult to access the vein, causing the patient discomfort and expense because of several cannulation attempts. Fluid overload is always a potential problem and allergic reactions can occur rapidly and without warning. While a medication administered by other routes takes longer to be absorbed and assimilated by the body, anything given intravenously exerts an immediate effect—a potentially fatal consequence if an incorrect drug or overdose is administered. As with any break in the body's skin barrier, the puncture of a vein can lead to a local or systemic infection and sepsis, especially if improper technique

Table 1-4	Advantages of Intravenous Infusion Therapy
Provides a route for emergency access	
Provides a route for the unconscious patient	
Provides a route for the patient who cannot take anything by mouth	
Provides a route during decompression of the stomach or bowel	
Provides a route for the patient with inflammatory bowel disease	
Provides a route to counteract the adverse reactions of other drugs or poisons	
Faster absorption than other routes	
Rapid distribution	
Maximum bioavailability	
Maintenance of controlled blood levels	
Less discomfort for the patient	
Saves time for the nurse	

Table 1-5 | Disadvantages of Intravenous Infusion Therapy

PROBLEM	DEFINITION
Local discomfort	Pain at site of needle or catheter insertion or in the vein from the infusate
Infiltration	The leakage of fluid outside the vein into the surrounding tissue
Needle or catheter displacement	Dislodgement of infusion device
Sepsis	Systemic circulatory infection
Thrombosis	Clot formation
Embolism	Solid, liquid, or gas traveling in the circulatory system
Fluid overload	More fluid than the circulatory system is able to handle
Rapid medication overdose	
Hypersensitivity	Allergic response
Precipitation	Formation of deposits that separate from a solution
Incompatibility with other medications or solutions	
Transmission of human immunodeficiency virus	
Transmission of hepatitis	

is used to initiate, maintain, or discontinue the infusion. There is always the possibility of venous thrombosis or embolism.

One of the greatest risks, for both the patient and the nurse, includes transmission of the hepatitis B, hepatitis C, or the human immunodeficiency virus (HIV) through blood contamination. Because blood is screened and tested prior to transfusion, the likelihood of exposure to these diseases through transfusion is minimal. The risk is greatest from inadvertent needlesticks or improper handling of blood and body fluids. (See Chapter 5 for risks and complications associated with intravenous therapy.)

Key Concepts

* Accountability is the act of being professionally responsible and answerable for one's actions, inactions, decisions, and judgments that are inherent in the practice of nursing.

* The nursing process is the organized and systematized approach to managing nursing care that is composed of five steps: assessment, nursing diagnosis, planning, implementation, and evaluation.

* Communication is the dynamic interchange of self-expression, emotions, beliefs, information, and knowledge between individuals. Therapeutic communication is the planned, goal-directed interchange between the patient and the nurse that results in a desired, mutually agreed-upon outcome.

* The nurse is expected to understand and utilize the concepts of teaching and learning in the practice of nursing. Teaching is the verbal, nonverbal, visual, or written act of transferring information from one person to another in order to impart knowledge and effect a desired change in behavior. Learning is the taking in and processing of information with a resultant change in behavior.

* The nurse who manages infusion therapy is expected to know what is ordered for the patient, why it is indicated, its expected impact, and any possible side effects or adverse reactions that may occur. She is required to prepare the patient physically and psychologically for all treatments and procedures, then carry them out in a safe and correct manner.

* There are numerous indications for venipuncture and intravenous therapy. Accompanying the need for such treatment are several advantages and disadvantages.

Review Questions and Activities

1. Define venipuncture and intravenous infusion therapy.
2. Make an outline of the nursing process. List its five steps and the nursing responsibilities that are associated with each step.
3. Compose a list of objective data and subjective data the nurse might use to assess a patient.
4. Write three nursing diagnoses that might be appropriate for a patient receiving intravenous infusion therapy.
5. Write two goals for each of the three diagnoses listed in the previous question.
6. Construct a flow sheet, diagram, or concept map of the communication process and show how each of the components interact. Illustrate how these can result in therapeutic communication between the patient and the nurse.
7. List three indications for intravenous infusion therapy.
8. Make a two-column list of the advantages and disadvantages of venipuncture and intravenous therapy as discussed in this chapter.

Chapter 2

Fluid and Electrolyte Fundamentals Related to Intravenous Infusion Therapy

COMPETENCIES

Upon completion of this chapter, the reader should be able to:

- Discuss the nurse's role in understanding fluid and electrolyte balance as a prerequisite to safely initiating, maintaining, and monitoring intravenous infusion.

- Define homeostasis.

- Differentiate among the structural and functional differences of the intracellular and extracellular fluid compartments.

- Explain the function of the cell and cell membrane in fluid and electrolyte balance.

- Relate how carbohydrates, lipids, and proteins contribute to cellular physiology.

- Describe the different mechanisms for cellular membrane transport.

- Illustrate the series of events that maintains the cellular membrane potential.

- Compare the three buffer systems in the body and their role in regulating acid-base balance.

- Interpret the physiology of the two acid-base imbalances in the body: respiratory and metabolic.

- Outline the functions of the electrolytes described in this chapter.

- Evaluate how imbalances in electrolyte concentrations in the body affect homeostasis.

KEY TERMS

absolute refractory period
acid
acid-base balance
acidosis
action potential
activator
active transport
adaptation
adenosine diphosphate (ADP)
adenosine triphosphate (ATP)
alkalosis
alopecia
amino acid
anion
baroreceptor
base
buffer
carrier-mediated diffusion
catabolism
catalyst
cation
chloride shift
Chvostek's sign
colloid osmotic pressure
complete protein
concentration gradient
crystalloid osmotic
    pressure
deaminization
dehydration
depolarization
disaccharide
endocytosis
endogenous
enzyme
excitability
exocytosis
exogenous
extracellular fluid
facilitated diffusion
filtration
fructose
galactose
glucose

glycogen
glyconeogenesis
homeostasis
hydraulic pressure
hydrogen ion acceptor
hydrogen ion donor
hydrophilic
hydrophobic
hydrostatic pressure
hypercalcemia
hypercapnia
hyperchloremia
hyperkalemia
hypermagnesemia
hypernatremia
hyperosmolar
hyperphsophatemia
hypertonic
hypertonic dehydration
hypocalcemia
hypochloremia
hypokalemia
hypomagnesemia
hyponatremia
hypophosphatemia
hyposmolar
hypotonic
hypotonic dehydration
incomplete protein
internal environment
interstitial fluid (ISF)
intracellular fluid (ICF)
intravascular fluid (IVF)
ion
ion channel
irritability
isosmolar
isosmotic
isotonic
isotonic dehydration

lipid
lymph
lysosome
membrane potential
milliequivalent
monosaccharide
net diffusion
net filtration
neutralization
noncarrier-mediated transport
nonelectrolyte
nonvolatile (fixed) acid
nucleolus
oliguria
oncotic pressure
osmolality
osmolarity
osmosis
osmotic pressure
oxidation
paresthesia
passive (simple) diffusion
passive transport
pH (potential of hydrogen)
phagocytosis
phosphorylation
pinocytosis
plasma
polar molecule
polydipsia
polysaccharide
polyuria
potential difference
protein
protoplasm
reaction-specific
relative refractory period
repolarization
resting membrane potential
salt

serum	solvent	Trousseau's sign
sodium-potassium gates	surfactant	vacuole
sodium-potassium pump	threshold potential	valence
solute	transcellular fluid (TSF)	vertigo
solution	transport proteins	volatile acid

Whenever the nurse is providing care to a patient, it is his duty to intervene in such a way so as to safely promote or restore her comfort and well-being. He is responsible for supporting her bio-psycho-social integrity through independent nursing actions, by carrying out dependent actions based on medical directives, and through interdependent actions.

When the patient's condition warrants intravenous medication and infusion therapy, the nurse is responsible for knowing why such interventions are necessary and how they will affect the patient. He is expected to understand the pathophysiology of her fluid and electrolyte and acid-base status and relate it to her need for intravenous intervention.

Under no circumstances should the nurse ever perform any procedure or administer any product unless he knows what it is, why it is ordered, and how it will affect the patient. Once treatment is initiated, he is responsible for continual assessment and evaluation of the patient's progress, the status of her laboratory and diagnostic results, and her response to treatment. Should there be any questions or concerns, the nurse must define the problem(s), consult his resources appropriately, and determine how to rectify the situation. He is responsible for documenting all care and patient responses and reporting and recording any untoward occurrences. The nurse is accountable to the patient and must provide for her comfort and safety at all times.

This chapter provides a review and overview of the basic principles of fluid and electrolyte balance and imbalance that serve as the basis for understanding and safely managing infusion therapy. The content contained herein integrates and builds on the knowledge learned in biology, anatomy, physiology, chemistry, and physics.

The nurse who initiates, maintains, and monitors intravenous infusions must comprehend the concepts and principles of fluids and electrolytes as well as their relationship to the physiology of health, illness, and disease processes. Such knowledge is a prerequisite for the provision of safe patient care. Because imbalances can occur suddenly, the nurse must be alert to such changes and intervene appropriately, in a timely manner. Communication with the patient, astute observation of her condition, knowledge of her history and disease, along with frequent review of laboratory values, diagnostic tests, medication, and parenteral fluid orders, are all critical assessment factors.

FLUIDS AND HOMEOSTASIS

The nineteenth-century French physiologist, Claude Bernard, originated the concept that the *milieu intérieur*, or **internal environment**, of the body, which remains relatively constant despite external environmental changes, is formed by the fluids that surround and bathe all body cells. These fluids, which make up the extracellular fluid, communicate with the body's organs, tissues, and structures to make exchanges with the body's external surroundings, thus contributing to a state of balance and stability.

The human body normally undergoes a continuous series of self-regulating adjustments to maintain a balance between its internal environment and the external forces that affect it. The physiologic term for this dynamic process that contributes to a state of internal constancy is called **homeostasis**. Homeostasis, along with **adaptation**, the process whereby the body adjusts to the ever-changing environment, serves to keep the human body functioning well despite changes in its surroundings. When any component of the internal environment deviates from its normal state, homeostasis is jeopardized and illness ensues.

The term *homeostasis*, when first introduced by the physiologist W. B. Cannon in 1926, referred to a relatively stable state of internal equilibrium as well as the coordination of all bodily processes that contribute to such balance. Since then, the definition of homeostasis has evolved to include the constancy and coordination of the human being as a dynamically integrated organism, encompassing the biologic, physiologic, psychologic, sociocultural, and religious aspects of the person.

Water

Water is the primary chemical component within the human organism and accounts for 50%–70% of adult body weight. It varies with differences in sex, weight, fat content, and age.

Individuals with a greater proportion of lean tissue mass have a higher percentage of body water than those whose bodies carry more fat. Neutral fat, most common in body tissues, contains very little water. Table 2-1 compares the approximate body water content among various age groups. Water serves as the vehicle for the delivery of chemicals and nutrients to body cells and tissues and for the excretion of waste products. It also is the medium in which biochemical reactions take place. In addition, water contributes to body temperature regulation, cushions organs and joints, and provides body contour and form through hydration of tissue structures. Homeostasis is preserved through the intake and output of water. Under normal circumstances water volume is regulated by fluids released during metabolic processes and by the intake of food and fluids. Water is the main substance the body is able to perceive a need for, being signaled through the mechanism of thirst.

Water balance is regulated through neurosecretions of the hypothalamus (where antidiuretic hormone [ADH], or vasopressin, is formed in the peraventricular and supraoptic nuclei) and via the actions of aldosterone (the mineralocorticoid secreted from the adrenal cortex). ADH acts directly on the collecting ducts and tubules of the kidneys to bring about water reabsorption. Aldosterone maintains water balance by regulating sodium metabolism in the kidneys. When there is decreased renal blood flow, aldosterone causes sodium retention, which, in turn, causes water retention.

Water Distribution

All fluids in the body are made up primarily of water, within which various materials are dissolved. The total volume of water in the body is distributed among two large compartments, the intracellular and the extracellular. The cell membrane, which is selectively permeable, separates these two areas. The extracellular compartment is further divided into subcompartments (Figure 2-1). Fluid composition within the two major compartments is unique in chemical formulation.

Although the two compartments are structurally different and carry out separate functions, they are in a constant state of interaction with each other. The amount of fluid as well as the manner in which it is distributed and used in these compartments is vital to homeostasis (Table 2-2). An understanding of the similarities and differences between these two areas and knowing how various illnesses and disease

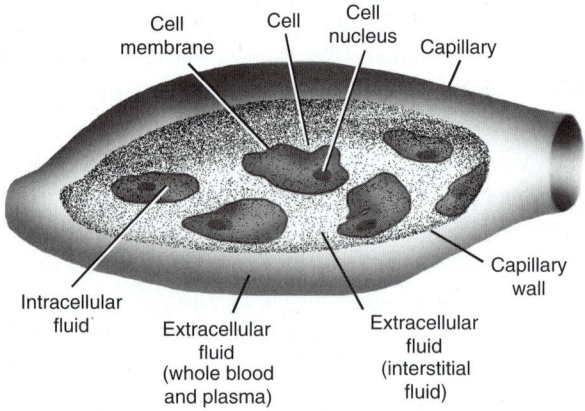

Figure 2-1 | Intracellular and extracellular fluids

Table 2-1 | Approximate Body Water Content as Percentage of Body Weight

	BODY WATER		
Age	Total	ECF	ICF
Children			
Newborn	79%	45%	34%
2–30 d	74%	40%	34%
1–12 m	63%	30%	33%
1–2 yr	59%	24%	35%
2–8 yr	62%	25%	37%
Men			
9–16 yr	59%	26%	33%
17–35 yr	60%	28%	32%
36–69 yr	55%	25%	30%
70+ yr	51%	25%	26%
Women			
9–15 yr	56%	25%	31%
16–35 yr	50%	25%	25%
36–59 yr	48%	23%	25%
l60+ yr	43%	21%	22%

Table 2-2 | Distribution of Body Water

	PERCENTAGE OF TOTAL BODY WEIGHT	
	Adult Male	Adult Female
Total body water	60.0%	50.0%
Intracellular fluid	45.0%	35.0%
Extracellular fluid	15.0%	15.0%
Interstitial fluid	11.0%	10.0%
Intravascular fluid	4.5%	4.3%

entities can bring about imbalances are of utmost importance for the nurse.

Intracellular Fluid

Intracellular fluid (**ICF**) is fluid contained within the cells of the body. It comprises approximately two-thirds of the total body fluid. Since the entire amount of fluid in the body comprises about 60% of total body weight, the ICF contributes to about 40% of that weight. The fluid within each cell is made up of materials individual to that cell. The concentration of these intracellular materials, potassium, magnesium, and phosphate ions, is much the same in the trillions of cells throughout the body. Because of this similarity, the intracellular fluid is classified as one large cellular component known as the intracellular fluid compartment.

Extracellular Fluid

The **extracellular fluid** (**ECF**) is fluid found in the spaces outside of the cells and comprises approximately one-third of the total body fluid, about 20% of total body weight. The ECF is rich in oxygen and carbon dioxide for nutrient and waste exchange, glucose for energy supply and demand, and amino acids and fatty acids for growth, repair, and health maintenance. It also contains large quantities of the electrolytes sodium, calcium, chloride, and bicarbonate. In addition, the ECF transports cholesterol, urea, lactate, creatinine, sulfates, and other products. The ECF is in constant movement within the systemic circulation, coming in contact with tissue fluids throughout the body. The ECF, as mentioned earlier, is referred to as the body's internal environment because it contributes to the homeostatic balance necessary to sustain a healthy human organism.

The two main functions of the ECF are (1) to maintain cell membrane permeability and membrane potential for appropriate membrane function, and (2) to serve as the vehicle for the movement of life-sustaining substances to and from various areas of the body.

The ECF compartment is divided into three subcomponents: the intravascular, the interstitial, and the transcellular compartments.

The Intravascular Compartment

The **intravascular fluid** (**IVF**) contained within the blood vessels of the body is also called plasma. Plasma is the liquid portion of blood and lymph and contains serum (the water portion of the blood left after coagulation), protein, and chemical products. The IVF serves as a vehicle for the transport and exchange of nutrients.

The Interstitial Compartment

Interstitial fluid (**ISF**) is the solution that exists in the small spaces and gaps between body structures, cells, and tissues. Lymph is formed in tissue spaces throughout the body and is the ISF that circulates within the lymphatic vessels; it varies in composition in different areas of the body. Lymph contains proteins, salts, organic substances (glucose, fats, urea, and creatinine), and water and is filtered in lymph nodes during its circulation throughout the lymphatic vessels. Toxins and foreign matter, such as bacteria, are filtered by the lymphatic system.

The Transcellular Compartment

Transcellular fluid (**TSF**) is formed as a by-product during the process of cellular activity. It consists of specialized fluids, which make up the smallest amount of ECF, and includes mucus, ocular fluids, sweat, secretions of the genitourinary tract, cerebrospinal fluid, and pleural, pericardial, and peritoneal secretions.

THE COMPOSITION OF BODY FLUIDS

Water is the main constituent of all body fluids. Within these fluids are numerous minerals and organic compounds. Water is a **polar molecule**: One part of its structure is negative and the other is positive, thus making it neutral as a whole (Figure 2-2). In the body, water acts as a **solvent**, able to hold substances and act to dissolve them. **Solutes** are the substances dissolved in the water (the solvent). The combination of the solute and the solvent forms a **solution**. Because water is polar, substances such as strong acids, bases, ions, and hydroxyl (-OH) groups gravitate around the water molecule, attach to it, and dissolve.

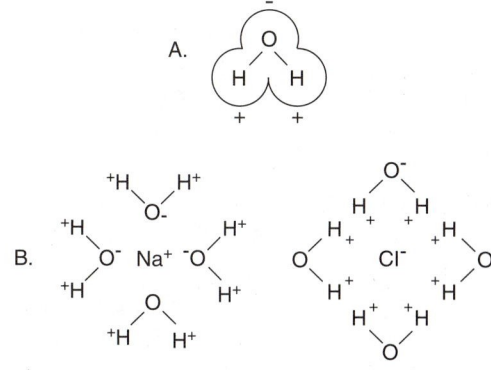

Figure 2-2 | A. Water is a polar molecule; B. Dissolution of ions in water

Two major categories of solutes exist in body fluids: electrolytes and nonelectrolytes. It is important to comprehend their differences in order to understand their interaction, their method of movement, and their utilization by the body.

Electrolytes

Electrolytes make up about 95% of the body's solute molecules and are chemicals that carry an electrical charge. Electrically charged molecules are called **ions**. When dispersed in fluid, electrolytes dissociate into constituent ions and convert the solution into a product capable of conducting electricity. Acids, bases, and salts that dissociate when dissolved in water are called electrolytes. Ions with a negative charge are called **anions**. Ions with a positive charge are called **cations**. The two are polar, meaning that they are attracted to each other, the anions gravitating toward the positive poles (cations) and vice versa. For chemical-combining activity to occur, there does not have to be the same number of anions and cations, but there must exist a balance in the number of positive and negative ions (charges). Because they separate into charged particles, electrolytes are expressed in milliequivalents per liter (mEq/L), or the number of electrical charges per liter of fluid. A **milliequivalent**, a measurement of the concentration of electrolytes in a volume of solution, refers to the ability of ions to combine chemically, which is dependent on the **valence** (electrical charge) of the ions. Electrolytes are sometimes measured in milligrams per deciliter (mg/dl).

Electrolytes are crucial to the body for the distribution and movement of water and for the maintenance of acid-base balance. They provide the chemicals needed to carry out cellular reactions and to regulate mechanisms at the cell membrane that allow transmission of electrochemical impulses in muscle and nerve fibers. It is very important to remember that any disruption of electrolyte balance can result in a pathophysiologic state.

In the intracellular compartment there are large amounts of potassium, magnesium, and phosphate, but small amounts of sodium, chloride, sulfate, and bicarbonate. By contrast, in the extracellular compartment, there are large concentrations of sodium, chlorides, and bicarbonate ions (Table 2-3). The difference between the two compartments is responsible for permeability of the cell membrane and for electrical potentials occurring across the cell membrane, which allow nerve fibers to conduct impulses and muscle fibers to contract. Since the electrical content between these two areas is different, the concentration is maintained by a mechanism known as the **sodium-potassium pump** (described later in the chapter). This pump, necessary for all cells, is present in cell membranes to draw

Table 2-3	Chemical Compositions of the Extracellular and Intracellular Fluid Compartments	
	EXTRA-CELLULAR FLUID	**INTRA-CELLULAR FLUID**
Sodium (Na^+)	142 mEq/L	10 mEq/L
Potassium (K^+)	5 mEq/L	141 mEq/L
Calcium (Ca^{++})	5 mEq/L	0–1 mEq/L
Magnesium (Mg^{++})	3 mEq/L	60 mEq/L
Chloride (Cl^-)	103 mEq/L	4 mEq/L
Bicarbonate (HCO_2^-)	28 mEq/L	10 mEq/L
Phosphate (PO_4)	4 mEq/L	75 mEq/L
Sulfate (SO_4)	1 mEq/L	2 mEq/L
Protein	17 mEq/L	60 mEq/L
Glucose	90 mg/dl	0–20 mg/dl
Partial pressure of oxygen (PO_2)	35 mm Hg	20 mm Hg
Partial pressure of carbon dioxide (PCO_2)	46 mm Hg	50 mm Hg
pH	7.4	7.0

sodium out of the cell and pull potassium in. It exists to maintain the balanced concentration of ions and is vital to cellular respiration and metabolism.

The calcium in the extracellular fluid is especially vital to homeostasis in regulating the degree of cell membrane permeability. The concentration of calcium is inversely proportionate to the permeability of the membrane; if the calcium level is high, permeability decreases, if the calcium level is low, permeability increases.

In caring for patients, the nurse must have a solid, working understanding of electrolytes and fluid balance and the factors affecting their gains or losses. He needs to monitor these levels and be alert to the signs and symptoms of changes. It is important not only to recognize problems and abnormalities that indicate an imbalance, but also to intervene quickly to correct the situation. When delivering infusion therapy, recognition and intervention become even more critical.

Nonelectrolytes

Nonelectrolytes present in body fluids are solutes that do not carry electrical charges, nor do they separate into particles when dispersed in fluid. Solutes incapable of dissociation include glucose, urea, creatinine, and bilirubin.

Glucose is a large, lipid-insoluble molecule that slowly crosses the cell membrane and affects water movement. It is normally present in both whole blood and plasma and cannot enter the cell unless it attaches to a carrier outside of the cell membrane that will render it lipid soluble.

Urea, a metabolic end-product of protein metabolism, is a small molecule that freely crosses the cell membrane. Urea quantities equalize between the intracellular and extracellular compartments. It has little effect on water movement.

Creatinine, a by-product of muscle catabolism, is derived from the breakdown of muscle creatine phosphate. Bilirubin, an end-product of red blood cell destruction and hemoglobin decomposition, circulates throughout the blood and interstitial fluid.

THE MOVEMENT OF BODY FLUIDS

Water, the principal component of all body fluids, is the medium in which most chemical reactions occur. Body fluids exist in a dynamic state with materials constantly moving into and out of cells. When the body is healthy, the movement of water is balanced among the fluid compartments. It is important to understand the mechanisms of fluid movement in the body in order to fully grasp the concepts of fluid and electrolyte balance and replacement during infusion therapy.

The Cell and the Cell Membrane

The cell is the structural and functional unit of all living organisms. It is composed of protoplasm, a complex mixture of organic and inorganic substances, and is surrounded by the cell membrane, a chemically active regulatory matrix.

Nucleus, Nucleolus, Protoplasm, Enzymes, and the Cell Membrane

The nucleus is the integral body in the protoplasm of the cell crucial for cell growth, metabolism, reproduction, and the transmission of cellular traits. The **nucleolus** is a spherical body of dense fibers and granules where ribonucleoprotein is formed. Ribonucleoproteins are composed of protein and ribonucleic acid, a substance that controls protein synthesis. **Protoplasm** refers to the substance of the cell and is made of five basic elements: water, electrolytes, carbohydrates,

lipids, and proteins. Protoplasm (99%) is composed chiefly of carbon, hydrogen, oxygen, and nitrogen. The remaining 1% is sodium, potassium, chlorine, phosphorus, calcium, magnesium, and sulfur, along with traces of copper, iodine, iron, and fluorine. The fluid medium of the protoplasm is water, in which some substances are dissolved in solution and others are suspended as small particles. The water allows the dissolved substances and the suspended particles to be transported from one part of the cell to another.

The protoplasm also contains **enzymes**, organic activators known as **catalysts**. Enzymes are highly specialized molecules that coordinate and control cellular chemical reactions and serve as activators for the timing or speed of cellular reactions. They initiate and carry out change in other substances, yet their individual composition is not altered; they can produce unlimited quantities of the end-products of reactions. They are **reaction-specific**, meaning they act only on certain substances or groups of closely related materials. Enzymes operate at individually optimum temperature ranges and specific degrees of acidity or alkalinity. They can be inactivated or inhibited by temperature extremes, states of dehydration, or by the presence of heavy metals or salts. They sometimes need the presence of other substances to activate their reactions. Specific substances that combine with enzymes and work only with certain enzymes are called **coenzymes**. Nonspecific substances that assist with enzymatic reactions are called **activators**.

In the body, as the extracellular fluid circulates among cells and permeates capillary walls, the cells are nourished with the materials they need to function. The cells, however, are unable to use these substances until they are transported through the cell membrane into the cell. The cell membrane (or plasma membrane) consists primarily of lipids (70% phospholipids, 25% cholesterol, and 5% glycolipids) and proteins, as well as minute water-filled pores.

Carbohydrates

Carbohydrates are organic compounds made up of carbon, hydrogen, and oxygen and are classified according to the amount of sugar in their chemical makeup. The **monosaccharides** are simple sugars whose structure cannot be further broken down by hydrolysis and include glucose, fructose, and galactose. **Disaccharides** are double sugars formed from two monosaccharides and include sucrose (table sugar), lactose (milk sugar), and maltose (malt sugar). **Polysaccharides** are large molecules made up of numerous glucose molecules and include starch (the stored form of glucose in plants), glycogen (the starch stored in the muscles and liver of vertebrates), and cellulose (the structural skeleton for plant cells such as wood and cotton).

Glucose, a monosaccharide, the most important carbohydrate in the body, is the main source of energy for cells and is transported in the blood. The concentration of glucose in the blood (approximately 0.1%) is maintained at a fairly constant range of 80 mg/dl to 120 mg/dl. Once in the cell it combines with oxygen (**oxidation**) to produce energy. Glucose not used by the cell is converted to **glycogen** by the liver and stored in all body tissues, but mainly in muscles and the liver. The stored glycogen is available for metabolism when needed. During periods of starvation, glycogen is formed from fat (**glyconeogenesis**) and acts as a protein sparer to prevent the use of protein for energy needs.

In the tissues, glucose may be used to form fat or may be oxidized to carbon dioxide and water. Free glucose cannot be used by the tissues until it undergoes a complex series of reactions. It must be penetrated with phosphorus (**phosphorylation**) by adenosine triphosphate (ATP) through the enzymatic action of hexokinase (which produces glucose-6-phosphate). Oxidation of glucose to carbon dioxide and water occurs after further enzymatic and hormonal action and the formation of intermediate components (lactic acid and pyruvic acid).

Fructose is the sweetest of the monosaccharides and is found in fruits, honey, sugar cane, and corn syrup. It is converted to glycogen and used by the body in the same manner as glucose.

Galactose is also a simple sugar. During metabolic processes, galactose and glucose are formed during the catabolism (breakdown) of lactose.

Lipids

Lipids are molecules that contain the elements carbon, hydrogen, and oxygen in the form of phospholipids, steroids, and fats. They are responsible for the structural integrity of the cell membrane and are categorized as **surfactants** (surface-active agents). Lipids have a dual nature because they are polar and charged (**hydrophilic**—attracted to water) on the phosphoric-acid portion of the molecule and nonpolar and uncharged (**hydrophobic**—repelled by water) on the fatty-acid portion. This makeup permits them to alter the interaction of molecules, therefore decreasing the surface tension of water. Because the cell membrane is surrounded by an aqueous environment on each side, the hydrophobic ends of the molecules group together in the middle of the membrane (Figure 2-3). The hydrophilic ends of the molecules exist on the cell membrane exposed to water on both surfaces of the membrane, producing a double layer of phospholipids within the cell membrane. The hydrophobic center of the membrane prevents water and water-soluble molecules from passing through. This structural makeup contributes to one of the most important functions of the membrane—making it nonpermeable to most

water-soluble molecules. Some of these molecules do pass through the cell membrane, however, because of the selective transport properties of the proteins. Even though membrane structure is maintained by the lipids, its functions are controlled by the proteins.

Proteins

Proteins, found in the cells of all living organisms, are organic compounds composed of carbon, hydrogen, oxygen, and nitrogen molecules, and usually phosphorus and sulfur as well. They are composed of molecular units called **amino acids**. These compounds serve as the building blocks of protein and are also the end-products of protein digestion. Of the amino acids required for human growth and repair, some are supplied by ingested food (essential amino acids) and others are produced by the body (nonessential amino acids). Proteins that contain all of the essential amino acids are called **complete proteins** and include meat, eggs, milk, and cheese. Those that do not contain all the essential amino acids, such as vegetables and grains, are called **incomplete proteins**.

Amino acids do not undergo any changes as they pass through the intestines, portal circulation, the liver, and into the general circulation. In the body, tissues are amino-acid specific; they absorb amino acids from the circulation according to which protein they need to manufacture. Any proteins that are not metabolized by the tissues are converted into urea (**deaminization**).

Proteins provide several important functions within the cell membrane. In addition to transporting molecules across the membrane, they provide for its structural support and control and act as enzymes to serve as pumps for the enzymatic regulation of chemical reactions on the cell surface. They function as receptors for hormones approaching the membrane surface, and work as antigens, which identify and recognize blood and tissue type.

Proteins also serve as transporters for amino acids and simple sugars and provide pores or channels for the passage of electrolytes. These protein pores in the cell membrane, which carry a positive charge, are lined with positively charged calcium ions. Because of this makeup, positively charged ions, such as sodium and potassium, have difficulty passing through the pores. Whenever they attempt passage, the two positive charges repel each other. Negatively charged ions pass through the membrane pores easily.

Mechanisms of Fluid Movement

Passage of substances across membranes is accomplished in one of two ways, depending on the substances being taken in or moved out. Passive transport, in which there is no expen-

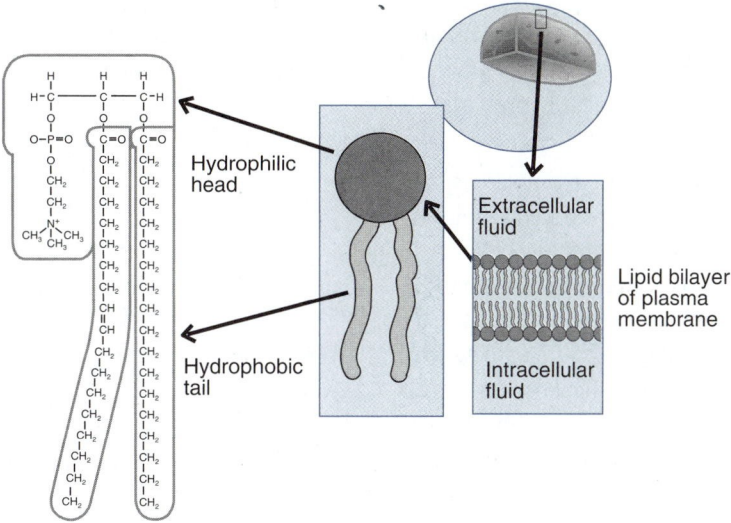

Figure 2-3 | Cell membrane phospholipids

diture of cellular energy, occurs spontaneously through any semipermeable layer. Biologic energy is not required for this process. Active transport requires a source of biologic activity and cellular metabolic energy for movement of particles across the cell membrane.

Passive Transport

Passive transport (or **noncarrier-mediated transport**) is the movement of solutes through membranes without the expenditure of energy. It includes passive diffusion, osmosis, facilitated diffusion, and filtration.

Passive Diffusion

Passive (**simple**) **diffusion** is the process in which ions, water, and lipid-soluble molecules move randomly in all directions from an area of high concentration to a lower solute concentration through the pores in the membrane or through the matrix of the membrane (Figure 2-4). The rate at which diffusion occurs depends on the variations in electrical potentials across membranes. For simple diffusion to occur, the particles must dissolve or be small enough to pass through the membrane. When in solution, particles move about randomly in any direction. If the molecules become more populous in one area of the solution than in another area, a concentration difference, or **concentration gradient**, results, and the particles will move to evenly redistribute themselves until they reach a state of equilibrium. This movement abolishes the concentration difference and is called **net diffusion**.

Net diffusion depends on membrane permeability, the differences in the concentrations on each side of the mem-

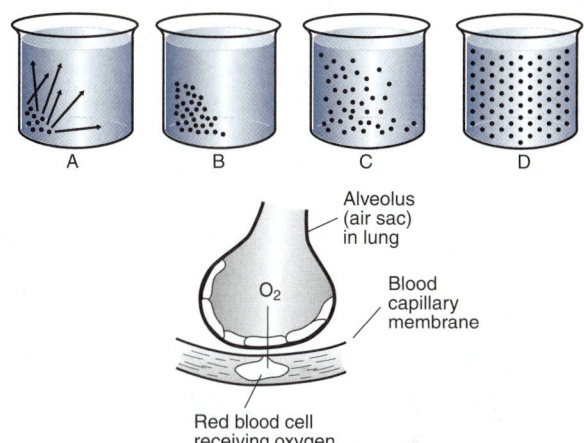

(A) A small lump of sugar is placed into a beaker of water; its molecules dissolve and begin to diffuse outward. (B and C) The sugar molecules continue to diffuse through the water from an area of greater concentration to an area of lesser concentration. (D) Over a long period of time, the sugar molecules are evenly distributed throughout the water, reaching a state of equilibrium.

Example of diffusion in the human body: Oxygen diffuses from an alveolus in a lung where it is in greater concentration, across the blood capillary membrane, into a red blood cell where it is in lesser concentration.

Figure 2-4 | Passive (simple) diffusion

brane, the differences in electric potentials, and differences in pressure across membranes. It is this passive movement from an area of higher concentration to lower concentration along a concentration gradient that results in simple diffusion. The random motion of molecules and ions in all directions occurs because of kinetic energy. As the movement continues, heat is produced and released, and diffusion continues. In diffusion, any substance that can move into the cell can move out. It is the net quantity of substances diffusing through the cell membrane, rather than the gross quantity, that is important to cellular function.

Osmosis

Osmosis is the passage of water through a semipermeable membrane from an area with a lower concentration of solutes to an area with a higher concentration of solutes (Figure 2-5). For a membrane to be semipermeable, it has to be more permeable to water than to solutes.

Osmosis governs the movement of body fluids between the intracellular and extracellular fluid compartments, thus affecting the volumes within each. The semipermeable membrane selectively controls the passage of solutes and serves to separate the major fluid compartments.

Through the process of osmosis, water flows through the semipermeable membrane to the side with the higher concentration of particles that cannot diffuse to the side with the lower concentration. It is the difference in the concentration of nondiffusable particles that controls water flow. Once the concentrations of solutes are equal on each side of the membrane, the flow of water stops and the solutions are **isosmotic** to each other, comparable in molecular concentration. Any change in the volume of solutes or water content in either compartment brings about an osmotic water shift.

Whereas diffusion is the passive flow of particles from an area of higher concentration to one of lower concentration, osmosis is the movement of water across a semipermeable membrane from an area of lower concentration to one of higher concentration. Both mechanisms involve movement across a concentration gradient, but diffusion moves solutes and osmosis moves water (solvent). Osmosis cannot occur

unless the membrane is more permeable to water than to solutes; water movement is enhanced because of the greater concentration of solutes.

Hydrostatic pressure refers to the physical force of water as it pushes against vessel walls or cellular membranes (Figure 2-6). **Hydraulic pressure** is the force of gravitational pressure that acts on hydrostatic pressure combined with the pumping pressure of the heart. **Osmotic pressure** is the amount of hydrostatic pressure needed to draw a solvent across a membrane and develops as a result of a high concentration of particles colliding with one another. As the number of solutes increases, there is less space for them to move, so they come in contact with one another more frequently. This results in increased osmotic pressure, which causes the movement of fluid (Figure 2-7). Total osmotic pressure in the extracellular fluid results from the movement of small molecules, ions, and proteins contained in it. The small molecules easily cross back and forth across membranes and have little effect on movement of water or osmotic pressure. The osmotic pressure created by the movement of dissolved ions is termed **crystalloid osmotic pressure**. The osmotic pressure that develops at a membrane because of proteins is the **colloid osmotic pressure** or **oncotic pressure**.

The osmotic activity of a solution is described according to its osmolarity, its osmolality, or both. **Osmolarity (tonicity)** refers to the concentration of solute particles

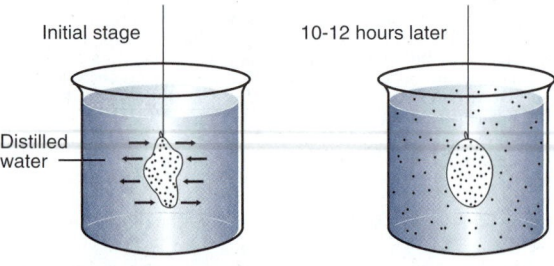

Initial stage   10-12 hours later

Distilled water

(A) Initially, the sausage casing contains a solution of gelatin, salt, and sucrose. The casing is permeable to water and salt molecules only. Since the concentration of water molecules is greater outside the casing, water molecules will diffuse into the casing. The opposite situation exists for the salt.

(B) The sausage casing swells due to the net movement of water molecules inward. However, the volume of distilled water in the beaker remains constant.

Figure 2-5 | Osmosis: A sausage casing as an example of a selective permeable membrane

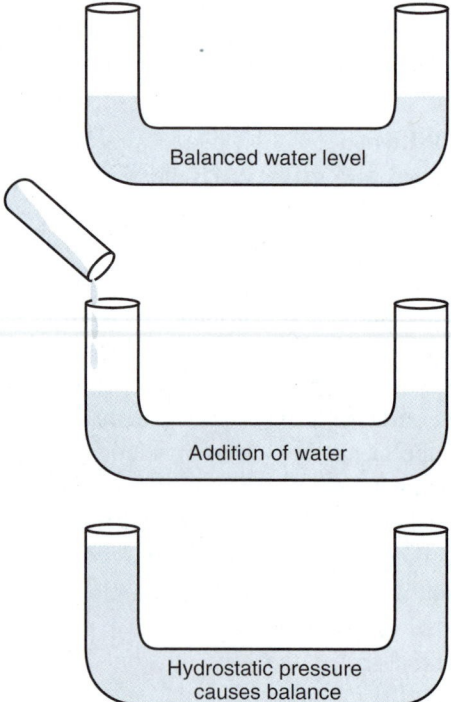

Balanced water level

Addition of water

Hydrostatic pressure causes balance

Figure 2-6 | Hydrostatic pressure

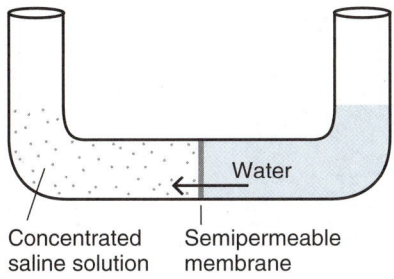

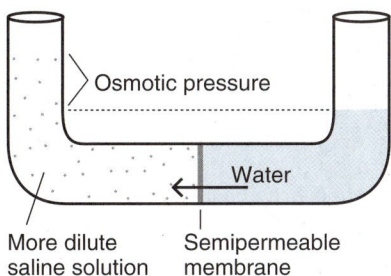

Figure 2-7 | Osmotic pressure

contained in a unit volume of solvent and is usually expressed as milliosmols per liter or mOsm/L. The osmolarity of a solution varies with changes in temperature because liquids expand with increasing temperature (Figure 2-8).

In contrast, **osmolality** (also called tonicity) describes the total number of solute particles in a unit weight of solvent and is usually expressed as milliosmols per kilogram or mOsm/kg. The osmol unit is used because osmotic pressure is determined by the number of particles, rather than the mass, of a solute. As a general rule, the osmol is too big a unit for describing osmotic activity in bodily solutes, so the milliosmol is used (1/1000 osmol). Both osmolarity and osmolality are used to characterize tonicity, but clinically, osmolality is the more commonly used system of fluid measurement because normal body solutions are very dilute. Temperature does not affect osmolality.

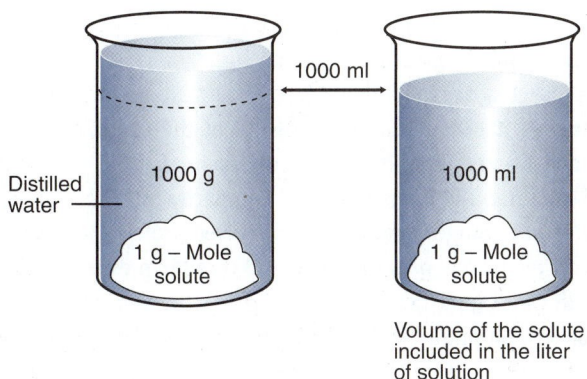

Figure 2-8 | Osmolality and osmolarity

An osmol equals the molecular weight in grams of the number of particles in one mole of a nonionizing material, such as sodium, calcium, urea, or glucose. One mole of such a substance, when added to water, results in a solution with one osmol or particle. Ionizing substances (capable of dissociating in solution and conducting electricity), when placed in water, result in the formation of a solution with more than one osmol. If a mole of potassium chloride is placed in water, there is a separation of ions resulting in a solution with two osmols, one of potassium and one of chloride.

Under normal circumstances body fluids are dilute solutions. Because of this characteristic, there is very little difference between the osmolarity and osmolality of body fluids. However, the fluid in the intravascular compartment is slightly greater than in other spaces because it contains plasma proteins.

A solution with an osmolality (or osmolarity) higher than another solution is considered **hypertonic (hyperosmolar)**. A cell placed in a hypertonic solution would shrink, or crenate, because water would be osmotically drawn from it. In contrast, a solution that has an osmolality lower than another solution is called a **hypotonic (hyposmolar) solution**. Pure water is hypotonic compared with body fluids, so if a cell is placed in it, the water is osmotically drawn across the membrane causing the cell to swell. A solution that is **isotonic (isosmolar)** has the same osmotic pressure as the comparison solution. The osmolality of plasma (approximately 290–300 mOsm/L) is generally used as the standard for comparison. The tonicity of plasma or extracellular fluid is clinically and physiologically significant with regard to the osmotic shift of water between the fluid compartments (Figure 2-9).

During illness it becomes a challenge to maintain the proper balance of fluids and electrolytes between the intracellular and extracellular compartments. When dealing with fluid replacement therapy, the nurse must understand the interrelationships that exist between these two compartments and the osmotic factors that contribute to fluid shifts.

Facilitated Diffusion

The cellular membrane allows free movement for the diffusion of lipid-soluble, nonpolar (uncharged) molecules, such as oxygen, the steroid hormones, and fatty acids. In addition, small molecules that have polar bonds but do not carry electrical charges, such as carbon dioxide, urea, and ethanol, are also able to pass with ease back and forth across the cell membrane. Water diffuses through because its molecules are small and uncharged. Charged inorganic ions can only pass through the membrane via **ion channels**, submicroscopic passageways present in the membrane matrix.

Lipid solubility determines whether a substance is able to pass through the cell membrane. Large polar (charged) lipid-insoluble materials cross the cell membrane only with the help of solute-specific carriers called **transport proteins** present

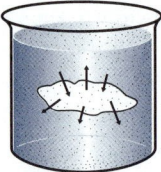
Hypertonic
solution

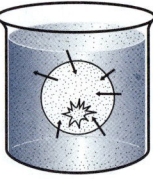
Hypotonic
solution

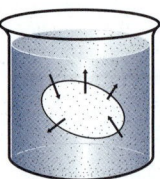
Isotonic
solution

**Hypertonic
solution
(seawater)**
A red blood cell will
shrink and wrinkle
up because water
molecules are
moving out of
the cell.

**Hypotonic
solution
(freshwater)**
A red blood cell
will swell and burst
because water
molecules are
moving into
the cell.

**Isotonic
solution (human
blood serum)**
A red blood cell
remains unchanged
because the movement
of water molecules into
and out of the cell is
the same.

Figure 2-9 | Movement of water molecules in hypertonic, hypotonic,
and isotonic solutions

within the cell membrane. The process by which material combines with carriers to cross the cell membrane is called **facilitated diffusion** or **carrier-mediated diffusion** (Figure 2-10). It is through this mechanism that amino acids and sugars, especially glucose, are transported into the cell. Once inside the cell, sugar molecules or amino acids break away from the carrier, and the carrier returns to the outside surface of the membrane to pick up more products for diffusion into the cell. The speed with which this process takes place depends on the amount of carrier present, the difference in the concentration of molecules on each side of the cell membrane, and the speed of the chemical reactions. In the case of glucose, the rate of transport by the carrier is increased because of the hormone insulin.

Facilitated diffusion is somewhat similar to active transport. In diffusion, the movement of molecules is from an area of higher concentration to one of a lower concentration, and in active transport the molecules move from an area of lower concentration through the membrane to an area of

higher concentration with the help of biologic, metabolic energy.

Filtration

Filtration is the movement of fluid and diffusible particles through a membrane from an area of greater hydrostatic pressure to one of lesser hydrostatic pressure. While diffusion moves in either direction across a membrane, filtration moves in one direction, owing to the mechanisms of hydrostatic, osmotic, and interstitial fluid pressures that expedite net fluid transport across the membrane. Filtration is similar to pouring a solution through a sieve. The size of the openings in the sieve determines the size of particle to be filtered (Figure 2-11).

In the body, arterial blood is transported via the arteries to the arterioles and then to the arterial capillary beds. From there the fluid enters the interstitial fluid where the cellular exchange of nutrients and wastes occurs. Once this exchange has taken place, the fluid returns to the venous circulation via the venous capillary beds, venules, and veins (Figure 2-12). Fluid movement from the arterial capillary beds into the interstitial compartment occurs through filtration. The mean capillary pressure is 17 mm Hg.

Proteins are abundant in the circulating plasma and serve to maintain osmotic pressure at the capillary membrane by not permitting the movement of fluid from the plasma into the interstitial fluid compartment. This osmotic pressure, brought about by the dissolved proteins (colloids), is called oncotic pressure or colloid osmotic pressure, which is 28 mm Hg in the plasma. In general, the size of capillary pores is too small to allow for the passage of plasma proteins into the interstitial fluid spaces. There are, however, some larger pores that allow very small amounts of plasma proteins to filter into the ISF compartment. This amounts to

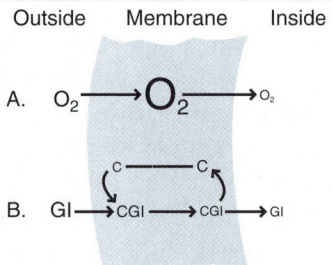

Outside   Membrane   Inside

A. $O_2 \longrightarrow O_2 \longrightarrow O_2$

B. $GI \longrightarrow CGI \longrightarrow CGI \longrightarrow GI$

Figure 2-10 | Facilitated diffusion: A. Free diffusion of oxygen through the lipid matrix of the cell membrane; B. Facilitated (carrier-mediated) diffusion of glucose through the membrane lipid matrix

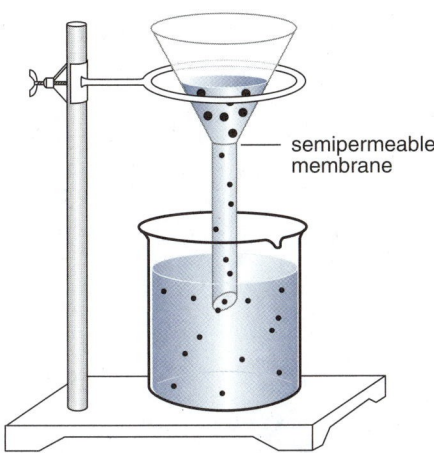

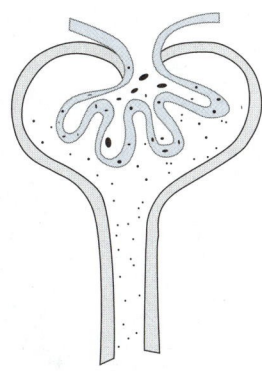

A. Filtration: Small molecules are filtered through the semipermeable membrane, while the large molecules remain in the funnel.

B. Example of filtration in the human body: Glomerulus of kidney; large particles like red blood cells and proteins remain in the blood, and small molecules like urea and water are excreted as a metabolic excretory product—urine.

Figure 2-11 | Filtration

about 0.3%, making the colloid osmotic pressure of the ISF about 5 mm Hg. The hydrostatic pressure in the ISF is about −6.3 mm Hg (or 6.3 mm Hg below atmospheric pressure).

The process of water and electrolyte filtration occurring through the capillary membranes is enhanced by the mechanical forces of blood pressure and gravity, so the capillary pressure at the arterial ends is ±15 mm Hg greater than at the venous ends, making the mean capillary pressure about ±17 mm Hg. As a result of this pressure difference, some fluid filters out of the arterial capillaries, flows through the interstitial spaces, and is reabsorbed into the venous capillary network.

Starling's law of capillaries (Figure 2-13) maintains that, under normal circumstances, fluid filtered out of the arterial end of the capillary bed and reabsorbed at the venous end is exactly the same, creating a state of near equilibrium. It is not exactly the same, however, because of the difference in hydrostatic pressure between the arterial and venous capillary beds. The forces that move fluid out of the arterial end of the network amount to a total of 28.3 mm Hg (mean capillary pressure of 17 mm Hg + negative interstitial pressure of 6.3 mm Hg + ISF colloid pressure 5 mm Hg). The forces that move fluid back into circulation at the venous capillary bed total 28 mm Hg (colloid osmotic or oncotic pressure). The small amount of excess filtration remaining in the interstitial compartment, referred to as **net filtration** (0.3 mm Hg), is returned to the circulation by way of the lymphatic system (Table 2-4).

Of major importance is that the lymphatics carry this excess fluid, proteins, and large particulate matter that cannot be reabsorbed by the venous capillary bed out of the ISF compartment. This minute excess or net filtration (that only amounts to about 0.3 mm Hg) accounts for

1.7 ml/min of fluid. If the lymphatics were not continually removing this small amount of fluid, there would be a buildup of 2,448 ml in the interstitial compartment over a 24-hour period, which would result in death.

Active Transport

Active transport is the process whereby molecules are moved against a concentration gradient, pressure gradient, or electrochemical gradient by utilizing cellular energy sources. As with facilitated diffusion, transport is through membranes by carriers. Active transport differs from diffusion, however, because substances are capable of crossing membranes even when there is a higher concentration on the side of the membrane the substance is transferring to, and because energy is needed to surpass the concentration gradient.

There exists some scientific debate regarding the details and intricacies of energy supply for the active transport system. What is known and agreed upon by the scientific community, however, is that ATP provides the energy for transport, that there is a chemical joining of the substance to be transported with a protein carrier, and that the process can be accomplished only with the assistance of enzymatic activity. Active transport carriers are sometimes referred to as pumps.

ATP

Every cell in the body contains enzymes for splitting proteins, fats, and carbohydrates into amino acids, fatty acids, and glucose, respectively. These chemicals are metabolized with oxygen to form carbon dioxide and water. In the process of

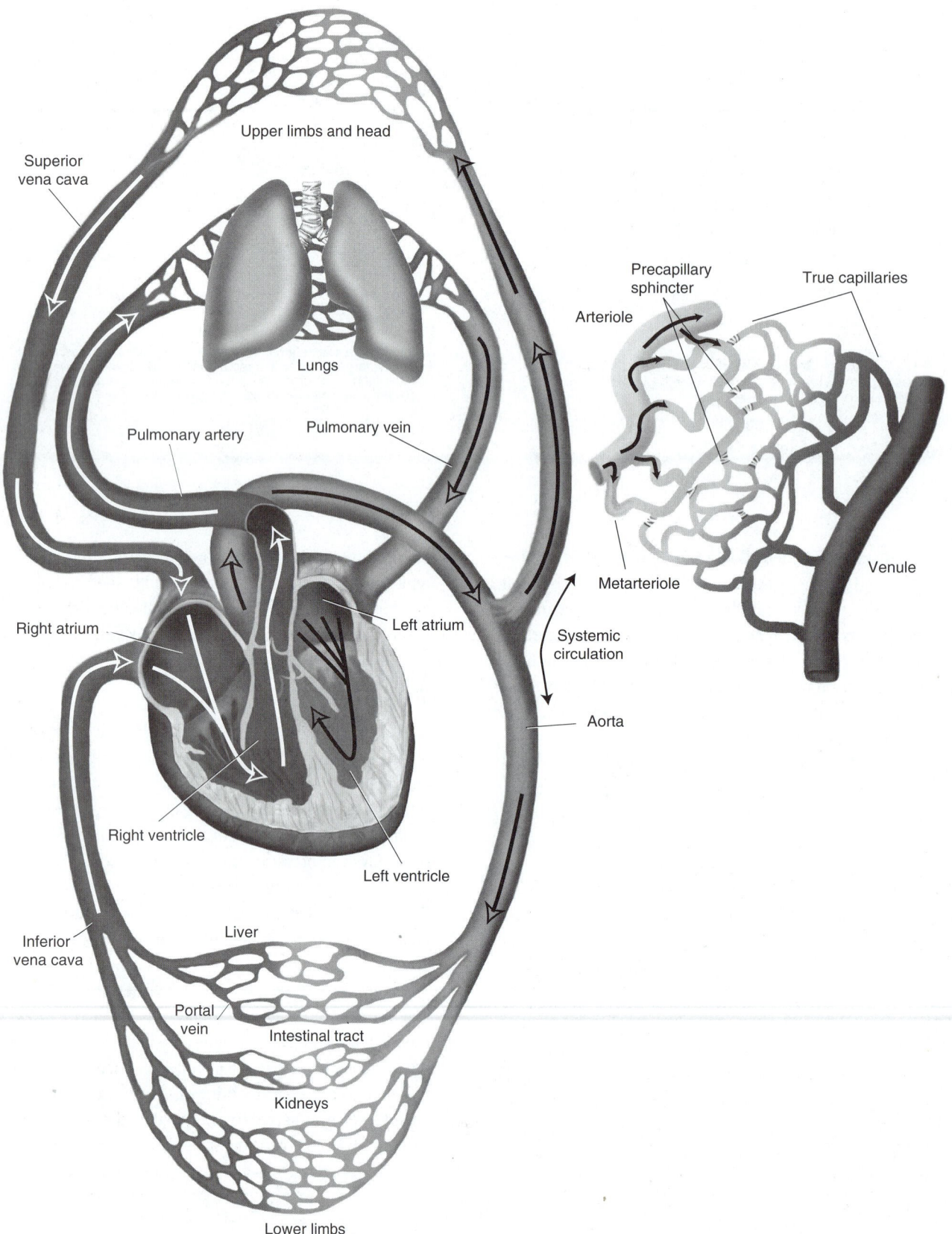

Figure 2-12 | Systemic circulation

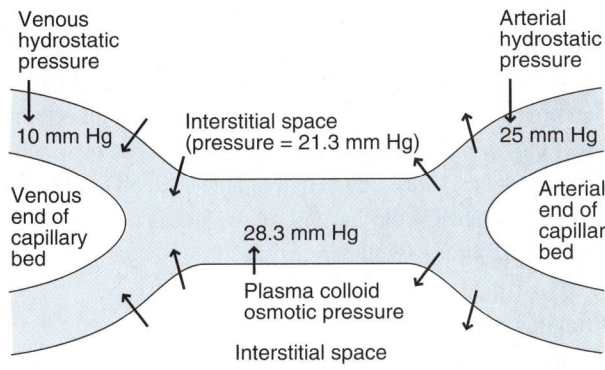

Figure 2-13 | Starling's Law of capillaries

Table 2-4 | Starling's Law of capillaries

SUMMATION OF FORCES	MILLIMETERS OF MERCURY (MM HG)
Forces Moving Fluid Out of the Capillary	
Mean arterial capillary pressure	17.0 mm Hg
Negative interstitial fluid pressure	+ 6.3 mm Hg
Interstitial fluid colloid osmotic pressure	+ 5.0 mm Hg
Total outward pressure	= 28.3 mm Hg
Forces Moving Fluid into the Capillary	
Plasma colloid osmotic pressure	28.0 mm Hg
Total inward pressure	= 28.0 mm Hg
	28.3 mm Hg
	− 28.0 mm Hg
Net outward pressure	= 0.3 mm Hg
(per minute filtration)	= 1.7 ml/min

1.7 ml × 60 min = 102 ml/hr × 24 hr = 2,448 ml/d
(Daily net filtration returned to circulation by the lymphatics)

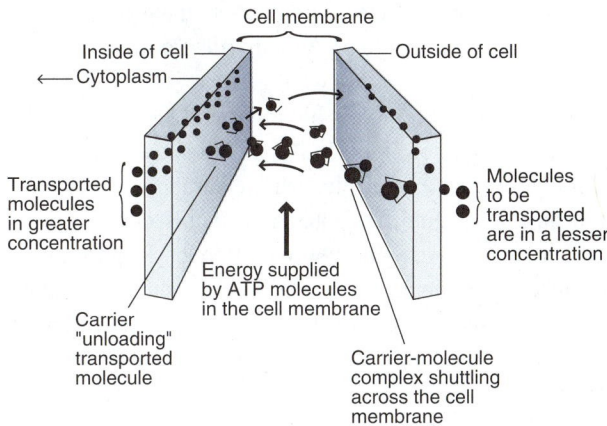

Figure 2-14 | Active transport

accomplishing this metabolic conversion, large amounts of energy are produced. The energy is used to convert **adenosine diphosphate** (**ADP**) to **adenosine triphosphate** (**ATP**), which then provides the energy needed for cellular chemical reactions to take place. ATP is present in all body cells but is especially abundant in muscle cells (Figure 2-14).

Active transport occurs when ATP hydrolysis energizes a protein carrier. As with facilitated diffusion, a carrier attaches to a substance crossing the cell membrane and the two diffuse into the cell. ATP is released on the inside of the cell membrane to trigger an enzyme-catalyzed reaction that causes the substance and carrier to lose their affinity for each other and to dissociate. The carrier diffuses out of the cell, and the substance that was split from the carrier, because of its membrane insolubility, remains.

Sodium-Potassium Pump

The sodium-potassium pump is an active transport system. It serves as a transport carrier to pick up and transport a substance across a membrane, detach from it, and then return to the outside to transport additional material. In addition, the sodium-potassium pump exchanges ions or molecules with other ions or molecules (Figure 2-15). It is present in all cells of the body, but is especially active in muscle and nerve cells and the cells of the kidney tubules.

The sodium-potassium pump is a mechanism that results in most of the body's potassium remaining in the intracellular fluid and most of the sodium remaining in the extracellular fluid. This pump is vital to physiologic functioning for

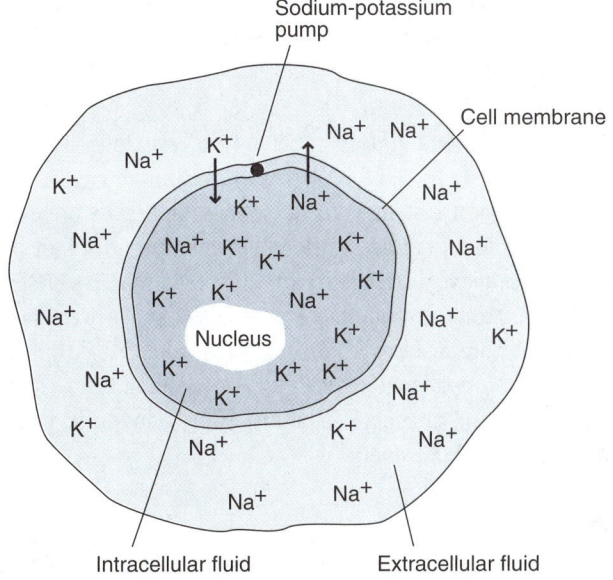

Figure 2-15 | Sodium-potassium pump

the transmission of electrical impulses, to the secretory functioning of glands, and to prevent all cells from swelling and bursting.

Sodium concentration is high in the ECF and low in the ICF. Potassium is low in the ECF and high in the ICF. Because of the pores that exist in the cell membrane, there is some diffusion of sodium and potassium. If this diffusion were allowed to continue, the concentration of sodium would equalize over time, and the cells would swell and rupture. The sodium-potassium pump is a carrier that transports sodium out of the cell and pumps potassium back into the cell. The concentrations of sodium and potassium do not change as a result of diffusion because of the sodium-potassium pump. The energy needed for this pump to work comes from the enzyme ATPase, which is present in the carrier itself, and acts to break down ATP.

The sodium-potassium pump is more effective in transporting sodium than potassium and usually carries three sodium ions for every two potassium ions. This contributes to a **potential difference** (charge separator) providing voltage across the membrane. The sodium-potassium pump contributes to the membrane by pumping more sodium out than potassium in. This promotes a constant membrane potential.

Transport by Vesicle Formation

In order for the cell to live and grow, it must maintain a source of nourishment from the surrounding fluids. It must also be able to excrete wastes and destroy and expel harmful and unnecessary substances.

In addition to the passive and active transport systems, a mechanism is required to move larger molecules that cannot pass through the cell membrane by these methods. These substances include certain fluids and larger extracellular molecules, such as proteins and polysaccharides.

Endocytosis

Endocytosis is a process whereby the cell ingests substances that are too large to be taken in through passive or active transport systems. Whenever these materials present themselves to the surface of the cell membrane, attributes of the surface tension change so that the membrane is able to fold inward and surround these materials. These invaginated areas then break away from the cell membrane and form individual vessels that travel into the cellular cytoplasm. Pinocytosis and phagocytosis are types of endocytosis, both requiring metabolic energy.

Pinocytosis

Pinocytosis is the endocytic process in which invagination of the cell membrane by the larger molecules occurs, and channels are made that encapsulate to form **vacuoles**, clear fluid or air-filled spaces in the protoplasm. Vacuoles break away from the cell membrane and combine with **lysosomes**, intracellular digestive systems containing hydrolytic enzymes that break down proteins and some carbohydrates for cellular use. Pinocytosis occurs in reaction to strong electrolyte solutions, proteins, and other macromolecules. Without this process, proteins would have no other means of penetrating the cell membrane (Figure 2-16).

Phagocytosis

Phagocytosis is the process whereby the cell selectively ingests large particles of material. The process is analogous to pinocytosis, but this system involves the taking in of bacteria, other cells, or particles of tissue degeneration. If the system were not selectively specific, phagocytes would ingest normal body structures as well.

As with pinocytosis, lysosomes act on phagocytic vesicles. Hydrolases are used to digest proteins, glycogen, nucleic acids, and other substances so the vesicles are able to function as digestive bodies. Any matter that is not broken down

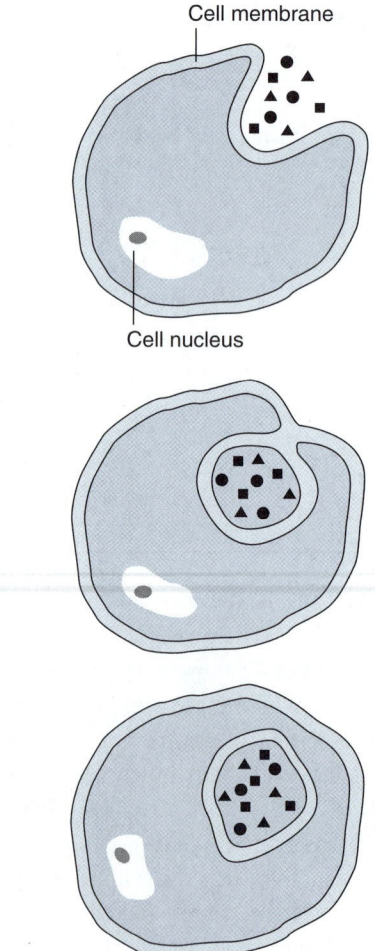

Figure 2-16 | Pinocytosis

and digested by lysosomal activity is transported out of the cell by the process of exocytosis.

Exocytosis

In some situations, intracellular molecules are too large to be transported out of the cell by active or passive transport. When this is the case, the molecules join with the cell membrane and exit the cell in the process of **exocytosis**, which is similar to pinocytosis, but a reverse form of it (Figure 2-17).

Movement of Electrical Potentials

It is extremely important for the nurse to fully understand the physiology and movement of electrical potentials across the cell membrane because so many medications administered to patients, especially via the IV route, affect the electrical activity of muscles and nerves. For example, the heart, a mass of cardiac muscle, is innervated and regulated by a nerve conduction system. The nurse employed in critical care specialty areas is often responsible for giving drugs according to changes in electrocardiograms (EKGs).

The capability of nerve and muscle to make and transmit membrane potential changes is called **excitability** or **irritability**. Neurons are able to transmit hundreds of impulses per second.

The inside of the cell carries a negative charge, while the outside is positively charged, resulting in the potential difference (voltage) called the **membrane potential**. These electrical charges, separated by the cell membrane, have the capability to work if they come together. This condition exists in all body cells. The difference in charge is the result of several factors: the negatively charged molecules inside the cell, the permeability properties of the cell membrane, and the action of the sodium-potassium pump that moves sodium and potassium against their concentration gradients.

Within the cell, proteins and organic substances carry negative charges. They do not leave the cell and are known as fixed anions. They do, however, attract small organic ions of sodium, potassium, and calcium, which are able to diffuse through from the extracellular fluid.

The cell membrane is more permeable to potassium than to other cations, so potassium is more concentrated in the intracellular compartment. The reason for this is the presence of polypeptide ion channels, known as **sodium-potassium gates**, which open and close under certain conditions. There are two different ionic channels for potassium, one that has no gates, thus always open, and another that has gates that close when the cell is at rest. Sodium channels have gates that are closed when the cell is at rest. The cell at rest is more permeable to potassium than sodium. Sodium and potassium gates are voltage regulated, opening or closing according to membrane potentials.

The inside of the cell is more negatively charged than the outside and creates a difference in electrical charges called the **resting membrane potential**, present when there is no cellular stimulation (Figure 2-18). The voltage difference is the result of the extracellular concentration of sodium ions and the intracellular concentration of potassium ions maintained by the sodium-potassium pump, which moves sodium out and potassium in. This resting membrane, one hundred times more permeable to potassium than to sodium, allows for some potassium diffusion into the ECF from its higher concentration in the ICF, thus leaving more negatively charged anions in the ICF to maintain the resting membrane potential. This resting membrane potential (-65 to -85 mV) occurs when there are more anions inside the cell and no impulses produced.

Stimulation by mechanical, chemical, or electrical means creates a change in the resting membrane potential of nerve and muscle cells, resulting in a nerve impulse or **action potential**. This is an electrical occurrence in which the polarity of the membrane potential is reversed rapidly and then restored. Any time a resting cell membrane is stimulated, it becomes more permeable to sodium, allowing sodium to move into the cell, thus decreasing the membrane potential from a negative value to zero. This reversal of membrane polarity during the production of action potentials is called **depolarization**. Depolarization occurs

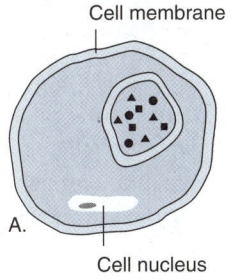 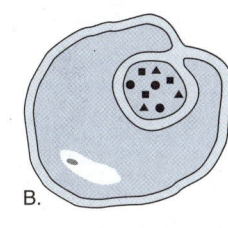 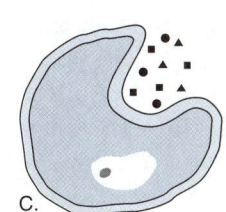 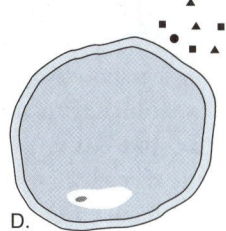

Cell membrane

Cell nucleus

A.   B.   C.   D.

Figure 2-17 | Exocytosis

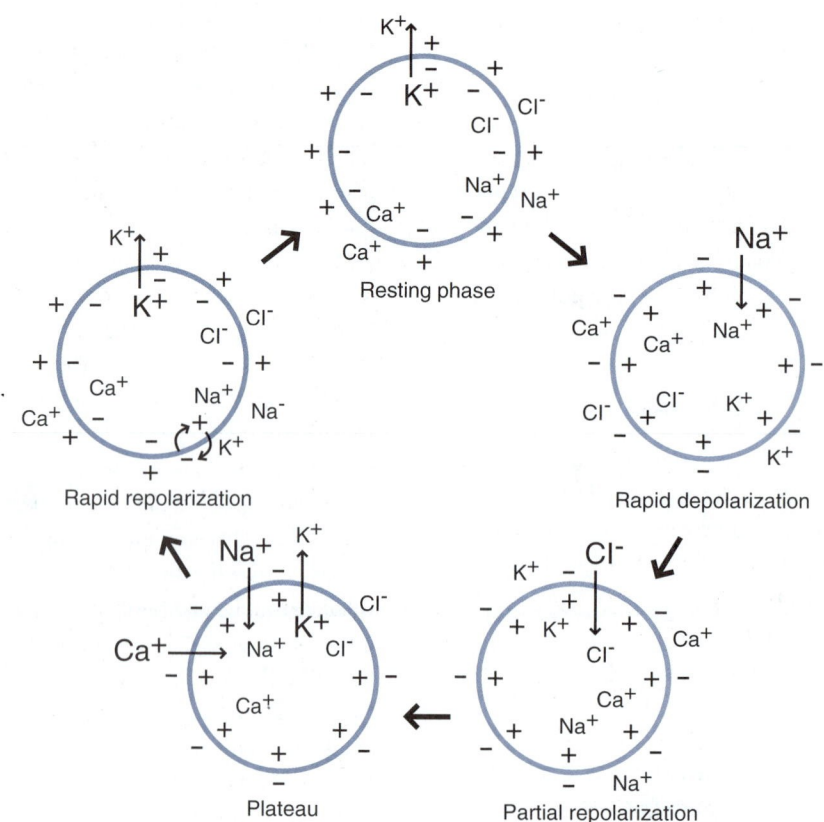

Figure 2-18 │ Cell membrane voltage

because large amounts of sodium are leaking into the cell, which the membrane cannot keep out. The intracellular side of the membrane becomes less negative than the outside. In order for the membrane potential to change and rapid polarity reversal to occur, a **threshold potential** of 15 mV–20 mV must be reached. Once reached, the cell continues to depolarize, even without additional stimulation. As sodium diffuses into the cell, the membrane potential falls to zero and then rapidly depolarizes, becoming positive (+40 mV). If a stimulus is weaker than the threshold potential, a nerve impulse (action potential) will not occur. This is known as the all-or-none law because an impulse is either propagated or not. There is no such entity as a partial impulse.

The cell membrane is not able to react to any other stimulation during most of an action potential because of changes occurring in membrane permeability. This time interval is known as the **absolute refractory period**. The **relative refractory period** occurs when potassium permeability increases toward the end of an action potential and only an extremely strong stimulus can generate another action potential. One action potential cannot begin until the one before it is finished. Each action potential serves as the stimulus for

another to occur, so there is a constant and continuous wavelike spread of action potentials across a membrane.

With depolarization, the sodium gates close, the potassium gates open, and potassium ions rapidly leave the cell and return the membrane interior to the normal negative state. This results in **repolarization**, the reestablishment of the resting membrane potential. It occurs in less than a millisecond (ms). The balance of sodium and potassium is not stabilized until the sodium-potassium pump, through active transport, removes excess sodium from the cell.

BODY SYSTEMS: FLUID AND ELECTROLYTE REGULATION

To fully comprehend body water content, its constituents, and its movement between compartments, it is necessary to review how balances are maintained and regulated. Fluid and electrolyte balance is maintained through the intake of food and fluids, known as **exogenous** sources, and the output of excess water and waste products. **Endogenous** production of water is that produced within the body through chemical oxidation processes. Endogenous sources of water are small compared with exogenous sources.

Regulation of body water occurs as the result of various organs and tissues working together to maintain a state of equilibrium. When the body is in a state of health, fluid intake and loss is about the same over a 72-hour period. Fluid intake and urine output are about equal, while water formed through the oxidation of food and fluid equals that lost through perspiration, respiration, and gastrointestinal excretion.

It is necessary for the nurse to understand the normal mechanisms of intake, output, and regulation in order to facilitate the identification of abnormalities and to intervene appropriately. When homeostasis is compromised and imbalances occur, the nurse is responsible for managing an important exogenous source of fluid replacement, intravenous infusions.

The Renal System

When addressing water balance in the body, the kidneys play a major role in controlling output, regulating fluid and electrolyte balance, and adjusting acid-base balance. Urine, formed by means of reabsorption and filtration, is composed of 95% water and 5% organic and inorganic material removed from the blood. In the glomeruli, where plasma filtration occurs, the rate of filtration is determined by systemic arterial pressure and plasma oncotic (colloid) pressure, as well as the hydrostatic pressure in the Bowman's capsule. Under normal conditions, the glomerular membrane prevents passage of large molecules, such as proteins and blood cells.

The renal tubules reabsorb 99% of the glomerular filtrate and return it to the extracellular fluid. The 1% that remains is excreted in the form of urine as a mixture of water, solutes, and wastes.

The Cardiovascular System

In order for the kidneys to reabsorb and secrete properly, the heart and blood vessels must be capable of pumping adequately. This driving force enables plasma filtration to occur across the glomerular membrane, resulting in the formation of urine. The cardiovascular system pumps to distribute water and nutrients to all organs and tissues and to remove waste products.

The Lymphatic System

The lymphatic system serves as an adjunct to the cardiovascular system by removing excess interstitial fluid, in the form of lymph, and returning it to the circulatory system. If it were not for the lymphatics, the inward force at the arterial capillary bed into the interstitial fluid compartment, which exceeds the outgoing force at the venous end, would result in fluid overload in the interstitial fluid. This would bring about a state of edema that would prove to be fatal within a matter of hours.

The Nervous System

The nervous system masterminds fluid and electrolyte balance through the regulation of sodium and water. It does this by stimulating the secretions of various endocrine glands.

Baroreceptors, pressure-sensitive nerve endings in the aortic arch, arteries, veins, atria of the heart, and carotid sinuses, respond to changes in volume in the extracellular fluid. Therefore, with overhydration or underhydration, they affect blood flow. They signal receptors in the brain to stimulate the posterior pituitary gland to secrete stored antidiuretic hormone. The hypothalamus triggers the sensation of thirst as a result of the baroreceptor responses to changes in osmolality, prompts fluid intake, and thus increases fluid volume.

The Endocrine System

The endocrine system responds selectively to the regulation and maintenance of fluid and electrolyte balance through hormonal production. Endocrine secretion is controlled by the nervous system, by chemicals in the blood, or through the action of other hormones.

Antidiuretic Hormone (ADH)

Antidiuretic hormone (ADH), also called vasopressin, is secreted by the posterior pituitary gland and regulates water retention and excretion. When there is an excess of sodium in the extracellular fluid or reduced blood volume, hypertonicity or diminished circulation signals the release of ADH by the posterior lobe of the pituitary gland. This results in the sensation of thirst while conserving body water through reabsorption (Figure 2-19). ADH is released in response to physical and emotional stressors, excessive physical activity, some anesthetics, morphine, barbiturates, and pain.

In contrast, when the extracellular fluid becomes hypotonic, if there is increased blood volume, or if the body becomes hypothermic, the pituitary is signaled to inhibit the release of ADH. This, in turn, stimulates the excretion of urine. Alcohol acts as a diuretic in this manner. ADH, therefore, regulates extracellular osmolality while aldosterone regulates extracellular volume.

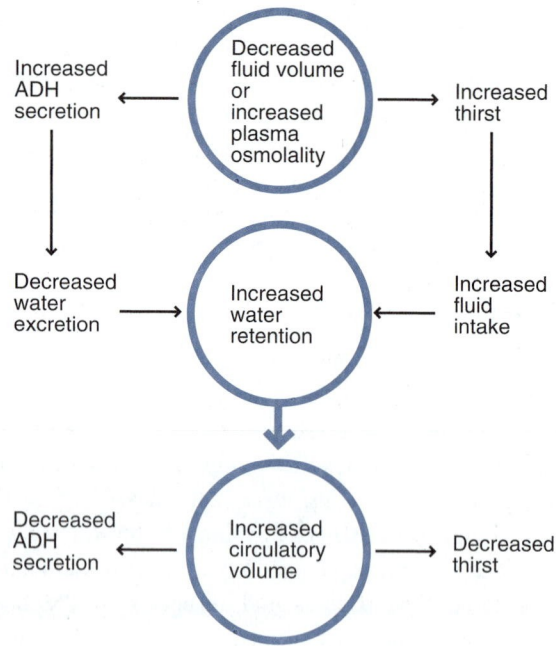

Figure 2-19 | Thirst mechanism and ADH secretion

Aldosterone

Aldosterone, a mineralocorticoid secreted by the adrenal glands, plays a major role in regulating distal tubular reabsorption of sodium in the kidneys, thus promoting water reabsorption and increasing blood volume. It regulates potassium concentrations by stimulating potassium secretion into the distal tubules and collecting ducts of the kidneys.

When the body is exposed to physical and psychic stress, has diminished sodium levels, or when the extracellular volume decreases, aldosterone is secreted to promote the reabsorption of water and sodium by the kidneys. It also promotes sodium retention (and potassium excretion) through its action on the gastrointestinal tract, salivary glands, and sweat glands.

Thyroid Hormone

The thyroid gland stores and secretes thyroid hormone, which influences metabolic rate and blood flow. Increased blood flow results in satisfactory renal perfusion and enhances urinary output. The thyroid also stores and releases calcitonin, which assists in the regulation of calcium levels in the blood and bones.

Parathyroid Hormone (PTH)

The level of calcium and phosphate is regulated by parathyroid hormone (parathormone) secretions. Calcium and phosphate homeostasis is physiologically necessary for bone and tooth formation, acid-base balance, cell membrane permeability, nerve and muscle functioning (especially the myocardium), and for enzyme activation.

Serum calcium homeostasis is achieved through a specialized parathyroid feedback system. When extracellular calcium levels drop, the parathyroid glands are stimulated to secrete parathormone, which acts on the bones to move calcium into the blood. Should the bones be deficient in calcium, the hormone stimulates the kidney tubules and the intestinal tract to reabsorb calcium. If blood levels of phosphate drop, the hormone stimulates its reabsorption in the kidney tubules. If abnormal increases occur, urinary excretion balances the excess of phosphates.

The Respiratory System

The lungs, through the process of internal and external respiration, regulate the exchange of oxygen and carbon dioxide in the body. The lungs also control acid-base balance through the production of carbonic acid. The carbonic acid–sodium bicarbonate system is the body's most important buffer system. In addition, the lungs control fluid balance by removing water from the body through the process of external respiration.

The Gastrointestinal System

The gastrointestinal tract absorbs nutrients and water, and serves as the main reservoir for the intake of fluids. It also removes a small portion of body water in feces. Many illnesses and diseases contribute to large body water loss through the gastrointestinal tract.

The Integumentary System

Body water is lost through the skin in the form of perspiration, or sensible loss. Insensible losses of water occur continuously, and cannot be felt or seen, but can amount to a minimum of a pint of fluid per day. Loss of body water through the skin can vary greatly, depending on such variables as internal body temperature, external environmental temperature, physical exertion, illness, or injury.

ACID-BASE BALANCE

In order for homeostasis to be maintained, an equalization must exist between the acidity and alkalinity of body fluids, known as **acid-base balance**. Whether a solution is acid or alkaline depends on its concentration of hydrogen and hydroxyl ions.

An **acid** is any substance that releases hydrogen ions (**hydrogen ion donor**) when placed in a solution. Within the body are **nonvolatile** (**fixed**) **acids** derived from the metabolic breakdown (**catabolism**) of proteins and fats. The fixed acids that result from protein catabolism are lactic and sulfuric acids, and acetoacetic acid from fat metabolism. Hydrogen ions that come from fixed acids are excreted by the kidneys. Carbonic acid is a volatile or nonfixed acid that is reciprocal with carbon dioxide and water in the body and dissociates into hydrogen and bicarbonate ions. A **volatile acid** can be vaporized or evaporated and is the means by which carbon dioxide in the ECF is transformed in the lungs to be removed during the expiratory phase of respiration.

A **base**, or alkali, is any substance that releases hydroxyl ions (**hydrogen ion acceptor**) in a solution and is able to accept and combine with hydrogen ions. Bases are derived from the metabolic breakdown of citrate, lactate, and isocitrate to carbon dioxide and water. They are found in most foods but are predominant in fruits and vegetables.

A **salt** is made up of the negative ion of any acid (except hydroxyl) and the positive ion of any base (except hydrogen). It results from the chemical interaction within a solution where the acid and base neutralize each other. **Neutralization** is the process whereby opposing forces balance each other so that neither force dominates.

The chemical unit of measurement used to describe the degree of acidity or alkalinity of a substance is known as the **potential of hydrogen** or **pH**. The degree of pH is gauged on a scale of zero to fourteen, with seven indicating neutrality. The neutrality of a solution means that its concentration of opposing forces balance each other, making it neither acid nor alkaline. Pure water has a pH of 7.0. It can dissociate into hydrogen and hydroxyl ions and act as both an acid and a base (Figure 2-20).

There is an inverse correlation between acid-base properties: As the hydrogen ion concentration increases, the pH decreases (acidity); as the concentration of hydrogen ions decreases, the pH rises (alkalinity). Acids are neutralized with bases and vice versa. As the acidity of a solution increases, with an increase in the number of hydrogen ions, the pH level drops below 7.0, and as alkalinity increases, and hydroxyl ions exceed the concentration of hydrogen ions, the

pH rises above 7.0. **Acidosis** is the accumulation of excess acids (hydrogen ions) or a deficiency of base (bicarbonate ions), resulting in a pH less than 7.0. **Alkalosis** is the reduction of acids (hydrogen ions) and an increase of base (bicarbonate ions), resulting in a pH greater than 7.0. The pH of plasma is maintained within the slightly alkaline range of 7.35 to 7.45.

Buffer Systems

Fluids within the intracellular and extracellular spaces must be equalized in terms of acidity and alkalinity. In order for this balance to remain, chemical and physiologic buffers exist. A **buffer** is a substance that maintains the body's acid-base balance by regulating hydrogen ion concentration. It is reaction-specific and only comes into action in response to abnormal changes in acidity or alkalinity. A buffer system is the combination of an acid and a base, and is sometimes referred to as a buffer pair.

For normal cellular activity to occur, the hydrogen ion concentration of the body's fluid must be sustained within a very limited range. This concentration is carefully controlled by three major buffer systems that work to maintain acid-base balance: (1) the carbonic acid-bicarbonate system, (2) the phosphate buffer system, and (3) the protein buffer system. They are extremely important in maintaining homeostasis and any deviation from the normal pH range can cause major disturbances in cellular, enzymatic, and neuromuscular activity within the body.

The Carbonic Acid-Bicarbonate Buffer System

The most important buffering system, which exists in the extracellular fluid compartment and serves to maintain acid-base balance, is the carbonic acid-sodium bicarbonate buffer system, which operates in the lungs and kidneys. Under normal circumstances, the body maintains a balanced ratio of one part carbonic acid (1.2 mmol/L) to twenty parts bicarbonate (24 mEq/L) in order to maintain a pH of 7.40 (Figure 2-21).

The carbonic acid supply is regulated by the respiratory system. Carbon dioxide, as it is formed during cellular metabolic processes, is returned to the extracellular fluid where the enzyme carbonic anhydrase acts on the water and carbon dioxide to form volatile carbonic acid. At the alveolar capillary bed, carbon dioxide is exchanged for oxygen during internal respiration. The lungs remove the carbon dioxide from the body by means of external respiration. Whenever the carbon dioxide level rises, the respiratory center of the brain in the medulla is stimulated. It signals the lungs to increase the rate and depth of respirations and rid the body of excess carbon dioxide. When carbon dioxide levels drop too low, the same mechanisms trigger a decrease in the rate

Acid $\longrightarrow$ OH$^-$

Base $\longrightarrow$ H$^+$

Water $\longrightarrow$ H$_2$O or HOH

Dissociates into hydrogen and hydroxyl ions

$$H_2O + H_2O = H_3O^+ + OH^-$$

Figure 2-20 | Water as an acid and a base

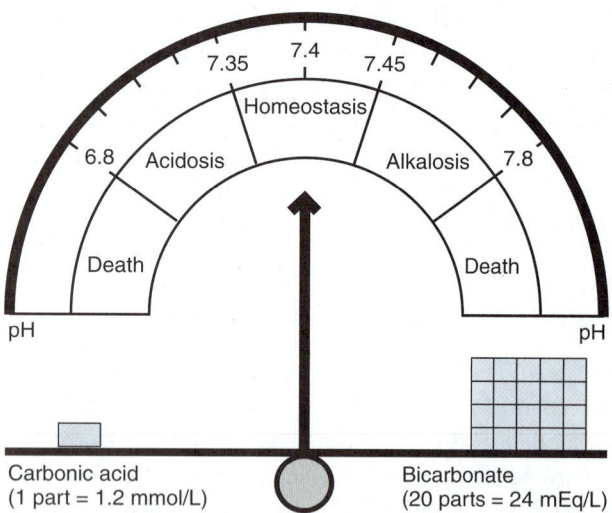

Figure 2-21 | Acid-base scale

and depth of respirations so that the 1:20 carbonic acid-bicarbonate ratio is maintained by holding back carbon dioxide so it can be transformed into carbonic acid.

The kidneys fine-tune the pH by supporting respiratory regulation of acid-base balance. In the renal tubules of the kidneys, nonvolatile acids are removed. During the formation of urine, acid and alkaline phosphates are altered to produce an acid urine. This mechanism conserves sodium, potassium, magnesium, and calcium, all of which maintain the body's fixed base. In the presence of acidosis, the kidneys assist in the regulation of acid-base balance through the excretion of hydrogen ions and the retention of bicarbonate ions. They also manufacture bicarbonate from carbon dioxide and water. In alkalotic situations the kidneys retain hydrogen ions and excrete bicarbonate ions.

The kidneys and lungs function as compensatory systems in balancing acids and bases, maintaining the 1:20 ratio of carbonic acid to bicarbonate. While the respiratory adjustments of acid-base balance occur rapidly, renal mechanisms take longer to restore pH neutrality (up to 72 hr).

The Phosphate Buffer System

Phosphates serve as intracellular and extracellular buffers. The concentration of phosphates is greatest within the cell, making phosphates powerful intracellular buffers. Because of this, the normal hydrogen ion concentrations within the cell can be maintained, which results in acid-base balance.

The Protein Buffer System

The protein buffer system, the largest and strongest buffer system in the body, exists in both the intracellular and extracellular compartments, but is mainly a mechanism of the intracellular fluid. It is able to maintain acid-base balance because the proteins carry numerous negative charges that can buffer positively charged hydrogen ions. Some proteins are unique, however, in that one part of their molecule is able to accept hydrogen ions, while another portion can release hydrogen ions.

Hemoglobin, which carries a negative charge, acts as a strong protein buffer. When carbon dioxide diffuses into a red blood cell, it reacts with part of the hemoglobin molecule to form carbaminohemoglobin, which combines with water to form carbonic acid. The carbonic acid is catalyzed by the enzyme carbonic anhydrase to dissociate into hydrogen and bicarbonate ions. The negatively charged bicarbonate ions diffuse out of the red blood cell into the plasma, allowing negatively charged chloride ions to diffuse into the cell in their place. This phenomenon is known as the **chloride shift**. The hydrogen ions derived from the carbonic acid dissociation are buffered because they combine with the negatively charged hemoglobin.

Acid-Base Imbalances

Whenever there is a change in the hydrogen ion concentration of the blood, acid-base imbalances can occur. The imbalances that relate to alterations in carbonic acid levels are referred to as respiratory disturbances, and those imbalances that are directed toward changes in bicarbonate ratios are considered metabolic disturbances. Any malfunction of the buffer systems results in respiratory acidosis or alkalosis, metabolic acidosis or alkalosis, or a combination.

Respiratory Acidosis (Carbonic Acid Excess)

Respiratory acidosis is the acid-base imbalance with an abnormally elevated hydrogen ion concentration and an excess of carbonic acid. This is the most common of the acid-base imbalances and refers to acidosis caused by a buildup of carbon dioxide in the body. The carbonic acid accumulation is the result of pulmonary hypoventilation. **Hypercapnia**, the increase of carbon dioxide in the blood, with resultant increase in the partial pressure of carbon dioxide (PCO_2) in the plasma, results from the retention of carbon dioxide by the lungs.

In respiratory acidosis, the excess carbon dioxide in the extracellular fluid lowers the carbonic acid-bicarbonate ratio. The kidneys compensate for respiratory alkalosis by increasing the plasma bicarbonate concentration, which helps return the carbonic acid-sodium bicarbonate ratio to normal, thus restoring the pH to normal (Figure 2-22).

Etiology and Contributing Factors

Respiratory acidosis, which may be acute or chronic, is usually the result of altered pulmonary ventilation owing to disease of the respiratory tract. It occurs with asthma, chronic obstructive pulmonary disease (COPD), pneumonia, bronchiectasis, and cardiopulmonary arrest. It is also associated with extreme abdominal pain, disorders that affect the respiratory muscles, pneumothorax, extreme obesity, and inadequate ventilation. In some instances anesthetics, sedatives (including alcohol), hypnotics, and barbiturates contribute to this problem. Respiratory acidosis may be compensated by the kidneys or uncompensated.

Clinical Manifestations and Defining Characteristics

Clinically, the individual with respiratory acidosis may be weak and sluggish, and experience confusion and disorientation, which are signs of central nervous system depression. There may be a productive cough, dyspnea, and cyanosis, along with a barrel chest in patients with chronic lung disease.

If there is no renal compensation for the respiratory acidosis, the partial pressure of carbon dioxide rises abnormally (>45 mm Hg). The plasma pH is low (<7.35) and the plasma bicarbonate levels are normal. If the kidneys compensate for the respiratory acidosis, the plasma bicarbonate concentration will rise (>28 mEq/L) and the plasma pH will return to normal.

Intravenous Infusion Implications

The goal of treatment is to return the pH and the carbonic acid-bicarbonate ratio to normal, if the underlying cause of the acidosis can be corrected. If there is chronic lung disease, the intention is to enhance ventilation as much as possible.

Parenteral infusion therapy is not a primary treatment modality, although intravenous antibiotics and bronchodilators may be indicated. In this situation an intravenous infusion is usually in place to access the systemic circulation should the need arise. In severe cases, bicarbonate or one of its precursors (gluconate or lactate) may be required.

Respiratory Alkalosis (Carbonic Acid Deficit)

Respiratory alkalosis is an acid-base imbalance when plasma pH is high and the hydrogen ion concentration is abnormally low, with a deficiency of carbonic acid. This condition results in an increased carbonic acid-bicarbonate ratio and is relatively uncommon.

The kidneys are the only compensatory mechanism for respiratory alkalosis, and lowering the bicarbonate concentration restores the normal carbonic acid-bicarbonate ratio, thus returning the pH to normal (Figure 2-22).

Etiology and Contributing Factors

Respiratory alkalosis is caused by hyperventilation and the excessive loss of carbon dioxide. There is a decrease in the partial pressure of plasma carbon dioxide that results in hypocapnia. Both the rate and depth of respirations increase.

It can occur as a secondary compensatory mechanism for metabolic acidosis.

The most common etiology is hyperventilation brought on by anxiety and tension. High altitudes induce hyperventilation owing to decreased atmospheric oxygen. Physical disorders and illnesses such as liver cirrhosis, hyperthyroidism, gram-negative sepsis, fever, and peritonitis, and some cardiopulmonary maladies, such as pulmonary edema or pulmonary embolism, are associated with hyperventilation. Central nervous system lesions, in which the respiratory center in the brain is affected, induce respiratory alkalosis. These include tumors, trauma, encephalitis, and neurosurgery. Salicylate poisoning in its early stages induces hyperventilation. Asthmatic individuals often hyperventilate in response to air-hunger anxiety.

Clinical Manifestations and Defining Characteristics

Hyperventilation, with deep respirations, rapid respirations, or both, is the chief sign of respiratory alkalosis. Patients often complain of **paresthesias**, sensations of numbness or tingling, especially in the extremities. They often experience light-headedness, sweating, heart palpitations, and muscle cramping. Agitation and mental restlessness occur and may progress to hysteria and a state of temporary unconsciousness. In severe cases there can be tetany, convulsions, and coma, as seen in alcohol withdrawal (delirium tremens).

The levels of plasma pH (>7.45) and urine pH (>7.0) rise, while the partial pressure of carbon dioxide (<35 mm Hg) and the level of plasma bicarbonate fall (<21 mEq/L).

Intravenous Infusion Implications

As with all acid-base imbalances, the goal of treatment is to correct the underlying cause of the respiratory alkalosis and return the carbonic acid-sodium bicarbonate ratio to 1:20. Parenteral therapy is not a primary intervention, although it is used to support the kidneys in their compensatory attempts to retain chloride ions and excrete bicarbonate ions.

Intravenous infusions are used to replace the water lost during hyperventilation and to provide the nonbicarbonate chloride ions needed to replace lost bicarbonate ions. Even though the total concentration of calcium may be normal on laboratory reports, the nurse must be alert to the onset of tetany, which might occur in respiratory alkalosis because of a reduction in ionized calcium. Sodium and potassium ions are lost with increased chloride concentrations and need to be replaced. If calcium levels are replenished too rapidly, tetany may be induced.

Metabolic Acidosis (Base Bicarbonate Deficit)

Metabolic acidosis describes any acidotic condition related to an excess of noncarbonic acid concentrations and

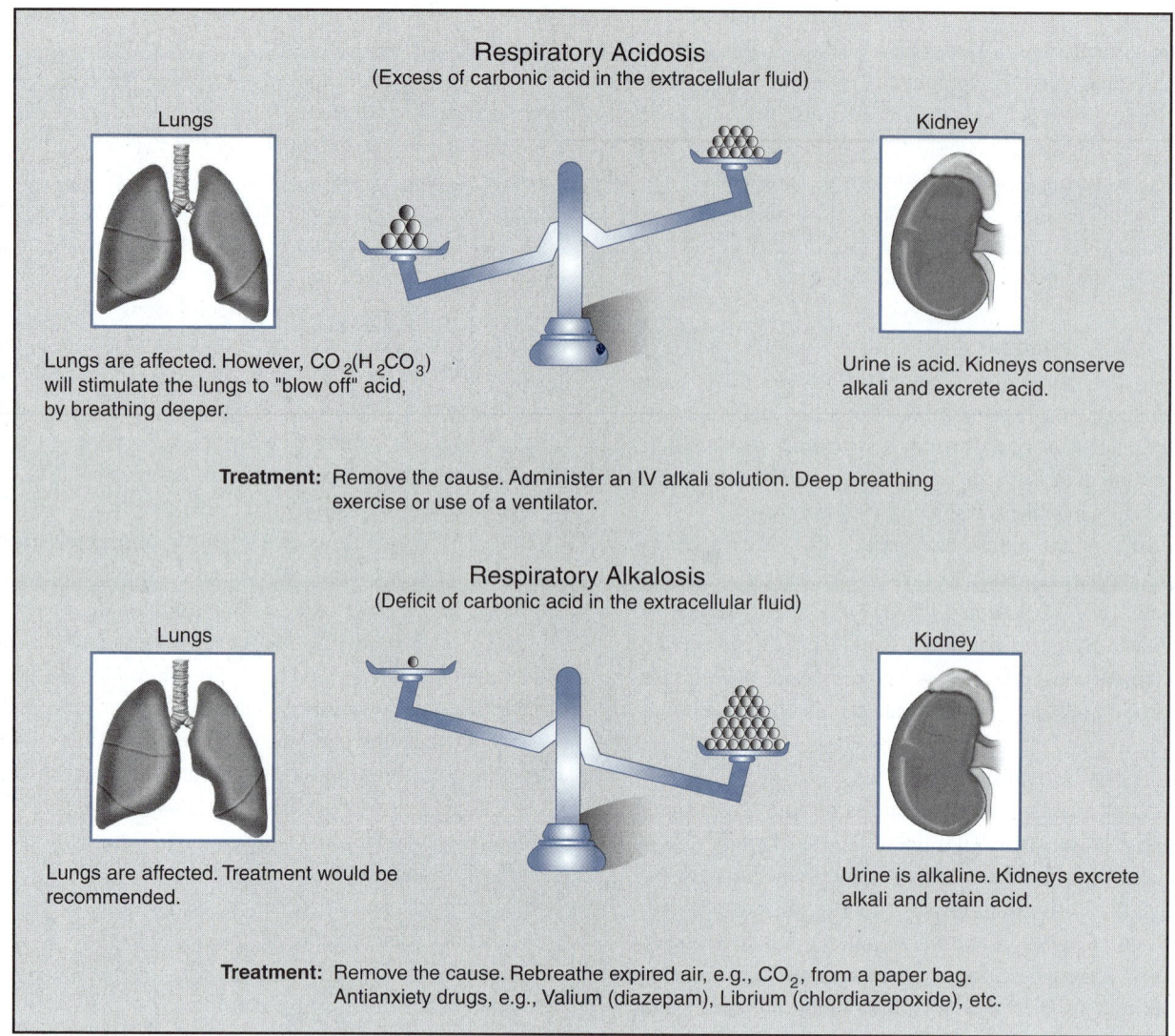

Respiratory Acidosis
(Excess of carbonic acid in the extracellular fluid)

Lungs

Kidney

Lungs are affected. However, $CO_2(H_2CO_3)$ will stimulate the lungs to "blow off" acid, by breathing deeper.

Urine is acid. Kidneys conserve alkali and excrete acid.

Treatment: Remove the cause. Administer an IV alkali solution. Deep breathing exercise or use of a ventilator.

Respiratory Alkalosis
(Deficit of carbonic acid in the extracellular fluid)

Lungs

Kidney

Lungs are affected. Treatment would be recommended.

Urine is alkaline. Kidneys excrete alkali and retain acid.

Treatment: Remove the cause. Rebreathe expired air, e.g., CO_2, from a paper bag. Antianxiety drugs, e.g., Valium (diazepam), Librium (chlordiazepoxide), etc.

Figure 2-22 | Respiratory acidosis and respiratory alkalosis

is characterized by a deficiency of base bicarbonate. Both the lungs and the kidneys compensate for this situation (Figure 2-23).

Etiology and Contributing Factors

There are several factors that contribute to the development of metabolic acidosis, and any one factor or a combination of factors can precipitate the disturbance. Whenever there is an abnormal increase in acid production, it can lead to a bicarbonate ion deficiency, a decrease in the carbonic acid-sodium bicarbonate ratio, an elevated hydrogen ion concentration, and a lowering of the pH.

Conditions that increase acid production are fever, infection, renal impairment, shock, salicylate poisoning, starvation, and impaired metabolic activity. The ketoacidosis that occurs in uncontrolled diabetes mellitus is a major cause of metabolic acidosis. Impaired cellular metabolism

that occurs with fever and infectious processes, anesthesia, and circulatory failure contribute. In liver diseases such as hepatitis and cirrhosis, acidosis occurs as well. Other causes are disturbances in dietary intake associated with starvation, increased fat intake, or reduced carbohydrate intake. Situations when acids remain in the body are diarrhea, from loss of base in the stool, and renal insufficiency, when the kidneys are unable to rid the body of acids.

Clinical Manifestations and Defining Characteristics

Individuals with mild metabolic acidosis can be asymptomatic. As the situation worsens there may be weakness, malaise, nausea, vomiting, and abdominal pain. There is often deep, rapid breathing or shortness of breath with air hunger. If the condition becomes severe, the patient becomes stuporous and may lapse into coma. The pH of the urine

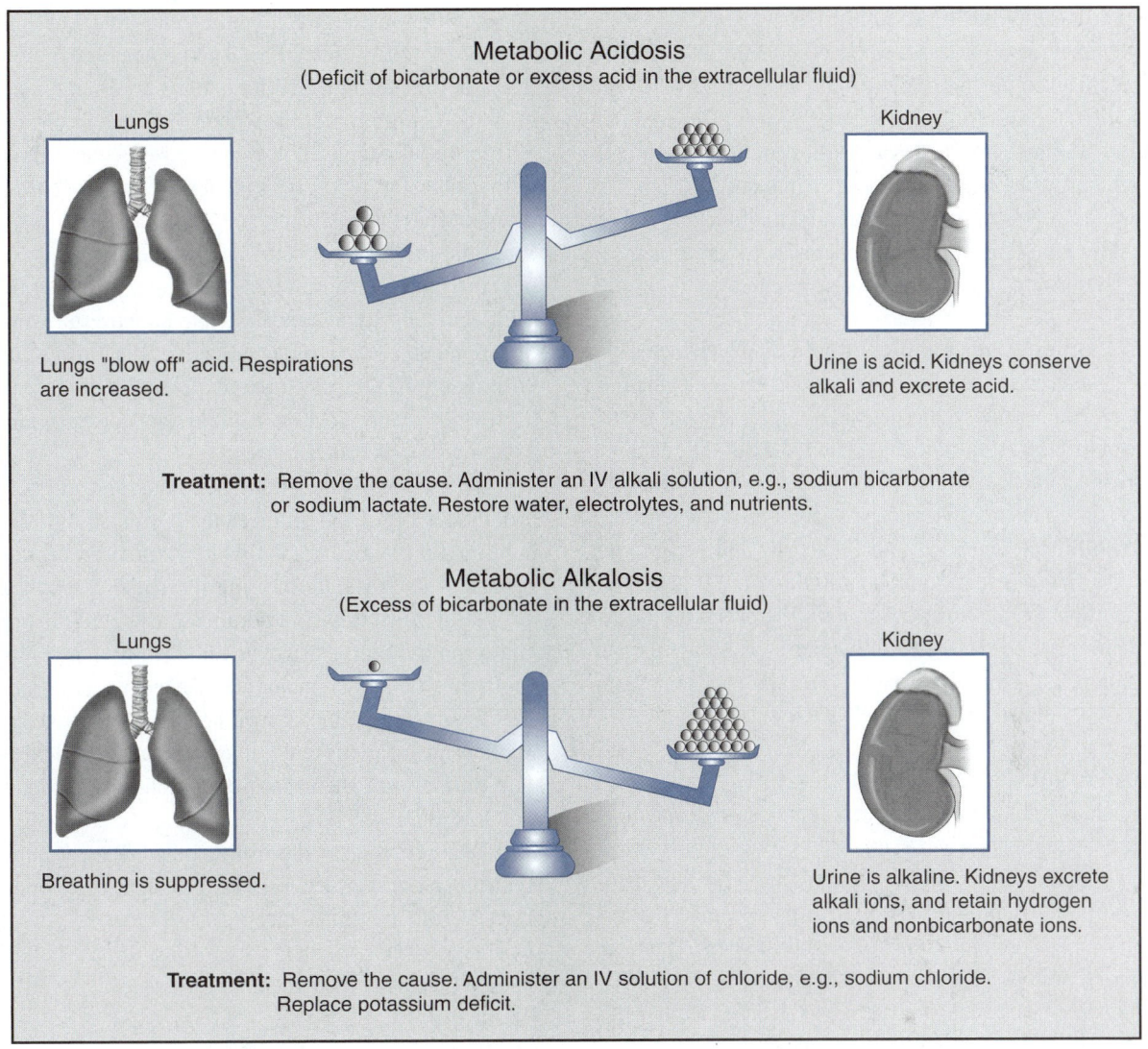

Figure 2-23 | Metabolic acidosis and metabolic alkalosis

(<6.0) and plasma (<7.35) is low as are plasma bicarbonate concentrations (<21 mEq/L). Depending on compensatory mechanisms, the partial pressure of carbon dioxide (PCO_2) is normal or low.

Intravenous Infusion Implications

The primary concern is to correct the acidosis, identify and remove the underlying causes, and prevent both from recurring. Metabolic acidosis can be produced by the parenteral administration of acidifying salts. If there is excessive delivery of sodium chloride and ammonium chloride, the extracellular fluid may become overloaded with chloride, thus lowering the concentration of bicarbonate.

Fluid volume deficits and electrolyte imbalances that coexist with metabolic acidosis must be adjusted with intravenous fluids and electrolytes and monitored carefully.

Special attention to potassium levels is critical. The nurse may be directed to administer sodium bicarbonate or sodium lactate if the acidosis is severe, or if interventions fail to treat the underlying cause.

Metabolic Alkalosis (Bicarbonate Excess)

Metabolic alkalosis describes all cases of alkalosis not caused by a carbonic-acid deficit. It occurs when the level of base bicarbonate is abnormally high or there is a decrease in the hydrogen ion concentration. With an excess of bicarbonate, there is an elevation in the carbonic acid-bicarbonate ratio.

Metabolic alkalosis is compensated for by the lungs and by the kidneys, but a compensatory respiratory acidosis usually occurs to restore the plasma pH by realigning the carbonic acid-bicarbonate ratio (Figure 2-23).

Etiology and Contributing Factors

Metabolic alkalosis occurs as a result of excessive intake of alkalis, such as sodium bicarbonate (baking soda) or the loss of acid, which results in an increased bicarbonate level. Vomiting and diarrhea can result in a loss of chloride and hydrogen ions, which causes an increase in blood bicarbonate, as well as a potassium deficit. Adrenal malfunction and renal failure can cause metabolic alkalosis, as can potent diuretics, tissue destruction, and hypercalcemia.

Clinical Manifestations and Defining Characteristics

Breathing patterns are depressed both in rate and in depth, a respiratory compensatory mechanism to raise the partial pressure of carbon dioxide and thus restore the carbonic acid-bicarbonate ratio. In contrast to metabolic acidosis, where there is central nervous system depression, there is hyperexcitability with hypertonicity of muscle activity and hyperactive reflexes. In severe metabolic alkalosis there may be tetany and convulsions because of calcium loss. The plasma bicarbonate concentration is elevated (>28 mEq/L) as is the pH of the plasma (>7.45) and the urine (>7.0). The plasma concentrations of potassium and chloride are low.

Intravenous Infusion Implications

As with acidosis, treatment for metabolic alkalosis involves correcting the underlying cause, if possible. Infusion therapy often includes the administration of electrolytes. Since bicarbonate excess is usually associated with potassium deficit, the hypokalemic condition must be alleviated. The administration of chloride ions, which are retained by the body in place of excess bicarbonate ions, relieves the base bicarbonate excess characteristic of metabolic alkalosis. Fluid and electrolyte therapy is usually a necessary component of treatment. In severe cases, the careful administration of ammonium chloride, an acidifying salt, may be necessary. Whenever electrolyte solutions are administered intravenously, the nurse must be vigilant to thoroughly assess the patient's general condition, intake and output, and related laboratory values, in addition to monitoring and maintaining the infusions.

ELECTROLYTE BALANCES AND IMBALANCES

Fluid and electrolytes must be balanced within a narrow margin for homeostasis to be sustained. Illness and disease processes can easily disrupt this balance, often placing the patient in jeopardy.

For the nurse to provide safe care and effectively manage patient situations, it is necessary to understand the underlying concepts of electrolytes and their role in supporting homeostasis. He must be able to identify the causes of fluid-electrolyte and acid-base imbalances and recognize them in the clinical setting. When imbalances occur, not only is the nurse responsible for recognizing them, he is also responsible for reporting and intervening to correct any irregularities discovered.

While possessing a sound understanding of body fluids and their mechanisms of movement, the nurse also needs to fully comprehend the role of each major electrolyte and how it is regulated. By comprehending how electrolytes function to promote health, the nurse is able to identify how electrolyte imbalance relates to illness and disease, and thus intervene appropriately.

In managing intravenous infusions, the nurse is confronted with several interrelated responsibilities: maintaining fluid regulation so that a balance between loss and replacement exists, monitoring the patient's physical and psychological status, and administrating various products that promote fluid-electrolyte and acid-base equilibrium.

In this chapter the major electrolyte imbalances and general treatment parameters will be addressed. Nursing interventions with various replacement modalities will be covered later in the text, when specific solutions and guidelines for administration will be covered.

When referring to electrolyte imbalances, it should be remembered that they can be primary or secondary in nature. Primary imbalances exist in and of themselves, whereas secondary imbalances occur as a result of another pathophysiologic phenomenon.

Sodium

Sodium is the major cation (Na^+) of the extracellular fluid compartment and is regulated by ADH and aldosterone. Sodium is one of the primary regulators of fluid balance in the body. Sodium is excreted mainly by the kidneys, which regulate its reabsorption and excretion, depending on sodium intake. Sodium concentration in the plasma is maintained at a constant level and averages 135–145 mEq/L.

Purpose

As discussed earlier, sodium plays a primary role in the transmission of neuromuscular impulses and the maintenance of the cellular membrane potential. It is the principal regulator of osmotic pressure in the extracellular fluid.

Sodium Deficit

Primary sodium deficit results in the redistribution of water between the fluid compartments and changes in extracellular osmolality. **Hyponatremia** is an abnormal decrease in plasma sodium levels. When sodium output exceeds its intake, a deficit results. Any abnormal loss of body water produces a state of **dehydration**. **Hypertonic dehydration** occurs when there is a greater loss of water than salt, which leads to increased sodium concentration and increased osmolality of the extracellular fluid. When salt loss exceeds water loss, **hypotonic dehydration** occurs; **isotonic dehydration** is the result of a proportional loss of water and sodium.

Etiology and Contributing Factors

Hyponatremia can be caused by inadequate dietary intake of sodium or from excessive loss. Salt is lost from body fluids through several routes: urine, perspiration, vomiting, diarrhea, gastric suction, and potent diuretic therapy. If there is adrenal malfunction, the lack of aldosterone impairs kidney tubule reabsorption of sodium. In renal disease, acute or chronic, sodium loss in the urine is common. The administration of large volumes of intravenous 5% Dextrose in water or excessive drinking of pure (electrolyte-free) water can aggravate hyponatremia. When there is excessive sodium loss, replacement must come, not from pure water, but from fluids with sodium and chlorides because chloride loss accompanies sodium loss.

Clinical Manifestations and Defining Characteristics

The signs and symptoms associated with sodium deficiency, depending on its severity, can range anywhere from mild cramping to cardiovascular collapse. In severe hyponatremia, lethargy and stupor are the result of increased water uptake by the cells in the central nervous system. There may be fatigue, headache, muscle weakness, nausea, vomiting, abdominal cramping, and seizures. Postural hypotension, reduced urine output, and tachycardia are secondary to hypovolemia. The patient may go into a state of shock, manifested by signs of cold, clammy skin, diaphoresis, and cyanosis.

Interventions and Treatment

Prevention of hyponatremia is most important and results from a thorough nursing history along with observation and assessment of the patient's physical findings. The most important prevention mechanism is the oral or parenteral administration of salt to maintain sodium balance.

Once hyponatremia occurs, treatment is guided by serum sodium levels with the goal of restoring the normal sodium concentration of the extracellular fluid, of reestablishing normal osmolality, and correcting fluid shift to the intracellular compartment. If losses occur, they should be replaced with solutions containing sodium and other electrolytes based on the extent of deficit.

Sodium Excess

Hypernatremia is an excess of sodium in the blood, resulting from positive sodium balance, and occurs when sodium intake exceeds loss. Primary hypernatremia is not a common electrolyte imbalance. Under normal circumstances, since sodium and water follow each other, an excess of sodium does not usually occur because water is retained to dilute the sodium.

Etiology and Contributing Factors

The cause of primary hypernatremia relates to excessive ingestion of salt without a corresponding water intake. The intravenous administration of excessive volumes of isotonic or hypertonic saline solutions leads to salt intoxication.

In primary sodium excess, there is salt intoxication with hypernatremia, an increase of fluid osmolality, and redistribution of water between the intracellular and extracellular fluids. Because of the elevated concentration of sodium in the extracellular compartment, water shifts out of the cell in order to promote osmotic balance. While this movement promotes extracellular volume, it does so at the expense of the intracellular fluid.

Clinical Manifestations and Defining Characteristics

The patient with hypernatremia is extremely thirsty with dry mucous membranes. The tongue is dry, red, and edematous, and the body temperature is elevated. As hypernatremia becomes more severe, the patient may become depressed, fatigued, and lapse into coma. Intracranial hemorrhage can occur. The serum sodium concentration (>145 mEq/L) and serum osmolality (>295 mOsm/kg) rise.

Interventions and Treatment

The primary treatment consists of removing the excess sodium from the body by limiting dietary and parenteral sources of intake. In addition, sodium-free fluids are infused to lower the serum sodium concentration and osmolality. In doing this, however, the extracellular compartment may expand. This fluid volume overload can result in pulmonary edema and heart failure. Sometimes dialysis may be the only recourse to lower serum sodium levels.

Potassium

Potassium (K^+) is the major cation of the intracellular compartment; its concentration is 3.5–5.0 mEq/L. Most of the body's potassium is found in voluntary muscle groups, with a substantial amount present in the skin, superficial tissues, and the red blood cells.

Potassium is regulated by the kidney tubules, where potassium ions exchange with sodium ions, and by the secretion of aldosterone, which controls potassium concentrations in the extracellular compartment. Aldosterone enhances renal tubular reabsorption of sodium and promotes the renal excretion of potassium and hydrogen ions. Gastrointestinal secretions of potassium are high, so a large amount is passed out through the feces. Because of the excretion through the renal and gastrointestinal systems, potassium must be replaced daily through dietary intake. If vomiting or diarrhea occurs, large amounts of these electrolytes are lost. Potassium is excreted through perspiration and is rapidly lost whenever there is tissue damage.

Purpose

Potassium maintains intracellular homeostasis and determines the cell's resting membrane potential. It assists various enzyme systems in catalyzing reactions and participates in protein synthesis and carbohydrate metabolism. Potassium is of vital importance in the transmission of electrical impulses in the cardiovascular, respiratory, and gastrointestinal systems.

Potassium Deficit

Hypokalemia is an abnormally low serum concentration of potassium that reflects an extracellular deficiency of the electrolyte. This is a fairly common deficiency, especially in hospitalized individuals. In some instances the levels can drop dangerously low before the imbalance is recognized. It is important to remember that, under normal conditions, losses of 25–50 mEq per day are expected.

Etiology and Contributing Factors

Several factors contribute to hypokalemia. Decreased dietary intake, especially in the older person, is common. During periods of fasting as much as 40–50 mEq can be lost per day. Impaired potassium conservation occurs when sodium needs to be retained, as in periods of alkalosis or acidosis. The hydrogen ion deficit of alkalosis interferes with potassium conservation because there is a greater secretion of potassium into the distal portion of the renal tubules rather than hydrogen ions. With acidosis, potassium excretion is increased because of the mobilization of potassium from the intracellular compartment to the extracellular compartment.

Diuretic therapy is a very common cause of hypokalemia, especially when there are dietary restrictions of sodium. Vomiting, diarrhea, disease (e.g., inflammatory bowel disorder), and surgical procedures (e.g., ileostomy) of the gastrointestinal tract, where potassium levels are usually high, can deplete potassium stores rapidly. Other situations that precipitate the condition are tissue destruction (e.g., burns or crushing injuries), diabetes insipidus, hyperinsulinism, and malnutrition.

Clinical Manifestations and Defining Characteristics

Many of the signs and symptoms of hypokalemia are nonspecific and can relate to many different illnesses. The clinical picture of potassium deficiency is evidenced by an alteration in cardiovascular, respiratory, gastrointestinal, renal, and neuromuscular activity. Pulses are weak, heart sounds are faint, and the patient is prone to dysrhythmias. Respirations are shallow, and there is mental depression. There may be muscle weakness, depressed or absent reflexes, and paralysis. The patient complains of excessive thirst (**polydipsia**), excessive urination (**polyuria**), and may be anorexic. There is often nausea, vomiting, and diarrhea.

NURSING TIP

Adding Potassium to an Infusion Container

Always check agency policy regarding the amount of potassium that can be added to an infusion container. The amount may vary from one nursing unit to another, based

---

The EKG will exhibit flattened or inverted T waves and S-T segment depression as well as premature ventricular contractions (PVCs). Serum concentration levels of potassium fall below normal (<3.5 mEq/L) and arterial blood gases show an increase in pH and bicarbonate levels.

Interventions and Treatment

Once the diagnosis of hypokalemia is made, oral replacement, parenteral potassium replacement, or both, must be undertaken, depending on the patient's condition. It is also necessary to determine the underlying cause of the deficit so that future losses can be prevented.

Potassium deficit is not usually an isolated imbalance, so the administration of water and other electrolytes may be needed. Before replacement therapy is started, it is necessary to determine renal function, since potassium is mainly excreted by the kidneys. If there is renal impairment, a buildup of potassium in the body can be toxic.

Replacement therapy for severe hypokalemia is undertaken with intravenous supplementations, under very close supervision, to prevent acute potassium intoxication. The dose should never exceed 80 mEq/L of potassium, and 40 mEq/L is preferable. Potassium must never be administered intravenously without diluting it in adequate volumes of fluid. Direct, undiluted administration usually results in cardiac arrest. The rate of administration should not exceed 20 mEq per minute.

N U R S I N G   A L E R T

Potassium Dilution

Potassium must always be adequately diluted prior to intravenous administration to prevent cardiac dysrhythmias or even cardiac arrest. The maximum dose should be 80 mEq/L and must be administered only with caution and meticulous supervision. Never administer IV potassium by direct IV bolus.

During potassium replacement serum electrolyte levels must be evaluated frequently. The patient must be meticulously observed for manifestations of both deficit and excess.

Potassium Excess

Hyperkalemia is an abnormal excess of potassium in the blood, mainly limited to the extracellular fluid. This condition is not as common as hypokalemia but must be treated quickly because it is potentially life threatening.

Etiology and Contributing Factors

Hyperkalemia usually results from an increase in potassium intake without a corresponding excretion, but it can also occur because of a redistribution of the electrolyte from intracellular fluid to extracellular fluid. In general, excess dietary intake of potassium is not a cause of hyperkalemia unless there is altered renal function to impede its excretion in the urine.

Excessive oral or intravenous administration of potassium supplements contributes to hyperkalemia, as does the intake of potassium-sparing diuretics. Whenever there is tissue trauma from burns or crushing injuries, potassium leaks out of the cells and into the extracellular compartment, resulting in hyperkalemia. It is also associated with adrenal cortical insufficiency, such as Addison's disease, and a deficiency of aldosterone. Hyperkalemia occurs with diminished urinary output (**oliguria**) or total absence of urinary output (anuria) seen in renal failure.

Clinical Manifestations and Defining Characteristics

Hyperkalemia occurs when the serum potassium level rises (>5.0 mEq/L). The patient presents with muscle weakness, paresthesia, and even paralysis. There is often dizziness (**vertigo**) and painful muscle cramps. Gastrointestinal hyperactivity is usually present with nausea, intestinal colic, and diarrhea. The EKG shows peaked T waves and depressed S-T segments. If hyperkalemia is severe, the P wave flattens and the QRS complex widens.

Interventions and Treatment

The first step in treatment comes with the recognition of precipitating factors of hyperkalemia so that life-threatening situations of severe potassium excess are avoided. The goal of treatment is to remove the extracellular overload of the electrolyte. This can be accomplished through dietary restriction of potassium (in mild cases) or through the administration of oral or parenteral sodium chloride (to individuals who can tolerate the sodium load), which enhances urinary loss of potassium. If renal function is inadequate, potassium-free hydrating solutions can be given.

In hyperkalemic emergencies the most rapid method of correction comes with the administration of glucose, insulin, and sodium polystyrene sulfonate, which promotes extracellular potassium movement into the cell. If acidosis is the problem, intravenous administration of sodium bicarbonate will move the potassium in the same manner. Diuretics may be given. Cardiac toxicity from elevated potassium levels may be alleviated by administering calcium gluconate or calcium carbonate. If renal insufficiency is present, dialysis may be needed to lower potassium levels.

Calcium

Calcium (Ca^+) is the most plentiful electrolyte in the body, with 99% of it stored in the bones and teeth. The 1% in the extracellular fluid is a minute amount, but maintenance of that concentration is of physiologic significance. Normal serum levels range between 4.4 mEq/L and 5.5 mEq/L.

Dietary calcium is absorbed in the small intestine (depending on pH and the presence of vitamin D), with about 80% excreted in the feces and the rest excreted in the urine. A very small amount can be lost through the skin with hyperthyroidism. Under normal conditions, urinary loss of calcium should balance its gastrointestinal absorption. With decreasing acidity, calcium is less readily absorbed in the bowel.

Purpose

Calcium is necessary for the strength and rigidity of bones and for normal coagulation of blood. It is extremely important for neuromuscular activity, especially myocardial stimulation. It has a role in cell membrane behavior by activating or inhibiting enzymatic activity.

Although the amount of calcium in the extracellular fluid is small, it is a vital component. Fifty percent is ionized and diffusible and governs parathormone secretion. The nonionized amount of serum calcium is bound to plasma proteins, mainly albumin.

The ionizing ability of the extracellular calcium is affected by acid-base balance. The increased pH of alkalosis decreases the serum concentration of ionized calcium, whereas the decreased pH of acidosis results in an increase of ionized calcium, at the expense of protein-bound nonionized calcium. A patient in acidosis may have a normal ionized calcium concentration while the total serum concentration will be low. For this reason, the determination of total serum calcium concentration must include serum albumin levels.

Calcium Deficit

Hypocalcemia is an abnormally low concentration of calcium in the blood. It is usually reflected in extracellular deficiency with the main problem a reduction of ionized calcium.

Etiology and Contributing Factors
There are numerous mechanisms that contribute to the development of hypocalcemia and a variety of illnesses and disease processes that cause the condition. One of the most common causes is hypoparathyroidism, where the mechanisms that regulate serum calcium concentrations are disrupted.

Nondietary vitamin D deficiency, due to pancreatitis, small bowel malabsorption, gastrointestinal shunt operations, or other intestinal disorders, is a cause, along with inadequate sun exposure. Because milk and many other food sources are fortified with vitamin D, dietary deficiency is rarely a problem in developed countries of the world. Burns and massive subcutaneous tissue infections induce calcium loss. Hypocalcemia can be induced through the administration of phosphate salts and alkalizing agents used to counteract acidosis, along with other drugs.

Clinical Manifestations and Contributing Factors
The extent of hypocalcemia necessary to elicit symptoms varies greatly among individuals. The EKG shows a normal T wave, but a prolonged Q-T interval because of a lengthened S-T segment. There is commonly the sensation of tingling and numbness of the circumoral area and the fingers. There can be abdominal and muscle cramps as well as spasm of both smooth (involuntary) and striated (voluntary, skeletal) muscles. Spasms of muscles in the face, larynx, bronchi, gastrointestinal tract, and the hands and feet can occur. Tetany is evidenced by a positive **Chvostek's sign** (unilateral facial muscle spasms when the 7th cranial or facial nerve is tapped anterior to the ear) and a positive **Trousseau's sign** (spasmodic contractions of the hands elicited by inflating a blood pressure cuff above systolic pressure for three minutes). There can be hyperactive deep tendon reflexes, depression, mood swings, memory impairment, hallucinations, and seizures.

Individuals with hypoparathyroidism and chronic hypocalcemia tend to have very dry skin, coarse hair with **alopecia** (hair loss), deformed nails, and poorly developed teeth. Cataracts are often a problem. An accompanying hyperphosphatemia may occur, with decreased urinary excretion of both calcium and phosphate.

Interventions and Treatment
In order to reestablish a normal serum concentration of ionized calcium, the underlying cause must be identified and treated. Increased dietary intake of calcium-rich foods is necessary along with oral calcium supplements. In emergency situations, with severe tetany and convulsions, intravenous calcium gluconate is usually administered. When the cause of an individual's hypocalcemia cannot be removed or controlled, continuous calcium salt infusions are given. If there is no response, low magnesium levels may be the problem, something common in patients with malabsorption syndromes, malnutrition, and alcoholism. Vitamin D supplements are administered to facilitate the absorption of calcium from the bowel.

Calcium Excess

Hypercalcemia is an abnormal excess of extracellular calcium. The main alteration is an excess of the ionized portion of calcium; serum levels exceed 5.3 mEq/L.

Etiology and Contributing Factors
Hypercalcemia results from several diseases and conditions. It occurs as a result of primary hyperparathyroidism where there is excessive parathormone secretion. A condition known as hypervitaminosis D occurs when there is increased bone resorption of the nutrient.

Hypercalcemia is a common complication associated with various malignant processes, including breast carcinoma, multiple myeloma, leukemia, and lymphoma, as well as lung and kidney neoplasms.

During periods of immobilization there is decreased bone formation and bone resorption. Hypercalcemia occurs when the rate of demineralization exceeds the ability of the kidney to excrete the excess calcium.

Clinical Manifestations and Defining Characteristics
In hypercalcemia, there is a decrease in neuromuscular excitability, with reduced muscle tone and fatigue. Nausea,

vomiting, anorexia, and weight loss are common. There is often deep bone pain related to pathologic fractures, and flank pain associated with the development of calcium renal stones because the kidneys cannot function appropriately with the increased calcium load.

In addition to increased serum calcium levels, the Q-T interval on the EKG is prolonged. In hyperparathyroidism, there is radiologic evidence of bone demineralization with cavitation.

When acute hypercalcemic crisis occurs, serum calcium levels rise drastically, resulting in a potentially fatal situation. There is intractable nausea, vomiting, polydipsia, polyuria, and dehydration, which lead to electrolyte imbalances. Delirium and coma usually follow.

Interventions and Treatment

If a patient has mild calcium elevation and is free of symptoms, treatment is conservative while its cause is determined. With acute hypercalcemic crisis, emergency measures must be initiated. Treatment of the underlying cause of excess calcium is directed toward lowering its concentration. Hypercalcemia with hypoparathyroidism may require surgical excision of the glands. Ambulation of an immobilized person often corrects hypercalcemia. Administration of sufficient fluids, while restricting calcium intake, is usually effective. Steroid treatment helps to counteract the hypercalcemia associated with malignancies.

Calcium-free fluid infusions are indicated in acute hypercalcemic crisis to hydrate the patient and promote urinary loss of calcium. Use of infusions containing calcium and phosphorus must be avoided. With extremely severe cases, dialysis is indicated to rid the body of excess calcium.

N U R S I N G   A L E R T

Hypercalcemic Patients

In patients with hypercalcemia, intravenous fluids must not contain calcium or phosphorus.

Magnesium

Magnesium (Mg^{++}) is exceeded only by potassium in abundance in the intracellular compartment. It is regulated, with calcium, by the parathyroids. Approximately 50% is found in the bones, with the rest present in various organs, especially the heart, liver, and skeletal muscle. Most of the body's magnesium is ionized, while only about 30% is bound to protein.

So, like calcium, albumin levels must be considered when assessing magnesium levels in the body.

The kidneys provide the main route for excretion of magnesium. When there is a deficiency, the kidneys conserve magnesium by excreting more potassium. Absorption of magnesium occurs in the small intestine. The body absorbs less than half of the magnesium ingested, unless more is needed, and excretes the excess in the stool. Normal blood magnesium level is 1.5–2.5 mEq/L.

Purpose

One of the main functions of magnesium is enzymatic cellular activation, especially for protein and carbohydrate metabolism. It is needed by nerve tissue, skeletal muscles, and the heart. Magnesium activates the sodium-potassium pump and is needed to maintain calcium levels within the cell.

Magnesium Deficit

Hypomagnesemia is an abnormal decrease in the serum concentration of magnesium. The condition reflects a deficiency in the ionized portion of the cation in the extracellular fluid.

Etiology and Contributing Factors

The causes of hypomagnesemia include decreased dietary intake, impaired absorption, excessive loss, or excessive use of magnesium-free infusions and thiazide diuretics. Vomiting, diarrhea, and intestinal surgeries contribute to magnesium loss as do malabsorption syndromes, parathyroid disease, alcoholism, and malnutrition. Cirrhosis, pancreatitis, vitamin D intoxication, chronic renal diseases, and diabetic acidosis also cause magnesium loss.

Clinical Manifestations and Defining Characteristics

Because magnesium deficits are accompanied by other electrolyte imbalances, the clinical picture of hypomagnesemia may mimic other situations, especially hypocalcemia. Hypomagnesemia leads to corresponding losses of sodium, calcium, and phosphorus. Until levels drop below 1.0 mEq/L, there may be no evidence of a problem.

The main nonspecific signs and symptoms of magnesium deficiency relate to increased neuromuscular irritability. Nonspecific T-wave alterations on the EKG may be present. There is usually confusion, agitation, hyperactive deep tendon reflexes, **nystagmus** (involuntary, slow or rapid rhythmical eyeball oscillations that may be rotary [counterclockwise] or vertical [up-down motion]), painful paresthesias, tetany, and seizure disorders.

There may be tachycardia, dysrhythmias, and blood pressure deviations. Nausea, vomiting, anorexia, and abdominal distention occur.

Interventions and Treatment

Administration of oral, intramuscular, and intravenous magnesium salts is the main treatment modality. When seizures or dysrhythmias occur, high doses are given rapidly by the intravenous route.

Magnesium Excess

Hypermagnesemia is an abnormally high serum concentration of magnesium. This is a very rare imbalance.

Etiology and Contributing Factors

Renal failure, in which the kidneys fail to rid the body of excess magnesium (and other compounds) is the major cause of magnesium excess. Hypermagnesemia can also result from diabetic acidosis, hyperparathyroidism, and toxemia of pregnancy.

Clinical Manifestations and Defining Characteristics

There is usually neuromuscular depression that can lead to peripheral muscle paralysis, respiratory depression, hypotension, and cardiac arrest. The EKG shows a prolonged QRS interval with atrioventricular block. There is central nervous system depression that results in drowsiness progressing to coma, and the patient complains of feeling hot and thirsty. Nausea and vomiting are usually present.

Interventions and Treatment

Since most situations of excess magnesium are the result of renal failure, magnesium compounds must be avoided and parenteral magnesium solutions should not be used. Calcium gluconate is used to reverse the depressant effects caused by excess magnesium. Respiratory support may be needed.

Chloride

Chloride is the major extracellular anion (Cl^-), joining with sodium to make saline. Most of it is present in the interstitial fluid, the lymph, and blood, with a very small amount present inside the cell. The normal serum concentration of chloride is 100–110 mEq/L.

Purpose

Chloride serves to maintain the osmotic pressure of the blood. Chloride levels decline in relationship to decreases in sodium, a result of water excess or deficit. Whenever a sodium ion is reabsorbed by the kidneys, a chloride (or bicarbonate) ion is also reabsorbed to preserve acid-base neutrality. The ratio of sodium to chloride is normally 3:2. As discussed earlier, chloride plays a major role in acid-base balance.

Chloride Deficit and Excess

An abnormal decrease in serum chloride is called **hypochloremia**. When chloride levels fall, there is a compensatory rise in bicarbonate levels so that the number of anions and cations in the extracellular fluid balance. Hypochloremia can result from hypokalemic compensation and from diuretic loss of chloride over sodium. During vomiting and diarrhea, chloride is lost with sodium. **Hyperchloremia** is the abnormal elevation of serum chloride concentrations.

Clinical manifestations and treatment of hypochloremia and hyperchloremia are basically those associated with metabolic alkalosis and acidosis. (See Acid-Base Imbalances.)

Phosphorus (Phosphate)

Phosphorus (P^+) exists in the body as organic and inorganic salts with the bulk (85%) of it present in the bones as cellular organic salts. Most of the element exists in the body as phosphate (PO_4^-), making it the major ion of the intracellular compartment. It is well absorbed by the intestine and excreted by the kidneys. The normal serum concentration is 1.7–2.6 mEq/L or 2.5–4.5 mg/dl.

Purpose

Together with calcium, phosphate is regulated by parathormone, and plays an integral part in bone and tooth development. It is necessary for protein, fat, and carbohydrate metabolism and for the production and storage of ATP. Most of the B vitamins must combine with phosphorus in order to work. Phosphorus is needed for nerve and muscle functions and helps maintain the body's acid-base balance.

Phosphorus Deficit

An abnormal decrease in serum phosphorus is called **hypophosphatemia**. Under normal conditions the kidneys reabsorb about 88% of ingested phosphorus. The intestine absorbs phosphorus more readily than it does calcium, so the kidneys excrete it more readily.

Etiology and Contributing Factors

Hypophosphatemia is usually related to deficient dietary intake or faulty absorption from the bowel because of vomiting, diarrhea, or vitamin D deficiency. Whenever there is a disruption of carbohydrate metabolism, as in diabetic acidosis or fever, phosphorus levels decline. Thiazide diuretics and hypoparathyroidism increase the loss of phosphorus from the kidney. Loss also occurs in the presence of potassium and magnesium deficiencies. Frequent ingestion of antacids, which are not absorbed, contributes to phosphorus depletion.

Clinical Manifestations and Defining Characteristics

The usual symptoms of acute phosphorus deficiency are muscle weakness and skeletal soreness, with progression to confusion and disorientation, convulsions, and coma. If the condition is chronic, there is memory loss, anorexia, and malaise, along with bone pain and joint stiffness.

Interventions and Treatment

As with all imbalances, prevention is the best treatment. Dietary supplementation is recommended for mild deficiency, and oral supplements are recommended for moderate deficiencies. In severe loss or when there is inadequate bowel function, intravenous sodium or potassium phosphate is used.

Phosphorus Excess

Hyperphosphatemia is the abnormal excess of serum phosphorus. The kidneys, when functioning normally, excrete excess phosphorus on a continual basis.

Etiology and Contributing Factors

Renal failure, acute and chronic, is the main cause of phosphorus excess. Hyperphosphatemia occurs with hyperthyroidism, excessive bone growth, or excessive doses of vitamin D. Some forms of cancer chemotherapy destroy cells, resulting in the release of large amounts of phosphorus into the circulation.

Clinical Manifestations and Defining Characteristics

There is little subjective evidence of transient phosphorus excess, and the symptoms that exist vary among patients. If the condition is severe, nausea, vomiting, and anorexia may occur. There may be digital and circumoral numbness, tingling, muscle spasms, and tetany. Tachycardia may be present and the EKG will record shortened S-T and Q-T intervals.

With chronic hyperphosphatemia, the kidneys and other soft tissues of the body are compromised. Calcium phosphate builds up in the kidneys, joints, and skin. The arteries, heart, gastric mucosa, and eyes may be affected.

Interventions and Treatment

Treatment, unless phosphorus excess results from dietary or drug sources, is aimed at remediating or controlling the underlying disorder. For hyperparathyroidism, surgical removal of the glands may be indicated. Dialysis is indicated for individuals with renal failure. In acute situations, intravenous administration of calcium may be necessary.

The usual treatment is dietary restriction of phosphorus and the administration of magnesium, calcium, or aluminum antacids that bind the phosphorus to solids in the intestine, thus removing it in the stools.

Key Concepts

* The nurse who initiates, monitors, and maintains intravenous infusions must be secure in his knowledge of the physiology and clinical implications associated with fluid and electrolyte acid-base balance in order to provide a safe level of care.

* Homeostasis is the balance that exists, under normal circumstances, between the body's internal and external environment. Any disruption of this equilibrium is indicative of illness and disease processes.

* Water is the primary chemical component within the human body and is the medium for exchange and regulation between the intracellular and extracellular fluid compartments.

* The fluid compartments of the body and balance of compounds within them provide the environment for cellular metabolic activity and the exchange of nutrients and wastes.

* Electrolytes, which make up 95% of the body's solute molecules, carry electrical charges, dissociate in water, and are crucial to body water distribution.

* The mechanisms of passive transport, active transport, and vesicle formation regulate water, electrolyte, and nonelectrolyte movement in the body and maintain the concentration of intracellular and extracellular components.

* Cellular membrane potentials serve to control the electrical activity of nerves and muscles, especially the heart.

* Each body system has a role in the movement of water and electrolytes throughout the body and works together with the other systems to maintain equilibrium.

* In order for homeostasis to be maintained, an equalization must be regulated between the acidity and alkalinity of body fluids (pH), known as acid-base balance.

✳ Acid-base balance is maintained through three major reaction-specific buffer systems that regulate hydrogen ion concentration: the carbonic acid-bicarbonate system, the phosphate buffer system, and the protein buffer system.

✳ The four major acid-base imbalances in the body are respiratory acidosis (carbonic acid excess), respiratory alkalosis (carbonic acid deficit), metabolic acidosis (base bicarbonate deficit), and metabolic alkalosis (bicarbonate excess).

✳ Fluids and electrolytes must be maintained within a narrow margin to achieve homeostasis. Primary and secondary electrolyte imbalances occur when there is a disruption in the interactions among sodium, potassium, calcium, magnesium, chloride, and phosphorus.

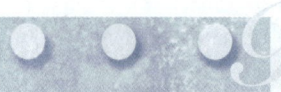

Review Questions and Activities

1. Why is it necessary for the nurse to understand fluid and electrolyte acid-base balance?
2. Make a two-column list and put the components of the intracellular fluid compartment in one column and the components of the extracellular compartment in the other column.
3. What is the function of the cell membrane in maintaining electrolyte balance?
4. What are the differences among the passive transport, active transport, and vesicle transport of substances into and out of the cell?
5. Diagram the series of events that occur in the cell membrane to illustrate the membrane at rest, at depolarization, and at repolarization.

6. What is the difference between respiratory and metabolic acidosis and between respiratory and metabolic alkalosis?
7. How does each of the three buffer systems of the body maintain acid-base balance?
8. Make a table listing the electrolytes sodium, potassium, calcium, magnesium, chloride, and phosphate. In the appropriate columns write two functions of each electrolyte, and two physiologic occurrences that result from (1) a deficiency, and (2) an excess of the electrolyte.
9. Create a physiologic flow sheet that illustrates how fluid and electrolyte acid-base balance contributes to homeostasis.

Chapter 3

Legal Implications of Intravenous Infusion Therapy

COMPETENCIES

Upon completion of this chapter, the reader should be able to:

✳ Define the terms *law* and *liability*.

✳ Discuss the four main sources of law and how they differ.

✳ Explain what a nurse practice act is.

✳ Describe the role of a state board of nursing.

✳ Define standard of care and describe how it relates to the practice of nursing.

✳ Differentiate between the two classifications of law: criminal and civil, and how they relate to the practice of nursing.

✳ Define malpractice.

✳ List the four elements needed to establish malpractice and discuss how they apply to intravenous infusion therapy.

✳ Discuss the Five Rights and the Three Checks of medication administration as tools to avoid making medication errors.

✳ Explain how patient-family teaching is a duty inherent to the delivery of nursing care.

✳ Examine how continuing education for the nurse relates to personal, professional, and public accountability.

✳ Discuss the legal implications encountered when the nurse delegates authority.

✳ Explain what the nurse can do to avoid litigation.

KEY TERMS

administrative law
assault
battery
breach of duty
causation
certification
civil law
constitutional law
crime
criminal law
duty

Five Rights of Medication
Administration
foreseeability
harm
injury
judicial law
legal precedent
liability
liable
litigation
malpractice

manslaughter
negligence
nurse practice act
precipitation
reasonableness
slander
standard
standard of care
state board of nursing
statute
tort

It is expected that the nurse, in any setting, practices with a patient-centered focus using the steps of the nursing process as the foundaiton of all of her actions. She must continually update her nursing knowledge, use scientific principles with sound rationales, and strive for optimum communication skills. The nurse should also be aware of the legal implications of intravenous infusion therapy. Because health care providers are often the subject of litigation, which is the act or process of carrying on a lawsuit, the nurse should possess a basic knowledge of the law and liability. It is not recommended that the nurse look at every clinical situation as a potential for litigation, but rather acknowledge the possibility that she could be involved in a suit. "Defensive practice" needs to be part of the nurse's commitment to rendering care.

LAW

The term *law* encompasses a wide spectrum of definitions depending on the context in which it is used. In a broad sense, law refers to a rule or group of rules and regulations that are man-made and which are established in order for individuals to live and work together within a society. The laws are enforced through an organized penal system. **Liability** refers to a person's individual responsibility for her own conduct. One is **liable** or accountable under the terms of current law.

The nurse should be aware that there are four main sources of law that concern society: constitutional law, statutory law, administrative law, and judicial or decisional law, often referred to as common law or legal precedents.

Constitutional Law

Constitutional law addresses the issues of governance and is the basis upon which our country is ruled. It is the highest level of law and is directed at the powers and limitations of the federal government. The Bill of Rights, which constitutes the first ten amendments to the Constitution, protects the citizens of the United States in terms of their basic rights or freedoms (Table 3-1). Every nurse should familiarize herself with these amendments, especially the last seven, since cases of negligence and malpractice often concern violations of the rights addressed in them. Individual states have their own constitutions that grant powers and limitations as well, which protect the citizens of those particular states. The nurse should be aware of laws that apply to the state where she practices.

Statutory Law

Statutes are laws enacted by legislative bodies that constitute the basic rules that govern society. They may be drawn up by the U.S. Senate or the House of Representatives, state legislatures, or city and county governing bodies. Statutes provide the basic, written directives of society. Once established, they cannot be changed unless they are amended or repealed.

Nurse Practice Acts

Nurse practice acts, rules that govern the practice of nursing, are examples of statutory laws. They define the parame-

Table 3-1 | The Bill of Rights

First Amendment	Congress shall make no law respecting an establishment of religion, or prohibiting the free exercise thereof; or abridging the freedom of speech, or of the press; or the right of the people peaceably to assemble, and to petition the Government for a redress of grievances.
Second Amendment	A well regulated Militia, being necessary to the security of a free State, the right of the people to keep and bear Arms, shall not be infringed.
Third Amendment	No Soldier shall, in time of peace be quartered in any house, without the consent of the Owner, nor in time of war, but in a manner to be prescribed by law.
Fourth Amendment	The right of the people to be secure in their persons, houses, papers, and effects, against unreasonable searches and seizures, shall not be violated, and no Warrants shall issue, but upon probable cause, supported by Oath or affirmation, and particularly describing the place to be searched, and the persons or things to be seized.
Fifth Amendment	No person shall be held to answer for a capital, or otherwise infamous crime, unless on a presentment or indictment of a Grand Jury, except in cases arising in the land or naval forces, or in the Militia, when in actual service in time of War or public danger; nor shall any person be subject for the same offence to be twice put in jeopardy of life or limb; nor shall be compelled in any criminal case to be a witness against himself, nor be deprived of life, liberty, or property, without due process of law; nor shall private property be taken for public use, without just compensation.
Sixth Amendment	In all criminal prosecutions, the accused shall enjoy the right to a speedy and public trial, by an impartial jury of the State and district wherein the crime shall have been committed, which district shall have been previously ascertained by law, and to be informed of the nature and cause of the accusation; to be confronted with the witnesses against him; to have compulsory process for obtaining witnesses in his favor, and to have the Assistance of Counsel for his defense.
Seventh Amendment	In suits at common law, where the value in controversy shall exceed twenty dollars, the right of trial by jury shall be preserved, and no fact tried by a jury, shall be otherwise reexamined in any Court of the United States, than according to the rules of the common law.
Eighth Amendment	Excessive bail shall not be required, nor excessive fines imposed, nor cruel and unusual punishments inflicted.
Ninth Amendment	The enumeration in the Constitution, of certain rights, shall not be construed to deny or disparage others retained by the people.
Tenth Amendment	The powers not delegated to the United States by the Constitution, nor prohibited by it to the States, are reserved to the States respectively, or to the people.

Source: U.S. National Archives and Records Administration, Washington, D.C.

ters within which individuals are qualified and licensed to practice nursing in a particular state and serve to codify nursing's obligation to act in the best interest of society. These acts vary from state to state. They confer upon nurses the authority to practice and grant society the power to sanction nurses who violate the standards of the profession by acting in any manner that threatens public safety (ANA, 1995). It was not until 1938 that the state of New York mandated the first nurse practice act, thus integrating nursing and the law. Later, other states initiated statutory laws to give the nursing profession the right to exist on the basis of licensure. It is critical that the nurse fully comprehend the licensure stipulations and scope of nursing practice for the state in which she lives and works. Most states use the American Nurses Association model nurse practice act in formulating their individual acts. The critical components of all nurse practice acts include a definition of nursing, the criteria for licensure, conditions for suspension and revocation of licensure, and creation of an agency that governs licensure, usually a board of nurse examiners or state board of nursing.

Administrative Law

Administrative law, also referred to as executive or regulatory law, covers laws made by administrative agencies or governing bodies. Such agencies are appointed by the executive branch of the government, the president, members of state legislature or state governor. There are numerous administrative agencies dealing with particular areas of concentration. Nursing boards, usually appointed by the governor, are administrative agencies at the state level.

State Boards of Nursing

Members of **state boards of nursing** regulate the practice of professional and vocational or practical nursing through enforcement of nurse practice acts. The board consists primarily of nurses actively involved in nursing education programs and clinical practice settings and consumer members from the general public. The state boards of nursing review applications, grant and renew licenses, conduct hearings, investigate complaints or problems, and participate in disciplinary proceedings. They also write or revise rules and regulations that affect nursing and institute standards for nursing education programs so nursing students are prepared to pass the licensure examination. All of these functions are directed ultimately at protecting the public—members of society served by the profession of nursing.

Standards of Nursing Care

A **standard** is an established reference criterion used as a basis for comparison in evaluating the outcome of a performance. In the profession of nursing, **standards of care** describe the minimum acceptable level of nursing care in various settings and determine whether consumers of nursing services receive adequate care. They are authoritative statements by which the nursing profession describes the responsibilities for which its practitioners are accountable.

Standards may be internal, such as job descriptions and employer policy and procedure manuals, or external, such as those set by the state nursing boards to ensure that the nurse practice act is enforced. The American Nurses Association has published *Standards of Clinical Nursing Practice*, a list of external standards that apply to care provided to anyone for whom the nurse is providing formally specified services as sanctioned by nursing practice acts (ANA, 1991). *Standards of Clinical Nursing Practice* is generic in nature and applies to all RNs engaged in clinical practice, regardless of clinical specialty practice setting or educational program. The National League for Nursing has also established external standards that apply to nursing education programs. The Intravenous Nurses Society has standards of practice that are revised, as needed, to define the responsibilities of nurses engaged in the specialty practice of IV therapy. Many health care institutions draw from these standards and from federal guidelines described by the Centers for Disease Control and Prevention (CDC) to formulate intravenous standards, policies, and procedures.

The board of nurse examiners of each state composes a list of current standards of nursing practice for registered, practical, or vocational nurses practicing within that state's jurisdiction. These standards identify the roles and responsibilities of the nurse as well as the degree of quality in administering care. The standards vary from state to state. The steps of the **nursing process**, assessment, nursing diagnosis, planning, implementation, and evaluation, are generally used as the basis for formulating standards of care. Practice guidelines usually accompany standards. Guidelines are more specific than standards—usually referring to clinical conditions, and serve to assist the nurse in making decisions. Guidelines describe recommended courses of action for var-

ious clinical situations or specific patient conditions or populations and serve as links among diagnoses, clinical situations, interventions, and outcomes.

Judicial Law

Judicial law, called decisional or common law, is the result of disputed legal issues. Statutes and regulations are interpreted from which rulings are made. The outcome of such disputes may be termed **legal precedents**. Court-determined law usually encompasses the area known as malpractice. Each issue of malpractice is addressed individually by the court. When evaluating malpractice, the court often looks at comparable cases whose outcomes serve to guide in making decisions. When a decision is made for the first time and sets a legal precedent, it is referred to as a landmark ruling.

CLASSIFICATIONS OF LAW

Laws are classified as either criminal or civil. Criminal law addresses the relationship between an individual person and the state and areas of conduct that are harmful to society. Civil law concerns the relationships of private individuals.

Criminal Law

Criminal law, also called penal law, is directed toward the actions of an individual that are harmful to society and ranges from minor traffic violations to murder. A **crime** is an act, either by commission or omission, of violating a written law or statute, and is punishable by imposed fines, restrictions, imprisonment, or, in some states, the death penalty.

Violation of a state nurse practice act may be a violation of criminal law and can result in probationary stipulations, as well as suspension or revocation of licensure. Infractions of a nurse practice act and violation of safe nursing practice may include improper administration of prescription medications, unlawful killing (such as euthanasia), failure to follow prescribed treatment protocols, or deviation from standards of practice.

CRITICAL THINKING

Nursing Error as Criminal and Civil Wrong

Can you think of any situations in which a nursing action can be both a criminal and civil wrong? Here is an example:

Mr. Lawton, a 54-year-old male, is admitted to the emergency department at 0600 hours on 9/14 with a medical diagnosis of gastroenteritis and dehydration. He has been complaining of nausea, vomiting, and diarrhea for the past 36 hours. Dr. Anderly orders the patient NPO and starts him on an intravenous infusion of 1000 cc 5% dextrose in 0.9% normal saline. Serum electrolytes reveal a potassium level of 3.1 mEq/L. The doctor orders "Add 30 mEq of KCl to the present IV solution" and "Transfer the patient to a medical nursing unit." The nurse erroneously administers the potassium, undiluted, IV push. Mr. Lawton suffers a cardiac arrest. Attempts to counteract the bolus dose of potassium and resuscitate the patient fail and he expires.

The nurse practice act states that the nurse must "know the rationale for, the effects of, and the proper administration of the medications she administers"; therefore, the nurse is in violation of the nurse practice act. She may also be held liable for the crime of involuntary **manslaughter**: killing that is both unintentional and without malice.

The civil wrong the nurse may be liable for is the tort of malpractice resulting in the wrongful death of a patient.

Civil Law

Civil law, also termed private or common law, involves the rights of private individuals and is subdivided into categories such as tort law, labor law, and contract law, among others. It relates to any legal actions associated with the rights and duties of private individuals within a society. Penalties for breach of such laws are enforced through the court system and often include payment or compensation for damages, performance of a prescribed course of action, or both, not fines or imprisonment. The word **tort** refers to a wrongful act, injury, or damage to an individual that can result in a civil action.

LIABILITY AND INFUSION THERAPY

A reasonably prudent adult of legal age is liable, or responsible for and answerable to authority, for her actions as well as the actions of individuals over whom she has custody, especially minors. It may also extend to employees who are assigned to her and supervised by her.

Negligence

Negligence is a general term that refers to carelessness on the part of an individual. When an adult is careless or fails to act as a reasonably prudent person would act, the conduct is labeled negligent. An act of negligence includes any action or inaction that can wrong another individual or cause that person harm.

Malpractice

Malpractice is negligence as it applies to professional behavior. Whereas negligence covers the imprudent actions or inactions of any adult in society (and those in her charge), malpractice is more specific because it is targeted at the professional person: one who is educated, trained, licensed or registered, and held accountable to the standards of a profession.

The focus in determining malpractice is usually that of **reasonableness**—the consideration regarding whether or not the nurse acted as any reasonably prudent nurse would have acted in the same or similar situation, having the same background, education, and experience. Reasonableness also seeks to verify that standards of care were followed. Expert witnesses are often called upon to help determine whether the nurse acted in a reasonable manner. Professional negligence or malpractice can be established and damages recovered only if four specific elements are present and proven: duty to care, breach of duty, causation, and injury or harm.

Duty to Care

Duty is the initial element to be established to prove a claim of malpractice. The nurse has a duty to render care to an individual, to apply knowledge, experience, and skill, and to act as any reasonably prudent nurse would act in a similar situation. The nurse is held accountable to the standards of care of the profession of nursing. A nursing student, although not yet licensed and registered, owes a duty to the patient as well. Once the student has studied the theoretical and clinical aspects of a subject area, she is held to the same standards as a graduate nurse. The LVN or LPN is also held accountable to the standards set by the state. The patient has the right to expect that both the nurse and the nursing student will act in his best interest. The nurse practice act of each state defines duty.

In dealing with intravenous infusion therapy, the nurse has the duty to be sure the medical order is correct and appropriate and to prepare the patient physically and psychologically. She must use principles of asepsis and infection control, then initiate, maintain, and monitor the patient and the infusion. She is duty-bound to know the side effects of all medications and fluids given, and to take necessary steps to avoid untoward reactions. It is her obligation to assess and evaluate the patient and the infusion, then appropriately document her actions and the patient's responses.

Breach of Duty

Breach of duty is the second element to be determined to establish malpractice. It is the failure on the part of the nurse to carry out the duty or care owed the patient. It may be an action, such as administering the incorrect intravenous solution, or an inaction, such as failing to assess and discontinue an infiltrated infusion, that is a digression from a standard of care. In determining breach of duty, the question of reasonableness is again the focus.

The subject of foreseeability is inherent in establishing breach of duty. **Foreseeability** implies the notion of cause and effect, and means that a nurse is expected to know that if something is done or not done, a particular outcome is likely to occur. For example, if the nurse fails to regulate the flow control clamp on the tubing of an intravenous infusion, the fluid will (foreseeably) enter and perfuse the circulatory system at a rapid, uncontrolled rate, which could result in fluid volume overload for the patient. In planning and implementing care, the nurse must look at the possible outcomes of her actions and their effect on the patient's well-being.

Causation

The third component of malpractice addresses the issue of causation, an area that is somewhat ambiguous and difficult to prove in some situations. **Causation** means that the damage or harm to the patient resulted from a breach of duty on the part of the nurse. The injury would not have happened if the nurse did not breach her duty to the patient. It must be established that the harm or injury to the patient was a result of the negligent action on the part of the nurse. The cardiac arrest and death that followed the intravenous bolus administration of potassium by the nurse, cited earlier, depicts an example of when the nurse owed the patient the duty to know the correct method of drug administration. Her breach of duty caused the patient's death.

Injury

The final element to be demonstrated in establishing malpractice is that of injury or harm. Even if negligence is demon-

strated yet there is no manifest injury, malpractice cannot be established. The words **injury** and **harm** are used interchangeably and can mean physical damages such as disability, disfigurement, pain, suffering, or wrongful death. Also included are loss of reputation, emotional pain, and financial harm, such as loss of wages (past, present, and future).

In the example where the nurse incorrectly administered the potassium, the injury that resulted from her breach of duty was the wrongful death of the patient. Harm in this case may include the pain and emotional suffering of the family as well as the loss of the deceased's present and future income.

THE LAW: IMPLICATIONS FOR IV NURSING PRACTICE

A **tort** is a civil wrong resulting from a breach of duty. Tort law covers intentional acts such as assault and battery, libel or slander, invasion of privacy, as well as negligent or unintentional actions. For the purpose of this text, only the torts that deal with aspects of intravenous therapy will be discussed. A focus on specific examples of nursing negligence will alert the reader to areas of personal liability that may occur as a result of administering intravenous infusions.

Intravenous Medication Errors

It is a primary duty of the nurse to administer medications to patients. Since this responsibility takes up a great deal of the nurse's time and involves handling numerous drugs, the potential for error is always present. Although an error in the administration of any medication by any route can be dangerous, the incorrect administration of an intravenous medication or fluid holds an even greater potential for a serious—even fatal—outcome. Once injected, an intravenous medication perfuses the circulatory system, is rapidly absorbed and metabolized by the body, and cannot be retrieved.

It is important that the nurse know the policies and procedures of her employer regarding medication administration. Most agencies require that certain intravenous drugs and infusions, such as chemotherapeutic agents, heparin drips, and blood products, be given only after they are checked and verified by two licensed nurses. This is a common policy in many health care institutions that ensures patient safety and reduces medication errors.

Medication errors double a person's risk of dying in the hospital. One study found that 2.3 errors occur for every 100 admissions, costing an estimated $2 billion per year. Errors most often occur with very ill patients who take more than one drug. Errors are most frequent with antibiotics and analgesics (Friend, 1997).

In dispensing medications, adherence to the age-old rules of the Five Rights and the Three Checks of medication administration are still the greatest safeguards to avoiding mistakes. If the nurse is conscientious in following these rules, it is less likely that she will make a medication error.

The Five Rights of Medication Administration

When administering drugs, it is critical that the nurse follow the **Five Rights of Medication Administration** to verify that she has identified the right patient to receive the right drug with the right dose by the right route at the right time. These rules are to be followed *without exception for each and every medication a nurse administers.*

Right Patient

Patient identification is vitally important, but is often overlooked. Before administering medications the nurse should ask the patient to state his name, if he is able to do so, then always, without fail, check the identification bracelet. It is wise to realize that several patients may have the same first or last name. If this is the case, extra care and diligence must be used to identify patients by comparing hospital identification numbers on the chart with identification bracelets and the medication administration records (MARs). The nurse who assumes that she knows all of the patients in her care without having properly identified them is falsely confident and is setting herself up to make a mistake. A large number of medication errors occur because of failure of nurses to correctly identify patients.

Right Medication

There are so many medications on the market today that have similar names and appearances that the nurse is constantly exposed to the possibility of making an error. With intravenous fluids and medications, the risk of error is even greater because the containers look the same or are very similar. Drugs are delivered in premixed bags or bottles, vials, ampules, and prefilled syringes. Each can contain one of a variety of medications that looks similar. A good example is the 50 ml or 100 ml piggyback bags of 5% dextrose in water used to dilute antibiotics and other solutes. The bags look alike but may have any variety of medications contained in them, or they may have attached vials with different types of medications available for reconstitution. The nurse must carefully read each label to ascertain the contents. Another example of misidentification is the closed injection system of single-use cartridge needle units (Figure 3-1). Unless the nurse carefully checks the label, she might easily inject the wrong medication intravenously, such as heparin sodium

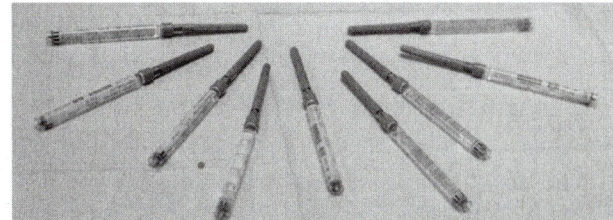

Figure 3-1 | Prefilled syringes for intravenous delivery, direct injection, or reconstitution with infusate diluents; each type used for a wide variety of medication classifications

rather than sodium chloride or meperidine hydrochloride rather than morphine sulphate.

Before preparing to administer any drug to a patient, the nurse must verify the physician's order for the correct drug and dosage and check for allergies. Even though the physician writes a medication order, the nurse is still responsible for its administration. It is up to her to know that the drug is appropriate for the patient. A nurse should never give a medication if she doesn't know what it is, its usual dosage, side effects, and any other properties of the drug. She also needs to check for compatibility with other medications the patient is receiving. If in doubt about any aspect of a medication, the nurse should question and verify what is correct by looking the drug up in the *Physician's Desk Reference*®, a drug handbook for nurses, or by consulting with a pharmacist. If she is still concerned that the drug is inappropriate for the patient, she must notify the physician.

When administering the correct drug to a patient, the nurse must also assess him for side effects and allergic reactions. A patient may not remember an allergy or be aware of a medication allergy until he receives the drug. It is the responsibility of the nurse who discovers a patient's untoward reaction to a medication to discontinue it, take the appropriate steps to counteract the reaction, then communicate this information, in verbal and written form, to all other members of the health team involved in his care. The patient and his family need to be informed to prevent future exposure to the substance.

With the intravenous administration of fluids and medications, the nurse must also be knowledgeable of any untoward local reactions that may occur if the infusion infiltrates. Extravasation of some medications can result in pain and burning at the site as well as permanent scarring and disfigurement. A paramount example of this problem occurs with the drug dopamine.

NURSING ALERT

Dopamine Administration

Dopamine is used in critical care units, under close nursing supervision, to counteract extreme hypotension. It is also used in small doses as a continuous IV drip for patients on general medical-surgical nursing units to enhance the perfusion of vital organs. If this drug infiltrates, it must be immediately discontinued, followed within 12 hours by the administration of a Regitine (phentolamine mesylate) and normal saline solution to the area of extravasation. If measures to counteract the escape of the dopamine infusion are not initiated, dermal sloughing and necrosis at the site of leakage will occur, resulting in permanent disfigurement.

Right Dose

Giving the correct dose of an intravenous medication to a patient is a critical safety factor. Giving too small a dose may inhibit attainment of the therapeutic blood level needed for the drug to exert its desired effect. Administering too much may result in an overdose that could be serious or potentially fatal.

A prerequisite for safe dosage administration is the ability to convert equivalencies between the metric, apothecaries', and household systems of measurement. Accuracy in computing drug dosage calculations using whole numbers, fractions, and decimals is important. Decimal points are especially critical because their movement one place to the left or right can alter a dosage tenfold. If there is any doubt about a dosage calculation, the nurse must verify accuracy by checking with another nurse or, preferably, a pharmacist.

NURSING TIP

Use Decimal Points and Zeros Carefully

When writing, interpreting, or implementing any dosage using decimal points or zeros, it is important to be extremely careful. The movement of a decimal point one place to the left or right can change a dosage tenfold. The addition or deletion of a zero can greatly alter a dosage. To safeguard your patients:

- Do not use a decimal when a whole number can be used. For example: Write 500 mg instead of 0.5 g or 500 mcg rather than 0.5 mg.

- Always place a zero before the decimal point when a fraction is expressed. For example: Write 0.5 mg instead of .5 mg (to avoid overlooking the decimal point or interpreting it as the number one).

- Never use trailing zeros after a round number. For example: Write 5 mg, not 5.0 mg (which could be interpreted as 50 mg).

It is also important when considering drug dosages for the nurse to take into account the functional capabilities of the patient's major organ systems as determined by laboratory tests. Poor kidney function, for example, can turn a normal dose into an overdose. Impaired liver function can alter dosages as well.

Right Route

Medications are given intravenously to exert a rapid effect and to initiate and maintain therapeutic blood levels. Since many medications can be given by different routes, it is extremely important that the nurse read every label carefully and ascertain that the drug to be administered is indicated for intravenous infusion. A drug must never be administered intravenously if it is not so indicated, or if the nurse has any doubt regarding the correctness of the dose and route.

When using the intravenous route, the nurse must also take into consideration how the drug is to be given: by direct IV push, by bolus into an injection port in the tubing of an existing infusion, via an intermittent infusion plug, a piggyback, or added to a bag or bottle of primary infusion fluid. Compatibility with other solutions must be evaluated to avoid **precipitation** (the suspension or crystallization of particles that occurs because incompatible agents are mixed), which results in the occlusion of an intravenous line. Properties of the drug that cause undesirable side effects such as local pain, burning, or irritation to the vein wall must be considered for patient comfort and safety.

There have been serious implications regarding the administration of medications by the incorrect route. Within a five-year period in one state, a board of nursing investigated four situations in which oral medications were injected into subclavian-line infusions. In one case, an oral tablet of Bactrim DS was crushed and injected into the IV line. Another case involved dissolving Mexitil in Maalox and injecting it. In both cases the infusion lines became clogged so the patients were spared the foreseeable fatal outcomes of receiving these oral drugs intravenously. In another incident, the oral/topical antacid Mylanta was injected intravenously, and the patient died. In another case, a graduate nurse injected a Mycostatin Swish and Swallow suspension and Mexitil into the subclavian line of one patient and Megace through the line of another patient. One wonders how incidents of this magnitude could happen, but public record shows that in fact they did occur as a result of failure to use the correct route of medication administration.

Right Time

For a routinely ordered drug to be given on time, the nurse must administer it within one half hour of the indicated time (30 minutes before or 30 minutes after). With the exception of prn or stat medications, most intravenous drugs are delivered at equally spaced intervals over a 24-hr period. It is important to give medications on time in order to reach and maintain therapeutic blood levels.

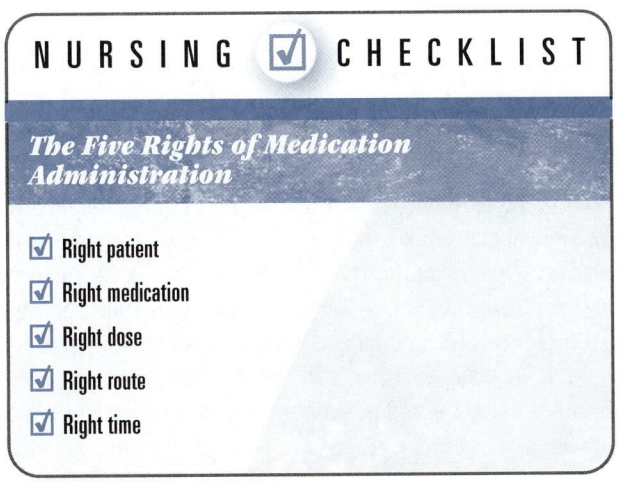

NURSING ☑ CHECKLIST

The Five Rights of Medication Administration

- ☑ Right patient
- ☑ Right medication
- ☑ Right dose
- ☑ Right route
- ☑ Right time

The Three Checks of Medication Administration

Prior to giving a drug, the nurse must carry out the Three Checks of medication administration in order to avoid an error. This involves looking at the label for verification of the drug name, its dosage, the route, and the expiration date. If the medication is contained in an intravenous bag or bottle, the nurse also must verify the patient's name and the time of administration. These checks, as they relate to intravenous administration, require the nurse to do the following:

1. Read the label of the medication as it is removed from a shelf, a unit dose medication cart, a refrigerator, or a dispensing system.
2. Read the label of the medication when comparing it with the MAR.
3. Read the medication label once again before administering the drug to the patient.

Even when the nurse is very busy or rushed, following the Three Checks along with the Five Rights helps to avoid medication errors. Shortcuts must never be taken. The nurse owes the patient the duty to administer drugs in a safe, accurate, and timely manner.

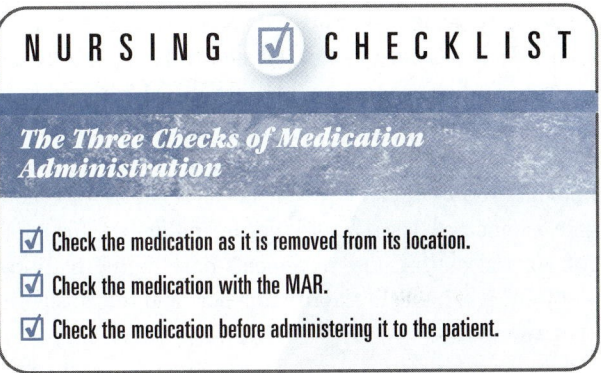

NURSING ☑ CHECKLIST

The Three Checks of Medication Administration

- ☑ Check the medication as it is removed from its location.
- ☑ Check the medication with the MAR.
- ☑ Check the medication before administering it to the patient.

The Human Element

As mentioned earlier, following the Five Rights and the Three Checks of medication administration reduces the likelihood a medication error will occur. In reality, however, mistakes do occur. The nurse may be overworked or the nursing unit understaffed. The human element is always present; the nurse is vulnerable to error. If an error occurs, the nurse must never ignore it or try to conceal it. The patient's safety must be her first concern so that measures to counteract the error can be initiated. The physician must be notified, the appropriate forms and documentation must be completed, and all employer protocols regarding a medication error must be followed. The patient also has the right to know about the error. Remember, to make an error is human, to conceal or lie about it is dishonest and a breach of duty owed to the patient.

Communication and the Law

All essential patient information must be communicated through verbal reports, by written documentation in the medical record, and on any checklists required by the nurse's employing institution. The statement, "If it was not reported and recorded, it wasn't done," still holds true today. The nurse is liable for communicating all data received from and about the patient that may alter his well-being or hinder his progress. Verbal reports and written records go hand in hand to confirm that a reasonable level of care, or lack of care, is rendered. Legal records document the fact that court rulings and out-of-court settlements have found the nurse negligent and liable for failure to report and record significant information.

Reporting

The nurse owes the patient the duty to utilize the steps of the nursing process in providing care for him. Special attention must be directed toward complete and continuous assessment and evaluation of his physical and psychological condition. Any alterations in his status must be reported expediently and accurately to the attending physician as well as to any consultants or specialists involved in the management of his medical care. Failure to report significant patient changes or situations may constitute negligence on the part of the nurse.

Reporting also entails apprising all members of the nursing staff and supervisory personnel of any information needed to maintain safe and efficient patient-oriented care. Utilization of both verbal reports and written notations on forms standard-

ized by the nurse's employer may be used. The data passed on during nursing rounds as well as intra-shift and change-of-shift reports must be clear and accurate to prevent communication gaps that may hinder the patient's well-being.

Any breach in communication among the staff administering nursing care to the patient undergoing intravenous infusion therapy may result in complications or untoward reactions. Areas that bear special relevance to reporting are listed in the Nursing Checklist.

Documentation

In addition to astute observation, timely reporting, and the provision of safe care, clear and accurate documentation is a major nursing responsibility. Not only does it reflect in writing that a reasonable level of care was rendered, it also provides a legal record, in case of litigation, that supports or refutes negligence. "Documentation in the patient's medical record shall contain complete information regarding infusion therapy and vascular access" (INS, 2000, Standard 17, S21).

Nursing care is based on adherence to standards of care and accepted protocols, which utilize the steps of the nursing process. Documentation related to care must be factual, accurate, thorough, and objective. "Documentation shall be legible, accessible to qualified personnel, and readily retrievable" (INS, 2000, Standard 17, S21). The nurse should record information as soon as possible after signs and symptoms are observed, assessments are made, and interventions are carried out. The nurse who waits until later or until the end of the shift to make chart entries is risking omitting critical information.

Initiating the invasive procedure of intravenous infusion therapy requires the documentation of:

- Solution ordered
- Type of venous access device used, including length and gauge
- Site of initiation and the type of dressing used
- Patient's physical and psychological response to the procedure
- Time of initiation
- Rate of infusion
- Site and condition of any unsuccessful sticks
- Use of an electronic infusion device
- Patient teaching associated with the procedure and therapy and the patient's understanding of the teaching

At the initiation of intravenous therapy, the access site, the infusion tubing, and the solution container must be labeled appropriately. The nurse must document when the site or dressing is changed, the tubing is replaced, or additional solutions are started.

Documentation must be objective, nonjudgmental, and unbiased, and describe behaviors and events. Only the specific observations and facts must be written. An entry may read in the chart nursing notes, "Patient pulled IV out," when in fact the tubing caught on the bed rail during sleep or on a door knob when the patient ambulated to the bathroom. The nurse who does not observe this act may jump to a false conclusion. Since she did not witness the IV coming out, such a false statement may libel (the act of falsely defaming a person in writing) the patient by accusing him of noncompliance when in fact it is not true. **Slander** is the verbal defamation of a person.

Documentation of allergies and interventions used to counteract them is a crucial nursing responsibility. With intravenous infusions and medication administration, a reaction can occur rapidly and result in a critical situation. For known allergies, the chart, chart forms, nursing care plan, and any other records must be labeled clearly. Once an allergy previously unknown to the patient is discovered, the information must be verbally communicated and documented on all necessary forms. The nurse who administers a medication intravenously to a patient for the first time is obliged to stay with the patient for a prescribed period to make sure that there is no untoward reaction.

When discovering any situation in which a patient's care or progress may be compromised and require medical intervention, the nurse is required to notify the physician expeditiously. She must document the time of notifica-

tion, the pertinent information included in her communication with him, and his responses. If unable to contact him directly she will have to go through office personnel, an answering service, or medical exchange. When this is the case, the nurse must get the name of the person to whom she speaks (or operator's number in the case of an exchange or service) and document it in the chart along with the time called and the message given. Each time a call is placed the same information must be documented. If the physician does not call back within a prescribed time frame, the call must continue to be placed until there is a response, and a nursing supervisor notified of the failure of the physician to return the call. Once the nurse has spoken with the physician, she is obliged to document her nursing actions and the patient's response. In recording the time of day, the 24-hour clock (military or universal time) is to be used, to avoid errors and confusion (Figure 3-2).

In her documentation, the nurse must use abbreviations approved by her employer, appropriate medical terminology, and correct grammar and spelling. It is also important to write or print legibly so that the information presented is clear to anyone who reads the chart.

Patient-Family Teaching

Teaching the patient about his health care, explaining all procedures, and honestly answering his questions are required nursing functions that serve to foster a therapeutic

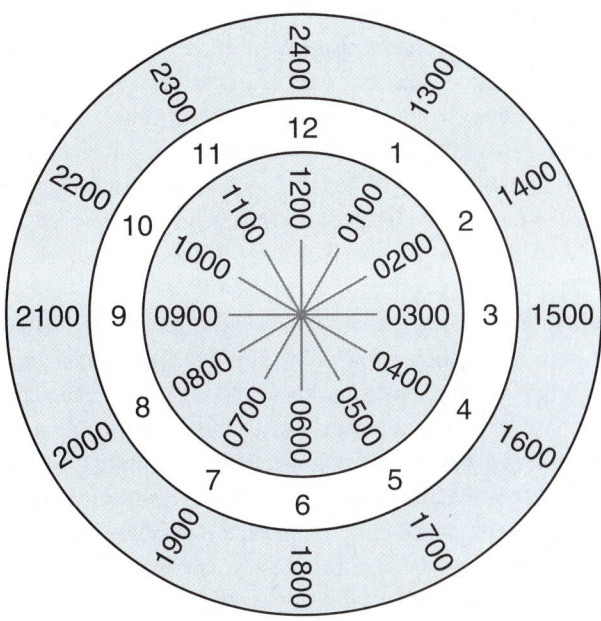

Figure 3-2 | The 24-hour clock (military or universal time)

relationship between the patient and the nurse. "The patient, caregiver, or a representative legally authorized to act on the patient's behalf shall receive instruction and education relative to the prescribed infusion therapy and care plan" (INS, 2000, Standard 12, S19). The nurse who fails to educate her patient regarding his health and illness patterns is remiss in her duty to care and may be deemed negligent. Most state nursing boards mandate patient education by including it in their rules and regulations. Failure to adhere to these stipulations constitutes a violation of state law.

Nearly every interaction with a patient provides the nurse with the opportunity to teach. It is wise to take advantage of any chance to explain and answer questions. The patient must be an equal partner in his health care plan and has the right to participate in setting realistic goals. The nurse is obligated to explain all nursing procedures and treatment protocols. The patient's knowledge base and level of comprehension must be evaluated frequently. It is important for the nurse to take into consideration how the patient feels—pain, anxiety, fatigue, medication side effects, mental state—when evaluating the teaching-learning process.

The nurse must assess a patient's ability to understand, then communicate with him on a level that he can comprehend. To be most effective, the nurse should review periodically the principles of teaching, learning, and therapeutic communication. The patient who is well informed and knowledgeable about his health and illness tends to comply with the regimen necessary for his care. In addition, he becomes an active partner in his health care and participates in his provider's plan of care.

Prior to initiating intravenous infusion therapy, the nurse must explain the necessity for it and describe the procedures involved even if the physician has already done so. She is expected to tell the patient about any anticipated discomfort and discuss any physical restrictions or inconveniences he may encounter as a result of the treatment. She also needs to inform him of any safety precautions or side effects involved. "The patient, caregiver, or legally authorized representative should be informed in clear and concise terminology of all aspects of the therapy including physical and psychological effects, side effects, risks, and benefits" (INS, 2000, Standard 12, S19). The patient must understand that he should notify the nursing staff if he has any questions, concerns, or discomfort so that the appropriate nursing assessments and interventions can be initiated as soon as possible.

Even though detailed instructions and explanations are presented, the patient may refuse treatment. The nurse should attempt to determine the reason for refusal in order to clarify or reinforce any needed information; but she should never coerce him. If a nurse threatens to perform a procedure against a patient's will, she may be liable for the intentional tort of **assault**. If she carries out the procedure, she may be liable for **battery**, the unlawful touching of a person without his consent. The patient has the right to refuse. The nurse must document the refusal and notify the physician. A nursing student should notify her clinical instructor and a staff nurse.

Delegation of Authority and Assignments

The RN is responsible for making nursing decisions, formulating hospital and unit assignments, and delegating authority to other members of the health care team according to the chain-of-command protocols of the employing agency. Medicare, prospective payment systems, new insurance guidelines for hospital admissions, health care down-sizing, managed care, nursing shortages, and the increase of lawsuits have complicated the process of delegation.

The LPN/LVN, depending on state licensure regulations and agency policy, may be permitted to perform venipuncture, monitor intravenous administration and sites, perform dressing changes, and administer specific solutions according to state nurse practice acts. Because some nurse practice acts are less specific than others in stating what a nurse may or may not do while on duty, making and delegating assignments may be confusing. In some states the LVN or LPN is not permitted to handle intravenous infusions, whereas in other states she may, even though the practice acts do not address the issue of intravenous infusion therapy per se. Instead, the nurse must follow her employer's guidelines, which may include external education programs followed by internal preceptorships under the guidance of a registered nurse. Other employers provide a course of in-house study with on-the-job training and some supervision. Delegation of responsibility for initiating and monitoring infusion therapy to an LVN or LPN is a gray area, and many registered nurses are uncomfortable allowing them to perform such skills even though the employer has authorized it. Most practical or vocational educational programs do not provide adequate background in anatomy and physiology or pharmacology to support these skills, yet their graduates are expected to do them.

Whenever a nurse delegates authority to another employee she is legally responsible for her assessment of the individual's competency and willingness to accept the assignment. If a nurse considers herself incapable of an assignment because of a lack of skill or experience, she is obliged to make her concerns known and explain why she feels incapable of the assignment. She should document her objections in writing, forward a copy to the nurse manager or nursing supervisor, and keep a copy for herself. Both the person delegating the assignment and the one accepting it must thoroughly understand the type of assignment, the unit routines, any procedures involved, and who will be supervising. Once an assignment is accepted, the person taking it is legally accountable for carrying it out and is responsible for its outcome.

In some areas, due to a nursing shortage or understaffing, the registered nurse delegates responsibilities to the LVN or LPN who does not have the education, scientific background, or skill to safely carry out such assignments. The LPN or LVN is put in charge at night and told to call a supervisor or registered nurse on another unit if help is needed. Some acute care facilities and nursing homes assign the LVN or LPN who has taken a prescribed course of study to initiate and maintain intravenous infusions and monitor and discontinue blood or blood-product transfusions. Situations of this nature set the stage for potential lawsuits because of inadequate background, training, and practice.

The same situations often arise when nurses float to other units. The regular staff nurse may see that these individuals are not competent, yet keeps them due to short staffing. If a patient is injured while under the care of a float nurse, the regular nursing staff on that unit could be held liable. The 1992 *Nursing Service Organization Risk Advisor* says the following:

> Don't ever consider yourself in such a pinch that you must accept an incompetent nurse—you're just asking for trouble. Most reasonably prudent nurses wouldn't agree to work with such a nurse. So if you do, you're breaching the standard of care. And that means you could be found liable if a patient is harmed and sues.
>
> When you know another nurse isn't capable of providing good care, notify your nurse manager immediately. Objectively describe the situation, giving examples of problems you've observed. Follow up with a written memo and keep a copy for your records. Your nurse-manager is then responsible for sharing your concerns with the appropriate people.
>
> Meanwhile, assign the nurse only those tasks you know she can handle. Give her clear directions, and ask her for feedback so you know she understands. Finally, make sure you stop in to see her patients. (Nurses Service Organization, 1992)

Fortunately, many nurse practice acts have been specifically amended to define the parameters concerning delegation of authority and supervision. If a nurse practices in a state in which the nurse practice act does not cover these areas, she must be very selective in delegating authority and assignments. If a patient is harmed as a result of her erro-

neous judgment, she could be held liable. Likewise, if a nurse accepts an assignment or position of responsibility, making it known to her supervisor that she is capable of the assignment, she may be held liable if a patient is injured.

Continuing Education

Even though many nurse practice acts mandate continuing education, each nurse is individually accountable to her profession and to the public for voluntarily maintaining updated knowledge and safe skills. With the constant emergence of advanced technology and sophisticated equipment, the nurse cannot practice safely and efficiently and adhere to standards of care without her education remaining current. The nurse who believes that day-to-day experience and on-the-job training are enough is misinformed and may be negligent in her duty to the patient.

There is a vast store of information available to keep the nurse up to date. In addition to seminars, books, computer adaptive programs, and videotapes, nursing journals and courses are available for home study to earn continuing education credit. Many universities and community colleges offer courses containing current nursing information. With all that is available, there are numerous opportunities to increase one's knowledge base and maintain a safe level of care. Every nurse should voluntarily embrace any channel that will increase her knowledge and enhance her expertise.

For the nurse who practices predominantly in the area of infusion therapy in the acute care setting or in the community, certification is advisable. **Certification** is the granting of special recognition to the nurse who has practiced and pursued an advanced role in a particular area of nursing. It is conferred by a nongovernmental agency or private organization (e.g., American Nurses Credentialing Center [ANCC]) on the nurse who has a higher level of competency than that mandated by state licensure. Membership in the Infusion Nurses Society (INS) and certification (CRNI) by the Intravenous Nurses Certification Corporation (INCC) are options to be considered by any nurse whose work focuses on intravenous infusion therapy.

In the legal sense, continuing education credit may be valuable to the nurse who becomes involved in a malpractice case. If her continuing education records are requested, and she is unable to provide them, the nurse may be deemed negligent in her duty to maintain the knowledge and skills needed to practice safely.

Aside from mandated continuing education or fear of litigation, it is hoped that the nurse will see continued learning as a lifelong endeavor to assist her in providing the best possible care to her patients, to impart her knowledge to other nurses, and thus improve the profession of nursing.

Florence Nightingale saw the need for continued learning on the part of the nurse over a century ago. Her words are still alive and current today:

Nursing is a progressive art, in which to stand still is to go back. A woman who thinks of herself, 'Now I am a full nurse, a skilled nurse, I have learnt all there is to be learnt,' take my word for it, she does not know what a nurse is, and never will know; she is gone back already. Progress can never end but with a nurse's life. (Kelly & Joel, 1999)

AVOIDING LITIGATION

As the nurse takes on more responsibility and practices in a number of extended roles, she is more at risk for becoming involved in a lawsuit than the nurse of years gone by. Today's nurse is more autonomous than ever before and will continue to be so with advances in science and technology. Some of the issues facing the nurse of today were unheard of even ten years ago.

NURSING ALERT

Patients Considering Litigation

Patients who are considering litigation may indicate their intentions by:

- Habitual complaining
- Questioning everything
- Open expressions of hostility toward the nurse and other health care providers
- Overreacting to any perceived neglect or negative comment—real or imagined
- Asking for names of nurses and health care personnel
- Taking notes of discussions with nurses, physicians, and health care personnel
- Exhibiting combative, noncompliant, or uncooperative behaviors
- Requesting chart prior to or upon discharge

When caring for such patients, maintain a polite, calm, professional demeanor and make every effort to meet the patient's needs. Patients are less likely to sue when their complaints and fears are acknowledged and dealt with promptly and courteously (NSO, 1992).

As discussed earlier, one of the best means of avoiding litigation is to communicate openly and honestly, verbally and

---

NURSING ☑ CHECKLIST

Situations That Reflect Nursing Negligence

- ☑ Poor nursing judgment
- ☑ Failure to assess a patient properly
- ☑ Failure to foresee the outcome of an action or inaction
- ☑ Failure to supervise and monitor a patient
- ☑ Improper administration of medications
- ☑ Errors in communication (observing, reporting, recording, and documentation)
- ☑ Lack of updated knowledge and skill regarding treatments, medications, and procedures
- ☑ Failure to question medical orders that are incorrect or inappropriate
- ☑ Failure to provide for patient safety
- ☑ Thermal or chemical burns
- ☑ Failure to monitor a patient postoperatively or following the delivery of an infant
- ☑ Failure to educate a patient and his family regarding his care, medications, treatment, and any necessary follow-up
- ☑ Failure to report the incompetence of another health care provider

---

nonverbally, to all concerned. When communicating with a patient, the nurse must be receptive, be sincere, and take the time to listen and respond to his needs. Honesty and empathy on the part of the nurse may be as important as any procedure she carries out. The patient who is treated with sensitivity and consideration believes that the nurse has his best interest at heart and that she truly cares about his feelings and needs. The nurse who cares for another as she would like to be cared for in the same or similar situation is giving the highest degree of respect to that patient and his family. In addition, she helps relieve the fears and anxieties associated with his health impairment.

Unbiased regard for the patient, his religious and cultural beliefs, and his concerns and needs can never be underestimated. The nurse who sees each and every patient as a unique human being is imparting a sense of caring that makes the patient a partner in his treatment.

When the nurse recognizes the nursing process as the basis for all of her interactions with the patient, family, and other health care professionals, she puts the patient at the best advantage, and he receives optimum care. From the first contact with a patient as a nursing student and continuing throughout her professional life, the nurse must use the nursing process as the underlying principle for everything she does.

As previously discussed, the nurse must maintain her skills and continually update her knowledge. She is obliged to meet the standards of care of the profession and those of the state in which she is licensed to practice, as well as any standards that apply to the specialty in which she works. If a lawsuit is initiated, the standards of care, the concept of reasonableness, and the employer's policies and procedures are often used in court to determine any deviation from the law. Each nurse is also wise to carry professional liability insurance to cover the cost of litigation.

The courts have revealed that the most common examples of nursing negligence involve situations when the nurse acted inappropriately or failed to act when she should have. The Nursing Checklist highlights some examples of action or inaction.

The malpractice crisis of the 1970s has continued to escalate over the years, resulting in numerous lawsuits involving nurses, physicians, allied health care workers, and health care institutions. The best protection the nurse can afford herself is knowledge of nursing and the law and being alert to any situation that may instigate litigation. This, along with a strong sense of accountability to the nursing profession and the public served by it, is the optimal means of practicing safely within the confines of the law.

Key Concepts

- ✳ It is necessary to have a basic understanding of the United States legal system and the sources of law in order to fully comprehend how the nurse practice act and the state board of nursing regulate the practice of nursing.

- ✳ The nurse is accountable to external and internal standards of care in the practice of nursing.

- ✳ The two main classifications of law, criminal and civil, directly relate to nursing practice.

- ✳ The nurse must be knowledgeable of the elements that establish malpractice (duty, breach of duty, causation, and harm) in order to recognize situations of liability and litigation.

- ✳ When dispensing medications, the best safeguard to avoid errors is adhering to the Five Rights and the Three Checks of medication administration.

- ✳ Verbal, nonverbal, and written communication among the nurse, the patient and his family, and all members of the health care team is essential to safe nursing care.

- ✳ The nursing process—assessment, nursing diagnosis, planning, implementation, and evaluation—underlies all activities of the nurse.

- ✳ Intravenous infusion therapy is a broad and complex area that requires by law a high degree of expertise to maintain patient safety and avoid litigation.

- ✳ Patient-family teaching is required professionally and legally to ensure that safe care is provided.

- ✳ When delegating and assuming authority or making and accepting assignments, the nurse is liable for her own actions and in many situations those of others.

- ✳ Continuing education is necessary for the nurse to remain knowledgeable and current in her skills. She is accountable to the public, to the nursing profession, and to her employer to remain current in her education and skills. Her failure to be so prepared may find her negligent in a court of law.

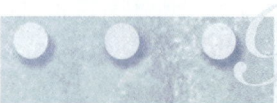

Review Questions and Activities

1. Why do you need to know what your state nurse practice act and board of nursing rules and regulations dictate when practicing nursing? What does your state mandate regarding intravenous infusion therapy and delegation of this responsibility to other health care providers?

2. How are the steps of the nursing process and standards of care related in the administration of infusion therapy?

3. What types of intravenous infusion procedures may put you at risk for litigation if you perform them improperly?

4. List the Five Rights and the Three Checks of medication administration and explain why they are so important when giving drugs, but even more critical when administering intravenous fluids and medications.

5. In the administration of intravenous therapy, name the actions or inactions of the nurse that may lead to a malpractice lawsuit.

6. Discuss some procedural and societal changes that have occurred over the last two decades that may pose a risk for litigation.

7. What are your best legal defenses to avoid litigation when practicing nursing? List as many as you can think of and discuss each one.

Chapter 4

Infection Control and Safety Measures Related to Intravenous Infusion Therapy

C O M P E T E N C I E S

Upon completion of this chapter, the reader should be able to:

✸ Define epidemiology and its relationship to infection control.

✸ Explain the components of the epidemiologic triangle.

✸ Discuss the process of infection and pathogenesis.

✸ Differentiate between local and systemic infections as they relate to intravenous infusion therapy.

✸ Analyze the components of the chain of infection.

✸ Explain why hand hygiene is the single most important means of preventing the spread of infection.

✸ Interpret the guidelines for Standard Precautions as recommended by the Centers for Disease Control and Prevention.

✸ State the CDC-recommended guidelines regarding postexposure prophylaxis following occupational exposure to HIV.

✸ Examine the rulings of the Occupational Safety and Health Administration as they pertain to health care personnel.

✸ Compare and contrast the advantages and disadvantages of the antiseptic agents used most often for intravenous therapy.

✸ Describe the recommended dressings available for intravenous infusion sites.

✸ Outline the approved protocols for intravenous tubing care.

✸ Evaluate the role of the nurse in preventing nosocomial infections as they apply to intravenous infusion therapy.

KEY TERMS

agent	epidemiologic triangle	onycholysis
antimicrobial	epidemiology	pathogen
antiseptic	fistula	pathology
asepsis	flora	percutaneous contact
autoinfection	fomites	portal of exit
bacteremia	germicide	reservoir
bactericidal	health care personnel	resident flora
carrier	hematogenous spread	resistance
causative agent	host	sepsis
colonize	infection	surgical asepsis
communicable	local infection	susceptible
community-acquired infection	medical asepsis	systemic infection
contagious	morbidity	transient flora
disease	mortality	vector
environment	nosocomial infection	virulence

With the rapid and continuous advances that are emerging in health care, the nurse is challenged by illnesses and infections occurring in patients receiving intravenous infusion therapy. Whereas the use of parenteral intervention is directed toward the alleviation and control of disease processes, it also poses associated risks and complications that can be serious—even life-threatening. The nurse who practices in this area needs to be knowledgeable of all aspects involved in the safe administration, management, and maintenance of IV therapy. The foundation for this knowledge involves an understanding of the principles of epidemiology, infectious disease processes, the body's immune system, and policies and procedures related to infection control.

EPIDEMIOLOGY AND INFECTION

Infusion therapy is essential to modern-day health care, since it is used in a wide variety of health care settings. With direct access to the vascular system, there is the constant potential for microbial introduction. It is imperative for the nurse to understand the basic concepts of epidemiology and the common causative organisms that are related to infusion therapy. **Epidemiology** is the scientific study of disease, injury, and other human conditions, their causes and determinants, their distribution within a population, and their control and surveillance. It is measured before, during, and after preventive and other interventions. Epidemiology is activated and managed through individuals and agencies operating at local, state, national, and international levels to promote and maintain conditions that protect the health and welfare of people everywhere. **Disease** is the term that refers to any combination of objective and subjective evidence that constitutes an abnormal infectious or noninfectious health process in the human organism. **Pathology** is the basic study of disease processes, a less encompassing term than epidemiology.

In the United States, the Centers for Disease Control and Prevention (CDC) in Atlanta, Georgia, is the agency that investigates, develops, recommends, and sets standards for infection control practices. The CDC is a division of the Department of Health and Human Services (DHHS), formerly the U.S. Public Health Service. The Occupational Safety and Health Administration (OSHA) is the enforcing agency that provides the mandates to protect employees in all fields. Its policies regarding health care personnel are aligned closely with the guidelines set forth by the CDC. It is the guidelines set forth by the CDC, along with those from the Infusion Nurses Society (INS), the National Association of Vascular Access Network (NAVAN), and The Association of Practitioners in Infection Control and Epidemiology, Inc. (APIC), as well as the directives of OSHA that are most often used in developing procedures and setting policies regarding the practice of intravenous infusion therapy.

The term **health care personnel**, according to the CDC, "refers to all paid and unpaid persons working in health care settings who have the potential for exposure to infectious materials, including body substances, contaminated medical supplies and equipment, contaminated environmental surfaces, or contaminated air." (CDC *Guidelines for Infection Control in Healthcare Personnel*, 1998e). Remember, the health care setting refers to any area in which the nurse practices—the hospital, community, or the home. Every week the CDC publishes the *Morbidity and Mortality Weekly Report*, which discloses and describes illnesses and communicable diseases, the deaths that result from them, and the statistics related to them. This valuable source of information keeps the public aware of health care situations on national and international levels. It is of special interest and value to all health care personnel, especially practitioners of intravenous infusion therapy. The new committee established by the DHHS, called the CDC Hospital Infection Control Practices Advisory Committee (HICPAC), meets annually and updates health care information in areas such as intravascular practice and hand hygiene procedures.

The Epidemiologic Triangle

In the epidemiologic sense, three interacting factors are addressed in the prevention, control, and eradication of disease. These include the host, the agent, and the environment—a dynamic interacting triad often referred to as the **epidemiologic triangle** (Figure 4-1). The **host** is the living organism (person or animal) that provides the structure in which other organisms are able to live. The **agent** refers to any organism (bacteria, viruses, rickettsiae, chlamydiae, spirochetes, fungi [molds and yeast], and protozoa) that is capable of eliciting an effect or a disease process. The **environment** is an interacting group of conditions, surroundings, and influences in which the host

and agent coexist. A change in any of the components alters the existing equilibrium and thereby increases or decreases the frequency of disease.

Infection and the Epidemiologic Triangle

Infection is the process in which a host is invaded by microorganisms that grow, reproduce, and cause injury. A **pathogen** is a substance that is capable of producing disease. The result of infection is usually disease. If a disease does not occur, the invading microorganisms may **colonize** (reside) in the host, and make the host a carrier of the microorganism without causing adverse clinical signs or symptoms. Infections develop as a consequence of the microorganism's strength and ability to produce disease (**virulence**) as well as the inability of the host to defend itself against the invader. For infection to occur there must be an imbalanced interplay among the host, the agent, and the environment.

INFECTION

Infection is the condition or state in which the body (host), or part of it, is invaded by a pathogen that, under favorable conditions, can multiply and cause injury to the host. There are many variables that are considered in terms of the host (Table

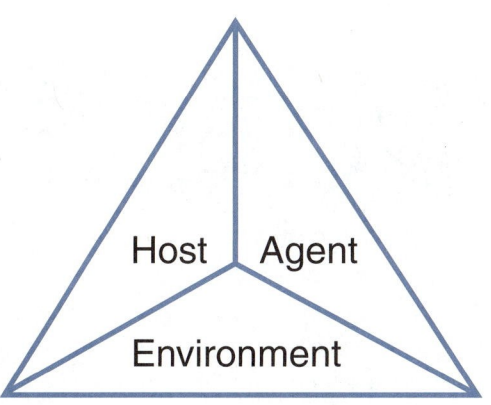

Figure 4-1 | The epidemiologic triangle

Table 4-1 | Host Factors Affecting the Disease Process

Age
Body weight
State of nutrition and hydration
Coexisting disease process
Ability to adapt to the external environment
Stress
Immune competence
Length of exposure to microorganism(s)
Amount of exposure to microorganism(s)
Medications (antibiotics, chemotherapy, corticosteroids)
Indwelling body-cavity devices
Skin integrity
Mucous membrane integrity
Body system functioning
Mental outlook
Social and psychological support

Table 4-2 | Microbial Factors Affecting the Disease Process

Ability to adhere to the skin
Ability to penetrate the skin
Ability to adhere to mucous membranes
Ability to penetrate mucous membranes
Ability to adhere to inanimate objects
Ability to proliferate on inanimate devices
Ability to exude toxic substances
Ability to resist phagocytosis
Ability to multiply within the host
Ability to mutate
Unique characteristics of the organism(s)
Virulence of the organism(s)
Ability to grow and multiply in the presence of certain antibiotics and other medications

4-1) as well as the invading organism (Table 4-2) that determine whether infection and disease will occur.

Classifications of Infection

Once the body is invaded by a pathogen and infection occurs, the effect is evidenced or classified as local or systemic. A **local infection** is one in which microorganisms penetrate the tissues of a specific area of the body, then grow, multiply, and exert their effect there, rather than migrate to other parts of the body. A **systemic infection** is one in which the microorganisms travel freely throughout the host's body and exert their effect on several, or all, body systems. **Sepsis** is the term used to describe the pathologic condition resulting from the spread of microorganisms or their toxins through the circulatory system, the lymphatic system, or both. Sepsis is the leading cause of death in ICUs, with 65% to 70% of the cases caused by gram-negative pathogens (e.g., *E. coli* and the *Pseudomonas* and *Klebsiella* species) (White, 1997). Local infections from strains such as *Candida*, *Streptococcus*, and others can initially exert a local effect. Given the proper conditions in the host, these pathogens can progress to systemic invasions. The nurse must always keep in mind that what may start out as a mild local infection can progress to a full-blown systemic **bacteremia** (bacteria in the bloodstream), as in the example of the nurse who sticks

the patient with a contaminated needle. Whenever pathogens are introduced into the blood or lymphatic circulation, they take free reign of the host's body, through the process of **hematogenous spread**, sometimes exerting disastrous systemic effects.

NURSING ALERT

Sepsis

Sepsis is on the rise as more and more pathogens become antibiotic resistant. An estimated 600,000 people, mostly those who are at risk due to multiple medical problems or advanced age, develop sepsis or septic shock. Only 50% to 60% survive, even with aggressive treatment (White, 1997).

NURSING TIP

Spread of Microorganisms

Colonized patients are those who harbor microorganisms (as evidenced by positive culture analysis) but do not show other signs or symptoms of infection. Always remember that organisms can be spread from contact with infected and colonized patients or from contact with contaminated objects.

The Chain of Infection

In order for an infection to occur, the three components of the epidemiologic triangle must be present—the host, the agent, and the environment. In addition, there is an interacting chain of events that must occur for disease transmission. The saying, "A chain is only as strong as its weakest link" applies to the transmission process for infectious disease. If the chain is interrupted at one or more of its links, infection will not be transmitted. The six links in this chain consist of the causative agent, its reservoir, its portal of exit, the method of transmission, its portal of entry, and the susceptible host (Figure 4-2).

The Causative Infectious Agent

The **causative agent** in the transmission of infection is the biologic, chemical, or physical entity that is capable of producing an infection. The biologic agents are the numerous microorganisms present in the environment. Depending on the circumstances, they may be beneficial, potentially harmful, or harmful.

The patient receiving intravenous therapy is at risk for becoming infected with any number of organisms. Every human being has both resident and transient microbiologic flora on and in her body. **Resident flora** are microorganisms that are indigenous to each individual and are present mainly on the skin and in the respiratory, gastrointestinal, and reproductive systems. **Transient flora** are microorganisms that are picked up, usually on the skin, that can be removed fairly easily with hand hygiene or bathing. In general, resident flora serve as a protective device. If an infection does occur from resident flora (as in the case of a patient with a compromised immune system), it is said to be an **endogenous** infection or an **autoinfection**. **Exogenous** infections are the result of invasion by nonresident flora.

A common microbe that is constantly present on the skin and poses a threat to a client receiving infusion therapy is one belonging to the genus of coagulase-negative *Staphylococcus* organisms. *Staphylococcus* is a predominant organism on the skin and a major cause of intravenous catheter-related infections and septicemia. The bacteria can collect on clothing, blankets, walls, and medical equipment. Coagulase-negative staphylococci account for 37% and *Staphylococcus aureus* account for 12.6% of reported hospital-acquired bloodstream infections BSIs (CDC, 2002). Some strains of this organism produce a capsule of slimy mucoid material (glycocalyx) that prevents the body's internal defenses from destroying it. This slime also has an affinity to intravenous catheters, allowing the organism to adhere tightly to them. Coagulase-negative staphylococci, followed by enterococci, are the most frequently isolated causes of hospital-acquired BSIs (CDC, 2002a, *Guidelines for the Prevention of Intravascular Catheter-Related Infections*).

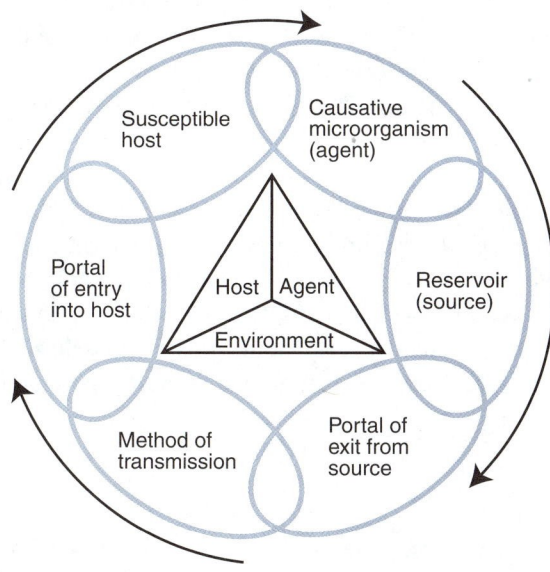

Figure 4-2 | The chain of infection

Because of the evolving ability of *Staphylococcus* strains to become antibiotic resistant (as with methicillin-resistant *S. aureus* [MRSA], an organism that can survive on hands for three hours), many previously effective antibiotics are now useless (with vancomycin now being the only option for treatment in many instances). MRSA has become endemic in hospitals, long-term care facilities, and in the home care setting. Should MRSA become resistant to vancomycin, many patients will succumb to septicemia, endocarditis, pneumonia, and wound infections.

Widespread use of vancomycin, in response to concerns over MRSA and for the treatment of vascular catheter-associated infections by resistant coagulase-negative staphylococci, is now of great alarm since vancomycin-resistant enterococci (VRE) surfaced. Now, of even greater concern is the appearance of a strain of *S. aureus* that is resistant to vancomycin (VRSA).

The Reservoir

The **reservoir**, or source of infection, refers to the environment (human, animal, fomite) in which microorganisms are able to live and grow. It provides the nutritional and environmental conditions necessary for microbial survival. Such sources may be animate or inanimate.

Animate Reservoirs

Human beings are the major source of animate contamination in the health care setting. Individuals may be ill with an identified disease or may be transmitting pathogens before any distinguishable signs or symptoms are evident (as is often the case with persons with tuberculosis). Many individuals serve as **carriers** for disease as well—those who harbor pathogens and transmit them to others without having the disease themselves.

NURSING ALERT

Potentially Hazardous Body Fluids

Blood serves as the reservoir for countless pathogenic organisms, the most lethal being the hepatitis viruses that cause hepatitis B (HBV), C (HCV), D (HDV), E (HDE) and the human immunodeficiency virus (HIV), responsible for advanced HIV disease (AIDS). Any contact with bodily secretions from the eye, ear, nose, and mouth and drainage from the urogenital tract, gastrointestinal tract, burns and wounds are potentially dangerous. Body cavity fluids such as pleural, peritoneal, amniotic, synovial, and cerebrospinal can pose a daily threat for health care personnel and patients.

In humans, the skin as well as bodily fluids emitted from any of the body's systems provide major pathogenic sources of contamination. The skin is usually the primary source of microorganisms responsible for intravenous-associated infections. Numerous cutaneous organisms are harbored on the skin of all people. Hospitalized individuals and health care personnel who are in contact with a broad spectrum of disease processes harbor an even greater number of microbes that are potentially pathogenic.

Animals, birds, fish, insects, and plants serve as living or dead reservoirs for organisms that can be harmful, even lethal, to members of their own species and humans. This has become especially evident with outbreaks of bovine spongiform (mad cow) disease and West Nile virus. Health care personnel often care for patients who have been attacked by rabid animals or bitten or stung by insects that are **vectors**, the intermediate animate carriers, or reservoirs of disease. In many circumstances, once infected, these individuals become highly contagious to others.

NURSING TIP

Using Gloves as Protection

All body substances from all individuals are potential reservoirs of infection. Always wear gloves and other protective devices as needed and recommended by the CDC and mandated by OSHA and the employing agency when physical contact with pathogenic agents is a possibility.

Inanimate Reservoirs

Inanimate reservoirs of infection include the air, soil, food products, water, and articles used in day-to-day living or in the workplace. Once removed from the living reservoir, some organisms are able to live for extended periods of time, depending on the environment. Body substances such as urine, sputum, feces, or blood can pose a threat as inanimate objects that harbor microorganisms. The term **fomites** refers to inanimate objects that may be contaminated, harbor organisms, and serve as sources of transmission. Microorganisms thrive especially well in moist, warm environments. In the health care setting, common fomites include utility room counters, sinks, faucets, charts, the patients' linens, drinking cups, urinals, and bed pans. For the patient who is ill, almost anything she comes in contact with can serve as a reservoir for infection.

The Portal of Exit

The **portal of exit** refers to the site where a pathogen leaves its reservoir. In humans, those organisms that reside in the blood can exit via the hollow bore of needles, as well as cuts, abrasions, and wounds that result in a break of the skin or mucous membranes. The mouth and anus are the usual portals of exit from the gastrointestinal tract. Patients who are ill, however, may have tubes, drains, ostomies, and decompression devices from which pathogens can depart their reservoir. Organisms that are harbored in the respiratory tract may exit through the nose and mouth during the normal processes of breathing, coughing, or sneezing, as well as through oral or nasal airways, endotracheal tubes, and tracheostomies. Semen and vaginal drainage serve as exit sites for blood and fluid escaping through the reproductive tract. The urinary meatus and urinary ostomy diversions, as well as catheters, allow for drainage from the urinary tract. **Fistulas**, the abnormal tubelike passages between normal cavities or tubes to free surfaces or other cavities, may serve as the portals of exit for organisms among one or more body systems. It is extremely important that the nurse assess all body secretions and intervene to handle and dispose of them properly, following approved guidelines.

Mode of Transmission

The next link in the chain of infection lies in the mode of transmission, the mechanism for transfer of the agent. Any disease that can be passed from one person or object to another person is said to be **communicable**. Pathogens are passed through direct or indirect contact with another person.

For direct transmission to occur there must be actual physical contact between the agent and the host, such as the mouth-to-mouth passage of pathogens during kissing or organisms in blood escaping from a patient's needle puncture site into a cut on the nurse's hand. A disease that spreads easily from one person to another is said to be **contagious**. The usual methods of direct contact include oral, fecal-oral, sexual, tactile, and airborne, the spread of droplets transferred during talking, coughing, and sneezing.

> ### N U R S I N G   A L E R T
>
> #### Spread of Infections
>
> In the health care setting, infections are often spread directly, from the hands of personnel, or indirectly, through contact with fomites—inanimate objects on which organisms live and thrive.

Any time an intermediate object is contaminated by an agent, and a host comes in contact with that object, the means of transmission is indirect. Inanimate objects are often the intermediate articles responsible for the indirect spread of infection. A common example of indirect spread

occurs when a person passes pathogens from her mouth onto a drinking glass and another person drinks from the same glass, thus picking up the organisms. This, of course, can occur only if the agent is able to live on the inanimate object (fomite) once it leaves the host. As mentioned previously, a vector is a carrier that can transfer an agent between hosts or to an inanimate object that a host then picks up.

In the health care setting, much of the spread of infection occurs via the indirect route, most of which could be stopped with the use of good hand hygiene and proper technique in handling patients and equipment.

The Portal of Entry

Once an organism or agent escapes from its host, it must find a portal of entry into another host. In many cases of infection, the portal of entry into a new host is the same as the portal of exit from the prior host, or between the same body system. A prime example is the venereal route. To gain entry, the agent must be able to permeate the first lines of defense—the skin or mucous membranes—of the receiving host. In the case of intravenous therapy, the skin is punctured deliberately, making the patient vulnerable to the bloodborne spread of organisms from the patient's skin, the nurse's hands, or contaminated equipment.

The Susceptible Host

Resistance is the combination of internal and external barriers that prevent the invasion, reproduction, and impairment caused by invading pathogens (agents). **Susceptible** means to have little resistance to an invading agent.

Whether an agent gains entry into a host depends on many host-related factors. The competence of the major body systems, the skin and mucous membrane barriers, and the general state of health and nutrition are all important. In addition, age, the presence of disease and pre-existing illness, medication and treatment regimens contribute to the possibility of host invasion. In the health care setting, patients may be deficient in one or more areas that predispose them to diminishing resistance against pathogenic assault.

INFECTION CONTROL

The goal of infection control is to break the chain of infection at any link that will bring about the prevention of disease or its transmission. By following the guidelines of the CDC and enforcement directives from OSHA and APIC, and adhering to professional standards of care and practice, the goal of infection control can be achieved for both the patient and health care personnel.

When infection occurs, it is important to identify it as soon as possible, determine the circumstances that precipitated it, use the most efficient means to eradicate it, and alter conditions in such a way so as to prevent its recurrence (Figure 4-3).

Nosocomial Infections

An infection that develops in a patient during or after and as a result of a stay in a health care setting is called a **nosocomial infection**. It is distinctly different from a **community-acquired infection**, which is acquired or incubating prior to an admission to a health care facility.

Nosocomial infections and medical errors, collectively referred to as preventable "adverse health events," are responsible for 44,000 to 98,000 deaths per year at a cost of $17–$29 billion (Institute of Medicine, 1999). Hospital-acquired infections affect approximately two million persons each year (Gaynes et al., 2001). There are three major influences related to nosocomial infections: overuse of antimicrobial products (which decrease resistance), failure of hospital personnel to follow basic infection control practices (especially proper hand hygiene), and an increase in the immuno-compromised patient population (Weinstein, 1998).

An estimated 200,000 nosocomial BSIs occur each year, most of which are related to the use of an intravascular device (CDC, Guideline for Prevention of Intravascular Device-Related Infections, 2001a). Intravascular catheter-related infections are a major cause of morbidity and mortality in the United States. Coagulase-negative staphylococci, *S. aureus*, aerobic gram-negative bacilli, and *Candida albicans* most commonly cause catheter-related BSIs (Mermel et al., 2001). The CDC estimates that one-third of all nosocomial infections are preventable.

Nosocomial infections usually target those who are immunocompromised as a result of advanced age, underlying disease processes, or medical/surgical interventions.

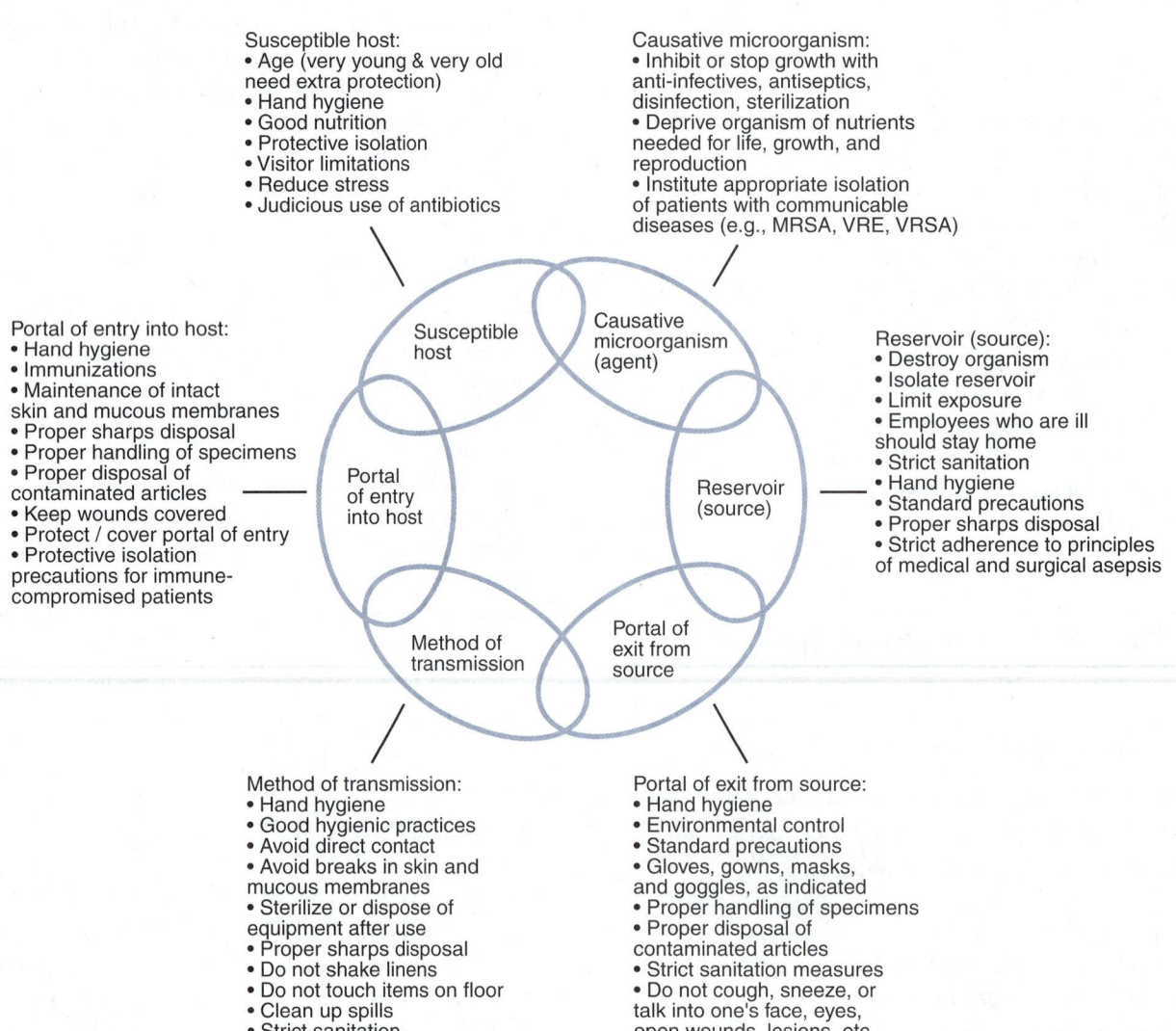

Figure 4-3 | Methods to break the chain of infection

Nosocomial infection rates in intensive care units (ICUs) occur at three times the rate of other areas within a hospital, with the sites of infection and the pathogens involved being directly related to ICU treatment (Weinstein, 1998). ICU patients, with invasive vascular catheters and monitoring devices have the highest incidence of BSIs.

The predominant organism that is responsible for intravenous catheter infections and the main organism that resides on the skin is *S. aureus*, which enters the bloodstream from the catheter lumen or the outside of the catheter surface (Sadovsky, 2000). *S. aureus* is capable of collecting on clothing, blankets, walls, and medical equipment. It is the number one cause of hospital infections, is blamed for about 13% of the nation's nosocomial infections, and kills over 80,000 people annually (CDC, *CDC Guideline for Prevention of Intravascular Device-Related Infections*, 2002).

Nosocomial infections present a major health care problem, with serious consequences in terms of **morbidity** (the incidence of illness), **mortality** (the incidence of deaths), and the millions of dollars spent each year on diagnosing and treating nosocomial infections. In addition, there are major legal ramifications for health care personnel and their employers whenever nosocomial infections occur. The public has the right to a safe level of care when entering any health care setting and at the very least should be protected from infection occurring as a direct result of care in such an environment.

The most common organisms responsible for nosocomial infections are *Escherichia coli*, *Pseudomonas aeruginosa*, enterococci, and staphylococci. *Staphylococcus epidermidis* accounts for the majority of intravenous cannula-related nosocomial infections (CDC, 1995). Contamination from the patient's own skin or that of the nurse (with eventual cannula colonization) accounted for 28% of all BSIs reported to the National Nosocomial Infection Surveillance System (NNISS). Since the mid-1980s there has been an increase in the proportion of nosocomial BSIs due to gram-positive, rather than gram-negative, species (CDC, 1995). The major portion of the overall increase in nosocomial BSIs has been due to four pathogens: coagulase-negative staphylococci (CoNS), *Candida spp.*, enterococci, and *Staphylococcus aureus*. Fungal pathogens account for an increasing proportion of BSIs as well. Between 1980 and 1990, in reports to NNIS, there had been nearly a fivefold increase in the rate of nosocomial fungal BSIs, with *Candida spp.* (particularly *Candida albicans*) accounting for more than 75% of all reported infections (CDC, 1995). It was hypothesized that candidemia arises from the endogenous flora of colonized patients. Recent epidemiologic investigations, however, point to exogenous infection resulting from the "administration of contaminated fluids, use of contaminated equipment, cross-infection, and the colonized hands of health care workers" (CDC, 1995).

In the past, people were admitted to health care facilities, especially hospitals, for conditions that today are treated largely on an outpatient basis or at home. With the changes in technology, Medicare, and the insurance industry, patients admitted to hospitals are "sicker and leave quicker" than ever before. Because of this, patients are susceptible to contracting nosocomial infections through exposure to numerous sources of contamination—other patients, health care personnel, visitors, equipment, machinery, treatment modalities—all harboring potential pathogens. This is especially true if the patients are immunocompromised, very old, or very young. The population at large is living longer with an upward trend in the number of senior citizens. Infants and children who in the past did not survive because of prematurity, low birth weights, and exposure to communicable diseases are now kept alive by advanced technology. The elderly, who often have pre-existing illness, multiple disease processes, and are on numerous medications, are much more susceptible to infection than the general adult population, as are the very young (see Chapters 15 and 16). Part of the treatment regimens for such patients often includes the intravenous administration of fluids, nutrients, blood products, and lifesaving medications. Nosocomial infections that are contracted as a result of intravenous infusion can be prevented or reduced considerably through diligent infection control practices.

CRITICAL THINKING

Reporting Infection in the Home Care Environment

As the life expectancy in the population increases, patients with chronic illnesses live longer and home care will continue to expand. In the U.S., approximately 1,000 agencies provide home care to patients (National Association for Home Care, 1999). Infection surveillance, prevention, and control have been acute-care oriented for the past 50 years. In home care, the diagnosis of infection is usually made on an empiric basis. Current reimbursement does not support the use of cultures and laboratory tests in the home. It is the responsibility of the home care nurse to assess, identify, and report infection.

Nosocomial infections must be prevented at all costs by carefully observing every patient for any signs or symptoms of infection. For the patient undergoing infusion therapy, any untoward reactions should be immediately evaluated and the necessary measures taken to prevent complications. Health care personnel must utilize standard precautions or body substance isolation (BSI) and follow all required isolation protocols and infection control policies and procedures. Documentation must be accurate and individualized for every patient.

Hand Hygiene

Clean hands, achieved through proper hand hygiene, are the single most important factor in preventing the spread of dangerous germs and antibiotic resistance in health care settings. Good hand hygiene can be achieved through the use of either a waterless, alcohol-based product or appropriate handwashing (Table 4-3) with an antibacterial soap and water with adequate rinsing (CDC, Centers for Disease Control: MMWR—Morbidity and Mortality Weekly Report—Recommendations and Reports. October 25, 2002/Vol. 51/No RR-216. *Guideline for Hand Hygiene in Health-Care Settings Recommendations of the Healthcare Infection Control Practices Advisory Committee and the HICPAC/SHEA/APIC/IDSA Hand Hygiene Task Force.* 2002d).

Hand hygiene by washing must be carried out properly by washing with running water, soap (an emulsifier), and vigorous friction for a period of at least 10–15 seconds, covering all hand surfaces, followed by thorough rinsing and drying. For routine patient care, there are no specific guidelines that dictate what type of soap is to be used by health care personnel for hand hygiene. Employer guidelines should be followed. Prior to invasive procedures, such as the insertion of intravenous devices or before manipulating central venous access lines, many practitioners of infection control recommend handwashing using antiseptic or antimicrobial compounds that contain germicidal properties, such as chlorhexidine gluconate or iodine. A **germicide** is an agent capable of killing germs. The germicides contained in any handwashing agents must be those listed as safe by the Environmental Protection Agency (EPA). Plain soap mechanically removes transient bacteria from the skin but does not kill the bacteria released by the shedding of dead skin cells. The term **antimicrobial** refers to any product that hinders the pathogenic activity of microorganisms on any surface. Antimicrobial soap products mechanically remove, kill, or inhibit bacterial growth. They have varying levels of action and may display bactericidal activity (killing of organisms), bacteriostatic activity (inhibition of organisms), or persistent activity (sustained reduction or inhibition of organisms over time). An **antiseptic** is a product that can safely be applied to the skin or the surface of mucous membranes, thus inhibiting microbial growth or destroying organisms. Antiseptic hand rubs, which have varying levels of activity, may kill or inhibit bacteria but do not remove soil.

Hand hygiene must be performed before and after each patient contact, after contact with patient belongings, after con-

tact with blood and body substances, before setting up equipment, before and after performing patient-related procedures, before eating, and after performing personal hygiene measures (e.g., toilet use). Hand hygiene is a medical aseptic technique that removes infectious organisms. **Asepsis** means the absence of infectious organisms. **Medical asepsis** (clean technique) refers to the absence of pathogenic organisms, whereas **surgical asepsis** (sterile technique) describes the removal of all microorganisms, pathogenic or nonpathogenic.

When in doubt, carry out proper hand hygiene thoroughly and frequently! The wearing of gloves does not preclude the need for hand hygiene. When health care personnel clean their hands frequently and correctly, they lower the populations of transient flora on their hands and inhibit the shedding of resident flora. Inherent in the practice of hand hygiene is educating others (health care personnel, students, patients, family members, and visitors) in the use of infection control protocols. In addition to hand hygiene, good personal hygiene must be maintained and fingernails should be kept clean and short. If nail polish is worn, it should be clear (so as not to obliterate visible dirt under nails) and free of chips so particles do not come off during patient care procedures. Artificial fingernails should not be worn because they increase the growth of gram-negative bacteria and fungus and may also breach the integrity of gloves (Larson, 1996).

Long natural nails and artificial nails harbor significantly more bacteria—both before and after handwashing—than do short natural nails. Both the CDC and APIC recommend that surgical and perioperative personnel wear short, natural nails due to the fact that handwashing is less effective at reducing bacterial colonization on hands with artificial nails. A study of 27 people with artificial nails colonized with gram-negative rods showed that the nails remained colonized with the organism following a five-minute surgical scrub (APIC, 2000). The most noteworthy link between long and artificial nails and a major *Pseudomonas aeruginosa* outbreak was published by the CDC in February 2000. Over a 15-month period, 16 neonate deaths were attributed to infant exposure to two nurses—one with long natural nails and a nurse with long artificial nails—in a newborn nursery. Both nurses harbored the *Pseudomonas* organism under their fingernails (Moolenaar et al., 2000). Another report confirms that three patients who acquired post-laminectomy deep-wound *Candida albicans* were linked to an operating room technician with artificial nails (Parry et al, 2001).

"Short" is a term used to describe nail length, but what does it mean? As a general guide, a fingernail that extends beyond the fingertip is considered too long. When gloves are routinely worn, tears occur in the glove's fingertips if the nails protrude over the edge of the fingertip, thus compromising barrier protection. In addition, patients can be

Table 4-3 | Hand Hygiene Guidelines

Hand hygiene can be accomplished with proper handwashing or with the use of alcohol-based handrubs.

WHEN
Upon arrival…
Before preparing….
Before preparing medications
Before and after…
Before donning gloves
(Gloves are *not* a substitute for handwashing or hand antisepsis with alcohol-based handrubs.)
After removing gloves (as mandated by OSHA)
Before and after personal…
Before and after eating
Before leaving work
After any exposure…
Handwashing is to be carried out

WITH
Running water at a comfortable temperature
Soap (emulsifier) (Use the correct kind, depending on the degree of contamination and the level and type of antimicrobial effectiveness required. Plain soap mechanically removes transient bacteria from the skin but does not kill the bacteria released by the shedding of dead skin cells. Antimicrobial soap mechanically removes, kills, or inhibits bacteria, depending on the levels of product activity. Antiseptic hand rubs kill or inhibit bacteria, depending on the levels of product activity, but don't remove soil.)
Friction (vigorous rubbing)
Towels (paper, from dispenser) or warm air dryer for drying

HOW
Wet hands and wrists…
Apply the correct soap or antiseptic
Apply vigorous friction, and maintain the vigorous rubbing for 10 to 15 seconds (longer if hands are visibly soiled), covering all hand surfaces, including thumbs and between the backs of fingers, with particular attention to fingertips and nails.
Rinse, in a flowing stream of water, from the wrists to finger tips. In the absence of water, use alternative agents (detergent-based towelettes to remove light soil; alcohol-based to reduce microbial flora)
Dry wrists and hands thoroughly with paper towel from wrists to finger tips (while water is still running) or with automated dryers. Activate lever-operated towel dispensers before washing and activate hand dryers with elbow.
Drop towel into waste container (without touching the container).
Obtain a dry paper towel and turn off the faucets (unless automated sinks are available). The dry towel is a more effective barrier to use to touch the contaminated faucet; a used towel is a weak barrier and bacteria may be "wicked" back onto the hand.

harmed during routine care when nails are too long. "A sign of healthy fingernails is well-manicured nails—clean, short, with jagged nail tips smoothed away and with surrounding skin intact" (Wen-Tsung et al., 2002).

Some policy manuals recommend that nail polish, if worn, should be clear (so as not to obliterate visible dirt under nails) and free of chips so particles do not come off during patient-care procedures. Although this is considered safe by some, small polish chips may not be obvious to the wearer. Nail polish deteriorates, chips, and breaks away from the nail surface. The time it takes varies, based on the age of the polish, its adherence characteristics, the health of the nail, and the wearer's activity. Polish fragments are foreign bodies that can potentially cause a reaction when deposited in wounds through glove tears. Dermatologists report that reactions to nail hardeners and laquers cause **onycholysis**, or loosening or detachment of the nail from the nailbed (Berger et al., 2000). "Studies have documented that subungual areas of the hand harbor high concentrations of bacteria, most frequently coagulase-negative staphylococci, gram-negative rods (including Pseudomonas spp.), Corynebacteria, and yeasts. . . . Even after careful handwashing or the use of surgical scrubs, personnel often harbor substantial numbers of potential pathogens in the subungual spaces" (CDC, 2002d, *Guideline for Hand Hygiene in Health-Care Settings*). Even though rings do not interfere with handwashing, they should be avoided in high-risk patient care areas because bacterial counts increase under rings (Jacobson, 1985).

Standard Precautions

In 1987 the CDC published *Recommendations for prevention of HIV transmission in health care settings*. This was an update of its 1983 guidelines for handling blood and body fluids in which precautions were listed for only those patients who were known to have, or were suspected of having, infected bloodborne pathogens. Because of the AIDS epidemic, the 1987 document "emphasizes the need for health care workers to consider *all* patients as potentially infected with HIV and/or other bloodborne pathogens and to adhere rigorously to infection-control precautions for minimizing the risk of exposure to blood and body fluids of all patients." Under Standard Precautions, blood and certain other bodily fluids of all patients are considered potentially infectious for human immunodeficiency virus (HIV), hepatitis viruses, and other bloodborne pathogens.

Standard Precautions pertain to blood and any other body fluids containing visible blood, as well as semen and vaginal secretions. Since the risk of transmission of HIV and hepatitis viruses is not known fully, and research is ongoing in this area, the CDC extends Standard Precautions to cerebrospinal, synovial, pleural, peritoneal, pericardial, and amniotic fluids.

Unless there is visible blood, Standard Precautions do not apply to feces, urine, vomitus, nasal secretions, saliva, sputum, tears, and perspiration. Although the risk of transmitting HIV and hepatitis from these fluids is very low,

common sense should be used in handling such materials. Health care personnel must remember that these may be sources of contamination from other organisms. Breast milk, although implicated in the perinatal transmission of HIV and the hepatitis B-specific antigen (HBsAG), is not considered an occupational threat to health care personnel.

Standard Precautions are not considered to be a replacement for routine infection control protocols, but serve as a supplement to them. The need for other disease category-specific isolation procedures, such as respiratory or enteric precautions, still prevails. Good judgment must always be used, along with good hand hygiene and the wearing of gloves (Table 4-4), to prevent contamination of hands.

Occupational Safety and Health Administration Guidelines

Blood and other potentially infectious materials have long been recognized as a potential threat to the health of employees who are exposed to these materials by **percutaneous contact** (penetration of the skin). Injuries from contaminated needles and other sharps have been associated with an increased risk of disease from more than 20 infectious agents. The primary agents of concern in current occupational settings are the human immunodeficiency virus (HIV), hepatitis B virus (HBV), and hepatitis C virus (HCV) (OSHA, 2001).

The CDC has estimated that health care personnel in hospital settings sustain 384,325 percutaneous injuries involving contaminated sharps annually. When non-hospital health care personnel are included, the best estimate of the number of percutaneous injuries involving contaminated sharps is 590,164 per year (CDC, 2001a, Guidelines for Prevention of Intravascular Device-Related Infections). When these injuries involve exposure to infectious agents, the affected workers are at risk of contracting disease. Workers may also suffer from adverse side effects of drugs used for postexposure prophylaxis and from psychological stress due to the threat of infection following an exposure incident.

Table 4-4 | Glove Guidelines (Source: APIC, 1999)

GLOVE GUIDELINES

Type to use:	**Medical grade examination (nonsterile) or surgical (sterile)**
	Natural rubber latex. The natural rubber provides dexterity, durability, flexibility, and tactile sensitivity and is preferred for procedures that are moderate-to-high risk for exposure to blood and other potentially infectious materials and when nonsterile hand protection is indicated. Change every 15–30 minutes, depending on the procedure, the amount of blood/fluid exposure, and contact with sharps.
	Nitrile. The preferred choice for latex-sensitive individuals and those with moderate-to-high risk for exposure to blood and other potential contaminants. Higher chemical resistance than latex to hydrocarbon-based products (lanolin, mineral oil, petrolatum).
	Vinyl synthetic. Appropriate for short-term use involving minimal stress on the glove and low risk of exposure to blood and other potentially infectious materials.
When to wear:	• Handling contaminants • Reasonable likelihood for contact with blood, potentially infectious materials, mucous membranes, and non-intact skin • Touching potentially contaminated items or surfaces • Vascular access procedures
What to do:	• Wear correct size • Keep fingernails short to prevent tears • Wash hands before and after use • Change frequently, depending on length of exposure to blood, potential sources of infection, contaminants, and procedure length • Change between patients • Change between tasks on same patient • Change both gloves (if double-gloving for safety) and wash hands before starting another task • Generously use water-soluble lotions/moisturizers (approved for health care use) to prevent skin abraisions
What not to do:	• Use nonmedical-grade gloves for direct patient care • Use gloves when there is no potential for contact with blood or contaminants (such as taking vital signs or charting) • Use hydrocarbon-based hand products with natural rubber latex gloves (which will cause gloves to break down within minutes of exposure) • Use fragranced hand-care products (which will cause chemical irritation to hands) • Store gloves near heat, sunlight, electrical machines, or areas of temperature extremes

To reduce the health risk to personnel whose duties involve exposure to blood or other potentially infectious materials, OSHA promulgated the Blood Borne Pathogen (BBP) standard on December 6, 1991. The provisions of the standard were based on the Agency's determination that a combination of engineering and work practice controls, personal protective equipment, training, medical surveillance, hepatitis B vaccination, signs and labels, and other requirements would minimize the risk of disease transmission. Since the inception of this standard, needlesticks and other percutaneous injuries resulting in exposure to blood or other potentially infectious materials continue to be of concern due to the high frequency of their occurrence and the severity of the health effects associated with exposure.

Since publication of the BBP standard, a wide variety of medical devices have been developed to reduce the risk of needlesticks and other sharps injuries. These "safer medical devices" replace sharps with non-needle devices or incorporate safety features designed to reduce the likelihood of injury. In 1998, OSHA solicited information on occupational exposure to bloodborne pathogens due to percutaneous injury. Based in part on the information received, OSHA pur-

sued an approach to minimize the risk of occupational exposure to BBP that involves (1) a revised recordkeeping mechanism requiring that all percutaneous injuries from contaminated needles and other sharps be recorded on OSHA logs, (2) a revised compliance directive for the BBP standard (November 5, 1999), and (3) the placing of an amendment of the BBP standard on its regulatory agenda to more effectively address sharps injuries.

In response to OSHA's findings, the growing concern over bloodborne pathogen exposures from sharps injuries, and technological developments that increase employee protection, Congress was prompted to take action. On November 6, 2000, the Needlestick Safety and Prevention Act (Pub. L. 106-430) was signed into law by President Clinton. The Act required OSHA to revise the Blood Borne Pathogen standard, with specific language included in the Act, within six months of the enactment.

The revised Blood Borne Pathogen standard took effect on April 18, 2001. The revised definitions do not reflect any new requirements being placed on employers with regard to protecting workers from sharps injuries, but are meant only to clarify the original standard of 1991 and to reflect the development of new, safer medical devices since that time.

The revisions to OSHA's BBP Standard required under the Needlestick Safety and Prevention Act are broadly categorized into the following four areas:

1. Modification of definitions relating to engineering controls.

   The revised standard adds "Sharps with Engineered Sharps Injury Protections" and defines this term as "a nonneedle sharp or a needle device used for withdrawing body fluids, accessing a vein or artery, or administering medications or other fluids, with a built-in safety feature or mechanism that effectively reduces the risk of an exposure incident." This term encompasses a broad array of devices that make injury involving a contaminated sharp less likely, and includes, but is not limited to, syringes with a sliding sheath that shields the attached needle after use; needles that retract into a syringe after use; shielded or retracting catheters used to access the bloodstream for intravenous administration of medication or fluids; and intravenous medication delivery systems that administer medication or fluids through a catheter port or connector site using a needle that is housed in a protective covering.

   The revised standard also adds the term "Needleless Systems," which is defined as "a device that does not use needles for: (A) The collection of bodily fluids or withdrawal of body fluids after initial venous or arterial access is established; (B) the administration of medication or fluids; or (C) any other procedure involving the potential for occupational exposure to bloodborne pathogens due to percutaneous injuries from contaminated sharps." "Needleless Systems" provide an alternative to needles for the specified procedures, thereby reducing the risk of percutaneous injury involving contaminated sharps. Examples of needleless systems include, but are not limited to, intravenous medication delivery systems that administer medication or fluids through a catheter port or connector site using a blunt cannula or other non-needle connection, and jet injection systems that deliver subcutaneous or intramuscular injections of liquid medication through the skin without use of a needle.

   The definition of "Engineering Controls" has been modified to include "safer medical devices, such as sharps with engineered sharps injury protections and needleless systems." This change clarifies that safer medical devices are considered to be engineering controls under the standard. The term "Engineering Controls" includes all control measures that isolate or remove a hazard from the workplace, encompassing not only sharps with engineered sharps injury protections and needleless systems but also other medical devices designed to reduce the risk of percutaneous exposure to bloodborne pathogens. Examples include blunt suture needles and plastic or mylar-wrapped glass capillary tubes, as well as controls that are not medical devices, such as sharps disposal containers and biosafety cabinets.

2. Revision and updating of the Exposure Control Plans.

   The review and update of the plan is now required to "(A) reflect changes in technology that eliminate or reduce exposure to bloodborne pathogens; and (B) document annually consideration and implementation of appropriate commercially available and effective safer medical devices designed to eliminate or minimize occupational exposure." Thus, the additional provisions require that employers, in their written Exposure Control Plans, account for innovations in procedure and technological developments that reduce the risk of exposure incidents. The revised Exposure Control Plan requirements make clear that employers must implement the safer medical devices that are appropriate, commercially available, and effective.

3. Solicitation of employee input.

   The revised standard now requires that "An employer, who is required to establish an Exposure Control Plan shall solicit input from non-managerial employees responsible for direct patient care who are potentially exposed to injuries from contaminated sharps in the identification, evaluation, and selection of effective engineering and work practice controls and shall document the solicitation in the Exposure Control Plan." This change represents a new requirement, which is performance-oriented. No specific procedures for obtaining employee input are prescribed. This provides the employer with flexibility to solicit employee input in any manner appropriate to the circumstances of the workplace. The revised standard requires that solicitation of input from employees be documented in the Exposure Control Plan.

4. Recordkeeping.

   The recordkeeping requirements of the standard have been amended to add the paragraph that now states, "The employer shall establish and maintain a sharps injury log for the recording of percutaneous injuries from contaminated sharps. The information in the sharps injury log shall be recorded and maintained in such manner as to protect the confidentiality of the injured employee. The sharps injury log shall contain, at a minimum: (A) The type and brand of device involved in the incident, (B) the department or work area where the exposure incident occurred, and (C) an explanation of how the incident occurred." The level of detail presented should be sufficient to allow ready identification of the device, location, and circumstances surrounding an exposure incident (e.g., the procedure being performed, the body part affected, objects or substances involved and how they were involved) so that the intended evaluation of risk and device effectiveness can be accomplished.

If data from the log are made available to other parties, any information that directly identifies an employee (e.g., name, address, social security number, payroll number) or information that could reasonably be used to identify indirectly a specific employee (e.g., exact age, date of initial employment) must be withheld.

Guidelines for Intravenous Care

The CDC estimates that, each year, nearly two million patients in the United States get an infection in hospitals, and about 90,000 of these patients die as a result of their infections. Infections are also a complication of care in other settings, including long-term care facilities, clinics, and dialysis centers (CDC, Guidelines for the Prevention of Intravascular Catheter-Related Infections, 2002a).

The patient undergoing infusion therapy is exposed to the risk of infection because the skin barrier is intentionally broken with an IV device, thus allowing for the free flow of organisms into the circulatory system. The incidence of catheter-related bloodstream infection (CRBSI) varies considerably by type of catheter, frequency of catheter manipulation, and patient-related factors, such as underlying disease and acuteness of illness (CDC, Guidelines for the Prevention of Intravascular Catheter-Related Infections, 2002a). The nurse is in a critical position to prevent infections from occurring. He does this through good and frequent hand hygiene and aseptic practices while caring for patients and by performing procedures correctly and in a safe manner.

One of the most serious complications of IV therapy involves sepsis, a pathologic state, usually with fever, that is the result of microorganisms in the bloodstream. Microorganisms usually gain access to the blood at the catheter or needle insertion site, but they can also enter via contaminated tubing and fluid. For the patient who is receiving several different medications and fluids intravenously, organisms can enter through injection ports, the fluid, or the filter systems.

Because the nurse has many responsibilities in his day-to-day routine, it is easy to overlook areas of infection control. Unfortunately, and all too often in health care, asepsis is neglected in the interest of saving time. This trend has evolved as a result of the numerous antibiotics available to "chase infections," so prevention of infection has become less important than fixing it after the fact. This negligent

mindset needs to be replaced with the philosophy that an ounce of prevention is worth a pound of cure. This is especially important because the excessive use of antibiotics in a patient weakens her response to them over time. Because society has become so litigious, physicians often prescribe antibiotics prophylactically or unnecessarily (such as for colds, which are nonbacterial), to appease the patient or "just to be safe." Physicians should responsibly prescribe antibiotics only where needed and not use powerful broad-spectrum agents if a lesser, precisely indicated agent will suffice (Zuger, 1995).

> ### N U R S I N G   A L E R T
>
> #### *Nosocomial Infection from Resistant Organisms*
>
> In principle, it may be possible for a patient who develops a nosocomial infection caused by a resistant organism to recover damages resulting from the organism's resistance if he or she can prove that the resistance was caused by the physician's or hospital's indiscriminate use of antibiotics. (Kaunitz, 1996)

As discussed earlier, microbiologists are witnessing the emergence of bacterial strains that are developing resistance to many of the antibiotics available. With each new generation they are becoming more virulent and more resistant to treatment. Bacteria responsible for hospital-acquired infections have gradually developed resistance to common antibiotics; although MRSA was initially the multidrug-resistant organism of concern, now others have emerged.

Because of developing problems of drug resistance, in 1995, the HICPAC issued recommendations for preventing the spread of vancomycin resistance. Along with the many advisements in this document, which include specifics regarding gloves, gowns, masks, and isolation procedures, it emphasizes that proper hand hygiene is still the most important method to stop the spread of infection—a concept that goes back to basics.

A great deal of research has been done (and continues to be done) regarding the safest and best protocols for infusion therapy. The studies look at the devices used, the antiseptic preparation and site care, dressing changes, patient comfort, nursing time, and cost effectiveness. The nurse who is primarily responsible for initiating, monitoring, maintaining, and discontinuing intravenous treatment makes use of the research by following the guidelines provided by the CDC and protocols mandated by OSHA and HICPAC, and by adhering to the employer policies and procedures that apply to the area where he works.

NURSING ALERT

Preventing Antimicrobial Resistance

The Centers for Disease Control and Prevention (CDC) has launched a campaign aimed at clinicians called the "Prevent Antimicrobial Resistance." The campaign focuses on four key strategies for preventing antimicrobial resistance in healthcare settings:

1. Preventing infection
2. Diagnosing and treating infection effectively
3. Using antimicrobials wisely
4. Preventing transmission of drug-resistant pathogens

Within these strategies are 12 action steps derived from evidenced-based guidelines and recommendations developed by the CDC that clinicians can take to prevent antimicrobial resistance in hospitalized adults.

These action steps include:

Action Step 1: Vaccinate

Action Step 2: Get the catheters out

Action Step 3: Target the pathogen

Action Step 4: Access the experts

Action Step 5: Practice antimircobial control

Action Step 6: Use local data

Action Step 7: Treat infection, not contamination

Action Step 8: Treat infection, not colonization

Action Step 9: Know when to say "no" to vanco(mycin)

Action Step 10: Stop antimicrobial treatment when infection is treated or unlikely

Action Step 11: Isolate the pathogen

Action Step 12: Break the chain of contagion

CDC is partnering with professional medical organizations, including the Infectious Diseases Society of America, the American Society for Microbiology, the National Foundation for Infectious Diseases, national medical centers and other health care institutions to distribute, implement and evaluate campaign materials. The materials include a slide set, posters, brochures and a pocket-sized clinician reminder card listing the 12 action steps. The campaign also features a Web site (www.cdc.gov/drugresistance/healthcare).

NURSING TIP

Patient Teaching and Antibiotics

The nurse plays a major role in slowing the epidemic of drug-resistant infections by teaching patients about the judicious use of antibiotics. Teaching should include the following:

- Advise patients to comply with physician directives when antibiotics are not prescribed for the common cold or flu—viral infections for which antibiotics are ineffective.
- Caution patients not to push their physicians to prescribe antibiotics "just in case."
- Remind patients that it is important when antibiotics are ordered for bacterial infections to take the prescribed dose at the proper time intervals for the full duration of treatment and to follow guidelines regarding food and fluid intake that may affect the drug's efficacy.
- Explain that taking antibiotics according to prescription guidelines may prevent reinfection and future resistance to lifesaving antimicrobials.

NURSING ALERT

The Consequences of Carelessness

The nurse must always keep in mind that carelessness and failure to follow proper protocols can cause a patient a great deal of discomfort, extend treatment time, and increase health care costs. The worst-case scenario is when a nosocomial infection results in disability or death. In spite of strict adherence to principles of asepsis and infection control, some patients still contract nosocomial infections.

Antiseptic Agents

An antiseptic is an agent that, when applied topically, is capable of killing microorganisms on the skin or inhibiting their growth. An antiseptic works by interrupting the cell's metabolic activity by chemically destroying cellular components, by interfering with the cell's protein structure, or by weakening the cell membrane so that the cell's contents are able to escape, thus destroying the organism. Proper skin cleansing and antisepsis of the cannula-insertion site and surrounding area is considered one of the most important measures for preventing catheter-related infections, and reducing the numbers of resident and transient skin organisms (CDC, 2002a).

The antiseptic products most often studied and compared in recent years are alcohol, iodine/iodophors, and chlorhexidine gluconate. These three, employed alone or in combination with other products, are often used for skin antisepsis during intravenous therapy. The CDC recommendations regarding cutaneous antisepsis are as follows:

Disinfect clean skin with an appropriate antiseptic before catheter insertion and during dressing changes. Although a 2% chlorhexidine-based preparation is preferred, tincture of iodine, iodophor, or 70% alcohol can be used . . . Allow the antiseptic to remain on the insertion site and to air dry before catheter insertion. Allow povidone iodine to remain on the skin for at least 2 minutes, or longer if it is not yet dry before insertion. Do not apply organic solvents (e.g., acetone and ether) to the skin before insertion of catheters or during dressing changes. (CDC, *Guidelines for the Prevention of Intravascular Catheter-Related Infections*, 2002a)

NURSING TIP

Ensuring the Efficacy of Antiseptics

Prior to the application of any antiseptic, the skin must be physically clean because organic matter can inactivate the efficacy of antiseptics.

70% Isopropyl Alcohol

70% isopropyl alcohol (isopropanol) or ETOH (ethyl alcohol) inhibits bacterial growth and is often used as a topical skin disinfectant. Alcohol is a good fat solvent; it exerts its effect by denaturing protein. It is one of the safest products for the purpose of antisepsis and is cost effective. (Toxic reactions have occurred in children following full body sponging for fever.) It is the antiseptic of choice when patients are allergic to iodine-containing products.

NURSING TIP

Proper Application of Alcohol and Iodine

When alcohol and iodine preparations are used together for skin antisepsis prior to IV cannulation, the procedure for applying them is as follows:

1. Vigorously apply the alcohol to the site, using enough alcohol to keep the site wet for one minute. Alcohol is applied first because it does not exert a residual effect.
2. Allow the site to air dry.
3. Apply the iodine to the site.

If applied to the skin with friction and allowed to air dry isopropanol is able to kill bacteria (**bactericidal**) within two minutes. (The nurse must never blow on the site or fan the area with his hand.) While it is rapid-acting, it does not exert a residual antiseptic effect. Alcohol is effective against most gram-negative and gram-positive organisms, tubercle bacilli, and many fungi and viruses (including HIV), but it is not effective against spores.

NURSING ALERT

Be Aware of the Effects of Alcohol

Alcohol causes a burning sensation with discomfort when applied to open wounds or cuts. When used on intact skin, it may cause drying and irritation on some patients. When applied as a skin prep, alcohol causes subcutaneous vasodilation, which enhances the ability to see the veins prior to needle or catheter insertion. Because of this vasodilating effect, alcohol should not be used to discontinue an IV infusion because vasodilation enhances bleeding; a 2 × 2-inch gauze should be used instead.

Commercially packaged skin wipes saturated with 70% isopropyl alcohol for one-time use are commonly used instead of multiuse containers, which may become contaminated. Also available for cleansing the site (usually on central line insertions) are cotton-tipped alcohol applicator sticks.

Alcohol is often used in combination with iodine as a skin prep prior to IV insertions. When used in tandem, the alcohol should be applied first and allowed to air dry, followed by the iodine preparation. (In some institutions, alcohol is used after the iodine preparation has been applied in order to de-color the area and allow for better vein visibility during venipuncture. This is not a good practice and should be avoided because the alcohol negates the residual effect of the other products and alcohol does not provide a prolonged cutaneous antiseptic effect. The INS recommends that "Antimicrobial solutions that should be used for site care include 2% tincture of iodine, 10% povidone-iodine, alcohol, or chlorhexidine, as single agents or in combination" (INS, 2000, Standard 57, S55).

Iodine Preparations

Iodine solutions are frequently used for skin preparation prior to venipuncture. Iodine is a potent antimicrobial, exerting its effects on gram-negative and gram-positive bacteria, viruses, fungi, yeasts, and protozoa. It penetrates the cell wall, causing intracellular oxidation with resultant release of free iodine within the microbial contents to (probably) disrupt protein and nucleic acid structure and synthesis. It is also cost effective, while producing minimal toxicity (although prolonged use of iodine can result in systemic absorption). Incidences of hypothyroidism have occurred in newborn infants treated topically with iodine. Iodine also stains the skin, interfering with the ability to see deep veins.

Tincture of iodine is a simple solution of 2% iodine and sodium iodide in dilute alcohol. It is capable of killing all bacteria present on the skin within 1.5 minutes. It causes less stinging than alcohol when applied to broken skin. Bandaging over tincture of iodine is not recommended as it may cause skin irritation and discomfort.

NURSING TIP

Iodine Allergies

Before using any iodine-containing product on a patient, it is very important for the nurse to find out if the patient is allergic to iodine or has had any unusual reaction (local or systemic) from its use. If the patient doesn't know if she is allergic to iodine, the nurse should ask her if she is allergic to shellfish (which contain iodine). As with all medications, the nurse must watch for hypersensitivity reactions.

Iodophors, such as povidone-iodine (the most common iodophor), are concentrations of iodine mixed with other substances that act as carriers to produce a substantial release of iodine on the skin, providing longer germicidal activity. Because they are weaker than other iodine compounds, there is reduced toxicity and less irritation and staining of the skin. Because the iodine is released gradually, a contact time of two minutes is necessary to allow for optimum microbial kill. If adequate time is not allowed for iodophor action, the use of tincture of iodine, with its more rapid action, should be considered. The site area may be covered with a dressing because there is less skin irritation. Iodophors burn less than alcohol or other iodine compounds, but they are not as effective as iodine solutions and iodine tinctures. Povidone-iodine is available in several forms—saturated disks, swabs, cotton-tipped applicator sticks, and cotton-tipped plastic ampules.

A shortcoming of iodophors is that their antimicrobial properties are neutralized in the presence of proteinaceous material such as blood and pus.

Chlorhexidine Gluconate

Chlorhexidine gluconate (CHG) is a potent broad-spectrum cationic biguanide antiseptic available in various strengths.

Clinical trials have shown that CHG is bactericidal on contact (through cell wall disruption) and displays persistent antimicrobial activity against a wide range of gram-positive and gram-negative bacteria, having residual antibacterial properties that last for hours after application. Organic material has little effect on CHG. CHG has a minimal effect on tubercle bacilli, is less active against fungi, but is active against many viruses. The major advantage of CHG is its ability to bind to skin protein, leaving a residue with persistent antimicrobial effects for up to six hours after application. In a randomized clinical trial using 70% alcohol, 10% povidone-iodine, and 2% CHG (as cutaneous antiseptics for the prevention of catheter-related infections [CRI] in central venous and arterial catheters), the rate of catheter-related BSIs, when CHG was used, was 84% lower than the rates when the other two regimens were used (Maki, Ringer, & Alvarado, 1991). In July 2000 the U.S. Food and Drug Administration (FDA) approved a 2% tincture of chlorhexidine preparation for skin antisepsis. CHG rarely produces reactions and is not absorbed through the skin. CHG has, however, been reported to cause deafness when instilled into the middle ear through a perforated ear drum. If it enters the eye, it must be flushed out immediately, as prolonged contact can cause serious and permanent eye injury.

Because of its properties, CHG is approved by the Food and Drug Administration (FDA) as a preoperative skin prep in a 4% strength (for areas other than the face and head), as a skin wound cleanser, for use as a surgical scrub, as a handwashing agent for health care personnel, and for preoperative showering or bathing for the patient.

Numerous studies have compared the efficacy of the three antiseptics discussed in this chapter, along with others that are available and approved by the FDA. The "perfect" agent has not been found—one that would kill all microorganisms on the skin, inhibit regrowth, be nontoxic and nonirritating to the patient, be convenient to use and nonstaining, save time, and be cost effective. In terms of antimicrobial efficacy and infection control, all of the research substantiates three very important facts: (1) hand hygiene continues to be the most important factor in preventing the spread of infection, (2) the proper application of an antiseptic to the intravenous insertion site prior to venipuncture and routinely thereafter with dressing changes is needed, and (3) dressings and tubing should be changed at specified, CDC-approved intervals using aseptic technique.

Antimicrobial Ointments

Studies regarding the application of antimicrobial ointments to the catheter insertion site at the time of placement and during dressing changes have produced conflicting results over the years. "The rates of catheter colonization with *Candida spp.* might be increased with the use of antibiotic ointments that have no fungicidal activity." Current CDC guidelines state, "Do not use topical antibiotic ointment or creams on insertion sites (except when using dialysis catheters) because of their potential to promote fungal infections and antimicrobial resistance." Studies conclude that mupirocin ointment is effective at reducing the risk for CRBSI but its use has also been associated with mupirocin resistance. In addition, the ointment may adversely affect the integrity of polyurethane catheters: "To avoid compromising the integrity of the catheter, any ointment that is applied to the catheter insertion site should be checked against the catheter and ointment manufacturers' recommendations regarding the compatibility" (CDC, 2002b).

Catheter-related bloodstream infections are more commonly associated with the use of central venous catheters than with small peripheral catheters. The microbes that colonize the catheter hub and the skin area surrounding the insertion site are the source of most catheter-related infections. Preventive strategies must be aimed at reducing microbial colonization at the insertion site and hub and minimizing the bacterial spread extraluminally (from the skin) or intraluminally (from the hub toward the catheter tip lying in the bloodstream) (Mermel, 2000).

The factors most obviously associated with the increased risk of catheter-related infection include prolonged duration of placement, frequent manipulation, use of thrombogenic catheter materials, an inadequate sterile barrier protecting the catheter insertion site, and inadequate sterile technique during catheter insertion. Some experts suggest, above and beyond what the CDC recommends, that preventive strategies to preclude infection incorporate enhanced skill and care during catheter placement, maximal sterile barriers, the use of antimicrobial catheters, the (preferable) use of the CHG for topical antisepsis, and flushing the catheter with antimicrobial and antiatherogenic agents (Sadovsky, 2000). The development of protocols to ensure that the proper technique is followed and that adequate catheter maintenance is performed should be a priority in all patient care settings.

Alcohol Gels

The spread of microbes in hospitals is making patients who are already ill even worse, with a resultant estimated 20,000 deaths each year (Haney, 2002). One feasible solution appears to be the use of waterless, alcohol-based disinfectants. Hospitals are placing dispensers of alcohol gels either near patient beds or outside patient rooms, where nurses and other health care personnel can apply and rub the solution on while on the move. The disinfectant dries as the skin absorbs it. Research findings, as presented by the American Society for Microbiology in September 2002, suggest that alcohol-based rinses kill more germs, require no sink or

water, and are easier to use than soap and water. The alcohol formulas are available as rinses, foams, gels, or lotions. The procedure for use is to place a dime-size spot of the material on one palm, then rub the hands together until it dries — which takes about 15 seconds. The solutions contain moisturizers, so they do not dry the skin.

Recent guidelines from the CDC recommend the use of sinkless alcohol-based hand degerming gels exclusively, except when workers' hands are visibly soiled—or use of the gels in conjunction with the traditional soap-and-water treatment (CDC, 2002d, Guideline for Hand Hygiene).

In 2000, researchers at the Veterans Administration Medical Center in Washington, DC measured the effects of switching to the alcohol rinses. Dispensers were put in all patient rooms and outpatient facilities. New cases of nosocomial drug-resistant staphylococcal infections decreased 21%, while resistant enterococcus dropped 43%. After four years of use at the University of Geneva Hospital in Switzerland, hospital-acquired infections were cut in half (Haney, 2002).

Dressings and Intravenous Site Maintenance

As previously discussed, preventing infections related to intravascular access depends on the aseptic practices and precautions used prior to and during the insertion of an IV device. Once in place, the entry site of the needle or catheter must be properly secured and maintained. In forthcoming chapters, the techniques for site preparation and maintenance will be covered in detail. From an infection control standpoint, it is important to review accepted dressing change and site maintenance protocols here.

There has been much discussion over IV site dressings in terms of safety and efficacy in preventing infections, durability, patient comfort, practitioner convenience, and cost effectiveness. The types of protective coverings used as recommended by the CDC are "either sterile gauze or sterile, transparent, semipermeable membrane dressings to cover the catheter site" (CDC, 2002b).

Transparent dressings vary among manufacturers in terms of their physical properties. Although their appearances are similar, there are differences regarding the transmission of oxygen and moisture vapor, as well as their ability to adhere to the skin. These dressings are reliable in securing the cannula, provide a means for continuous visual inspection and palpation of the IV site (thus allowing for quick assessment and identification of redness, swelling, warmth, or dislodgement even before the patient may sense any discomfort), and allow patients to bathe and shower without saturating the dressing. They also require less frequent changes than do gauze and tape dressings, thereby saving personnel time. Many IV practitioners prefer transparent dressings because they can be placed directly over the hub of the needle or catheter, thus stabilizing the IV device. When using these dressings, it is very important not to cover them with tape or other dressing materials that would obliterate the IV insertion site. "Products employed to stabilize the catheter should include sterile tapes, transparent semipermeable membrane (TSM) dressings, sutures, manufactured catheter securement devices, and sterile surgical strips" (INS, Standard 49, S 43, 2000).

When using a gauze dressing, the hub of the needle or catheter must still be stabilized in a sterile manner. As soon as the IV device is in place, tape must be used to prevent dislodgement and movement. Once the IV device is adequately secured, the sterile gauze may be applied. A major advantage of this type of dressing is that the patient who may be uncomfortable about seeing a needle or catheter in her body is spared from looking at it.

With either type of dressing, it is always important to note on the dressing the type and size of the needle or catheter, the date and time of insertion, and the initials of the person who inserted it. This should be placed to the side of the insertion site, so as not to manipulate the IV device or obliterate visualization of the insertion site. This is an excellent communication tool for everyone who assesses the dressing, because at a glance all of the important information about the IV device is available.

Studies have shown that the type of dressings used may not be as important as the manner in which they are applied, maintained, and monitored. In the largest controlled trial of dressing regimens (on more than 2000 peripheral catheters) done thus far, the findings of Dr. Maki and associates suggest that the rate of catheter colonization among IV sites dressed with transparent dressings (5.7%) is comparable to that of those dressed with gauze (4.6%) and there are no clinically significant differences in either the incidences of catheter-site colonization or phlebitis between the two groups (CDC, 2002).

A meta-analysis has assessed studies that compared the risk for catheter-related BSIs for groups using transparent dressings versus groups using gauze dressing. The risk for CRBSIs did not differ between the groups. The choice of dressing can be a matter of preference. If blood is oozing from the catheter insertion site, gauze dressing might be preferred . . . . Data suggest that transparent dressing can be safely left on peripheral venous catheters for the duration of catheter insertion . . . . (CDC, 2002a).

The monitoring of intravascular devices and dressings should be done on a daily basis (CDC, 2002) and they should be manipulated as little as possible. Patient complaints must always be thoroughly investigated and resolved.

The CDC (2002) recommends that the IV dressing be left in place until the catheter is removed or changed or it

becomes damp, loosened, or soiled. IV site dressings need to be changed more frequently in diaphoretic patients.

The dressing must be securely applied so as to prevent dislodgement of the intravascular device. The nurse must be careful not to manipulate the catheter as this irritates the intima of the vein and increases the risk of phlebitis and infection. He must also take precautions to prevent inadvertent removal of the cannula during dressing changes.

Intravascular Catheters

An intravenous catheter usually remains in place longer than a needle because it is used for prolonged therapy. The patient's risk for developing an infection depends on the manner of site preparation and insertion, the site location, the size of the catheter, the patient's condition, and the length of time the IV device remains in place. Any time the skin is punctured, for any reason, one of the body's natural defenses is to prevent blood loss, so the process of clot formation begins. Fibrin, a protein, develops in the process of blood clotting. Fibrin forms around (fibrin sheath) and on the tip of the catheter, sometimes forming a tail protruding from the tip of the catheter. Microorganisms have an affinity to this fibrin sheath, which generally develops within 48 hours of catheter insertion.

The correlation between infectious morbidity and the IV cannula makeup has been studied extensively. Peripheral cannulas made with Teflon® or polyurethane are associated with fewer infectious complications than those composed of polyvinyl chloride (PVC) or polyethylene. In one major study, polyurethane catheters were associated with nearly a 30% lower risk of phlebitis when compared with those made of Teflon®, yet neither was associated with bloodstream infections (while PVC and polyethylene cannulas were affiliated with BSI rates up to 5%). The CDC recommends cannula selection "based on the intended purpose, duration of use, known complications, and experience at the institution . . . (using) a Teflon® catheter, polyurethane catheter, or a steel needle" (CDC, 2002).

Certain types of catheters and cuffs that are coated with or impregnated with antimicrobial or antiseptic agents, although more costly, have been shown to decrease the risk for CRBSIs and have the potential to decrease hospital costs associated with treating CRBSIs. Catheters coated with chlorhexidine/silver sulfadiazine only on the external lumen surface have been studied as a means to reduce CRBSI (and) . . . reduced the risk for CRBSI compared with standard noncoated catheters. A second-generation catheter has been developed with chlorhexidine coating on both the internal and external luminal surfaces, with the external surface having three times the amount of chlorhexidine and extended release of the surface-bound antiseptics than that in the first-generation products. Preliminary studies indicate that prolonged anti-infective activity provides improved efficacy in preventing infection (CDC, 2002a).

Ionic platinum/silver metals have broad antimicrobial activity and have been FDA-approved for use on catheters and cuffs in the United States. Further studies need to be done to support their prolonged antimicrobial effect. Ionic silver has also been used in subcutaneous collagen cuffs attached to CVCs. The ionic silver provides antimicrobial activity and the cuff provides a mechanical barrier to the migration of microorganisms along the external surface of the catheter. Further studies are needed on these as well, to determine long-term efficacy.

Changing Regimens for Intravascular Devices and Administration Sets

An important consideration in the prevention of phlebitis and catheter-related infections, is the routine replacement of intravascular catheters. Although studies of short peripheral catheters indicate that the incidence of thrombophlebitis and bacterial colonization increases when they are left in place longer than 72 hours, the rates of phlebitis are not substantially different when left in place for 96 hours. "Because phlebitis and catheter colonization have been associated with an increased risk for catheter-related infection, short peripheral catheter sites commonly are rotated at 72- to 96-hour intervals to reduce both the risk for infection and client discomfort associated with phlebitis" (CDC, 2002a). Additional CDC (2002a) guidelines include the following:

1. Prompt removal of any intravascular catheter that is no longer essential
2. No routine replacement of central venous or arterial catheters solely for the purpose of reducing the incidence of infection
3. Leaving peripheral venous catheters in place in children until IV therapy is completed, unless complications occur
4. Replacement of catheters when adherence to aseptic technique cannot be ensured (i.e., when inserted during a medical emergency), as soon as possible and after no longer than 48 hours
5. Use of clinical judgment to determine when to replace a catheter that could be a source of infection (e.g., do not routinely replace venous catheters in clients whose only indication of infection is fever)
6. No routine replacement of venous catheters in clients who are bacteremic or fungemic if the source of infection is unlikely to be the catheter
7. Replacement of any short-term CVC if purulence is observed at the insertion site, which indicates infection;
8. Replacement of all CVCs if the client is hemodynamically unstable and CRBSI is suspected
9. Avoidance of the use of the guidewire technique to replace catheters in clients suspected of having catheter-related infection

The data from several well-controlled studies regarding the optimal interval for changing IV administration sets (not used for blood or blood products, lipids, or TPN) has resulted in the conclusion that it is both safe and cost effective to change them no more frequently than at 72-hour intervals unless catheter-related infection is suspected or documented (CDC, 2002). Tubings used to administer blood, blood products, or lipid emulsions (those combined with amino acids and glucose in a 3-in-1 admixture or infused separately) within 24 hours of initiating the infusion. When the solution contains only dextrose and amino acids, the administration set does not need to be replaced more frequently than 72 hours. Tubing used to administer propofol infusions is to be replaced every 6 or 12 hours, depending on its use, and according to recommendations from the manufacturer (CDC, 2002). Parenteral nutrition and any infusates that, if contaminated, may support microbial growth, may necessitate more frequent tubing changes. In this situation it is important for the nurse to follow institutional guidelines and INS standards. When blood and blood products are administered, many institutions advise that the tubing should be changed with every unit infused. Fat emulsions usually have special tubing that can only be used with lipids. The tubing is generally changed every 24 hours if the solution is infused continuously. If used intermittently, the tubing is changed at the start of each new unit.

Filters

Filters were once used extensively in the practice of IV therapy (when nurses performed admixture procedures) to reduce the risk of infection from infusate contamination, for the removal of particulate matter, as well as to reduce the risk of phlebitis in clients receiving high doses of IV medication. Because of the potential undesirable effects of blockage (which increases line manipulation) and reduction of drug dosage, filters are no longer advocated by the CDC (CDC, 2002). It has been suggested that the routine use of in-line filters actually may contribute to infection (because when the bacteria are trapped and die, their toxins can escape the filter and circulate in the bloodstream) and increase cost and personnel time. Pre-use filtration by the pharmacy is safer, more practical, and cost-effective.

Policies and procedures regarding the use of filters vary among employment settings. Many institutions use some type of filter for total parenteral nutrition (TPN) and there is a special lipid filter, with larger pores, that is available for use with some fat emulsions. The nurse is expected to know and follow the protocols set forth by his employer. According to the INS, "the indications and protocol for the use of bacterial/particulate-retentive, air-eliminating, and blood and blood component filters should be established in organizational policies and procedures" (INS, Standard 38, S33, 2000). If filters are used, they should be replaced with each new administration set, or sooner if they become occluded or do not allow the infusion to be delivered at the scheduled rate.

Fluids

The 2002 CDC guidelines regarding the "hang time" of parenteral fluids are as follows:

1. Lipid-containing solutions (such as 3-in-1) should be completed within 24 hours of hanging the solution.
2. Lipid emulsions, when administered alone, should be completed within 12 hours of hanging. If the client's fluid volume is a consideration, the infusion can be completed within 24 hours.
3. Blood and blood products are to be completed within 4 hours of hanging.

The CDC has not set forth recommendations regarding the "hang" time limit for other parenteral infusates. Most institutions dictate that the maximum time any infusate may hang at room temperature is not to exceed 24 hours.

If there is any suspicion that any infusion is contaminated, it must be discontinued immediately and saved for laboratory testing. Blood and blood products, which provide an excellent environment for microbial growth, should never stay at room temperature for more than 4 hours. If the nurse anticipates that a unit will take longer than that to infuse, he must notify the blood bank so smaller quantities can be dispensed.

Nursing Responsibilities

The nurse who initiates, monitors, and maintains IV infusion therapy is responsible for the patient's safety and comfort while strictly adhering to infection control measures. With the large number of patients receiving some type of IV therapy, the nurse must use all the necessary measures to prevent the occurrence of nosocomial infections. The nurse must follow the guidelines set forth by the CDC, the mandates of OSHA, and his employer's directives. He is also wise to incorporate the INS standards of practice in order to maintain the health and safety of his patients, their families, his coworkers, other health care personnel, and himself.

The nurse must be able to recognize the signs and symptoms of infection so that treatment can be initiated to avert the complications of infectious disease. Some infectious processes are easy to identify while others are more difficult to detect. Early recognition depends on the patient's general state of health, her age and nutritional status, her ability to communicate, the organism(s) involved, and the body system(s) affected.

NURSING TIP

CDC Definitions

According to the CDC the following definitions relate to intravenous cannula-related infection:

Colonized catheter growth of more than 15 colony-forming units from a proximal or distal catheter segment in the absence of accompanying clinical symptoms

Catheter-related bloodstream infection: isolation of the same organism ... from a ... culture of a catheter segment and from the blood ... of a patient with accompanying clinical symptoms of BSI and no other apparent source of infection ...

Infusate-related bloodstream infection: isolation of the same organism from infusate and from separate percutaneous blood cultures, with no other identifiable source of infection

Exit-site infection: erythema, tenderness, induration, or purulence within 2 cm of the skin at the exit site of the catheter

Pocket infection: erythema and necrosis of the skin over the reservoir of a totally implantable device or purulent exudate in the subcutaneous pocket containing the reservoir

Tunnel infection: erythema, tenderness, and induration in the tissues overlying the catheter and more than 2 cm from the exit site

From: *Federal Register,* Vol. 60 (Wednesday, September 27, 1995)

Fever is usually the first sign of infection, but that may not always be the case. Localized infection is usually recognized by inflammation (redness, heat, pain) and swelling. The inflammatory response is a protective mechanism the body uses in an attempt to protect itself from pathogenic invasion. Later in the text, when the complications of IV therapy are covered, the signs and symptoms of IV-related inflammatory responses and infection will be detailed.

Home parenteral therapy (HPT) has become a safe, effective, and economical alternative to prolonged hospitalization. It is one of the fastest-growing segments of the health care market, growing at an expected annual rate of 20% to 25% (National Alliance for Infusion Therapy, 1992). One of the biggest segments of the HPT market is infusion therapy (National Association for Home Care, 1999). Antibiotic, hydration, and parenteral nutrition therapy, which are often started at home (without prior hospitalization), are the three most common forms of home therapy (Masoorli, 1996). Others include pain management, chemotherapy, and dobutamine therapy for patients with severe refractory CHF or those awaiting heart transplant. With such a broad spectrum of home infusion, the nurse who works in this realm must have expert IV therapy skills. He needs to assess accurately, anticipate problems, and take charge when emergencies arise or are imminent. He must always keep in mind that pathogenic organisms can enter the body at any time, that patient morbidity and mortality are an ever-present risk (APIC, 1996), and that care and teaching must always be a priority to prevent the ill effects of HPT.

Although concern for the welfare of his patients is important, the nurse must also take the necessary measures to protect himself. He needs to take care of himself through rest, exercise, good hygienic practices, safe social interactions, and a healthy diet. If he is ill, he should not go to work because he will not only jeopardize his own health but endanger the patients in his care. If he has fever or is ill more than two days he should seek medical attention.

In the workplace the nurse is expected to follow procedures correctly and in a safe manner so as not to acquire diseases from the patients or transfer them to others. Proper hand hygiene remains the most important thing the nurse can do to prevent picking up an infection or communicating it to others. Appropriate hand hygiene and strict adherence to Standard Precautions are infection control procedures that must be practiced and taught in all settings, including the patient's home. It is essential that the nurse follow the guidelines for wearing gloves and other protective barriers such as gowns, masks, and goggles. A good way to remember when to wear gloves is to follow the advice of many infection control practitioners: If it's wet, wear gloves. As discussed earlier, Standard Precautions are mandated for all health care personnel.

It is important for the nurse to understand how disease is transmitted, but it is equally important that he teach others as well. Patients are often concerned that they might pick up a disease such as AIDS while in the hospital or health care environment. Many misinformed individuals are afraid to donate blood for fear of getting AIDS. It is important for the nurse to reassure patients that HIV can only be transmitted through intimate sexual contact, percutaneous exposure to blood, or through prenatal transmission from mother to infant. Whereas HIV does not survive well outside the body, it can remain viable in blood spills. If the nurse has a cut or open sore that comes in contact with HIV-positive blood, transmission of the virus can occur. The risk of HIV transmission is greater if there is contact with a large volume of blood and if the source patient is in the end stage of AIDS (CDC, 1995). Should occupational HIV exposure occur, prompt treatment is important to decrease the risk of HIV seroconversion. It is

NURSING TIP

Hand Hygiene

- Alcohol-based handrubs significantly reduce the number of microorganisms on skin, are fast acting, and cause less skin irritation.

- When using an alcohol-based handrub, apply product to palm of one hand and rub hands together, covering all surfaces of hands and fingers, until hands are dry. Note that the volume needed to reduce the number of bacteria on hands varies by product.

- Handwashing with soap and water remains a sensible strategy for hand hygiene in non-health care settings and is recommended by CDC and other experts.

- When health care personnel's hands are visibly soiled, they should wash with soap and water.

- The use of gloves does not eliminate the need for hand hygiene. Likewise, the use of hand hygiene does not eliminate the need for gloves. Gloves reduce hand contamination by 70% to 80%, prevent cross-contamination, and protect clients and health care personnel from infection. Handrubs should be used before and after each client, just as gloves should be changed before and after each client.

- Health care personnel should avoid wearing artificial nails and keep natural nails less than one quarter of an inch long.

(CDC, 2002a)

essential for the nurse to wear gloves when handling blood and body fluids. Spills and splatters need to be cleaned up immediately. Gloves never take the place of hand hygiene, which is to be done immediately following removal of the gloves.

The hepatitis B and C viruses are far more resilient than HIV when they exit the body. HBV and HCV can survive outside the body on inanimate objects up to 2 weeks. They are serious diseases that can become chronic and progress to cirrhosis, liver cancer, and death. HBV can be prevented with a vaccine, available without cost (due to OSHA regulations) to all health care personnel by their employers. Everyone who works in the health care industry or any other occupation where the possibility of exposure to blood and body fluids is likely should be vaccinated.

Needlesticks continue to be a problem that wearing gloves does not safeguard against. The most frequent cause of

Initiate Prompt Treatment Following Exposure to HIV

The CDC (2001e) recommends that health care practitioners (HCP) occupationally exposed to HIV be treated within one to two hours of exposure. Postexposure prophylaxis (PEP) decreases the risk of HIV seroconversion by almost 70%. Most HIV exposures warrant a two-drug regimen using two nucleoside analogues, ziduvudine (ADV) and lamivudine (3TC), or 3TC and d4T, or d4T and ddl. The addition of a third drug should be considered for exposures that pose an increased risk for transmission. Selection of the PEP regimen should consider the comparative risk represented by the exposure and information about the exposure source, including history of and response to antiretroviral therapy based on clinical response, CD4+ T-cell counts, viral load measurements, and current disease stage. When the source person's virus is known or suspected to be resistant to one or more of the drugs considered for the PEP regimen, the selection of drugs to which the source person's virus is unlikely to be resistant is recommended; expert consultation is advised. If this information is not immediately available, initiation of PEP, if indicated, should not be delayed; changes in the PEP regimen can be made after PEP has been started, as appropriate. Reevaluation of the exposed person should be considered within 72 hours postexposure, especially as additional information about the exposure or source person becomes available.

PEP should be administered over 4 weeks, with follow-up counseling and medical evaluations for at least 6 months following exposure (at 6 weeks, 12 weeks, and 6 months).

For additional information, the following agencies should be contacted:

- CDC
- Hepatitis Hotline
- National AIDS Clearinghouse
- Needlestick! Web site
- PEPline

borne pathogens, studies show that, even when completely followed, they prevent only about one in three needlestick wounds (APIC, 2000) due to the fact that gloves and other barriers are not impermeable to sharp items.

Needleless systems and protective needle devices are, or should be, in effect in all clinical agencies. As stated earlier, the Needlestick Safety and Prevention Act was passed in the United States in November 2000 in the effort to eliminate needlestick injuries. Protective devices encompass two broad categories: (1) automatically-activated protection (where the device mechanizes at the appropriate point in time), and (2) user-activated protection (where the user must activate the safety device). The nurse must use extreme care in handling and disposing of needles, syringes, and other sharp items. Studies illustrate that as many as one-third of all reported sharps injuries are related to the disposal practices (APIC, 2000).

Even with advanced safety technology and improved protective needle devices, the use of sharps disposal containers remain the vanguard against injuries. Used needles are not to be recapped, broken, bent, or cut. Used syringes, needles, scalpel blades, and all disposable sharps, must be properly placed, immediately after use, in puncture-resistant containers for disposal. The blades of safety razors must be handled with care, and then discarded in sharps containers. Razor blades are not to be used between patients. The disposal containers for sharps must be in closest proximity, as is practical, to the area where sharp items are implemented. If a needle is used, and an appropriate disposal container is not nearby ("Point-of-Use Disposal"), the cap may be "scooped up" with the needle, using one hand, and then carried to the sharps container (Figure 4-4). The cap is not, under any circumstances, to be pushed into place over the needle. "Needles/stylets (sharps) shall be disposed of in nonpermeable tamper-proof containers. Needles/stylets (sharps) shall not be broken, bent, or recapped with two hands" (INS, 2000, standard 31, S29).

Don't Start or Promote Unsafe Habits

Glove layering, when the health care person puts on several pairs of gloves and removes one pair to attend to another patient or task without washing his hands, should never be permitted. New gloves are to be worn with each new patient or procedure, and hands must be washed as soon as the gloves are removed and discarded. You, the nurse, play a vital role in preventing bad habits from getting started and in stopping them once they are identified.

bloodborne infections in health care settings—with nurses sustaining the most—are needlesticks. While the use of Standard Precautions can help prevent the spread of blood-

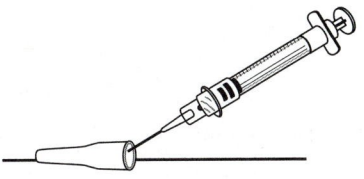

1. Scoop into cap using one hand. Do not touch the cap with the other hand.

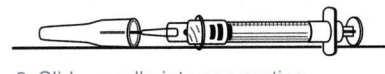

2. Slide needle into cap resting on table.

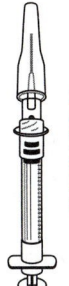

3. Holding the barrel of the syringe in one hand, carry to the sharps container. Do not push the cap onto the syringe.

Figure 4-4 | Scoop technique

Table 4-5	Infection Control and Safety Measures

Know where policy and procedure manuals are located in your agency and use them. Consult with the infection control practitioner in your agency whenever necessary.

Use the nursing process to assess your patient's level of consciousness, orientation, and ability to comprehend instructions.

Know and understand all procedures before performing them.

Know and understand the principles of use regarding safety-engineered devices in your agency. You should be trained in their use and have the opportunity to practice using such devices. Do not use any device if you haven't received sufficient instruction and the opportunity to perform, at the very least, one demonstration before a person who is knowledgeable regarding the product's use. Once trained, properly use safety devices—every time they are indicated.

Explain all procedures to your patient and explain her role in carrying out the procedures. Remember, a well-informed patient is more willing to become actively involved and comply.

Use proper hand hygiene before and after all physical patient contacts, patient care procedures, and donning and removing gloves.

Avoid eating and drinking in areas where blood or body fluids may be present.

Protect yourself. Do not touch your eyes, insert/remove contact lenses, or apply makeup in patient care areas.

Know where safety disposal containers for sharp items are located.

Never recap sharps (or use the one-handed technique when not in close proximity to an approved disposal container).

Dispose of sharp items immediately after use.

Whenever there is any doubt regarding infection control protocols, the nurse is expected to follow the guidelines set forth by the CDC, OSHA, the employer infection control department, and the agency-approved policy and procedure manuals (Table 4-5). If he is still not sure about something related to his safety or the safety of others, he should contact an infection control practitioner. Under no circumstances should he ever perform any task in a manner that could result in injury or the spread of infection.

NURSING TIP

Internet Resources on Infection Control

American Journal of Infection Control: http://www1.mosby.com/Mosby/Periodicals/Medical/AJIC/ict.html

Antibiotic Guide: Treatment Recommendations for Common Infections: http://www.intmed.mcw.edu/drug/InfectionRx.html

Association for Professionals in Infections Control and Epidemiology: http://www.apic.org

BroadStreetSolutions: http://broadstreetsolutions.com

Epidemiology and Prevention Program: http://epi-center.ucsf.edu

Hospital Infections Program: http://www.cdc.gov/ncidod/hip/hip.htm

Infection Control: http://www.md.ucl.ac.be/entities/esp/hosp/infcon.htm

Infection Control and Hospital Epidemiology: http://www.slackinc.com/general/iche/ichehome.htm

Infection Control Services: http://infectioncenter.com

Infectious Disease WebLink: http://pages.prodigy.net/pdeziel/

National Center for Infectious Diseases: http://www.cdc.gov/ncidod/ncid.htm

National Foundation for Infectious Diseases: http://www.nfid.org

Key Concepts

- Epidemiology is the study of disease and injury, their causes and determinants, their distribution within a population, and their control and surveillance.

- In the United States, CDC, a division of the Department of Health and Human Services, is the agency that investigates, develops, recommends, and sets standards for infection control practices.

- The epidemiologic triangle consists of (1) the host, the living person or animal that provides the atmosphere in which organisms are able to live; (2) the agent, the organism that is capable of eliciting a disease process; and (3) the environment, the interacting group of conditions, surroundings, and influences in which the host and agent are coexisting.

- Infection is the process whereby a host is invaded by microorganisms, which then grow, reproduce, and cause injury. A local infection is one in which microorganisms penetrate the tissues of a specific area of the body, then grow, multiply, and exert their effect there, rather than migrate to other parts of the body. A systemic infection is one in which the microorganisms travel freely throughout the host's body and exert their virulence on several or all body systems.

- The chain of infection consists of six links: the causative agent, its reservoir (animate or inanimate), its portal of exit, its means of transmission, its portal of entry, and the susceptible host. The goal of infection control is to break the chain of infection at any link that will bring about the prevention of disease or its transmission.

- A nosocomial infection is one which develops in a patient during or after, but as a result of, her stay in a health care setting. It is different from a community acquired infection which is picked up and present, or incubating, prior to one's admission to a health care facility.

- Proper hand hygiene is the single most important means of preventing the spread of infection. It must be carried out correctly with the use of handwashing—using running water, soap (an emulsifier), and friction for a period of at least ten seconds.

- The CDC recommends that health care personnel are to consider all patients potentially infected with HIV, AIDS, and other bloodborne pathogens. This infection control measure is referred to as Standard Precautions. It is enforced by OSHA of the U.S. Department of Labor, which surveys facilities for compliance.

- One of the main complications of intravenous infusion therapy is sepsis, a pathologic state, usually with fever, that is the result of microorganisms in the bloodstream. Such organisms usually gain access to the bloodstream at the needle or IV catheter insertion site. The staphylococci organisms are responsible for the majority of nosocomial IV infusion-related infections.

- An antiseptic is an agent that, when applied topically, is capable of killing microorganisms on the skin or inhibiting their growth. An antiseptic works by interrupting the microorganism's cellular metabolic activity, by chemically destroying its cellular components, by interfering with cellular protein structure, or by weakening the cell membrane to such an extent that the contents of the cell escape and destroy the organism. The antiseptics recommended for intravenous infusion therapy are 70% isopropyl alcohol, 10% povidone-iodine, and 2% tincture of iodine.

- The nurse who manages infusion therapy must be aware of and follow the guidelines recommended by the CDC, OSHA, the INS, the APIC, and current research findings. When in the workplace, the policies and procedures of the employer are to be followed regarding infection control practices dealing with IV therapy.

- The nurse is responsible for the patient's safety and comfort and must be able to recognize the signs and symptoms of inflammation and infection so that treatment can be initiated to avert the complications of infectious disease.

- Inherent in the practice of infection control is the need for the nurse to take all necessary measures to protect his own health and well-being as well as that of his patients, visitors, coworkers, and other health care personnel. He needs to take care of himself through rest, exercise, good hygienic practices, safe social interactions, and a healthy diet. In addition, he must have a thorough understanding of the process of disease transmission so he can protect himself and teach others to do the same.

Review Questions and Activities

1. List five major responsibilities of the nurse who manages intravenous infusion therapy.
2. Describe the function of the two governmental agencies, the CDC and OSHA, and how they operate to protect both the patient and the health care worker.
3. Make a two-column listing that enumerates the variables that affect the disease process from the standpoint of the host and the microorganism.
4. Outline the six links in the chain of infection, and for each link, list three things that might prevent the transmission of infection.
5. Identify 10 fomites that might be responsible for the inanimate spread of infection.
6. Make a chart of the process of handwashing that you could put by the sinks in your workplace. Be creative so it will be an attention-getter and promote good hand hygiene.
7. Contact the infection control practitioner in your workplace or clinical setting and find out which nosocomial infections occurred most frequently over the past year.
8. Describe what the term Standard Precautions means, why it came into existence, and list five substances that are addressed in this category.
9. List and compare the advantages and disadvantages of the three antiseptic agents discussed in this chapter.
10. Look up in your clinical agency's policy and procedure manual, the recommended infection control protocols regarding intravascular catheters, IV site dressings, administration sets, and IV line filters. Compare these guidelines with those of the CDC.
11. Describe the manner in which needles and sharps are to be handled so as to prevent injury to you, your patient, and other health care personnel.
12. What can you do to prevent the spread of infection?

II

The Practice of Intravenous
Infusion Therapy

Chapter 5

Risks, Complications, and Adverse Reactions Associated with Intravenous Infusion Therapy

COMPETENCIES

Upon completion of this chapter, the reader should be able to:

- Differentiate between local and systemic complications associated with intravenous infusion therapy.

- Describe the signs and symptoms of the following local complications of infusion therapy:

  - Pain and irritation

  - Infiltration and extravasation

  - Occlusion and loss of patency

  - Phlebitis

  - Thrombosis and thrombophlebitis

  - Hematoma formation

  - Venous spasm

  - Vessel collapse

  - Cellulitis

- Explain the nursing interventions for each of the local complications of infusion therapy listed.

- List five commonly used vesicant drugs that cause damage with extravasation.

- Outline the physiologic processes that occur with cellular and tissue damage.

- Interpret the sequence of events that reflects the progression of phlebitis to thrombophlebitis.

- Examine how nerve, tendon, ligament, and limb damage can occur as a result of intravenous therapy.

✴ Describe the signs and symptoms of the following systemic complications associated with intravenous infusion therapy:

– Contamination and infection

– Drug and fluid interactions

– Hypersensitivity reactions

– Sepsis

– Emboli (blood clot, air, and catheter)

– Speed shock

✴ Explain the nursing interventions associated with each of the systemic complications listed.

KEY TERMS

absorption	extravasation	phlebitis
allergen	hematoma	postinfusion phlebitis
allergy	homan's sign	precipitation
anaphylaxis	homotropic	protease
angina pectoris	idiosyncrasy	reagin
antagonism	incompatibility	red flare
antigen	indurated	sensitization
biotransformation	infarction	side effect
cellulitis	infiltration	speed shock
contamination	inflammation	superficial thrombophlebitis
cramp	inflammatory	suppurative
deep vein thrombosis (DVT)	interstice	synergism
displacement	intima	tachycardia
disseminated intravascular coagulation (DIC)	irrigate	thrombophlebitis
ecchymosis	irritation	thrombosis
elimination	ischemia	thrombus
emboli	myocardial infarction (MI)	venous spasm
embolus	necrosis	venous stasis
endogenous embolus	pain	vesicant
erythema	peau d'orange	vessel collapse
exogenous embolus		

Because intravenous infusion therapy breaks the skin barrier, one of the body's major natural defenses, and further invades and accesses the circulatory system, it carries with it numerous inherent risks and potential complications. To avoid complications associated with such therapy, the nurse should be knowledgeable of every likely complication that might develop. When a problem develops, however, it is important to recognize it as soon as possible so appropriate interventions can be taken.

The nurse must understand the signs and symptoms of each type of complication along with its etiology and defining characteristics. With this information, she can formulate a nursing diagnosis and responsibly carry out the nursing interventions that are germane to the complication. Complications of IV therapy can be classified as local, systemic, or a combination of the two.

LOCAL PROBLEMS AND COMPLICATIONS

Local complications are adverse reactions that occur at the insertion site of an IV device or close to the IV site. The majority of complications in IV therapy are local problems, and are usually less serious than systemic problems. This does not imply they can be taken lightly. The nurse must always keep in mind that she must intervene appropriately when local complications first arise to prevent progression to systemic complications that can further compromise the patient.

Localized infusion-related complications include pain and irritation at or near the IV site, infiltration and extravasation, cannula dislodgement, catheter or needle occlusion, and phlebitis. Also included are hematoma, venous spasm, vessel collapse, cellulitis, thrombosis and thrombophlebitis, and nerve, tendon, ligament, or limb damage. Each of these complications will be covered in detail throughout the course of this chapter.

Pain and Irritation

Pain, according to the International Association for the Study of Pain, is "the sensatory and emotional experience associated with actual or potential tissue damage . . . pain includes not only the perception of an uncomfortable stimulus but also the response to that perception" (Thomas, 2001). Pain at the intravenous site is **homotropic**, because the sensation of discomfort occurs at the point of injury. The insertion site of the IV device or the inner lining of the vein wall (**intima**) where the infusate comes in contact with it can cause homotropic pain. Pain can be **inflammatory**, which occurs with the increased pressure that accompanies the inflammatory response. **Irritation** is synonymous with tenderness.

Etiology and Defining Characteristics

With infusion therapy, pain can develop as a result of various physical and emotional situations. Pain that radiates proxi-

mally (upward) from the IV insertion site is usually a sensation of burning or stinging resulting from the infusion of a fluid or medication with a high or low osmolarity or pH. In addition, severe pain at the IV site can result from mechanical irritation by the IV device, or nerve, tendon, or ligament damage as well as venous spasm (Table 5-1).

Localized pain can be associated with or be a precursor to any of the intravenous complications discussed in this chapter. Because the symptom of pain can be related to numerous complications, the nurse must understand all the problems that might occur, know the assessment variables associated with such problems, and be able to intervene appropriately. Under no circumstances should patient complaints of pain be deferred or ignored. Pain is a warning sign that more serious problems might be developing.

When cellular or tissue injury occurs, pain-producing substances (bradykinin, histamine, and serotonin) and other products are produced and released by the body. These chemicals are responsible for the impulses that result in the sensation of pain. Once cell injury occurs, prostaglandins are synthesized and released to exert a local effect that activates pain receptors and augments histamine and bradykinin activity. The neurotransmitters epinephrine, norepinephrine, dopamine, and acetylcholine enhance pain transmission at the local level, but are released centrally.

Table 5-1 Pain Associated with Infusion Therapy	
SYMPTOM(S)	**ETIOLOGY/ CONTRIBUTING FACTORS**
Pain at insertion site	• Infiltration/extravasation • Phlebitis/thrombosis • Hematoma • Cellulitis • Type of insertion device • Method of insertion • Location of infusion site • Improperly secured IV device • Length of time device in place
Vein irritation (burning-stinging sensation)	• Type of insertion device • Method of insertion • Fluid pH • Fluid osmolality • Fluid temperature • Irritating medications • Length of time device in place • Infusate contamination • Rate of infusion
Severe pain radiating away from site, loss of sensation, or paralysis	• Damage to nerves, tendons, or ligaments from improper insertion or location of IV device • Pressure buildup from extravasation of fluid or irritating substances into surrounding area

Preventing a Systemic Complication

What starts out as a local infusion-related complication can quickly progress to one that is systemic if assessment, problem identification, and appropriate nursing interventions are not immediately taken to correct the situation.

Nursing Assessment and Interventions

Pain is evidenced by a sympathetic response, which brings about an increase in cardiac rate (**tachycardia**) and output, elevated blood pressure, and increased respiratory rate, sometimes with hyperventilation. The patient often experiences the fright–flight–fight (–freeze) response that brings with it pupil dilation, peripheral vasoconstriction, hypermotility, and excessive perspiration of the palms of the hands and the soles of the feet.

Since pain is subjective, it is extremely important for the nurse to assess, intervene, and evaluate each patient on an individual basis. She must never overlook the fact that there are psychological and emotional factors as well as physical components that influence pain. Religious, cultural, and social considerations must be incorporated into the assessment and evaluation, and it is important to be alert for both verbal and nonverbal indicators of pain. The inconveniences and interferences as well as the fear and anxiety associated with illness and disease are important considerations for the nurse. The nurse must make every attempt to evaluate the patient's pain through therapeutic communication skills (Table 5-2). In addition to the patient's verbalizations and actions, the nurse can recognize pain and irritation through touch and visual inspection of the IV site. Signs of blanching or redness over the vein and the sensation of warmth over the site validate the patient's complaints.

Once pain is properly assessed, the nurse must determine the most appropriate intervention(s). Depending on her findings, nursing actions might include discontinuing and restarting the present infusion, changing the position of the extremity, adjusting the flow rate, retaping the site, applying warm or cool compresses, or notifying the physician. She must know which fluids and medications cause pain or irritation during the process of infusion so she can take the necessary measures to prepare the patient and reduce the pain as much as possible (Table 5-3). A great deal of discomfort can be avoided by making changes in the amount of diluent used for some medications or by slowing the rate of infusion, if these measures are not contraindicated. The use of distraction, visualization, and other psychoemotional

A Patient's Descriptions of Pain

Pain associated with IV infusion therapy may be described by a patient as follows:

- A burning or stinging sensation at the IV site
- A dull, aching sensation with a feeling of tightness or hardness (induration) at the site
- A shooting pain that radiates upward along the vein wall
- Tenderness above the cannula insertion site
- A cramping or gripping sensation (venospasm)

Table 5-2 | Communication with the Patient: A Guideline for Pain Assessment

1. Tell me about the pain you are having.
2. Where does it hurt?
3. When did it start?
4. Is the pain in one spot, or does it radiate (move) to other places?
5. What kind of pain is it?

Aching?	Gnawing?
Burning?	Stabbing or piercing?
Dull?	Throbbing?

6. Does it hurt constantly, or at intervals?
7. When is the pain most severe?
8. Are there any other symptoms of discomfort?
9. Rate the pain on a scale of 1 to 10, with 0 to 1 indicating no pain and 10 being the worst pain.
10. Tell me anything else about your pain that is important to you.

NOTE: For patients with cognitive dysfunction or verbal or language barriers, a useful visual tool, such as the Wong-Baker Faces Rating Scale, may be used.

tools should not be forgotten when attempting to reduce the pain associated with IV therapy.

Many times a patient senses pain simply because the IV device is in place. This may occur because of anxiety and misconceptions regarding therapy. Thorough explanations along with reassurances from the nurse are very important in such cases. The patient often becomes more relaxed about having an IV device and infusion if he knows why it is needed, how it works to his benefit, and the estimated length

Table 5-3 | Pain Related to the Administration of some of the Commonly Used Medications and Infusates

MEDICATION OR INFUSATE	ASSOCIATED DISCOMFORT
Amino acids (proteins) in 10% dextrose	Venous inflammation
Ampicillins (antibiotics)	Infusion site pain; venous irritation
BCNU (carmustine) (alkylating agent)	Venous pain
Cephalosporins (antibiotics)	Infusion site pain; venous inflammation
Dextrose solutions (10% to 50%)	Venous irritation
Diazepam (depressant; sedative/hypnotic)	Infusion site pain; venous Inflammation
DTIC (dacarbazine) (alkylating agent)	Infusion site pain; venospasm
Erythromycins (antibiotics)	Venous pain; venous inflammation
Foscarnet sodium (antiviral)	Infusion site irritation
Ganciclovir sodium (antiviral)	Infusion site pain; venous inflammation
Imipenem-cilastin (antibacterial)	Infusion site pain; venous inflammation
Iron dextran	Infusion site inflammation
Lymphocyte immune globulin	Infusion site pain
Methocarbamol (skeletal muscle relaxant)	Infusion site pain
Miconazole (antifungal)	Venous inflammation
Mitomycin (antibiotic; antitumor)	Infusion site pain
Penicillins (antibiotics)	Infusion site pain; venous inflammation
Potassium acetate and potassium chloride (electrolytes)	Infusion site pain; venous burning
Ranitidine (histamine receptor antagonist)	Burning and itching at infusion site
Streptozocin (antibiotic; antitumor)	Venous irritation
Tetanus antitoxin (antitoxin)	Infusion site pain
Thiotepa (alkylating agent)	Infusion site pain
Vancomycin hydrochloride (antibiotic)	Infusion site pain
Vinblastine sulfate (alkaloid)	Venous inflammation

of time it will be in place. It cannot be stressed enough how important the nurse's interactions with the patient are in terms of his progress and response to care.

Infiltration and Extravasation

In the past the terms *infiltration* and *extravasation* were often used interchangeably. **Infiltration**, a broader term, is the process in which a substance enters or infuses into another substance or a surrounding area. Infiltration may be an intentional or unintentional process. **Extravasation**, a more specific term, refers to the actual (unintentional) escape or leakage of material from a vessel into the surrounding tissue. IV infiltration is defined as the escape, or outflow, of non-vesicant infusate from a vessel into the surrounding tissue. IV

NURSING TIP

The Well-Informed Patient

A patient who is well informed regarding his condition and treatment regimen perceives himself as an active participant in his care, thus making him more relaxed and better able to adapt to the stress of illness and therapy.

extravasation is the escape, or outflow, of a vesicant solution from a vessel into the surrounding tissue. A **vesicant** is an agent that is irritating and causes blistering.

Infiltration and extravasation are probably the most frequently encountered problems associated with infusion therapy. Unfortunately, because they are so common, they are sometimes overlooked or not addressed as soon as they should be, yet they can produce debilitating effects.

Etiology and Defining Characteristics

Infiltration and extravasation can arise from several situations (Table 5-4). Dislodgement of the catheter or needle cannula from the intima of the vein wall during venipuncture is a common occurrence. Puncture of the distal vein wall during venipuncture also occurs. Sometimes the infusate leaks into the surrounding tissue from the cannula's insertion site. This is usually related to the cannula being too large for the diameter of the vein (resulting from insertion of an oversized cannula), or the narrowing of the vein lumen from surrounding pressure (as with the edema accompanying the inflammatory response). In addition, the wall of the vein may weaken and rupture from the inappropriate choice of vein or site or from previous venipunctures. Irritating infusates can weaken the vein wall to the point of rupture as can the delivery of fluid under high pressure. Infiltration can occur because of mechanical pressure from the cannula against the vein wall that results in breakage (especially with steel needles). Any time an IV device is overmanipulated, the wall of the vein becomes compromised and infiltration can occur. Poor or improper taping is another problem. If enough tape is not applied or not placed in the right area, the vein can be irritated because the cannula is unstable. Tape applied too tightly to the skin above the cannula tip can act as a tourniquet, disrupt flow, and rupture the vein wall.

Table 5-4 | Major Causes of Infiltration or Extravasation

- Puncture of the distal vein wall during venipuncture
- Puncture of any portion of the vein wall by mechanical friction from the catheter/needle cannula
- Dislodgement of the catheter/needle cannula from the intima of the vein
- Poorly secured (taped) IV device (too loose, too tight, or secured incorrectly)
- Poor vein or site selection
- Improper cannula size
- High delivery rate or pressure of the infusate
- Overmanipulation of the IV device, the site, or both
- Irritating infusate that inflames the intima of the vein and causes it to weaken

NURSING TIP

Avoiding Infiltration or Extravasation

Prevention, a result of frequent assessment and good nurse–patient communication, is the best safeguard for avoiding infiltration or extravasation.

Nursing Assessment and Interventions

Pain at or near the IV site may or may not be present depending on the chemical nature of the infusate, the amount of infiltration, the patient's pain threshold, or his level of consciousness. This is why frequent nursing assessment is so important. The nurse must always keep in mind, too, that a minute amount of extravasation from a vesicant can be far more dangerous than a large amount of infiltrated isotonic infusate. The INS recommends that the Infiltration Scale (Table 5-5) "should be standardized and used in documenting the infiltration; infiltration should be graded according to the most severe presenting indicator" (INS, Standard 60, S57).

Depending on the amount of leakage, there might be swelling around the IV site (ventral or dorsal) or edema that extends proximal or distal to the IV site. Contingent on the

Table 5-5 | INS Infiltration Scale (INS, 2000)

GRADE	CLINICAL CRITERIA
0	No symptoms
1	Skin blanched Edema <1 inch in any direction Cool to touch With or without pain
2	Skin blanched Edema 1–6 inches in any direction Cool to touch With or without pain
3	Skin blanched, translucent Gross edema >6 inches in any direction Cool to touch Mild-moderate pain Possible numbness
4	Skin blanched, translucent Skin tight, leaking Skin discolored, bruised, swollen Gross edema >6 inches in any direction Deep pitting tissue edema Circulatory impairment Moderate-severe pain Infiltration of any amount of blood product, irritant, or vesicant

amount of fluid that escapes, the skin may be taut or rigid, with blanching and a sensation of coolness. The more infusate that is exuded, the tighter the skin becomes and the cooler the temperature. The dressing may be damp or wet. If an infiltration is left unchecked, the site may become dark in color owing to tissue injury.

NURSING TIP

Recognizing Infiltration

Because a fibrin sheath develops around the tip of the cannula, it may prevent the backflow of blood during aspiration, even though the IV fluid is infusing. Likewise, the presence of a blood return does not necessarily preclude infiltration.

Sometimes, before obvious signs and symptoms of infiltration are evident, the infusion may begin to run at a slower than prescribed rate or cease to flow. The backflow of blood into the tubing may or may not occur when checking for cannula placement in the vein, and therefore is not a reliable indicator of extravasation.

Another way to determine if infusate is leaking is to apply fingertip pressure to the vein just above the cannula tip or to briefly place a tourniquet above the IV site while the fluid is infusing. If the cannula is in place and there is no break in the patency of the vein, the infusate will stop dripping. If the infusion continues to drip when these measures are instituted, there is leakage into the surrounding tissue.

Once infiltration is determined, the infusion must be stopped, the catheter or needle removed, and pressure applied to the insertion site until bleeding is arrested. It is the responsibility of the nurse to initiate interventions that will reduce or avert tissue damage. Continued observation, assessment, and client education are critical to a positive outcome. Complete and accurate documentation in the medical record is necessary and all reports related to the incident must be completed per agency policy.

If there is only a small escape of fluid, the nurse may apply firm pressure to the site with a 2×2-inch gauze for a few minutes. If a large amount of fluid has escaped into the surrounding tissue, some seepage of serous-like fluid may continue from the puncture site. If this is the case, a light dressing should be applied. It is important to assess for circulatory competence by checking for capillary refill and checking pulses proximal and distal to the area of infiltration. The extremity, depending on individual patient circumstances, agency protocols, and medical orders, may be

NURSING TIP

Signs and Symptoms of Infiltration and Extravasation

- Pain at or near the insertion site
- Swelling proximal to or distal to the IV site
- Puffiness of the dependent part of limb or body
- Taut, rigid skin around IV site
- Blanching and coolness of skin around IV site
- Damp or wet dressing
- Slowed infusion rate
- No backflow of blood into IV tubing when clamp is fully opened and solution container is lowered below IV site
- No backflow of blood into IV tubing when tubing is pinched above cannula hub
- Infusion stops running
- The infusion continues to infuse when pressure is applied to the vein above the tip of the cannula

NURSING TIP

How to Treat Infiltration

The use of warm compresses to treat infiltration has become controversial. It has been found that cold compresses may be better for some infiltrated infusates and warm compresses may be more effective for others. It has also been documented that elevation of the infiltrated extremity may be painful for the patient (Masoorli, 1997). To act in the best interest of the patient, following IV infiltration, consult with the physician for orders regarding compresses and elevation.

elevated and the patient should be encouraged to actively move it to assist in the absorption and removal of the excess fluid. If infiltration is small, the intermittent application of ice packs may relieve swelling and discomfort. Ice is usually applied at 15- to 30-minute on/off intervals depending on agency policy. For larger infiltrations, the application of continuous warm compresses may be necessary to assist in the reabsorption of fluid, but only if agency approved and medically indicated.

If extravasation occurs, the IV must be stopped immediately or discontinued directly following the aspiration of drug left in the cannula and instillation of a prescribed antidote (anti-inflammatory or neutralizing agent) into the cannula, the notification of the physician, and the initiation of the appropriate antidote into the surrounding tissue, following the doctor's orders and institutional protocols. Whenever an antidote is administered by injection, it is important to use a small-gauge intradermal or subcutaneous needle (27–25ga) to minimize further tissue injury. It is also important to frequently check capillary refill and pulses to assess circulatory status in the extremity. Because procedural policies vary among agencies, it is the responsibility of the nurse to know and understand employer guidelines regarding extravasated drugs, the equipment needed, and the method(s) in which to utilize the counteragent(s) (Table 5-6).

If treatment is not promptly executed for extravasated irritants or vesicants, tissue sloughing or destruction may ensue. In addition, there may be nerve and blood vessel damage to the limb and loss of functional use. Severe pain and burning may be present. In some cases, surgical excision of large portions of the extremity—or even amputation—is the only alternative. The nurse must remember, too, that the antidotes for infiltration sometimes carry serious side effects that also need to be addressed. She must also understand that some of these remedies must be started within a certain time frame or they will not be effective. Table 5-6 lists the antidotes commonly used for extravasation. It is always important to follow agency protocols and medical directives when using them. Once treatment is initiated for extravasation, the nurse must restart the IV as soon as possible proximal to the previously cannulated site or in another location so as not to interrupt the scheduled rate of infusion.

Documentation must be thorough and accurate regarding all pertinent events regarding the signs and symptoms of the infiltration, written and verbal communications, nursing and medical interventions, and the patient response patterns.

Catheter and Needle Displacement

Displacement of the catheter or needle means that the cannula has shifted from its intended placement site in the vein. It also can mean that the cannula is inadvertently removed from the vein.

Etiology and Defining Characteristics

Catheter or needle displacement usually occurs because the cannula was inadequately secured after its insertion into the vein. It also occurs when the tape around the site becomes loose or detaches from the skin. Tape detachment occurs because the wrong type of tape was used, or the site becomes damp or wet from perspiration or contact with external sources of moisture. When infiltration occurs, the

cannula can be physically pushed out of its position in the vein from the pressure of the fluid in the tissues surrounding the needle or catheter.

Cannulas that are placed in the radial or metacarpal veins can easily become dislodged or pulled out during routine patient movements such as transfer from a bed to a chair, getting up for ambulation, or during the routine activities of daily living in which the hand and wrist are used. It is easy, too, for the IV device or tubing to get caught on clothing, bed linens, and side rails. Catheter dislodgement often happens while the patient is being transferred from his bed to a wheelchair or gurney for transport to other areas.

Nursing Assessment and Interventions

Prior to inserting an intravenous cannula, the nurse must make a detailed assessment of the patient's level of consciousness, activity, and movement so as to allow for as much freedom as possible without disturbing the IV device. It is also a good idea, if possible, to place the IV in the patient's nondominant hand if he is ambulatory and carrying out self-care activities.

By using the most appropriate site and the correct type of tape and dressing, the IV device should remain intact. The dressing should allow for frequent inspection of the site so that any change in cannula position can be expediently recognized.

The nurse should also explain to the patient his role in caring for the IV, if he is able to do so. He should be advised to call for assistance when carrying out activities that may compromise his IV and to call the nurse if he notices any change in the IV's placement or experiences any discomfort or change in sensation around the site.

A transparent dressing placed over the insertion site that covers the hub of the cannula is ideal for visually inspecting the insertion site for displacement. The hub and the IV tubing should be secured with tape placed in a chevron formation (Figure 5-1) and all loops of tubing should be secured so they do not catch on anything. Should the tape become loose, the nurse must re-secure the cannula and tubing immediately. If a portion of the cannula extrudes from the vein, it should not be pushed back into the vein. Rather, it should be checked for infiltration. If still in the vein and infusing properly, it may be further secured with tape to keep it in place and avoid further movement out of the vein.

Occlusion and Loss of Patency

Occlusion occurs when there is some type of blockage that interferes with the passage of infusate into the vein. It can occur at any point within the vein, the cannula, or the tubing. Loss of patency is probably one of the easiest complications to prevent.

Table 5-6 | Extravasion Antidotes for Irritating or Vesicant Drugs

The 15 antidotes listed in the table are to be used alone, or in combination, for extravasation of the following drugs, based on agency/institutional protocols and medical directives.

CLASSIFICATION	MEDICATION	ANTIDOTE(S)
Adrenergic Agents (sympathomimetics) (Generally cause sloughing and tissue necrosis with extravasation)*	Amrinone (Inocor)	1, 5, 11, 13
	Dobutamine HCl (Dobutrex)	1, 5, 11, 13
	Dopamine (Intropin)	1, 5, 11, 13
	Epinephrine (Adrenaline)	1, 5, 11, 13
	Isoproterenol (Isuprel)	1, 5, 11, 13
	Metaraminol bitartrate (Aramine)	1, 5, 11, 13
	Methoxamine HCl (Vasoxyl)	1, 5, 11, 13
	Norepinephrine (Levophed [levarterenol])	1, 5, 11, 13
	Phenylephrine HCl (Neo-Synephrine)	1, 5, 11, 13
Alkalinizing Agents (Generally cause ulceration, sloughing, cellulitis, and tissue necrosis with extravasation)	Sodium bicarbonate	1, 7 and/or 8, 11, + 13
	Tromethamine (Tham-E)	8 + 5 or 8 + 7
Alkylating Agents (Generally cause sloughing and tissue necrosis)	Carmustine (BCNU) [irritant]	1, 6 or 7, 11, 13
	Mechlorethamine (nitrogen mustard; mustargen) [vesicant]	1, 9, 12 (ice), 13
	Streptozocin (Zancosar) [vesicant]	1, 6 or 7, 11
Antihypertensives	Nitroprusside sodium (Nipride)	1, 9
Antineoplastic Agents (DNA/RNA inhibitors or mitotic inhibitors) (Generally cause severe tissue sloughing and necrosis with extravasation)	Dacarbazine (DTIC) [vesicant]	1, 6 or 7, 11, 13
	Etoposide (VePesid) [irritant]	1, 6, 11, 13
	Vinblastine sulfate (Velban) [vesicant]	1, 6 or 7, 13
	Vincristine sulfate (Oncovin) [vesicant]	1, 6 or 7, 11, 13
	Vindesine sulfate (Eldisine) [vesicant]	1, 6 or 7, 11, 13
Antibiotic Antineoplastic Agents (Generally cause stinging, burning, severe cellulitis, and tissue necrosis with extravasation)	Dactinomycin (Actinomycin D) [vesicant]	1, 4, 6 or 7, 12, 13
	Daunorubicin HCl (daunomycin, Cerubidine) [vesicant]	2, 4, 6 or 7, 12, 13, 15
	Doxorubicin HCl (Adriamycin)	2, 4, 6 or 7, 12, 13, 15
	Idarubicin HCl (Idamycin) [vesicant]	1, 3, 4, 6 or 7, 12 (ice), 13, 15
	Mitomycin C (Mutamycin) [vesicant]	2, 6, 13
	Plicamycin (Mithramycin) [vesicant]	1, 6, 11
Chemotherapy (others) [vesicants]	Bisantrene	2, 10
	Dacarbazine (DTIC-Dome)	2, 10
	Mitoxantrone (DHAD)	2, 10
Electrolytes (Vein irritants that generally cause necrosis, sloughing, cellulitis, and tissue necrosis with extravasation)	Calcium salts / Ca carbonate / Ca chloride / Ca gluconate / Ca lactate / Ca glucepate / Potassium salts	1, 7, or 8, 11, 13
Hypertonic (<10%)	Dextrose Solutions	1, 7, 11, 13
Penicillins (Some can cause sterile abscesses, thrombophlebitis, and severe pain with extravasation)	Nafcillin (Nafcil; Unipen) / Ampicillin sodium (Unasyn) / Azlocillin sodium (Azlin)	1, 7

ANTIDOTE KEY

1. Stop the infusion immediately. Aspirat any remaining drug in the cannula with a syringe. Administer antidote into the cannula per physician orders, then discontinue the IV.
2. Stop the infusion and aspirate any remaining drug in the cannula with a syringe. Administer sodium bicarbonate (neutralizing agent) or a corticosteroid (anti-inflammatory agent) into the cannula and discontinue the IV.
3. Aspirate as much of the extravasated drug as possible from the tissue.**
4. Flush the extravasated area with normal saline (0.9% NaCl).**
5. As soon as possible, liberally inject 5 to 10 mg of phentolamine mesylate into the extravasated area to prevent dermal necrosis and sloughing.**
6. Inject long-acting dexamethasone or other corticosteroid to produce anti-inflammatory effect.**
7. Inject hyaluronidase throughout the area to dilute the extravasated drug.**
8. Inject 1% procaine to reduce venospasm.*
9. Inject isotonic sodium thiosulfate into the indurated area.**
10. Inject 4% sodium bicarbonate.**
11. Apply warm, moist compresses to enhance blood flow and transport extravasate out of tissues.
12. Apply cold compresses or ice packs (20 min/hr until inflammation dissipates) to reduce inflammation and arrest tissue destruction.
13. Elevate extremity to enhance fluid drainage.
14. Actively move extremity to enhance fluid drainage.
15. Consult reconstructive surgeon. Excision of the involved area may be indicated for necrosis or persistent pain at the site.

*Antidotes for alkylating agents are ineffective if more than 12 hr have passed since the extravasation occurred.

**Always use a small-gauge (27 to 25 ga.) intradermal or subcutaneous needle.

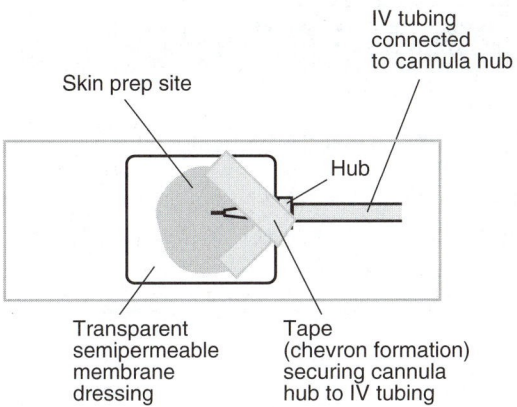

Figure 5-1 | Proper taping of IV site

Etiology and Defining Characteristics

Loss of patency can occur for reasons ranging from the simple to the more complex. Whatever the cause, measures must be taken as soon as the problem is identified so that the integrity of the infusion can be restored.

An easily identified and remedied problem is tubing that is kinked or bent because the patient has rolled over onto it. If an IV device is inserted near a joint, such as the antecubital space, the line may occlude when the patient flexes his arm. Sometimes the line is clamped off as a result of the patient, his visitors, or untrained personnel manipulating the line. Most often, however, flow is impeded when the IV line is changed from an electronic infusion device to gravity flow, such as during showering or ambulation when the flow rate is not properly maintained. Also, if a line is kept open at too slow a rate, the fluid flow may cease, especially if the patient is hypertensive.

If the infusate runs out and is not immediately replaced, occlusion can occur because of the backflow of venous blood into the cannula and tubing. This is caused by the loss of gravitational flow that is overtaken by venous pressure. If such a situation is left unchecked for even a short period of time, the backed-up blood will clot, thus obstructing the IV cannula as well as the infusion tubing.

The fibrin sheath that forms around and over the tip of a cannula can also disrupt the flow of fluid. Usually this does not cause obstruction unless the cannula is left in place longer than the recommended time. If during cannulation the intima of the vein is damaged, platelets may attach to the injured area and obstruct flow.

When too large a cannula is used to access the vein, the tip of the catheter may press against the vein wall, thus disrupting or inhibiting the prescribed rate of infusate flow. For a vein that is kept open with an intermittent infusion plug (saline or heparin lock), but not properly flushed at the prescribed intervals, occlusion can occur.

Nursing Assessment and Interventions

The first sign that there is obstruction of the IV line is a slowing or stopping of the infusate. There is often a backup of blood from the cannula into the IV tubing. The IV site usually appears normal.

Since loss of patency can easily be prevented, the nurse can usually maintain the integrity of the IV with thorough assessment of the patient, his position, his IV site, and the flow of infusate through the IV tubing. Patient teaching directed at maintaining the extremity properly positioned and keeping the tubing free of kinks is very important. The patient must not lie on the tubing or manipulate the tubing clamps or the controls on his electronic infusion device.

NURSING TIP

Signs and Symptoms of Occlusion and Loss of Patency

- Slowed rate of infusion even if clamp is opened or height of infusate is raised
- Infusion stops infusing
- Infusion site pain (with normal appearance)
- Blood backs up from the cannula into the IV tubing

NURSING ALERT

Veins That Are in Close Proximity to a Joint

If possible, the nurse should avoid cannulating veins that are in close proximity to joints. If a steel needle is used and the patient flexes his arm or wrist, the needle can puncture the vein wall and damage surrounding nerves, vessels, and tissues. Although somewhat flexible, an intravenous catheter can become occluded or break off with repeated movement or flexion of a joint. If veins near moveable joints cannot be avoided for use, the nurse must take measures to prevent flexure through patient compliance or the use of arm boards or soft splints.

Patients, visitors, and health care personnel must be advised that only properly trained personnel may handle IV products and equipment. The nurse must maintain the infusion rate at a flow that will keep the line open and prevent backflow of blood into the cannula and tubing. This is especially important for patients with hypertension when venous pressure may exceed gravitational flow. When the patient is receiving continuous infusions, the nurse must have the next container of infusate ready to hang in advance of the previous one running out.

Intermittent infusion devices (saline or heparin locks) are to be flushed routinely with normal saline or heparin (if ordered) according to protocols. If electronic infusion devices are used, the nurse must monitor them and determine whether the controller or pump mode of flow is to be used. Any time a patient is removed from these machines, the nurse must be careful to manually adjust the IV flow rate. The clamps should never be closed completely (to avoid occlusion), nor should they be left wide open (to avoid fluid overload).

Despite using all measures to prevent the loss of patency, if an obstruction occurs, the nurse must intervene accordingly. If there are no problems with the position of the cannula, the taping, the tubing, or height of the infusate (which should be approximately 36 inches above the IV site), but the flow rate is impeded, the nurse should suspect that the line is occluded and perform the following interventions:

1. Using the fingertips, pinch the IV tubing open and closed or gently milk it, in an attempt to free a cannula tip that is positioned against the vein wall and obstructing flow.
2. If the fluid still doesn't infuse properly, attempt to irrigate the line with normal saline in a 3- or 5-cc syringe (2 cc of normal saline in a 3-cc syringe; 3 to 4 cc in a 5-cc syringe). Should there be any resistance when light pressure is applied to the plunger, stop.

NURSING ALERT

The Importance of Gentle Flushing When Irrigating

When attempting to irrigate an IV, if there is any resistance when gentle pressure is exerted on the syringe plunger, STOP. The application of force could dislodge the obstruction and send it traveling in the circulatory system. Remember, the term **irrigate** means to cleanse a canal with *gentle* flushing. It does not mean to force fluid through the canal.

---

3. Try to aspirate, in an attempt to remove the obstruction. If this fails, stop.
4. Discontinue the IV and restart the infusion in another location.

NURSING ALERT

Syringe Sizes for Irrigating

Never use smaller than a 2-cc or 3-cc syringe to irrigate or aspirate clots in an IV line. A smaller syringe creates excess pressure that can damage the intima of the vein.

---

5. Document all assessment findings, interventions, and patient responses.

Phlebitis

Phlebitis is the inflammation of a vein. **Inflammation** is part of the body's normal immune response to any type of injury or invasion. Phlebitis, along with infiltration, is a fairly common complication of infusion therapy that can occur as a result of various situations. It can lead to permanent vein damage and other serious complications if left unchecked. Phlebitis can be caused by mechanical, bacterial, or chemical sources, or a combination of them.

Etiology and Defining Characteristics

Phlebitis occurs because of local vasodilation with increased blood flow, augmented vascular permeability, and the movement of white blood cells (especially the neutrophils) from the blood into the area of injury. Plasma moves from the capillaries into the surrounding tissues. This phenomenon results in localized swelling, which in turn results in pain from the pressure of the edema on surrounding nerve endings. As inflammation of the vein progresses, white blood cells (leukocytes) and tissue cells (histocytes) are destroyed by lysosomes emitted from macrophages. This action results in warmth and redness. Pus, the end-product of dead leukocytes, accumulates and can result in **suppurative** phlebitis. As inflammation progresses, the bacterial toxins and proteins released by the invading organisms signal the hypothalamus to elevate body temperature above normal. Prostaglandins are released from phospholipids in the cell membrane, which also contribute to the inflammatory processes of pain and fever.

There are several types of IV therapy-related phlebitis that the nurse must understand:

1. Bacterial phlebitis

    With the breakage of the skin's protective barrier and a portal of entry into the circulatory system that occurs with venipuncture, pathogenic organisms can gain access and stimulate inflammation, thus producing bacterial phlebitis. Phlebitis can also occur if a cannula is left in the vein longer than the prescribed or recommended time or if contaminated fluid or infusates are used.

2. Chemical phlebitis

When the vein becomes inflamed by irritating or vesicant solutions, chemical phlebitis occurs. This is the result of contact with infusates with high or low osmolarities or those with a high or low pH, especially if small veins are used for venous access.

3. Mechanical phlebitis

With mechanical phlebitis, the inflammation may develop as a result of the physical trauma from the skin puncture and the movement of the cannula into the vein during insertion. It can arise with any subsequent manipulation and movement of the cannula that alters the integrity of the internal vein wall. Sometimes it is caused by a clot at the tip of the catheter, the consequence of platelet aggregation around the injured vein wall. If a cannula is too large for the vein and prevents the free flow of blood around it, phlebitis can occur. The simple fact that a foreign object (the cannula) is present in the vein is enough to initiate an inflammatory response.

N U R S I N G   T I P

Signs and Symptoms of Phlebitis

- Erythema at the site
- Pain or burning at the site and along the length of the vein
- Warmth over the site
- Edema at the site
- Vein hard, red, and cordlike
- Slowed infusion rate
- Temperature elevation one degree or more above baseline

Nursing Assessment and Interventions

Prevention is the best intervention for phlebitis and other complications of IV therapy. Measures the nurse must take to prevent phlebitis begin before the IV infusion is even started. It is important to know what infusates will be administered and understand their expected therapeutic outcomes and side effects. Solution containers, tubings, and insertion devices must be checked to be sure there are no breaks in their integrity, and expiration dates must be verified. When preparing solutions, they must be checked for clarity, the

presence of particulate matter, and discoloration. When setting up the infusion and priming the tubing, measures must be taken to avoid contamination. Asepsis and good hand hygiene are vital to safe preparation.

N U R S I N G   T I P

Height of Infusion Container

To avoid mechanical irritation to the vein, the infusion container should never be hung higher than 36 inches above the IV site.

The nurse must properly assess the proposed IV site and determine that the vein intended for venous infusion is appropriate for the infusate that will be delivered. She must determine whether an IV catheter or needle should be used. Steel needles pose a greater chance for infiltration compared to catheters, but cause a lower incidence of phlebitis. The INS recommends that stainless steel needles be "limited to short-term or single-dose administration" (INS, 2000, Standard 44, S39). The nurse must select the smallest length and gauge cannula that will allow for the free flow of blood around it yet safely deliver the infusate. Veins in the legs should be avoided because of their propensity for phlebitis.

Prior to starting the infusion, the nurse must prepare the patient psychologically and physically. She needs to explain what will be done and why, and the approximate length of time the infusion will be in place. Patient teaching is so important at this time because the nurse can enlist the patient's help in troubleshooting potential problems, especially during home infusion therapy. It is wise to take the patient's temperature and record it in the chart to have as a preinfusion baseline.

N U R S I N G   T I P

Clipping Body Hair

If the patient has a lot of body hair over the intended IV site, it should be clipped short with scissors/clippers, not shaved. Shaving predisposes the skin to microabrasions, providing an ideal environment for bacterial contamination to set in (INS, 2000, Standard 45, S40).

Once the equipment is set up and the nurse is ready to cannulate the vein and start the infusion, she should wash her hands thoroughly, preferably with an antimicrobial emulsion, and don gloves. Following the institution or agency protocols, the nurse must use strict aseptic technique when starting the IV and dressing the site to prevent bacterial seeding. Tape should be applied to keep the IV secure but not so tight as to constrict circulation and interfere with the infusion. Once the infusion is running, there should be minimal manipulation of the cannula and site so as to avoid the mechanical trauma that predisposes to phlebitis.

If an additive is ordered for the infusate, the nurse should use a filter needle to draw it up into a syringe. Once drawn up, the needle is to be replaced with a regular needle (or appropriate needleless device) before injecting it into the IV solution. Using a filter needle followed by the regular needle reduces the chance for contamination of the IV infusate with particulate matter. When medications are given by direct intravenous injection, by bolus into the tubing, or by piggyback, it is important to administer them at the prescribed rate. If given too fast, the vein can become chemically damaged because the venous blood is unable to properly dilute them.

The nurse must be alert to the signs and symptoms of phlebitis. By recognizing them as early as possible, she can act to prevent further complications, especially the development of infection. Usually, the initial sign of phlebitis is **erythema** (redness) at the IV site with the patient complaining of pain or burning in that area. There may be edema. Upon palpation, the site feels warm and the patient experiences discomfort when the skin over the tip of the catheter is touched. The vein may feel **indurated** (hard) with a red streak on the skin that runs the length of the inflamed vein. The indurated vein may look and feel like a reddened cord. There may be temperature elevation and drainage from the IV site.

At the first sign of phlebitis, the IV infusion must be discontinued and the cannula removed. If there is fever and drainage at the site, especially if it is purulent, the physician must be notified. Depending on agency protocols, the infection control nurse should be notified and the site or cannula, or both, cultured. The appearance of the site and the patient's communications are to be thoroughly documented. When purulent drainage is present, or when "an infusion-related infection is suspected, the catheter, the delivery system, the access site, and/or the infusate shale be cultured using septic technique and observing Standard Precautions. The Semiquantitative culture technique should be used for obtaining a culture." (INS, 2000, Standard 63, S59).

There are various rating systems used to classify phlebitis. Agencies may use the INS-recommended phlebitis scale (Table 5-7), one of several scales developed by various IV product manufacturers, or they may develop their own. It is important to use the selected scale consistently in order to maintain a uniform tool for assessment, reporting, and documentation purposes.

After the IV is discontinued, warm compresses may be applied to the skin over the phlebitis, depending on agency protocols. The IV should be restarted in another place as soon as possible so as not to disrupt the infusion schedule. New tubing and infusate should be used. This is important because the phlebitis may have resulted from bacterial contamination that originated or migrated into the tubing or infusate.

Sometimes there are no signs or symptoms of phlebitis until after an IV or intermittent infusion device has been dis-

Table 5-7 | INS Phlebitis Grading Scale* (for infusion phelibitis and postinfusion phlebitis)

CRITERIA	GRADE 0	GRADE 1	GRADE 2	GRADE 3	GRADE 4
No symptoms	✳				
Erythema at access site with or without pain		✳			
Pain at access site with erythema and/or edema			✳		
Pain at access site with erythema and/or edema				✳	
Streak formation				✳	
Palpable venous cord				✳	
Pain at access site with erythema and/or edema					✳
Streak formation					✳
Palpable venous cord > 1 inch in length					✳
Purulent drainage					✳

* INS, 2000, standard 59, S56

continued. This is known as **postinfusion phlebitis** and it usually occurs within 48 hours of removal. Postinfusion phlebitis may be a delayed reaction or the result of improperly discontinuing an IV. The signs, symptoms, and treatment are the same as for phlebitis.

Thrombosis and Thrombophlebitis

Thrombophlebitis is the inflammation of a vessel due to the development of a **thrombus**, an abnormal blood clot, that obstructs or occludes the vessel. **Thrombosis** is the process whereby the clot develops. **Superficial thrombophlebitis** involves the subcutaneous vessels of the arms and legs that usually are cannulated for IV therapy. If left unchecked or inadequately treated, it may progress to **deep vein thrombosis** (**DVT**), which involves inflammation of the larger, deeper veins of the extremities, usually the legs. As blood flows past the clot, there is always the possibility that a portion of it will break away and travel throughout the circulatory system until it lodges in a major vessel and obstructs blood flow.

Etiology and Defining Characteristics

Thrombophlebitis is often the sequela of phlebitis (Figure 5-2). Its etiology as related to IV therapy is, therefore, usually the same. When the endothelial lining of a blood vessel becomes traumatized, as with phlebitis, the clotting process is initiated. Once a clot forms, blood flow is inhibited or stopped, a condition known as **venous stasis**. The clot then often continues to grow in the direction of the slow-moving blood.

Thrombophlebitis very often occurs when veins in the legs are used for IV therapy. Unless an emergency situation exists in which no other site is available, the leg veins should not be used in adults.

Nursing Assessment and Interventions

Since thrombophlebitis can result in serious complications, even death, prevention should always be the primary therapeutic regimen. The initial sign of thrombophlebitis is usually a slowing of the prescribed infusion rate, although the IV site may look and feel normal. As it persists, there may be pain and burning at the IV site with warmth, redness, cording, and induration of the vein. As inflammation progresses there is usually fever and malaise. As with phlebitis, baseline vital signs should be assessed prior to IV therapy and the patient's level of consciousness must be closely monitored so any untoward changes can be quickly identified.

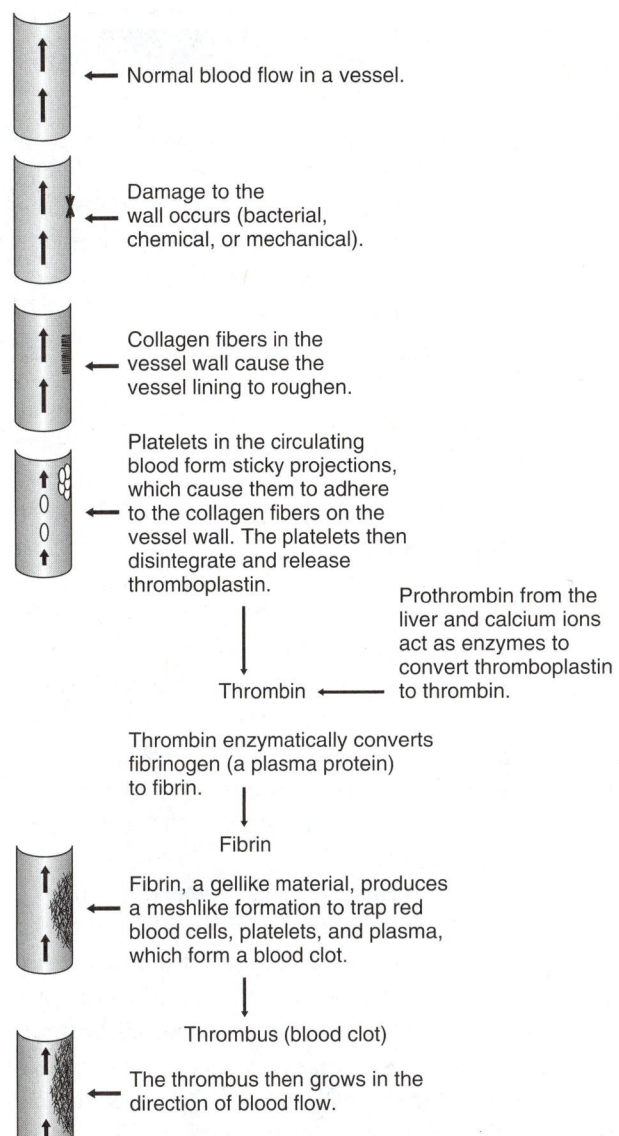

Normal blood flow in a vessel.

Damage to the wall occurs (bacterial, chemical, or mechanical).

Collagen fibers in the vessel wall cause the vessel lining to roughen.

Platelets in the circulating blood form sticky projections, which cause them to adhere to the collagen fibers on the vessel wall. The platelets then disintegrate and release thromboplastin.

Prothrombin from the liver and calcium ions act as enzymes to convert thromboplastin to thrombin.

Thrombin ◄——

Thrombin enzymatically converts fibrinogen (a plasma protein) to fibrin.

Fibrin

Fibrin, a gellike material, produces a meshlike formation to trap red blood cells, platelets, and plasma, which form a blood clot.

Thrombus (blood clot)

The thrombus then grows in the direction of blood flow.

Figure 5-2 | Progression of phlebitis to thrombophlebitis

Whenever hypertonic or highly acidic infusions are prescribed, the nurse must always be alert to the possibility of thrombophlebitis. If an infusion is discontinued and treatment is initiated at the first sign of superficial thrombophlebitis, further complications do not usually ensue and DVT does not develop.

When the lower extremities must be used for IV therapy, there is always the possibility that DVT will occur. If the leg veins must be used, the nurse must take precautions to avoid venous stasis. If possible, the patient should ambulate to promote venous return or perform active and passive range of motion (ROM) exercises in the extremity. Prolonged immobility or positioning the limb in a dependent position when sitting or standing must be avoided and the limb elevated when the patient is in bed.

NURSING ALERT

Avoiding DVT

Due to the possible development of DVT the leg veins should not be used for IV therapy, unless an emergency situation arises in which other veins are inaccessible. As soon as another site can be accessed, the site must be changed.

Unfortunately, the clinical signs and symptoms of DVT are nonspecific and there may be no warning until acute respiratory distress occurs when a clot breaks away and lodges in the lung. Since a slowing of the IV infusion rate and swelling of the extremity are the most reliable indicators of thrombophlebitis and further complications, the nurse should frequently assess the site and flow rate. If the area of inflammation is extensive there will be reduced venous return, resulting in mottling or cyanosis or both. The skin temperature can be increased and superficial veins may be dilated. Although not always a good indicator, if the IV is in the leg, there may be a positive **Homan's sign**—calf pain with dorsiflexion of the foot.

Once identified, thrombophlebitis must be treated expeditiously. The IV must be discontinued and restarted elsewhere. The physician should be consulted as to whether the extremity should be elevated and warm, moist compresses applied. The physician may order antiembolic stockings and/or the use of sequential compression devices (SCDs). The nurse must strictly follow the treatment regime, which usually includes the administration of anticoagulant and anti-inflammatory drugs and a balanced routine of active and passive activity and rest. Reporting and documentation must be thorough and accurate.

Hematoma

A **hematoma** is the accumulation of clotted blood in the tissue **interstices** (spaces). It results from the loss of integrity in a vessel wall due to disease or trauma that allows the escape of blood in the surrounding area. The result is **ecchymosis**—a black-and-blue skin discoloration.

Etiology and Defining Characteristics

Whenever a vessel is damaged, platelets migrate to the site to patch it and prevent blood loss. The presence of platelets also signals the activation of the clotting mechanism with the formation of fibrin from circulating fibrinogen.

NURSING TIP

Signs and Symptoms of Thrombophlebitis

- Slowed or stopped infusion rate
- Aching or burning sensation at the infusion site
- Elevation in temperature one degree or more above baseline
- Skin warm and red around IV site
- Cording of the infusion vein
- Malaise
- Swelling and edema of the extremity
- Throbbing pain in the limb
- Mottling and cyanosis of the extremity
- Diminished arterial pulses
- Pallor

The usual cause of hematoma formation is faulty venipuncture technique, where the cannula passes through the distal vein wall. It can also occur with infiltration following cannulation of a vein. Sometimes a hematoma develops following successful venipuncture when the flow control clamp for the infusion is opened before the tourniquet is removed. The fluid pressure distal to the tourniquet causes the vessel to rupture.

NURSING TIP

Releasing the Tourniquet after Cannulation

Once a vein is successfully cannulated for an infusion, release the tourniquet before opening the flow control clamp on the IV tubing. Failure to do so causes excess pressure to build up distal to the tourniquet and ruptures the vein.

If the lumen of the cannula is too large for the vein to accommodate it, vessel rupture can occur. If the cannula is too long for the vein, it may sever the vessel at a junction where the vein merges with another portion of the vein. For patients with fragile skin and veins, the pressure of the tourniquet, if applied too tightly, can cause a hematoma to form when the vein is punctured. Also, if venipuncture has been unsuccessful and the nurse attempts to start the IV in a nearby area, the application of the tourniquet can cause the first puncture site to break open and bleed.

A hematoma can form when inadequate pressure is applied following a blood sampling stick or the discontinuation of an infusion or heparin lock. Even though bleeding has been arrested, it can start again if the patient lowers the extremity too soon after the cannula has been removed, especially if a pressure dressing has not been applied.

NURSING TIP

Signs and Symptoms of Hematoma

- Ecchymosis over and around insertion area
- Pain at the site
- Swelling and hardness at the insertion site
- Inability to advance the cannula all the way into the vein during insertion
- Inability to flush the IV line

Nursing Assessment and Interventions

Although hematoma formation cannot always be avoided, the incidence can be reduced with thorough assessment of the patient's skin and vein integrity. The method of cannulation may need to be altered, especially for patients with fragile veins, paper-thin skin, or veins that roll—those that move laterally when manipulated. For patients with veins that tend to roll, rather than insert the cannula directly over the vein, it may be preferable to enter indirectly from the side and gently advance the cannula into the vein. This also decreases the chance of puncturing the opposite vein wall. For patients with very fragile veins, it is sometimes necessary to cannulate the vein bevel down, rather than the usual bevel-up method, as a means to prevent puncture of the opposite vein wall. It is also important to select a cannula that is not too large or too long for the vein. It may be beneficial to use a blood pressure cuff rather than a tourniquet to restrict venous flow during venipuncture. For patients with fragile veins, it is preferable not to use a tourniquet at all.

The tourniquet must never be applied above the site of a recent lab stick, unsuccessful venous cannulation (where the vessel has been nicked), or following the discontinuation of an IV. Once a vein is cannulated for an infusion, the tourniquet must be immediately removed.

A hematoma is fairly easy to identify because the area around the venipuncture site is usually ecchymotic. It may also be tender or painful and edematous. If a large amount of blood has escaped, the area will be raised and hard.

If these indicators are not evident, the nurse may suspect hematoma formation when she is unable to advance the cannula into the vein during insertion or meets with resistance when attempting to irrigate.

Once a hematoma is identified, the IV must be discontinued, and a 2 × 2-inch gauze pressure dressing applied. Alcohol should not be used when removing the cannula because it enhances bleeding and may cause stinging at the puncture site. Once bleeding has stopped, the extremity may be elevated and warm moist compresses applied, depending on the severity of the hematoma. The nurse should follow agency protocols and medical directives regarding treatment interventions.

Venous Spasm

Venous spasm is the sudden involuntary movement or contraction of a vessel wall. It occurs as a result of trauma or irritation from chemicals or temperature extremes and is usually painful. A strong, painful spasm is a **cramp**.

NURSING ALERT

Infusates That May Cause Venous Spasm

- Cold solutions
- Dextrose solutions with concentrations greater than 12.5%
- Infusates with a high or low pH
- Diazepam (Valium)
- Nafcillin sodium (Nafcil; Unipen)
- Phenytoin (Dilantin)
- Potassium chloride solutions
- Propofol (Diprivan)
- Vancomycin HCl

Etiology and Defining Characteristics

Venous spasm is usually caused by the administration of an irritating infusate with a high osmolarity or a high or low pH. The delivery of cold or viscous infusates can also precipitate venous spasm. For some patients, the entrance of the IV cannula into the vein can result in spasm, especially if the cannula is too large to allow for adequate hemodilution. Venous spasm often occurs if a solution is infused too rapidly, particularly with a small-gauge cannula. The vasovagal response resulting from pain or anxiety also contributes to venous spasm.

Nursing Assessment and Interventions

In most situations, venous spasm is a complication that can be prevented. When it does occur, it is identified by a slowing of the infusion rate due to the wavelike contractions of the vessel wall. The patient complains of a sharp, painful sensation that radiates from the IV site up the extremity. Some patients say it feels like an electric shock going up the arm. The skin over the vein may blanch or it can be red, an indication of phlebitis.

Venous spasm can be prevented by using a large vein and a small-gauge cannula so that blood flow is unrestricted and allows for dilution of the infusate. Fluids should be administered at room temperature. Refrigerated medications must be taken out of the refrigerator for the minimum time needed to get them to room temperature. A blood warmer can be used to prevent venous spasm during a transfusion. Irritating solutions should be well diluted. The nurse must assess the patient's anxiety level and his pain threshold, then take the necessary measures to help him relax.

Once venous spasm occurs, it can usually be reversed by decreasing the infusion rate. The application of warm compresses to the area surrounding the IV site can be used if the infusate is cold. If not contraindicated, and with a medical order, some irritating infusates can be buffered by adding sodium bicarbonate. A pharmacist should be consulted regarding the amount of buffer to add. When a vein continues to spasm in spite of these measures, the IV must be discontinued and restarted in a larger vein.

Vessel Collapse

When the walls of a vein or artery retract abnormally, **vessel collapse** occurs. This is one of the less commonly encountered complications of IV therapy.

Etiology and Defining Characteristics

Vessel collapse usually occurs as a result of decreased circulation, as seen with excessive blood or fluid loss and shock.

The veins in the extremities constrict in an attempt to shunt blood and oxygen to the brain and vital organs. When negative pressure is exerted on a vessel from aspiration of an IV line with a syringe, vessel collapse can occur.

Nursing Assessment and Interventions

When attempting to cannulate a vein, the nurse may identify that the vessel is collapsed because she cannot see or palpate the vein. If the vein is palpable, it has little elasticity and feels flaccid and flat. If an infusion is already running and the vessel collapses, the fluid flow will cease. When aspirating to check for patency or to remove a blockage, a vessel may collapse due to the negative pressure exerted on the vessel wall. This usually happens when a small-capacity syringe, 1 cc or smaller, is used.

Whatever the cause of the vessel collapse, the nurse must restart the IV elsewhere, preferably in a larger vein. If the patient is in shock, this may not be possible, and a physician may have to insert a central venous line. The nurse, then, must stay with the patient, provide reassurance, assist with the central venous cannulation, and keep the patient warm. She should lower his head and elevate his legs to promote venous return, and carefully monitor vital signs. Accurate reporting and documentation is critical in such a situation.

Cellulitis

Cellulitis is the diffuse inflammation and infection of cellular and subcutaneous connective tissue. It is bacterial in nature and, although localized, it has poorly defined borders and spreads to surrounding areas by way of watery seepage that extends along tissue spaces. If severe, cellulitis can lead to abscess formation and ulceration of the body's deeper tissues. It often spreads to the lymphatic system.

Etiology and Defining Characteristics

Cellulitis associated with IV therapy occurs in response to the invasion and multiplication of bacteria, usually the *Staphylococcus* and *Streptococcus* strains. The portal of entry is usually the IV puncture site. The organisms may come from the nurse during venipuncture or dressing changes or they may migrate to the IV insertion site from the patient's body. Poor aseptic technique and the failure to follow established infection control protocols are usually to blame for the development of cellulitis.

> ## NURSING TIP
>
> ### Signs and Symptoms of Cellulitis
>
> - Tenderness
> - Pain
> - Warmth
> - Edema
> - Induration
> - Red streaking on skin
> - *Peau d'orange*
> - Vesicles
> - Abscess formation with pus
> - Ulceration
> - Fever
> - Chills
> - Malaise

Nursing Assessment and Interventions

With cellulitis there is tenderness, pain, induration, and edema (pitting or nonpitting) when pressure is applied. The site feels warm and the skin has the roughened appearance of orange peel (**peau d'orange**). If the cellulitis has spread to the lymphatics, there may be red streaks on the skin over the vessels. Vesicles may form and there is often purulent exudate. The patient presents with fever, chills, and malaise.

The nursing intervention measures for cellulitis are similar to those for infiltration, extravasation, and phlebitis. The IV must be discontinued and started elsewhere. The nurse may have to assist the physician with the incision and drainage of an abscess. The limb may be elevated to reduce edema. Cool compresses to promote comfort are often alternated with warm, moist compresses to promote circulation, depending on medical directives and agency protocols. Hand hygiene must be meticulous and gloves are to be worn when tending to the cellulitis. Sterile dressings should be used. The nurse must assess for the signs and symptoms of systemic infection and sepsis. Antibiotics, analgesics, and antipyretics are generally administered.

Documentation must be thorough and accurate. It should reflect the signs and symptoms that led to the cellulitis as well as its progression, the description of the healing process, and the patient's response to treatment.

Nerve, Tendon, Ligament, and Limb Damage

In addition to the tissue damage already covered, there can be nerve, tendon, and ligament damage that can occur as a result of IV therapy. Some complications can progress to the loss of function in an extremity or to amputation of the limb.

Etiology and Defining Characteristics

The major causes of functional and structural damage are the incorrect insertion and placement of the IV cannula, or improper securing and stabilization of the cannula and IV line after insertion. Problems usually occur when the selected IV site is in close proximity to a joint and the IV site is not naturally splinted by bone. If the IV must be placed near a joint, problems occur because of failure to artificially splint the joint. Damage can also result from extravasated solution, from the pressure of infiltrated infusate, the pressure and anatomic displacement caused by a hematoma, or the sequelae of cellulitis.

> ## NURSING TIP
>
> ### Signs and Symptoms of Nerve, Tendon, Ligament, or Limb Damage
>
> - Tingling
> - Numbness
> - Loss of sensation
> - Loss of movement
> - Cyanosis
> - Pallor
> - Deformity
> - Paralysis

Nursing Assessment and Interventions

When starting an IV, the nurse must know the circulatory anatomy so the appropriate vein is properly accessed and damage is not done to the surrounding areas during cannulation. The cannula must never be moved back and forth in the subcutaneous tissue in an attempt to find a vein. Not only can damage be done to nerves, tendons, and ligaments, but an artery can be punctured.

The extremity in which the IV is placed must be frequently assessed and accurately documented. The skin should be warm and dry with normal color. The nurse must be alert to altered circulation, movement, and sensation. The patient should be able to move the extremity distal to the IV insertion site to promote circulation. In the home care setting, the nurse must teach the patient and his family what to look for and report.

SYSTEMIC COMPLICATIONS OF INFUSION THERAPY

Several of the local complications already covered can serve as warning signs for and precursors to the development of systemic problems of infusion therapy. Other systemic problems occur because of contamination, drug and fluid interactions, hypersensitivity reactions, sepsis, and emboli.

Contamination and Infection

Contamination is the introduction of microorganisms or particulate matter into a normally sterile environment. With intravenous therapy, the serious consequences of infection can result from a break in asepsis at any point in the manufacture of IV products or the delivery of infusion therapy.

Etiology and Defining Characteristics

Although the most infrequent cause, contamination can result from breaks in asepsis during the manufacture, packaging, and storage of infusates, medications, and delivery systems. It occurs most frequently, however, during the setup and administration of infusion therapy. During preparation, any break in aseptic technique on the part of the nurse can provide an entry port for microorganisms. The use of three-way stopcocks, which are frequently handled, often serve as the entry site for contaminants.

NURSING TIP

Signs and Symptoms of Infection

- Chills
- Malaise
- Fever
- Elevated leukocyte count
- Normal appearance of IV site

Nursing Assessment and Interventions

Although the nurse cannot be sure that the infusates and delivery systems are sterile, she must use every means to ensure that they are safe. Such measures include visually examining all containers and equipment for the presence of particulate matter, leaks or breaks, and discoloration along with verification of expiration dates. Following agency protocols, the cannula, tubings, and infusates must be changed on schedule. Filters and extension tubings should only be used when necessary and according to policy.

Frequent assessment of the patient and his IV site alert the nurse to any problems that might arise as the result of contamination. The first signs of contamination are the same as those with sepsis. There may be chills, malaise, a fever, and an elevated leukocyte count with no apparent etiology. The IV site will look normal, unless there is phlebitis.

NURSING TIP

Proper Site Preparation

Proper hand hygiene is always the single most important means of preventing the spread of infection. Proper site preparation is extremely important to ensure that organisms harbored on the patient's body or the nurse's hands do not migrate into the circulatory system. The IV site should be minimally manipulated and the cannula needs to be secured so it does not move around in the vein. All connections—the cannula hub and the tubing, the main tubing and piggyback attachments, and filters or extension tubings—must be well secured.

Once it is determined or suspected that contamination has occurred, the IV must be discontinued. The IV should be restarted at another site with new tubing and fresh infusate. The physician and the infection control department should be notified. The cannula, connection sites, tubing, and infusate should be cultured.

Sepsis

Sepsis is the (usually) febrile disease process that results from the presence of microorganisms or their toxic products in the circulatory system. Approximately 700,000 cases of severe sepsis (that associated with acute multiple organ dysfunction syndrome (MODS), hypoperfusion, and shock), occur in the U.S. annually (Linde-Zwirble et al., 1999). According to the Centers for Disease Control (CDC), it is the leading cause of death in noncoronary ICU patients in the U.S. (Sands et al., 1997) and the 11th leading cause of death overall (CDC, National Vital Statistics Report, 2000). On a worldwide scale, this amounts to several million cases annually. Sepsis results in mortality rates that range from 28% to 50% (Natanson et al., 1997; Zeni et al., 1997). The widespread use of broad-spectrum antibiotics, which has increased the rates of both antibiotic resistance and nosocomial infections, will have a direct impact on the rising incidence of sepsis (Opal and Cohen, 1999).

Etiology and Defining Characteristics

The organisms that are usually responsible for sepsis in the nonimmunocompromised adult are the gram-negative (*Escherichia*, *Klebsiella*, *Pseudomonas*, *Enterobacter*, *Serratia*, *Proteus*, and *Neisseria* species) and gram-positive (*Staphylococcus* and *Streptococcus* species) organisms, anaerobes, and the yeast *Candida* (Gorbach, Mensa, & Gatell, 1999). Sepsis is caused by the gram-negative *Escherichia coli*, *Pseudomonas*, and *Klebsiella* species 65% to 70% of the time (White, 1997).

IV infusion-related sepsis is most often attributed to *Staphylococcus aureus* and *S. epidermidis* bacteria, the *Candida albicans* yeast (Sanford, Gilbert, & Sande, 2002), and the coliform species *Escherichia*, *Enterobacter*, and *Klebsiella* (CDC, 2001). Vascular system septicemia, introduced by way of IV catheters, foreign bodies, and surgical interventions, is generally caused by the *Enterobacter*, *Serratia*, *S. epidermidis*, *Pseudomonas*, enterococci, and *Candida* pathogens (Myers, 1996).

Nursing Assessment and Interventions

Because of the widely disseminated infection that occurs with sepsis, fever develops (as the body's attempt to provide an unfavorable environment for organism growth and reproduction). The fever and toxins from the organisms stimulate cellular metabolism and vasodilation causing the patient to look flushed, with warm, dry skin. He has general malaise, chills, and headache.

With vasodilation there is decreased peripheral resistance causing a drop in blood pressure and reduced cardiac output. The heart compensates for loss of vascular volume by increasing its rate in order to shunt blood to the vital organs. Because of this, the extremities are somewhat dehydrated, pale in color, and cool to the touch. The patient complains of thirst. Renal compensation for decreased vascular volume results in oliguria.

When the bacterial toxins increase cellular metabolism, intravascular clotting may be stimulated, leading to the development of microclots throughout the body, a condition called **disseminated intravascular coagulation (DIC)**. The

clots clog capillaries, impair tissue profusion, and damage vital organs because they are deprived of nutrients. The DIC eventually uses up the available clotting factors in the blood, so hemorrhage into the tissues, especially those of the gastrointestinal tract, occurs.

The body will continue to compensate, but if sepsis is not halted, decompensation occurs. The metabolism of all cells shuts down and the vital organs are damaged. The patient becomes stuporous or comatose. The circulatory system becomes involved and circulatory collapse ensues. Despite adequate fluid resuscitation, severe hypotension occurs (systolic BP <90 mm Hg) and septic shock ensues. Simultaneous and progressive organ failure (CNS, lungs, liver, heart, GI tract, kidneys) or MODS occurs. Once this happens and cardiac output falls below 40% of normal, death soon follows.

Sepsis must be treated aggressively to prevent septic shock and death. Figure 5-3 illustrates the pathophysiology of the progression of sepsis from contamination through septic shock. Interventions are aimed at treating the cause of sepsis with antibiotic therapy and preventing or reversing shock. The patient should be kept flat with his legs elevated (modified Trendelenburg position). Oral fluids are given to relieve thirst and IV infusions must be maintained. Chilling must be

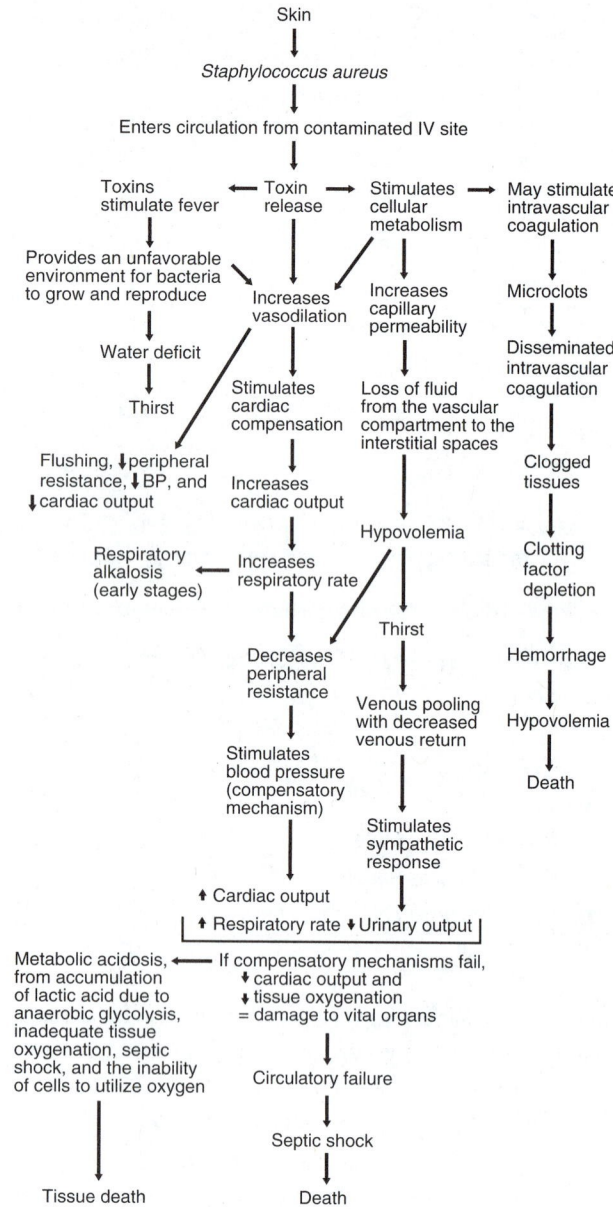

Figure 5-3 │ Progression of sepsis

Dyspnea and cyanosis require oxygen administration and positioning to assist the patient's breathing. Fever is treated with prescribed antipyretics, cool sponges, and fluid replacement. For muscle and joint pain, analgesics are administered and the patient must be positioned to minimize pressure on sore areas. It is important for the nurse to promote self-care within his limitations, encourage therapeutic communication, and support the patient and his family emotionally and psychologically.

Numerous investigational compounds have been studied for the treatment of sepsis (Natanson et al., 1998; Zeni, 1997). Many of these investigational therapies may have been unsuccessful because they modulated only a single pathophysiologic component of sepsis. Current research supports the use of recombinant human-activated protein C (drotrecogin alfa activated), the first drug found to fight sepsis. Those given this drug, a genetically engineered protein and natural blood product that helps prevent clotting and inflammation, have a 19% greater chance of survival. It is estimated that one life out of every sixteen patients with sepsis could be saved (Bernard et al., 2001).

Medication and Fluid Interactions

Many combinations of medication and fluid are delivered during the course of infusion therapy. The concurrent administration of some products can result in unintended or undesirable effects.

Etiology and Defining Characteristics

Incompatibility refers to the qualities of certain fluids and medications that cause unintended effects when they are mixed (drugs with drugs, drugs with fluids, or fluids with fluids). Refer to Table 5-8 for common drug–drug incompatibilities. When two or more agents are mixed, the intended action of either drug or fluid may be neutralized, intensified, or weakened. The mixture may form a **precipitation**—the suspension or crystallization of particles that occurs due to the mixing of incompatible solutions or adding solutes to incompatible solutions. Precipitation results in the occlusion of an intravenous line. **Antagonism** means that the combined effect of two or more agents is less than the sum of each one acting alone, while **synergism** means that the combined effect is greater than the sum of each one acting independently. **Idiosyncrasy** is an unusual or abnormal response to a medication or fluid. The interactions between some medications or fluids can also alter or distort laboratory tests.

An interaction occurring because a medication acts not only on the tissue or system it is targeted for but also on other structures is known as a **side effect**. A common

prevented, but the patient should not be kept so warm as to cause peripheral vasodilation. Medications are given as necessary to support blood pressure, circulation, and promote comfort. If the patient is disoriented, he must be protected from injury. Accurate monitoring of vital signs is necessary.

Since the patient is weak, nursing care is planned to conserve his strength and allow for frequent rest. Care is directed toward supporting the patient as symptoms develop. The patient must be observed for internal bleeding. If DIC occurs, there may be purpura or frank bleeding from mucous membranes, the IV site, and all body orifices. Pressure and cool compresses may be applied to sites of bleeding and the nurse will be involved in blood product replacement therapy.

Table 5-8 | Significant Drug–Drug Interactions

The following drugs are generally incompatible when combined with any other products:

- Aminoglycosides
- Chlordiazepoxide
- Diazepam
- Digitalis glycosides
- Pentobarbital
- Phenobarbital
- Phenytoin
- Secobarbital
- Sodium bicarbonate
- Theophylline derivatives

example is the IV administration of meperidine (Demerol) for the alleviation of postoperative pain, which also exerts a depressant effect on the central nervous system, resulting in drowsiness.

Absorption is the process in which a drug or fluid moves from the site of administration (such as the mouth, in the gastrointestinal system) to body fluids (blood, in the circulatory system) to the intended site of action (such as the heart) to elicit a therapeutic effect (e.g., increased cardiac output). With intravenous administration, the medication is directly absorbed into the blood and is immediately distributed to its target tissue. **Biotransformation** is the actual breakdown and metabolism of a drug; **elimination** is its removal from the body. Drug interactions can occur at any point during the processes of absorption, distribution, biotransformation, or elimination.

Nursing Assessment and Interventions

The nurse must never under any circumstance administer an intravenous medication or solution unless she knows what it is and its intended effect on the patient. This includes knowing whether it is compatible when mixed with other drugs or fluids. She must also know which drugs cannot be given by direct IV push because they need to be diluted with another fluid of a specified volume prior to intravenous administration (e.g., IV potassium supplements).

With the multitude of drugs and IV infusates on the market today, it is not possible for the nurse to know everything about every product. She is expected, however, to know where to find information about every medication and fluid to be given and refer to the source prior to administration.

Consultation with a pharmacist is necessary when any doubts regarding drug and fluid compatibilities exist. She should be familiar with the current *Physicians' Desk Reference* in order to understand the manufacturer's guidelines regarding medication use and admixture preparation. A drug compatibility chart should be available and it is recommended that the nurse refer to a nursing drug handbook or reference guide to understand the nursing implications associated with intravenous infusions. Whenever an IV medication or fluid is administered for the first time to a patient, the nurse is expected to stay with the patient long enough to determine if the patient will develop any untoward or unexpected reactions. (See Chapter 10.)

Hypersensitivity Reaction

A **hypersensitivity** reaction is the profound physiologic response of the body to an antigen. It is one of the most serious consequences of infusion therapy. It transpires when the immune system fails to protect the body against foreign materials. **Allergy** is the acquired abnormal immune response to an **allergen** (any substance that causes an immune response) following **sensitization**, or the first exposure to the allergen. More precisely, an allergen is an antigen that reacts specifically to a **reagin**—a type of immunoglobulin E (IgE). An **antigen** is an agent that is capable of stimulating antibodies. It is a protein that coats the surface of specific tissue cells (e.g., muscle, bone) and identifies them as part of the body, rather than as "strangers," or invaders.

Etiology and Defining Characteristics

Some individuals are more prone to allergic reactions because they carry in their systems large volumes of IgE antibodies, rather than IgG antibodies, which are more common in the general population. These people tend to be drug-sensitive. When an allergen enters the body, an allergen-reagin reaction occurs, which subsequently develops into an allergic reaction because the IgE antibodies bind to cells in the lungs and mucous membranes of the respiratory tract or skin cells.

IgE antibodies are attracted to basophils and mast cells, which can bind with up to a half million IgE molecules. Whenever allergens bind with these molecules, the cell membranes are altered and many of the basophils and masts rupture and release substances that cause blood vessel dilation and damage to tissues by enzymes (**proteases**) that break down proteins. There is increased capillary permeability, which allows fluid to leak into the tissues, and smooth muscle contraction occurs. These reactions are the result of histamine release, toxin secretions (called slow-reacting substance of anaphylaxis), heparin, and factors that activate platelets. Enzymes that are attracted to eosinophils and neutrophils are also released.

NURSING ALERT

Effects of Anaphylaxis

Anaphylaxis, also called anaphylactic shock, is a severe allergic reaction that results from an allergen moving throughout the circulatory system. The allergen comes in contact with the basophils in the blood and the mast cells that exist near the surface of small blood vessels, which results in a substantial release of histamine. This causes massive peripheral dilation, which deprives the vital organs of blood and oxygen, along with increased capillary permeability and plasma loss from the circulation. Shock and death can ensue within minutes if treatment is not initiated.

Nursing Assessment and Interventions

A thorough nursing history is very important in eliciting information regarding a patient's allergic status. Proper patient identification and assessment for allergies are crucial in both the acute care and home care settings. Immediately before medications are administered, especially those delivered intravenously, it is a good idea to question the patient again regarding allergies. In addition to prescription medications, the nurse needs to verify allergies to over-the-counter (OTC) medications, foods, topical preparations (especially iodine, if it is used as an IV site prep), and tape. If there is a known history of allergies, patient teaching should include recommending the use of a Medic Alert identification bracelet (Figure 5-4).

The signs and symptoms of a hypersensitivity reaction can range from mild to severe, can affect several body systems (Table 5-9), and may develop rapidly, gradually, or be delayed hours after the allergen has been delivered. There is often pain and edema around the IV site along with a characteristic **red flare**, due to the local release of histamine and resulting vaso-

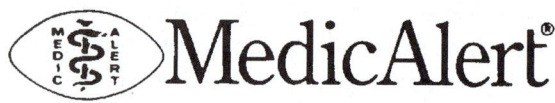

Figure 5-4 | Medic Alert logo
Reprinted with permission of Medic Alert Foundation

NURSING TIP

Hypersensitivity in Intravenous Infusions

With intravenous infusions, hypersensitivity to the infusate, its preservatives, or to IV medications can occur. The patient may be allergic to the cannula, skin antiseptic preparation, or tape. Depending on where a specific type of allergen-reagin reaction occurs, the result can be anything from rashes, itching, and hives, to bronchial spasm and anaphylaxis.

---

dilation. There is red streaking on the skin over venous routes and there may be a rash, with itching. Because of smooth muscle contractions, the patient often presents wheezing and bronchospasm, palpitations, gastric and intestinal cramping, and nausea with vomiting. The patient may have a headache, feel anxious or agitated, or be confused.

NURSING ALERT

Proper Actions in a Hypersensitivity Reaction

At the first indication of a hypersensitivity reaction, the nurse must either discontinue the infusion and keep the vein open with normal saline or, if the reaction is mild, slow the IV to a KVO (keep vein open) rate until further orders can be obtained. NEVER REMOVE THE CANNULA! Vital signs are to be taken and the physician notified. The nurse must stay with the patient, reassure him, and keep him warm. Emergency equipment must be readily available. Emergency drugs are administered according to agency policy and physician orders. Documentation must be complete, accurate, and reflect all necessary assessment data, problem identification, and nursing interventions.

Embolism

An **embolus** (plural: **emboli**) is an aggregate of undissolved material in the blood that is carried by circulatory flow. It may be solid, liquid, or gaseous. An **endogenous embolus** arises from within the body and usually consists of clotted blood (thrombus), tissue particles, tumor cell mass, or fat globules (that arise from skeletal trauma). An **exogenous embolus**

Table 5-9 | Systemic Signs and Symptoms of a Hypersensitivity Reaction

CARDIOVASCULAR/ CIRCULATORY SYSTEM	GASTROINTESTINAL/ DIGESTIVE SYSTEM	INTEGUMENTARY SYSTEM
• Facial edema	• Dysphagia (difficulty swallowing)	• Flushing
• Generalized edema	• Gastric cramping	• Red flare
• Erythema along veins	• Intestinal cramping	• Rash
• Palpitations	• Nausea	• IV site edema
• Hypotension	• Vomiting	• Pruritus (itching)
• Cardiac arrest		• Urticaria (hives)
NERVOUS SYSTEM	**RESPIRATORY SYSTEM**	**SPECIAL SENSES**
• Agitation	• Nasal congestion	• Pruritus (itching)
• Anxiety	• Rhinorrhea (runny nose)	• Watery eyes
• Confusion	• Cough	• Scratchy throat
• Disorientation	• Sensation of tightness in throat	• Tinnitus (ringing in ears)
• Headache	• Mucous membrane edema	• Buzzing sound in ears
• Paresthesias (loss of sensation or numbness/tingling)	• Wheezing	• Throbbing sensation in ears
• Vertigo	• Bronchospasm	• Tingling/numbness in fingers and/or toes
	• Respiratory obstruction	• Vertigo
	• Respiratory arrest	

originates outside of the body and is introduced into the bloodstream. It consists of particulate matter (such as hair, glass, or other particles), liquids, or gaseous material (such as room air). When an embolus meets with a vessel that is smaller than its diameter, it obstructs the vessel, blocks blood flow, and deprives the area distal to the embolism of blood and oxygen, a condition known as **ischemia**. The result is usually **infarction**—an area of **necrosis** (death of tissue) following the loss of blood supply. An embolus is named according to the vessel or organ it obstructs, usually cerebral, myocardial, pulmonary, or renal. Even the smallest embolus will be caught in a pulmonary vessel. Emboli that arise in veins, because of slower blood flow, are more common than those that arise in arteries.

Etiology and Contributing factors

Risk factors that predispose to embolic formation are impaired mobility and circulation, advanced age, recent surgery, obesity, and thrombophlebitis. In IV therapy, the emboli that most frequently occur result from dislodgement of a thrombus, the accidental admission of air into the circulatory system, or catheter embolism.

Blood Clot

The flow of blood past a thrombosis or any mechanical manipulation of the thrombotic area can cause a portion of the clot to break off and become an embolism, which can then break into multiple emboli. With IV therapy, the cause is usually the result of trauma to the intima of a vein. Bedridden patients are more prone to thromboembolic formation because of immobility (and the resulting venous stasis). About one in ten times an embolus travels through the right atrium and ventricle and lodges in the arterioles of the lung(s) resulting in massive pulmonary embolism (Guyton & Hall, 1997).

Just as a thrombus increases in size on a vein wall, the embolism, if not treated, continues to grow where it lodges in a pulmonary vessel, usually resulting in a fatal outcome. Small emboli may circulate until they become trapped in coronary vessels and cause a myocardial infarction, or lodge in cerebral vessels and effect a cerebral vascular accident, or stroke.

Air Embolism

Vessels can also be obstructed by air that enters the circulation through severed IV lines, tubings that are not primed with infusate, vented infusion containers that are allowed to run dry, or disconnected and loose tubing junctions. Piggyback lines that run dry can predispose to air entry if the primary tubing does not have a back-check valve proximal to the highest injection port. Air embolization occurs more frequently with improper handling of central venous catheters than with peripheral lines. (See Chapter 12.)

When air is present in the infusion line, it must be removed so it does not enter the patient's bloodstream. When clearing the line of air by using a syringe connected to an injection port, the plunger must not be removed prior to attachment to the infusion line. If the plunger is removed, air can enter the bloodstream when the flow control clamp is open and the tubing proximal to the cannula hub is not closed off. The plunger should always remain in the syringe barrel to assist with air removal by manually drawing back on the plunger.

Room air is approximately 70% nitrogen and, although blood is able to dissolve nitrogen relatively fast, it cannot do so rapidly enough when there is a large amount. As a result, the blood in the capillary beds and arterioles becomes displaced by the air, so there is ischemia and necrosis distal to the air blockage (Figure 5-5).

Catheter Embolism

When a portion of an IV catheter breaks off, it can become an embolism. This can occur when a through-the-needle catheter (TNC) is inserted and a portion of it is sheared off, usually because the catheter is moved back and forth through the needle. It also happens when an over-the-needle catheter (ONC) is in place and the stylet is advanced back into the catheter.

Other Causes for Embolic Formation

Any particle in the blood can initiate the coagulation process. Other sources of embolism can be hair from the patient's extremity, and cotton, gauze, or linen fibers that enter the blood during venous cannulation. A clot on the tip of a cannula can be propelled into the circulation with improper irrigation technique. Failure to use a filter needle when drawing up IV additives from an ampule or vial can result in the introduction of glass or rubber-stopper fragments. Inadequately diluted solute-solvent admixtures can introduce particles of undissolved medications, which can embolize or attract platelets, which will form an even larger embolism. Bacteria circulating independently do not act as emboli, but if clusters form (when there is contamination to a vein at an IV puncture site), they may deteriorate the vein intima and cause shreds of the vein to break off.

NURSING TIP

Signs and Symptoms of Pulmonary Embolism

- Dyspnea
- Tachypnea
- Cardiac arrhythmia
- Hypotension
- Diaphoresis
- Anxiety
- Substernal pressure
- Chest pain with inhalation and exhalation
- Localized decreased breath sounds
- Pleural friction rub
- Cough (often with hemoptysis)

Nursing Assessment and Interventions

Emboli, no matter how small, will cause pulmonary embolism. If large enough, death is usually instantaneous. Nursing care is primarily aimed at prevention of thrombosis and emboli.

Blood Clot

If a clot lodges in a small branch of the pulmonary artery, the patient usually is tachypneic, dyspneic, and has fever. He complains of chest pain and has a cough, which some-

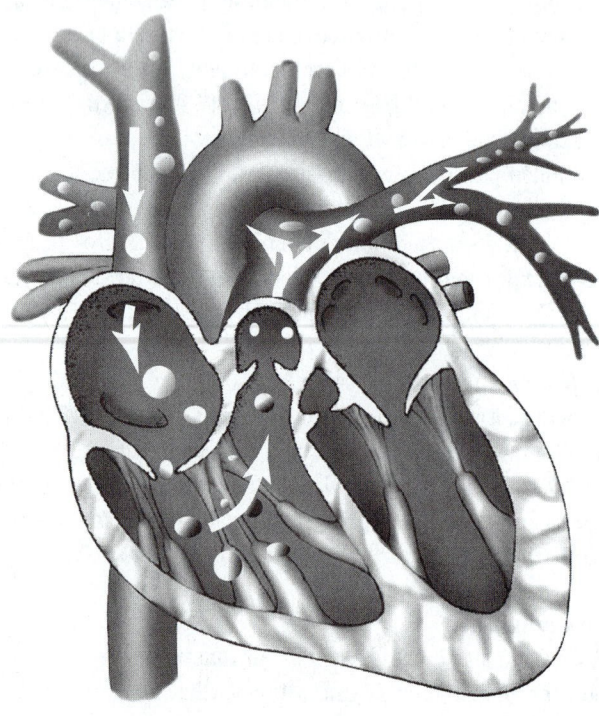

Figure 5-5 | Anatomy of an air embolism

times produces hemoptysis. Although a small embolism may not elicit any symptoms, it usually progresses to a larger one because its presence initiates the coagulation process.

CRITICAL THINKING

Discerning the Causes and Diagnosis of Chest Pain

Is your patient who is complaining of chest pain suffering from an infarction or something else? How do you know?

This is a frightening situation and can present a confusing dilemma. The nurse must be able to accurately assess the etiology of chest pain in any patient. This is especially important in the home care setting because of the potential need for emergency transport to a hospital. The nurse should remember that **angina pectoris** is chest pain caused by coronary artery spasm or constriction, not by an obstruction from a clot. The patient usually complains of substernal pressure that radiates to the neck, jaw, and down the right shoulder and arm. There may be dyspnea, diaphoresis, and pallor. It is usually temporary, reversible, and relieved with rest and nitroglycerin. A **myocardial infarction (MI)** results from prolonged ischemia from an infarcted vessel that causes hypoxia and irreversible damage to the myocardium if treatment is not initiated immediately. The symptoms may be similar to those of angina, or there may be no symptomatology (called silent heart attack). A patient having an MI does not experience relief of symptoms from rest and nitroglycerin.

When central organs are obstructed, pain and dysfunction result from infarction and necrosis. Renal vessel obstruction causes flank pain and oliguria. With mesenteric blockage, the patient has abdominal pain and cramping with impaired bowel mobility. Wherever blood flow is impeded, the necrotic tissue that results provides an ideal medium for bacterial growth and reproduction, which further compromises the patient.

Nursing care is primarily aimed at the prevention of thrombosis. For patients who are at risk for thrombus development, the nurse may be required to administer low-dose heparin or oral anticoagulants. She may need to plan activity and movement to discourage venous stasis. For IV therapy, leg veins must be avoided and it is important to use a cannula that is not too large for the vein. Blood products must be administered through appropriate filters. When checking for the patency of an IV line, fluid must never be

NURSING TIP

Instructing a Patient in the Valsalva Maneuver

Whenever a central venous line is accessed or changed, it is important to instruct the patient to perform a Valsalva maneuver. Ask him to take in a deep breath and, while holding it, bear down or push as if having a bowel movement.

forced into a line if there is any resistance to flow. Proper site preparation and cannulation technique must be used to prevent phlebitis, so that the sequence of events leading to embolization does not occur.

Should thrombosis occur, anticoagulants must be administered as ordered. It is important to give heparin (which rapidly acts to increase blood-clotting time) as scheduled to prevent the development of further thrombi. In some situations, the nurse may be required to administer thrombolytic drugs. Antiembolic stockings, or SCDs, are often used for both the prevention and treatment of thrombosis.

The nurse must promote comfort and gas exchange by elevating the head of the bed, assisting with coughing and deep breathing (unless contraindicated), administering analgesics, and maintaining a restful environment. To promote tissue perfusion, she must assist the patient with ROM exercises and active foot dorsiflexion. The leg must be inspected regularly but never massaged, to avoid breaking off a portion of the thrombus.

It is necessary to accurately document all signs and symptoms associated with thrombosis and monitor and report laboratory coagulation studies. The patency of the IV infusion must be maintained in case emergency venous access is needed.

Air Embolism

With infusion therapy, the possibility of air embolism is always present. The amount of air needed to cause death is not precisely known, but can occur with as little as 10 cc, depending the patient's size and condition. Once an air embolism occurs, the situation becomes very serious. Therefore, it is important to prevent the entry of air into the circulatory system.

The nurse can prevent air embolism by removing air from tubings and syringes prior to IV cannulation. It is important to secure all tubing junctions with tape and it is preferable to use Luer-lok connections as well. When accessing or changing lines on central venous infusions, the patient's head should be lowered (below the level of the heart) to raise thoracic venous pressure above atmospheric pressure, or instruct the patient to perform the Valsalva maneuver.

The signs and symptoms of air embolism are associated with vascular collapse and can be nonspecific. The patient may become extremely anxious and, if able, verbalize that death is approaching. There is dyspnea, hypotension, and tachypnea. The nurse, on auscultation, may hear a loud, churning sound over the heart, called a cog wheel murmur. It occurs because air and blood are obstructing ventricular output.

NURSING TIP

Signs and Symptoms of Air Embolism

- Extreme anxiety—fear of impending death
- Light-headedness and confusion
- Nausea
- Substernal pain
- Tachypnea
- Hypotension
- Cog wheel murmur

Treatment for air embolism is supportive, but the nurse must act quickly. If known, the source of air entry must be blocked. If cardiac arrest occurs, CPR must be initiated. Otherwise, the patient must be positioned on his left side with his head lowered below heart level (left lateral Trendelenburg). This traps air in the right atrium of the heart, keeping it from passing into the right ventricle and on to the pulmonary artery and lungs. 100% oxygen is delivered by mask to assist in reducing the embolism by assisting in the dissolution of nitrogen in the blood. If hemodynamic monitoring is being done and a lumen of the central line opens in the right atrium, medical or nursing intervention may include aspiration of air from the heart.

If the patient is conscious, he must be reassured and supported. Vital signs must be monitored and the patient observed for impending cardiac arrest. As with any situation, documentation must be thorough and accurate, and reflect the steps of the nursing process.

Catheter Embolism

With catheter embolism, the patient may complain of sudden, severe pain at the IV site and there will be a reduced or absent blood return upon checking for placement. If the catheter lodges in the pulmonary circulation or a chamber of the heart, there will be hypotension, tachycardia, chest pain, and cyanosis. The patient may lose consciousness. If the catheter does not migrate, the patient may be asymptomatic and the nurse will discover that the catheter is severed when she removes the cannula.

Catheter embolism can be prevented by inserting ONCs or TNCs according to procedure. As a general practice, infusions should never be started near a joint, where bending of the extremity could cause the catheter to break. If there is no other place, the joint must be prevented from flexure by placing it on an arm board.

Once it is ascertained that a catheter has broken, a tourniquet should be applied high on the extremity to limit venous flow and prevent embolism. Arterial circulation must not be impeded, so the nurse must be able to palpate a pulse distal to the tourniquet. The physician and radiologist must be notified and a new infusion must be started immediately. The patient must be kept on bed rest, receive cardiopulmonary support, and be prepared for x-ray or surgery. The catheter may have to be surgically removed or retrieved under angiography. The patient needs to be emotionally supported.

Documentation must include the patient's signs and symptoms, vital signs and level of consciousness, and the amount of catheter that is missing when the cannula is removed. The portion removed should be saved to determine the cause of breakage.

Other Causes of Embolic Formation

When embolism by thrombus, air, or catheter is ruled out, identification and treatment of other sources of embolism is usually symptomatic and supportive. Unless verified by x-ray or discovered during surgery or autopsy, other causes of embolism may not be determined.

Speed Shock

Speed shock is the systemic reaction to the rapid or excessive infusion of medication or infusate into the circulation. The body reacts by flushing, shock, or cardiac arrest.

Etiology and Defining Characteristics

With rapid administration of a fluid or medication, there is inadequate dilution with the circulating blood. The vital organs, therefore, are "shocked" by a toxic dose.

Speed shock can occur when a flow control clamp is inadvertently left completely open, allowing a large volume of fluid to infuse rapidly. It can also occur when an electronic infusion device (EID) is programmed incorrectly. Whenever an IV bolus or piggyback infusion of medication is given rapidly, plasma concentrations can reach unsafe or toxic proportions.

Nursing Assessment and Interventions

With speed shock, the first sign is usually flushing of the head and neck with the patient complaining of a severe,

NURSING TIP

Signs and Symptoms of Speed Shock

- Flushing of head and neck
- Feeling of apprehension
- Hypertension
- Pounding headache
- Dyspnea
- Chest pain
- Chills
- Loss of consciousness
- Cardiac arrest

pounding headache and a feeling of apprehension. (The patient may correlate the sensation, although more powerful, to that occurring when ice cream or a cold beverage is consumed too fast.) There is hypertension, tachycardia with arrhythmia, dyspnea, and loss of consciousness. Cardiac arrest can occur.

If cardiac arrest occurs, CPR must be initiated. The infusion must be slowed or stopped (and the vein kept open with another infusate), and the physician notified. Vital signs, level of consciousness, and neurologic checks must be evaluated and documented.

The best intervention for speed shock is prevention. A medication should never be given without reading and following the manufacturer's guidelines. For highly toxic medications, an EID or a volume-controlled set with microdrop delivery should be used.

Key Concepts

✳ Prevention is the best intervention for avoiding the complications of infusion therapy. Prior to initiating IV therapy, the nurse must make a detailed assessment of the patient, his level of consciousness, mental status, activity, and need for explanations, teaching, and reassurance.

✳ The nurse who administers infusion therapy must be fully knowledgeable of all the actual and potential complications that can arise and know how to prevent and treat such occurrences.

✳ The risks, complications, and adverse reactions associated with intravenous infusion therapy can exert a local and systemic effect on the patient. The nurse must always bear in mind that what starts out as a local complication can progress to a dangerous systemic process.

✳ Pain at the IV site is a primary warning that more serious complications may ensue. Since pain is subjective, it is extremely important for the nurse to assess, intervene, and evaluate each patient's discomfort on an

individual basis, always keeping in mind the emotional and psychological factors associated with pain.

✳ Infiltration is the most frequently encountered problem associated with infusion therapy. Because it is so common, it may sometimes be overlooked. Infiltration and extravasation can cause extreme discomfort, permanent damage, disfigurement, and loss of use in the extremity if left untreated.

✳ Phlebitis (bacterial, chemical, or mechanical) is a frequently encountered problem associated with infusion therapy that can lead to cellulitis, thromboembolic complications, sepsis, and death.

✳ It is important for the nurse to understand the pathophysiologic cascade effect of the clotting process that occurs in response to foreign material (solid, liquid, or gas) entering the circulatory system.

✳ The nurse who initiates, monitors, and maintains intravenous infusion therapy is responsible for following the established policies and procedures of the agency where she is employed.

Review Questions and Activities

1. List the local complications of infusion therapy and briefly outline how each one can progress to a systemic problem.

2. Formulate three nursing diagnoses (actual or potential problems) for each of the following:
   (a) Infiltration
   (b) Phlebitis
   (c) Cellulitis
   (d) Venous spasm

3. Name five commonly administered intravenous drugs that have vesicant properties.

4. Look up in your nurses' drug guide and your institution's procedure manual the antidotes for the five vesicants listed in the previous question.

5. Outline the sequence of events in the progression of phlebitis to thrombophlebitis and embolism.

6. Explain the variables that contribute to a hypersensitivity reaction.

7. Write a nursing care plan for a patient with sepsis that developed from contamination with *Staphylococcus aureus* during cannulation of the vein prior to an outpatient endoscopy.

8. List the nursing interventions, with rationales, used for a patient with an air embolism.

9. Describe the signs, symptoms, and nursing interventions for a patient with speed shock.

10. Develop a teaching plan for a patient who has just developed a generalized rash following the IV administration of penicillin.

Chapter 6

Intravenous Infusion Preparations

KEY TERMS

| colloid | crystallization | crystalloid |

In addition to having a substantial knowledge of the principles of fluid, electrolyte, and acid-base balance, the nurse must also understand the principles of fluid volume maintenance, replacement, and restoration in order to safely manage infusion therapy and promote a state of homeostasis for the patient. Although the physician prescribes infusions, the nurse must know what they are, confirm if they are appropriate for the patient, and administer them correctly.

Body water, which accounts for 50%–70% of adult body weight, is distributed between the ICF and the ECF compartments. The ECF is further divided into subcompartments, which are in a state of dynamic movement, constantly bathing the cells to maintain homeostasis (Figure 6-1). Electrolytes, which make up about 95% of the body's solute molecules, are crucial to the distribution and movement of water and for the maintenance of acid-base balance. They provide the chemicals needed to carry out cellular reactions and regulate vital cellular control mechanisms.

NURSING TIP

Approximate Intake Requirements

The approximate daily average intake requirements of a moderately active adult who weighs 145 lb (65.9 kg) is as follows:

Water	1974 ml
Calories	2174.5
Carbohydrates (46%)	1000.04 kcal
Fats (30%)	652.20 kcal
Proteins (24%)	521.76 kcal
Sodium	1100–3300 mg
Potassium	1875–5624 mg
Chloride	1700–5100 mg
Calcium	800–1200 mg
Magnesium	325 mg
Phosphorus	800–1200 mg

Plus vitamins, minerals, and trace elements (Dudek, 2001)

In the average adult, daily water requirements are approximately 30 ml/kg (13.6 ml/lb) of body weight. The recommended dietary allowances (RDA) in kilocalories (kcal) are estimated at 33 kilocalories per kilogram or 15 kilocalories per pound of ideal body weight, with 46% derived from carbohydrates, 30% from fat, and 24% from protein. In addition the body must be supplemented with electrolytes, vitamins, minerals, and various trace elements to maintain homeostasis (Dudek, 2001).

OSMOLALITY AND OSMOLARITY

Osmolality is the osmotic pull or pressure exerted by all particles per unit of water (expressed as milliosmoles per kilogram of water), and osmolarity is the osmotic pull (pressure) exerted by all particles per unit of solution (expressed as milliosmoles per liter of solution). A unit of osmotic pressure is the osmole (Osm) and the milliosmole (mOsm) is $1/1000$th of an osmole. Osmotic pressure determines osmotic activity (Kee & Paulanka, 2004).

Extracellular fluid compartment (ECF)

Cell	ECF is composed of:
(ICF) Intracellular fluid	Plasma (in the intravascular compartment)
	ISF (interstitial fluid) (in the space between the cells)
	Lymph (in lymphatic vessels)
	Bone (water bound to intracellular bone)
	Connective tissue (water bound to dense connective tissue)
	Transcellular fluids (formed as a result of cellular activity):
	Mucus
	Digestive juices
	Fluid in the lumen of the gastrointestinal tract
	Serous fluid
	Synovial fluid
	Cerebrospinal fluid (CSF)
	Ocular fluid
	Genitourinary secretions

Figure 6-1 | Total blood volume distribution between the ICF and ECF

Osmolality is influenced by the quantity of dissolved particles that exert an osmotic pull in the intracellular and extracellular fluids. The primary solutes are serum sodium, urea, and glucose. Under normal circumstances, as the nurse will recall, there is very little difference between the osmolality of body fluids. Plasma (in the intravascular compartment) contains proteins and has a slightly higher osmolality than fluid in other areas. The concentration of plasma, though, is only about 25% of that found in the ICF. Interstitial fluid has little to no protein.

NURSING TIP

Differentiating Osmolality and Osmolarity

Both osmolality and osmolarity are used to characterize tonicity. Since body solutions are very dilute, osmolality is the term used to clinically characterize tonicity. Osmolarity describes the tonicity of infusions that are administered intravenously.

It is the responsibility of the nurse to know whether a prescribed infusate is hypertonic, hypotonic, or isotonic, and to determine which route is appropriate for its administration. Plasma, under normal conditions, has approximately 280–300 mOsm/L and is isotonic (or isosmotic). Anything below this range is considered hypotonic, while anything above it is hypertonic. The normal isotonic plasma level is used as the standard for comparing the tonicity of intravenous infusions. With parenteral fluid administration, the IV infusion is determined by the average serum osmolality (290 mOsm). The normal osmolality range is +50 mOsm or −50 mOsm of 290 mOsm (Kee & Paulanka, 2004). An infusion with about the same osmolality of serum is categorized as isotonic. If it is +50 mOsm higher, it is hypertonic (340 mOsm or more), and if it is −50 mOsm below 290, it is hypotonic (240 mOsm or less).

NURSING TIP

Differentiating Plasma and Serum

Plasma is the liquid portion of the blood without corpuscles and consists of serum (plasma that has lost its fibrinogen, or Factor I, due to the clotting process), protein, and chemicals.

When the body is in a healthy state, there is a normal pattern of water intake and loss (Figure 6-2) and a balanced movement of water molecules back and forth between

Intake
Liquid 1200 ml
Food 1000 ml
Oxidation of food 300 ml

Output

Lungs 500 ml

Skin 500 ml

Urine 1400 ml

Feces 100 ml

Total 2500 ml

Total 2500 ml

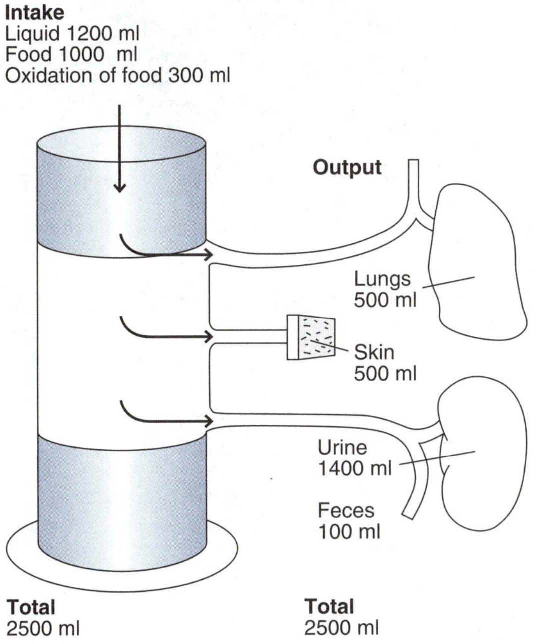

Figure 6-2 | Normal pattern of water intake and loss

the fluid compartments. This movement is controlled by colloid osmotic and hydrostatic pressures as well as the sodium-potassium pump and ATP.

NURSING TIP

Differentiating Hydrostatic Pressure and Osmotic Pressure

Hydrostatic pressure is regulated by the number of molecules contained in a given volume of fluid. Osmotic pressure is governed by the number of solutes contained in a volume of solution.

During illness and disease, physical and chemical alterations occur that impede the normal regulatory mechanisms that contribute to fluid balance (Table 6-1). When one or more of these controls falters, medical and nursing interventions are aimed at restoring and supporting homeostasis through the implementation of intravenous infusion therapy.

DETERMINATION OF FLUID BALANCE

Before IV therapy is initiated, it is necessary to determine if a fluid imbalance exists, and then attempt to identify what precipitated it. To do this it is essential to know what a patient's serum osmolality is, so the correct infusion can be administered to rectify an abnormal condition.

Table 6-1 | Regulators of Fluid Balance

REGULATORS	ACTIONS
Thirst	An indicator of fluid need.
Electrolytes Sodium (Na)	Sodium promotes water retention. With a water deficit, more sodium is reabsorbed from the renal tubules.
Protein, albumin	Protein and albumin promote body fluid retention. These nondiffusable substances increase the colloid osmotic (oncotic) pressure.
Hormones Antiduretic hormone (ADH)	ADH is produced by the hypothalamus and stored in the posterior pituitary gland (neurohypophysis). ADH is secreted when there is an ECF volume deficit. ADH promotes water reabsorption from the distal tubules of the kidneys.
Aldosterone	Aldosterone is secreted from the adrenal cortex. It promotes sodium reabsorption from the renal tubules.
Renin	Decreased renal blood flow increases the release of renin from the juxtaglomerular cells of the kidneys. Renin promotes peripheral vasoconstriction and the release of aldosterone (sodium and water retention).
Lymphatics	Plasma protein that shifts to the tissue spaces cannot be reabsorbed into the blood vessels. Thus, the lymphatic system promotes the return of water and protein from the interstitial spaces to the vascular spaces.
Skin	Skin excretes approximately 500 ml of water daily through normal perspiration.
Lungs	Lungs excrete approximately 500 ml of water daily with normal breathing.
Kidneys	The kidneys excrete 1200 to 1500 ml of body water daily. The amount of water excretion may vary according to fluid intake and fluid loss.

From *Fluids and Electrolytes with Clinical Applications: A Programmed Approach* (7th ed.), by J. L. Kee, B. J. Paulanka, & L. Purnell, 2004, Clifton Park, NY: Delmar Learning.

To accurately calculate serum osmolality, the following formula, based on the serum sodium, urea, and glucose levels (Kee & Paulanka, 2004) is used: multiply the serum sodium by two; add the BUN, which has been divided by 3; and add the glucose, which has been divided by 18 (Table 6-2).

Table 6-2 | Mathematical Formula for Calculating Serum Osmolality

$$2 \times \text{serum sodium} + \frac{\text{BUN}}{3} + \frac{\text{glucose}}{18} = \text{Serum osmality}$$

CLASSIFICATIONS OF INFUSATES

The five basic classifications of IV infusions are crystalloids, colloids, hydrating solutions (sources of free water and calories), hypertonic-hyperosmolar preparations, and blood or blood components (Kee & Paulanka, 2004). The first three are covered in this chapter; the other two are detailed in Chapters 13 and 14.

Crystalloids

Crystalloids are materials that are capable of **crystallization**, or have the ability to form crystals. Crystalloids are solutes that, when placed in a solvent, homogeneously mix with and dissolve into a solution and cannot be distinguished from the resultant solution. Because of this, crystalloid solutions are considered true solutions and are able to diffuse through membranes. Crystalloid infusions are usually electrolyte solutions that may be isotonic, hypotonic, or hypertonic.

Colloids

Colloids are glutinous substances whose particles, when submerged in a solvent, cannot form a true solution because their molecules, when thoroughly dispersed, do not dissolve, but remain uniformly suspended and distributed throughout the fluid. Because of this, such fluids have a cloudy appearance. The particles of colloidal dispersions are too large to pass through cell membranes.

Intravenous colloid infusions raise colloid osmotic pressure, thus they are often called plasma or volume expanders. When small amounts of plasma proteins are forced into the interstitium at the arterial end of the circulation, because of the increased pressure, they cannot return at the venous capillary end, so they are removed by way of lymph vessels. The colloid infusions that are commonly used consist of albumin, dextran, plasmanate, and the artificial blood substitute, hetastarch (see Chapter 14).

Hydrating Solutions

Various infusions are frequently administered to patients to supplement caloric intake, supply nutrients, provide free water for maintenance or rehydration, or promote effective renal output. When used, their chemical makeup or rate of administration is adjusted so the equilibria of body fluids are not disturbed. Glucose solutions are most often used. When glucose and other nutrients are administered in water, they are quickly metabolized, leaving an excess of water. This is why glucose solutions are often called hydrating solutions. Any water that is not needed by the body is excreted by the kidneys in the form of dilute urine.

> ## NURSING TIP
>
> ### Frequently Used Hydrating Solutions
>
> Hydrating solutions that are often infused for maintenance, rehydration, and to enhance renal output are as follows:
>
> Dextrose 2½% in 0.45% saline
> Dextrose 5% in water
> Dextrose 5% in 0.45% saline
> Sodium chloride 0.45%
> Dextrose 5% in 0.2% saline

DETERMINING TONICITY

Depending on the type of infusate, the addition of glucose and electrolytes determines the tonicity of the infusion. Just as the nurse can calculate the patient's serum osmolality, so can he determine the osmolarity of the infusion his patient is receiving. Osmotic pressure, remember, is determined by the measurement of the total number of particles in a volume of solution.

Electrolyte Solutions

One gram mole of a substance that is nonpermeable and non-ionizable equals one osmole. If the substance is capable of ionization, such as sodium chloride, 0.5 g of the mole of the substance equals one osmole. As discussed earlier, because the osmole unit is too big in relation to body fluid osmolality, the milliosmole unit is used. With electrolyte-containing infusates, each milliequivalent of an electrolyte equals one milliosmole. Milliequivalents measure how many chemically active ions are present in a solution.

When a monovalent electrolyte, such as normal saline, is placed in a solvent and ionized, or separated, the amount of electrolyte is equal to the sum of the separated ions. Sodium chloride contains 154 mEq/L of sodium and 154 mEq/L of chloride. The osmolarity, therefore, is about 308 mOsm/L. 0.45% NaCl (half-strength saline) has 77 mEq/L of sodium and 77 mEq/L of chloride, making the osmolarity 154 mEq/L.

Dextrose Solutions

Dextrose solutions, which are frequently used as infusates, are manufactured as percentage concentrations in water or sodium chloride. Remember that percentage solutions express the number of grams of solute per 100 g of solvent. A 5% dextrose in water (D_5W) infusion contains 5 g of dextrose in 100 ml of water. One ml of water equals one gram.

> ## NURSING TIP
>
> ### Percentage Solutions
>
> Percentage solutions express the number of grams of solute per 100 g (100 ml) of solvent.

To determine the osmolarity of dextrose infusions, it is necessary to know the caloric value of dextrose and the number of milligrams in one millimole of dextrose. The monohydrate form of dextrose used in parenteral solutions provides 3.4 kcal/g (dietary glucose contains 4 kcal/g). Table 6-3 illustrates how to calculate the number of calories in infusions containing varying percentages of dextrose.

Table 6-3 | Calculation of Kilocalories in Dextrose Infusions

STRENGTH	CALORIC VALUE
2%	6.8 kcal/100 ml (68 kcal/L)
2.5%	8.5 kcal/100 ml (85 kcal/L)
5%	17.0 kcal/100 ml (170 kcal/L)
10%	34.0 kcal/100 ml (340 kcal/L)
20%	68.0 kcal/100 ml (680 kcal/L)
25%	85.0 kcal/100 ml (850 kcal/L)
50%	170.0 kcal/100 ml (1,700 kcal/L)

Note:
1 ml of water	=	1 g
1 g	=	3.4 kcal
A 1% solution	=	1 g/100 ml
A 1% solution	=	3.4 kcal/100 ml

Table 6-4 │ Calculation of Osmolarity of Dextrose Infusions
STRENGTH

1%	=	1 g of dextrose/100ml
	=	10 g/L (10,000 mg/1000 ml)
		1 mmol of dextrose
	=	198 mg
		(10 mg = 1 ml)
		(10,000 mg = 1 L)
1%	=	$\dfrac{10,000}{198\ mg/mOsm}$ = 50.50 mOsm/L
2.5%	=	2.5 g of dextrose/100ml
	=	25 g/L (25,000 mg/ml)
		1 mmol of dextrose
	=	198 mg
		(25 mg = 1 ml)
		25,000 mg = 1 L)
		$\dfrac{25,000\ mg/L}{198\ mg/mOsm}$ = 126.26 mOsm/L
5%	=	5 g of dextrose/100ml
	=	50 g/L (50,000 mg/ml)
		1 mmol of dextrose
	=	198 mg
		(50 mg = 1 ml)
		50,000 mg = 1 L)
		$\dfrac{50,000\ mg/L}{198\ mg/mOsm}$ = 252.52 mOsm/L

Note: 1 millimole (weight in mg) of monohydrate dextrose = 198 mg of dextrose

1 millimole of monohydrate dextrose = 1 mOsm of osmotic pressure

1 milliliter of water = 1 gram

One millimole of dextrose contains 198 mg of dextrose. One milliosmole of dextrose equals 1 mOsm of osmotic pressure. There is 1 mg in 1 ml. Table 6-4 illustrates how to formulate the osmolarity of infusions with different percentages of dextrose.

INFUSATES: CATEGORIES OF TONICITY

When the body is in a state of homeostasis the serum osmolality is the same as that in other body fluids, approximately 280–300 mOsm/L. IV infusions are isotonic, hypotonic, or hypertonic when compared to serum osmolality.

It is important for the nurse to understand the tonicity of every infusion order so he can determine if it is safe for his patient, discern what type of vein to access for the infusion, and regulate the rate appropriately.

Isotonic Infusates

Isotonic or isosmotic infusates have the same tonicity as body fluids. Because of this, they do not alter osmolality and, once infused, they remain within the intravascular space because osmotic pressure is equal between the intracellular and extracellular compartments. For this reason, they are used to treat hypotension resulting from hypovolemia. Isotonic infusions, because they are compatible with the plasma, can be administered at a more rapid rate than hypo or hypertonic solutions. Figure 6-3 illustrates how red blood cells (RBCs) maintain their size and shape when placed in an isotonic solution of 0.9% NaCl. Isotonic infusions are primarily used to expand the intravascular compartment, as depicted in Figure 6-4. Table 6-5 outlines the various isotonic infusions available, their indications for use, and precautions associated with them.

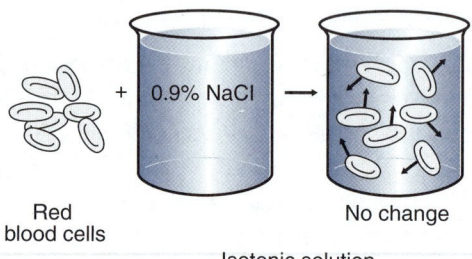

Red blood cells · + · 0.9% NaCl → · No change

Isotonic solution

Figure 6-3 │ Red blood cells maintain their size and shape in isotonic 0.9% NaCl.

Physiologic effect of an isotonic infusion

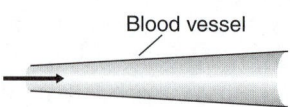

Blood vessel

Figure 6-4 │ Isotonic infusion expands the intravascular space because osmotic pressure is equal.

Table 6-5 | Isotonic Infusions: Indications for Use and Precautions

INFUSION	OSMO-LARITY	INDICATIONS AND INCOMPATIBILITIES	PRECAUTIONS, COMMENTS, CONTRAINDICATIONS
5% dextrose in water (D₅W) 50 g dextrose per liter pH 4.5 (3.5–6.5)	252.52 mOsm/L	**Indications:** Hydration: replaces water losses in dehydration Provides free water for the excretion of solutes Provides 20 kcal/100 ml (200 kcal/L) Diluent for medications **Incompatibilities:** Ampicillin sodium (after 2 hr) Diazepam Erythromycin lactobinate (after 6 hr) Fat emulsions Phenytoin sodium Procainamide Sodium bicarbonate Warfarin sodium Whole blood Vitamin B₁₂	D_5W is isotonic in the container. Once infused, the dextrose is rapidly metabolized and the infusion becomes hypotonic Do not administer to patients with increased intracranial pressure because it is hypotonic in the body and will increase edema D_5W does not contain electrolytes Because of excess ADH secretions, as a stress response to surgery, use cautiously in the early postoperative period to prevent water intoxication Hypokalemia can occur because, during the cellular use of glucose, potassium shifts from the ECF to the ICF Use cautiously in patients with signs of fluid overload and CHF Can cause dehydration from osmotic diuresis if infused too rapidly D_5W may alter insulin or oral hypoglycemic needs in diabetics Contraindicated in diabetic coma Contraindicated in patients allergic to corn and corn products
Normal saline (0.9% NaCl) Na 154 mEq/L Cl 154 mEq/L pH 5 (4.5–7.0)	308 mOsm/L	**Indications:** Replaces ECF losses by expanding the intravascular space when chloride loss is greater than sodium loss Corrects hyponatremia Corrects hypovolemia Replaces sodium losses Corrects mild metabolic acidosis Corrects metabolic alkalosis when fluid depletion exists because the chloride ions cause a decrease in bicarbonate ions Only infusate compatible with blood; used to initiate and follow transfusions Diluent for medications Used as an irrigant for intravascular devices Maintains patency of heparin locks **Incompatibilities:** Amphotericin B Chlordiazepoxide hydrochloride Diazepam Fat emulsions Levarterenol Mannitol Methylprednisolone sodium succinate Phenytoin sodium	Accurately monitor I & O Can cause intravascular overload Can cause hypokalemia because saline promotes potassium excretion Can cause hypernatremia Can induce hyperchloremic acidosis due to loss of bicarbonate ions Normal saline can cause sodium retention during the intraoperative and early postoperative periods. Does not provide free water Does not provide calories Use with caution in patients with decreased renal function Use with caution in patients with altered circulatory function Use with caution in the elderly Contraindicated in the presence of edema with sodium retention Causes excess sodium retention when used with glucocorticoids

continues

Table 6-5 | Isotonic Infusions: Indications for Use and Precautions (*continued*)

INFUSION	OSMO-LARITY	INDICATIONS AND INCOMPATIBILITIES	PRECAUTIONS, COMMENTS, CONTRAINDICATIONS
Dextrose in Saline Solutions		**Indications:**	To prevent circulatory overload, use with caution in the following:
0.2% dextrose in 0.9% NaCl	318.1 mOsm/L	Rehydration by replenishment of salt and water	patients with CHF
2 g dextrose per liter (10.1 mOsm/L)		Fluid replacement for burns	patients with pulmonary edema
Na 154 mEq/L		Supply calories	patients with edema with sodium retention
Cl 154 mEq/L		Reduce nitrogen depletion	patients undergoing corticosteroid therapy
pH 4.5 (3.5–6.5)		Used in place of plasma expanders (until they are available) to treat circulatory insufficiency and shock	patients with urinary obstruction
2.5% dextrose in 0.45% NaCl	264.86 mOsm/L	Hypotonic saline with dextrose infusions (2.5 % D in 0.45 NaCl and 5% D in 0.2% NaCl) are used to establish renal function prior to electrolyte administration	Maintain strict I & O
25 g dextrose per liter (126.26 mOsm/L)		D_5 in 0.2% NaCl is used as a maintenance infusion	Contraindicated in patients in diabetic coma
Na 69.3 mEq/L			Contraindicated in patients with allergies to corn and corn products
Cl 69.3 mEq/L		**Incompatibilities:**	May falsely elevate BUN laboratory reports
pH 4.0 (3.5–6.5)		Amphotericin B	Once renal function is assured, electrolytes must be supplemented to prevent hypokalemia
5% dextrose in 0.2% NaCl	314.12 mOsm/L	Ampicillin sodium	
50 g dextrose per liter (252.52 mOsm/L)		Diazepam	
Na 30.8 mEq/L		Erythromycin lactobinate	
Cl 30.8 mEq/L		Mannitol	
pH 4.0 (3.5–6.5)		Phenytoin	
		Warfarin sodium	
		Whole blood	
Ringer's solution	310 mOsm/L	**Indications:**	Provides no calories (When dextrose is added to Ringer's solution, the dextrose provides calories and spares protein loss)
Na 147 mEq/L		Restores fluid balance	
K 4 mEq/L		Restores electrolyte balance	May exacerbate the following:
Ca 4 mEq/L		Replaces ECF loss resulting from dehydration, gastrointestinal losses, and fistula drainage	sodium retention
Cl 155 mEq/L			CHF
pH 5.5 (5.0–7.5)		Used instead of lactated Ringer's when patients have liver disease and are unable to metabolize lactate	renal insufficiency
		May be used as a blood replacement for a short period of time	Maintain strict I & O
			Added potassium is needed to correct severe hypokalemia
		Incompatibilities:	Contraindicated in renal failure
		Ampicillin sodium	
		Cefamandole	
		Cyphradine	
		Chlordiazepoxide	
		Diazepam	
		Erythromycin lactobinate	
		Methicillin	
		Phenytoin	
		Potassium phosphate	
		Sodium bicarbonate	
		Whole blood	

continues

Table 6-5 | Isotonic Infusions: Indications for Use and Precautions (*continued*)

INFUSION	OSMO-LARITY	INDICATIONS AND INCOMPATIBILITIES	PRECAUTIONS, COMMENTS, CONTRAINDICATIONS

Lactated Ringer's (Hartmann's solution)
 	
Na 130 mEq/L
Cl 109 mEq/L
K 4 mEq/L
Ca 3 mEq/L
Lactate 28 mEq/L
pH 6.5
(6.0–7.5)
	274 mOsm/L	**Indications:**
		Restores fluid volume deficit
		Used for rehydration in *most* types of dehydration
		Replaces fluid lost as a result of *bile loss*, *burns*, or *diarrhea*
		Treats mild metabolic acidosis
		Treats diabetic ketoacidosis
		Treats salicylate overdose
		
		Incompatibilities:
		Amphotericin B
		Ampicillin sodium
		Cefamandole
		Cephradine
		Chlordiazepoxide
		Diazepam
		Erythromycin lactobinate
		Methicillin
		Methylprednisolone sodium succinate
		Oxytetracycline
		Phenytoin sodium
		Potassium phosphate
		Sodium bicarbonate
		Thiopental
		Warfarin
		Whole blood
			Resembles blood serum electrolyte content
			Provides 9 calories from lactate
			Lactate is metabolized to bicarbonate in the liver
			Does not provide free water for renal excretion
			Can precipitate hypernatremia because the amount of potassium is not sufficient for daily requirements
			Hyperkalemia can develop with use of potassium-sparing diuretics and potassium supplementation
			Contraindicated with severe metabolic acidosis and alkalosis
			Contraindicated in hypoxia
			Contraindicated with hepatic disease where the liver is unable to metabolize lactate
			May exacerbate the following:
			  CHF
			  edema
			  sodium retention

Multiple Electrolyte Solutions
Plasma-Lyte R® (Baxter)
Isolyte E® (McGaw)
Na 140 mEq/L
Cl 103 mEq/L
K 10 mEq/L
Ca 5 mEq/L
Mg 3 mEq/L
Acetate 47 mEq/L
Lactate 8 mEq/L
pH 5.5
(4.0–6.5)
	316 mOsm/L	**Indications:**
		Replace water and electrolytes caused by the following:
		  severe diarrhea
		  severe vomiting
		  gastric suctioning
			Monitor electrolytes because, once the deficits have been replaced, hyperkalemia can occur
			Monitor I & O
			Observe for signs of circulatory overload

Plasma-Lyte 148® Na 140 mEq/L Cl 98 mEq/L K 5 mEq/L Ca 0 Mg 3 mEq/L Acetate 27 mEq/L Gluconate 23 mEq/L pH 5.5 (4.0–6.5)	296 mOsm/L		
Plasma-Lyte A®	296 mOsm/L	Plasma-Lyte® has the same constituents as Plasma-Lyte 148,® but has a pH of 7.4 (6.5–8.0) and is used in anesthesia	
Gastric replacement solutions			In addition to the constituents in the electrolyte replacement solutions, gastric replacement fluids have the addition of ammonium ions

continues

Table 6-5   │   Isotonic Infusions: Indications for Use and Precautions (*continued*)

INFUSION	OSMO-LARITY	INDICATIONS AND INCOMPATIBILITIES	PRECAUTIONS, COMMENTS, CONTRAINDICATIONS
Alkalinizing Fluids **Sodium lactate ⅙ molar (M/6 sodium lactate)** Na 167 mEq/L Lactate 167 mEq/L pH 6.5 (6.0–7.3)	334 mOsm/L	**Indications:** Mild to moderate acidosis, not for the treatment of lactic acidosis Alkalinization of urine **Incompatibilities:** Oxytetracycline Sodium bicarbonate	Contraindicated in lactic acidosis Contraindicated with hypernatremia Contraindicated in hypoxic patients Can exacerbate respiratory or metabolic alkalosis Use with caution when administering to patients with conditions that increase lactate use, such as hepatic insufficiency Monitor glucose, electrolytes, and acid-base balance Strict I & O Daily weight Monitor for fluid retention Administer with caution to patients with altered (reduced) tissue perfusion
Sodium bicarbonate ⅙ molar (1.45% sodium bicarbonate) Na 166.70 mEq/L HCO₃ 166.70 mEq/L pH 8.0 (7.0–8.5)	333 mOsm/L	**Indications:** Treats systemic acidosis Increases serum bicarbonate and buffers excess hydrogen Alkalinization of urine **Incompatabilities:** Numerous; consult pharmacist **Drug Interactions:** Numerous; consult pharmacist	Contraindicated in chloride depletion from gastrointestinal losses Contraindicated in hypocalcemia Use with caution in patients with renal insufficiency Use extreme caution in patients with edema due to sodium retention Monitor for signs of alkalosis (overdose) Take precautions to prevent extravasation
Acidifying Fluids **0.9% sodium chloride**	308 mOsm/L	**Indications:** Corrects metabolic alkalosis when fluid depletion exists because the chloride ions cause a decrease in bicarbonate ions	See comments under normal saline
Ammonium chloride solution 0.9% NH₄ 168 mEq/L Cl 168 mEq/L	336 mOsm/L	Systemic acidifier indicated for severe metabolic alkalosis resulting from vomiting, gastric suctioning, or chloride depletion from diuretic use Rids body of excess hydrogen ions in metabolic acidosis and supplies chloride Ammonium ion is converted to hydrogen ion and ammonium then excreted as urea in the urine **Incompatibilities:** Alkalides and their carbonates Dimenhydrinate Levorphanol tartrate Methadone Potent oxidizing agents Warfarin	Can produce dangerous dysrhythmias Accurate I & O Accurate respiratory assessment Seizure precautions Contraindicated in severe liver disease because the liver is unable to convert ammonium ions to urea; ammonia retention results in hepatic coma Contraindicated in primary respiratory alkalosis due to chance of development of systemic acidosis

continues

Table 6-5 | Isotonic Infusions: Indications for Use and Precautions (*continued*)

INFUSION	OSMO-LARITY	INDICATIONS AND INCOMPATIBILITIES	PRECAUTIONS, COMMENTS, CONTRAINDICATIONS
Mannitol 5% in 0.45 NaCl (Osmitrol,® Resectisol®) pH 5.0 (4.5–7.0)	274 mOsm/L	**Indications:** Diuresis Treatment of oliguria Reduction of increased intracranial pressure Reduction of cerebrospinal fluid pressure Reduction of intraocular pressure **Incompatibilities:** Blood products Imipenem/cilastic sodium	Strict I & O Hourly vital signs Closely monitor BUN and electrolytes, especially sodium and potassium levels Contraindicated with anuria due to possibility of circulatory overload Can cause renal failure May induce dangerous dysrhythmias May exacerbate intracranial bleeding May cause congestive heart failure in patients with cardiopulmonary compromise May exacerbate electrolyte imbalances Monitor for rebound increase in intracranial, cerebrospinal, and intraocular pressures within 12 to 24 hours after administration
Plasma Volume Expanders **Dextran 70 and 0.9% NaCl (6% Gentran® 70 and 0.9% NaCl)** Na 154 mEq/L Cl 154 mEq/L pH 5.0 (4.0–6.5) **Dextran 40 and 0.9% NaCl (10% Gentran® and 0.9% NaCl)** Na 154 mEq/L Cl 154 mEq/L pH 5.0 (3.5–7.0) **Dextran 40 and D₅W (10% Gentran® and D₅W)** pH 4.0 (3.0–7.0)	 308 mOsm/L 308 mOsm/L 255 mOsm/L	**Indications:** Restoration of circulatory dynamics Fluid replacement Treatment of perioperative shock Used prophylactically in surgical patients at risk for acute thrombosis and embolization Hemorrhage Trauma Moves water from body tissues to increase urinary output **Incompatibilities:** Ascorbic acid Chlortetracycline Phytonadione Promethazine Protein hydrosylate	**Caution:** Never add any medications to dextran infusions. **Contraindicated with:** Cardiac decompensation Coagulation defects Corticosteroid therapy Hypersensitivity to dextran Hypervolemia Pulmonary edema Renal failure Severe bleeding disorders Monitor for any signs of allergic reaction Never administer near site of trauma or infection Monitor I & O hourly Monitor pulse, blood pressure, and central venous pressure (CVP) hourly Monitor specific gravity Monitor for fluid overload Monitor for signs of bleeding Monitor for exacerbation of bleeding Monitor site of infusion for venous thrombosis and phlebitis **Comments:** Solution must be clear—not cloudy Crystallization may occur; before administration, submerge bottle in warm water to dissolve crystals

continues

Table 6-5 │ Isotonic Infusions: Indications for Use and Precautions (*continued*)

INFUSION	OSMO-LARITY	INDICATIONS AND INCOMPATIBILITIES	PRECAUTIONS, COMMENTS, CONTRAINDICATIONS
Hetastarch (HES) 6% in 0.9% NaCl Na 154 mEq/L Cl 154 mEq/L pH 5.5	308 mOsm/L	**Indications:** Similar to dextran but causes fewer allergic reactions Used in shock due to sepsis, acute hemorrhage, or burns Similar to human albumin in colloidal properties **Incompatibilities:** Amikacin Ampicillin Cefamandol Cefazolin Cefonicid Cefoperazone Cefotaxime Cefoxitin Cephalothin Gentamicin Phenytoin Ranitidine Theophylline Tobramycin	Contraindicated with severe bleeding disorders Contraindicated in congestive and renal failure Maintain strict I & O Monitor CVP and PCWP (hemodynamic monitoring) to assess for circulatory overload

Hypotonic Infusions

Hypotonic infusions lower serum osmolality by causing fluid to shift out of the blood and into the cells and interstitial spaces. These solutions are used to hydrate the intracellular and interstitial compartments and lower sodium levels. The rate of administration of hypotonic infusions must be carefully controlled to prevent water from hemolyzing RBCs (rupture). Figure 6-5 illustrates how hemolysis occurs when RBCs are placed in hypotonic free water, with water passing from the blood vessels into the cells, causing the RBC to burst. Because hypotonic infusions hydrate the intracellular compartment, care must be taken to prevent circulatory depletion. They should not be administered to hypotensive

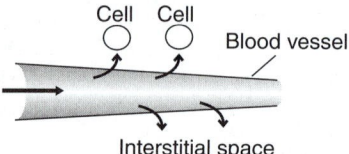

Physiologic effect of hypotonic infusion

Figure 6-6 │ Hypotonic infusion lowers serum osmolality by causing fluid to shift out of the intravascular space and into the cells and interstitial spaces.

patients, as this can further lower blood pressure. Figure 6-6 shows the physiologic effect of the administration of a hypotonic infusion. Table 6-6 lists the hypotonic infusions available, their indications for use, and the precautions associated with them.

Hypertonic Infusions

Hypertonic infusions raise serum osmolality by causing a pull of fluids from the intracellular and interstitial compartments into the blood vessels. They act to greatly expand the intravascular compartment and are administered when there is a serious saline depletion. Extreme caution must be exercised with hypertonic infusions to prevent cir-

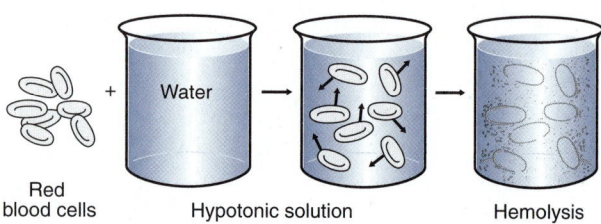

Figure 6-5 │ Red blood cells hemolyze when placed in hypotonic (free) water.

Table 6-6 | Hypotonic Infusions: Indications for Use and Precautions

INFUSION	OSMO-LARITY	INDICATIONS AND INCOMPATIBILITIES	PRECAUTIONS, COMMENTS, CONTRAINDICATIONS
Dextrose in Water Solutions **2.5% dextrose in water** **25 g dextrose per liter** pH 4.5 (3.6–6.5) **5% dextrose in water** (Reminder: D_5W is isotonic, but it becomes hypotonic when it is infused because the dextrose is metabolized rapidly.)	126 mOsm/L 252.52 mOsm/L	**Indications:** Provides 85 kcal/L Diluent for medications Provides hydration to cells in hyperglycemic situations and in cellular dehydration associated with diuretic administration Review Table 6-5: Isotonic Infusions **Incompatibilities:** Refer to isotonic dextrose in water above	Depletes intravascular compartment Monitor for signs of cardiovascular collapse from fluid volume depletion Contraindicated in patients with increased intracranial pressure Contraindicated in patients with decreased serum protein levels Assess for hypokalemia after prolonged use without potassium supplementation Review under isotonic infusions. D_5W is isotonic in the container. Once it is infused, the dextrose is rapidly metabolized, and the infusion becomes hypotonic. Review Table 6-5: Isotonic Infusions
Sodium Chloride Solutions **0.45% (half normal)** **saline** pH 5.0 (4.5–7.0)	154 mOsm/L	**Indications:** Used when fluid losses exceed electrolyte depletion Preferable to 0.9% NaCl for electrolyte restoration of sodium and chlorides Provides free water for the renal elimination of solutes Lowers serum osmolality by moving body fluid from the blood vessels into the cells and interstitium Used in hyperosmolar diabetes when dextrose is contraindicated, but fluid without excess sodium is indicated **Incompatibilities:** Amphotericin B Levarterenol Mannitol	Contraindicated in hypernatremia Use with caution in situations of fluid retention Assess for cellular dehydration
Dextrose in Sodium Chloride Solutions No hypotonic infusions			
Multiple Electrolyte Solutions **Plasma-Lyte 56® or Normosol R® injection** Na 40 mEq/L Cl 40 mEq/L K 13 mEq/L Mg 3 mEq/L Acetate 16 mEq/L pH 5.5 (4.0–6.0)	112 mOsm/L	**Indications:** Maintenance solution; provides free water and electrolytes Provides water for retention of needed electrolytes and the excretion of excesses **Incompatibilities:** Refer to isotonic multiple electrolyte solutions	Monitor I & O Monitor electrolyte levels Use with caution in patients with impaired renal function Observe for signs of hyperkalemia Weigh daily to assess for water retention and intoxication
Sterile water for injection pH 5.5 (5.0–7.0)	0 mOsm/L	**Indications:** Use as a diluent	Never administer free water alone, as it causes cell rupture

culatory overload. They also are irritating to the intima of veins. Figure 6-7 shows how RBCs crenate (shrink) when placed in a hypertonic solution. Figure 6-8 illustrates the physiologic effect of a hypertonic infusion. Table 6-7 lists the hypertonic infusates available, their indications, and the precautions associated withtheir use.

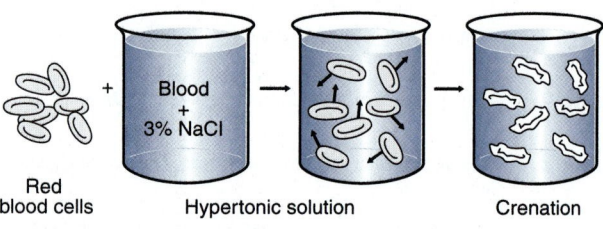

Figure 6-7 | Red blood cells crenate when placed in hypertonic 3% NaCl.

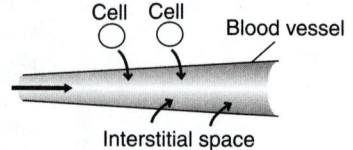

Figure 6-8 | Hypertonic infusion raises serum osmolality by causing a pull of fluids from the intracellular and interstitial compartments into the intravascular compartment.

Table 6-7 | Hypertonic Infusions: Indications for Use and Precautions

INFUSION	OSMO-LARITY	INDICATIONS AND INCOMPATIBILITIES	PRECAUTIONS, COMMENTS, CONTRAINDICATIONS
Dextrose in Water Solutions		**Indications:** Nonelectrolyte source of calories (protein-sparing) and water	Monitor for hyperglycemia and glycosuria Monitor for sepsis, with high glucose concentrations Accurate I & O
10% dextrose in water	505 mOsm/L	Provides 340 kcal/L	10% solution should be administered in a large arm vein. The site must be assessed frequently for pain, phlebitis, and thrombosis
20% dextrose in water	1,010 mOsm/L	Provides 680 kcal/L	
30% dextrose in water	1,510 mOsm/L	Provides 1,020 kcal/L	
40% dextrose in water	2,020 mOsm/L	Provides 1,360 kcal/L	Solutions over 10% must be delivered via a central line into a large vessel for adequate dilution and the prevention of peripheral vein sclerosis
50% dextrose in water	2,520 mOsm/L	Provides 1,700 kcal/L	
60% dextrose in water	3,030 mOsm/L	Provides 2,040 kcal/L	
70% dextrose in water	3,530 mOsm/L	Provides 2,380 kcal/L	
pH 4.5 for all strengths			
Sodium Chloride Solutions		**Indications:** Hypertonic NaCl injections are indicated for severe sodium depletion accompanied by abnormal neurologic functioning	Hypertonic saline solutions must be given with extreme care and should be administered only in critical care areas Strict I & O
2.225% NaCl	685.30 mOsm/L		Assess for fluid overload
Na 342.65 mEq/L		Used when sodium losses exceed fluid losses	Monitor renal function
Cl 342.65 mEq/L		Used in crisis associated with Addison's disease	Assess for hypernatremia
3.0% NaCl	924 mOsm/L		Contraindicated in CHF, fluid retention, impaired renal function, and hypernatremia
Na 462 mEq/L		Used in diabetic coma	
Cl 462 mEq/L			
5.0% NaCl	1,540 mOsm/L	**Incompatibilities:**	Do not administer more than 2 mEq/L/hr
Na 770 mEq/L		Amphotericin B	The strength and rate of administration of these infusions depends on the patient's age, weight, and clinical condition
Cl 770 mEq/L		Benzquinamide	
		Chlordiazepoxide	
pH 5.0		Diazepam	
(4.5–7.0) for all strengths		Fat emulsions	
		Levarterenol	
		Mannitol	
		Methylprednisolone sodium succinate	
		Phenytoin sodium	

continues

Table 6-7 | Hypertonic Infusions: Indications for Use and Precautions (*continued*)

INFUSION	OSMO-LARITY	INDICATIONS AND INCOMPATIBILITIES	PRECAUTIONS, COMMENTS, CONTRAINDICATIONS
Dextrose in Sodium Chloride Solutions		**Indications:**	Strict I & O
5% dextrose in 0.45 NaCl	391.12 mOsm/L	Indicated for shock and circulatory insufficiency until plasma volume expander is available	Daily weight
Dextrose 252.52 mOsm/L		Treats severe dehydration	Monitor for fluid overload
Na 69.3 mEq/L		Replaces fluid losses from burns	Monitor for electrolytes with prolonged therapy
Cl 69.3 mEq/L		With hypertonic dextrose in saline solutions, the concentrations and rate are determined by the patient's weight, circulatory status, and electrolyte-acid-base balance.	Use with caution in the elderly
5% dextrose in 0.9 NaCl	560.52 mOsm/L		Use with caution in patients with renal obstruction and patients with renal disease
Dextrose 252.52 mOsm/L			Contraindicated in conditions associated with fluid retention
Na 154 mEq/L			Use with extreme caution in patients with diabetes
Cl 154 mEq/L		**Incompatibilities:**	Contraindicated in diabetic coma
10% dextrose in 0.9 NaCl	813.04 mOsm/L	Amphotericin B	
Dextrose 505.04 mOsm/L		Ampicillin sodium	
Na 154 mEq/L		Amsacrine	
Cl 154 mEq/L		Diazepam	
pH 4.0		Erythromycin lactobinate	
(3.5–6.5) for all strengths		Mannitol	
		Phenytoin	
		Warfarin	
		Whole blood	
5% dextrose in Ringer's injection	564.52 mOsm/L	**Indications:**	Contraindicated in renal failure
Dextrose 252.52 mOsm/L		Provides calories from dextrose and spares protein with electrolyte composition similar to that of plasma	Use with caution in patients with CHF
Na 147.5 mEq/L			Monitor electrolytes
Cl 156 mEq/L		Replaces ECF losses and replaces electrolytes	Use with caution in hypernatremic and hypercalcemic patients
K 4 mEq/L			
Ca 4.5 mEq/L		**Incompatibilities:**	
pH 4.0		Refer to isotonic Ringer's solution	
5% dextrose and lactated Ringer's injection	526.52 mOsm/L	**Indications:**	Dextrose and lactated Ringer's infusions are contraindicated in lactic acidosis
Dextrose 252.52 mOsm/L		Treats mild metabolic acidosis	Use with caution in metabolic or respiratory alkalosis
Na 130 mEq/L		Provides 170 kcal from dextrose and 9 kcal from lactate per liter	Use with caution in patients with hepatic insufficiency
Cl 109 mEq/L		Replaces fluid losses from burns	Monitor for circulatory overload
K 4 mEq/L			Contraindicated in diabetic ketoacidosis
Ca 3 mEq/L			Because of lactate, excess administration could cause metabolic acidosis
Lactate 28 mEq/L			
pH 5.0			
10% dextrose and lactated Ringer's injection	779.04 mOsm/L	Treats mild metabolic acidosis	
Dextrose 505.04 mOsm/L		Provides 340 kcal from dextrose	
remaining constituents same as 5% solution		Spares protein	
		Replaces fluid losses from burns	
		Incompatibilities:	
		Refer to isotonic lactated Ringer's solution	

continues

Table 6-7 | Hypertonic Infusions: Indications for Use and Precautions (*continued*)

INFUSION	OSMO-LARITY	INDICATIONS AND INCOMPATIBILITIES	PRECAUTIONS, COMMENTS, CONTRAINDICATIONS
Electrolyte Solutions			With all electrolyte infusions, monitor electrolytes carefully, monitor for fluid overload; and perform hemodynamic monitoring in patients with renal, and cardiovascular impairment
5% dextrose and Electrolyte # 75 injection	410.52 mEq/L	**Indications:** Fluid replacement	
Dextrose 252.52 mOsm/L		Fluid and electrolyte maintenance	
Na 40 mEq/L		Treats mild metabolic acidosis	
Cl 48 mEq/L			
K 35 mEq/L			
Lactate 20 mEq/L			
Phosphate (as HPO_4^-) 15 mEq/L			
pH 5.0			
5% dextrose and Plasma-Lyte 56®	364.52 mOsm/L	Fluid replacement	
Dextrose 252.52 mOsm/L		Fluid and electrolyte maintenance	
Na 40 mEq/L			
Cl 40 mEq/L			
K 13 mEq/L			
Mg 3 mEq/L			
Acetate 16 mEq/L			
pH 5.5			
5% dextrose and Plasma-Lyte M®	380.52 mOsm/L	Fluid replacement	
Dextrose 252.52 mEq/L		Fluid and electrolyte maintenance	
Na 40 mEq/L		Treats very mild metabolic acidosis	
Cl 40 mEq/L			
K 16 mEq/L			
Ca 5 mEq/L			
Mg 3 mEq/L			
Acetate 12 mEq/L			
Lactate 12 mEq/L			
pH 5.0			
5% dextrose and Plasma-Lyte 148®	548.52 mOsm/L	Fluid replacement solution	With all electrolyte infusions, monitor electrolyte levels, maintain strict I & O, assess for hypernatremia, and monitor for fluid overload
Dextrose 252.52 mOsm/L		Electrolyte replacement	
Na 140 mEq/L			
Cl 98 mEq/L			
K 5 mEq/L			
Mg 3 mEq/L			
Acetate 27 mEq/L			
Gluconate 23 mEq/L			
pH 5.0			
5% dextrose and Plasma-Lyte R®	568.52 mOsm/L	Fluid replacement solution	Because of the addition of lactate, contraindicated in patients with liver impairment
Dextrose 252.52 mEq/L		Electrolyte replacement	
Na 140 mEq/L			
Cl 103 mEq/L			
K 10 mEq/L			
Ca 5 mEq/L			
Mg 3 mEq/L			
Acetate 47 mEq/L			
Lactate 8 mEq/L			
pH 5.0			

continues

Table 6-7 | Hypertonic Infusions: Indications for Use and Precautions (*continued*)

INFUSION	OSMO-LARITY	INDICATIONS AND INCOMPATIBILITIES	PRECAUTIONS, COMMENTS, CONTRAINDICATIONS
Invert Sugar as Fructose and Dextrose Solutions		**Indications:**	These infusions are equimolar mixtures of fructose and dextrose
5% Travert® and Electrolyte # 2 injection	433.02 mOsm/L	Provide calories in the form of carbohydrates	Contraindicated for patients with fructose intolerance
Dextrose 252.52 mOsm/L		More rapidly metabolized and can be administered more rapidly than dextrose	Strict I & O
Na 56 mEq/L		Use for diabetic patients because insulin is not required for the metabolism of these carbohydrate forms	Use with caution in patients with conditions associated with fluid overload
Cl 56 mEq/L			Do not use small peripheral veins for administration
K 25 mEq/L			Do not exceed 1g/kg/hr
Mg 6 mEq/L		Supply electrolytes at the maintenance level	Monitor for lactic acidosis
Lactate 25 mEq/L			Contraindicated in patients with gout because hyperuricemia may occur as an adverse reaction to the invert sugar
Phosphate (as HPO$_4^=$) 12.5 mEq/L		Provide fluid replacement and maintenance	
pH 4.5		**Incompatibilities:**	Assess for fluid overload
10% Travert® and Electrolyte # 2 injection	685.54 mOsm/L	Aminophylline	The 10% solution delivers more calories in less fluid (up to 3 L/day is safe and provides 340 kcal/L)
Dextrose 505.04 mOsm/L		Amobarbital	
Electrolytes are same as 5% solution		Ampicillin sodium	
		Blood products	
		Diazepam	
		Penicillin G	
		Phenytoin	
		Warfarin	
		Thiopental sodium	
Mannitol		**Indications:**	Contraindicated in anuria
10% mannitol solution	549 mOsm/L	Osmotic diuretic	Contraindicated in patients who are severely dehydrated
15% mannitol solution	823 mOsm/L	Reduces intraocular, intracranial, and intraspinal pressures by raising plasma osmolality and causing fluids in these areas to diffuse back into the plasma and intravascular space	Use with extreme caution in patients with congestive heart failure or pulmonary edema
20% mannitol solution	1,098 mOsm/L		Use filter with 15% and 20% solution
			Strict I & O with output measurements every 30 to 60 minutes
		Used to measure glomerular filtration rate	Hemodynamic monitoring
		Promotes excretion of toxic substances	Monitor electrolytes and BUN
		Promotes diuresis during oliguric phase of acute renal failure	Weigh daily, or more frequently
		Incompatibilities:	
		Refer to isotonic mannitol infusions	
Amino Acid (Protein) Solutions	Range from 400 mOsm/L to 1,600 mOsm/L	**Indications:**	There are numerous precautions and guidelines associated with use of these products; refer to Chapter 13, which covers various hyperalimentation and total parenteral nutrition formulas
Aminess®		These are nutritional agents indicated for use when oral routes of nutrition are not possible or are inadequate due to disease, surgery, severe infections, chemotherapy, or severe anorexia	
Aminosyn®			
Branch-Amin®			These hypertonic preparations range in amino acid content from 3.5% to 10%, with or without electrolytes. They also are available in preparations with 5% to 50% dextrose
FreAmine®		Refer to Chapter 13 for complete information on the use of these products	
HepaAmine®			
Nephramine®			
Novamine®		**Incompatibilities:**	
ProcalAmine®		Do not add anything without consultation with a pharmacist	
RenAmine®			
Travasol®			
TrophaAmine®			

continues

Table 6-7 | Hypertonic Infusions: Indications for Use and Precautions (*continued*)

INFUSION	OSMO-LARITY	INDICATIONS AND INCOMPATIBILITIES	PRECAUTIONS, COMMENTS, CONTRAINDICATIONS
Alcohol in Dextrose and Water Infusions		**Indications:**	Contraindicated in
5% alcohol and 5% dextrose in water	1,010.08 mOsm/L	Caloric provisions are: dextrose 3.4 kcal/g, alcohol 5.6 kcal/ml	alcoholism diabetic coma epilepsy
Alcohol 252.52 mOsm/L		Fluid replacement	urinary tract infections
Dextrose 252.52 mOsm/L		**Incompatibilities:**	Use with caution in diabetes mellitus
pH 4.5		Check with pharmacist before mixing anything with these infusions	Monitor for intoxication
10% alcohol and 5% dextrose in water	757.56 mOsm/L		Monitor for hyperglycemia
Alcohol 505.04 mOsm/L			Monitor for glycosuria
Dextrose 252.52 mOsm/L			Strict I & O
			Drug Interactions:
			There are many drug interactions because of the alcohol in these infusions. Many medications are potentiated or have a reduced effect when given concurrently with alcohol infusions. Note the medications the patient is taking and determine untoward interactions.
Alkalinizing Agents		**Indications:**	Contraindicated with
Sodium bicarbonate 5% 595 mEq/L (0.595/mL)	595 mOsm/L	Alkalinizing agent for temporary treatment of severe metabolic acidosis	acidosis (respiratory) alkalosis (metabolic and respiratory) edema
Sodium bicarbonate 7.5%	893 mOsm/L	Increases plasma bicarbonate and buffers excess hydrogen ion concentration	hypertension hypocalcemia
892.50 mEq/L (0.893/mL)		Dosage corresponds to degree of acidosis according to pH (<7.25), PO_2, PCO_2, and electrolytes	hypochloremia impaired renal function
Sodium bicarbonate 8.4%	1,000 mOsm/L		Use with extreme caution in patients with sodium retention
999.60 mEq/L (0.999/mL) pH 7.75 (7.0–8.5)		Treats hyperkalemia	Use with caution in patients on corticosteroids
		Used as a buffer to raise the pH of intravenous infusates	Excessive or rapid administration can result in intracranial hemorrhage
		Treatment for barbiturate and salicylate intoxication	Extravasation can result in severe tissue damage
		Incompatibilities:	Flush IV line before and after injection
		Numerous; consult pharmacist	

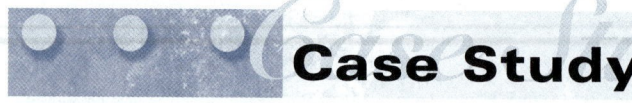

Case Study

HELPING A DEHYDRATED PATIENT BALANCE MEDICAL AND FAMILY PRIORITIES

Mrs. Diaz is a 46-year-old housewife with three young children. She is 5'6" tall and normally weighs 145–150 lbs. Her husband travels out of town on business during the week and returns on Friday evening.

Mrs. Diaz has been feeling weak and fatigued, with nausea, vomiting, abdominal cramping, and diarrhea for the past four days. She is thirsty but unable to keep oral fluids down. Her symptoms have become worse in the past 24 hours, with the addition of postural hypotension and vertigo when she is standing. Neither the over-the-counter medications nor the Phenergan suppositories and Bentyl prescribed by her physician have helped. Her husband brought her to the hospital late Friday evening, leaving the children with a neighbor.

Dr. Barbara Reed admits her to a general medical unit. Mrs. Diaz says, "Can't I be treated at home? I'm worried about leaving the children."

Admission Assessment Data

Vital Signs: Blood pressure: 80/40; Temperature: 101°; Pulse: 66 per minute and weak; Respirations: 26 per minute and shallow; Weight: 141 lbs.
Eyes appear sunken with dark circles around them.
Mucous membranes are dry and sticky.
Skin is dry with poor turgor.
Neck veins are flat.
Emesis: 60 ml dark orange fluid with mucus (sent to lab)
Stool: 140 ml brownish yellow liquid with mucus (sent to lab)
Urine: 30 ml dark amber urine with strong odor (sent to lab)

Diagnostic Studies

CBC Hgb: 15 g/dl; Hct: 45%; WBC: 6,000 mm^3
UA sp: 1.121; Na: 37 mEq
SMA Glucose: 90 mg/dl

BUN: 25 mg/dl
Creatinine: 1.3 mg/dl
Na: 130 mEq/L
Cl: 92 mEq/L
Ca: 4.2 mEq/L
K: 3.2 mEq/L

Medical Orders

2000 cc 0.9% NaCl @ 125 cc/hr (add 10 mEq KCl/L)
CBC and SMA in AM
Urine for C & S
Ice chips and sips of 7-Up, as tolerated
Try clear liquid diet in AM
BP lying and standing q 4 hr
Reglan 25 mg IVPB in 50 cc D$_5$W over 30 min. Repeat in 4 hr
Compazine 10 mg IM q 3–4h prn n/v
Once n/v relieved, start:
    Donnatal 2 tabs PO t.i.d.
    Lomotil 2.5 mg PO t.i.d.
    Motrin 400 mg prn aches/pains
Call me if n/v continues.

Nursing Care Plan

THE DEHYDRATED PATIENT

Nursing Diagnoses

Nursing diagnoses appropriate to this patient may include:

1. *Imbalanced nutrition less than body requirements*, related to nausea, vomiting, and inability to take food and fluid orally for five days
2. *Deficient fluid volume* related to gastrointestinal losses, as evidenced by nausea, vomiting, and diarrhea for five days
3. *Risk for trauma* related to weakness and fatigue, as evidenced by postural hypotension and vertigo when standing
4. *Anxiety* related to physical discomfort, separation from children, and unfamiliar environment
5. *Pain* related to abdominal cramps, nausea, and vomiting
6. *Impaired oral mucous membrane* related to deficient fluid volume, associated with increased gastrointestinal loss and decreased oral intake

Planning (Goals: desired outcome and evaluation criteria statement)

Mrs. Diaz will:

- Take ice chips or sips of 7-Up every 20 to 30 min while awake without further n/v
- Maintain improved fluid balance as evidenced by moist mucous membranes, normal skin turgor, and normal urine color and specific gravity
- Report anxiety is reduced and state she feels more relaxed
- Verbalize that abdominal discomfort is alleviated

Noncollaborative Nursing Actions and Interventions

1. Monitor vital signs. Take BP lying, sitting, and standing. Monitor temperature for elevation. Assess for chest pain with dyspnea and moist cough.
   Rationale: Deficient fluid volume contributes to hypotension and tachycardia. Fever contributes to additional fluid

loss by raising metabolic rate. There is a potential for the formation of thrombi and emboli due to hemoconcentration.

2. Provide for safety by keeping bed in low position and side rails up. Instruct patient to call for assistance when getting up.

   Rationale: Weakness, fatigue, and hypotension contribute to the possibility for falls and injury.

3. Monitor oral and IV intake and losses from all sources. Assess patient's oral fluid preferences and plan an intake schedule over a 24-hour period.

   Rationale: Fluid replacement must be based on previous and concurrent losses. Decreased urinary output can indicate decreased renal perfusion. Oral fluid intake relieves thirst, moistens mucous membranes, and contributes to fluid volume replacement. Providing beverages the patient prefers might encourage the patient to drink more.

4. Provide mouth care frequently.

   Rationale: Mucous membranes are dry, with little elasticity because of decreased fluid volume. Mouth care provides physical and aesthetic comfort, which may encourage the patient to drink more. It also enhances oral circulation.

5. Monitor intake and losses from all sources.

   Rationale: Replacement needs are based on losses.

6. Keep skin clean (with mild soap and thorough rinsing) and dry. Turn often and apply emollients to skin, with special attention to bony prominences.

Rationale: Because of hypovolemia, vasoconstriction, and decreased nutrition, there is cellular fragility and the tissues can break down easily. Bathing and massaging promote circulation and comfort.

7. Daily weight.

   Rationale: Replacement needs are based on losses.

Collaborative Nursing Actions and Interventions

1. Administer IV infusions as ordered.
2. Assist in identifying the underlying cause(s) of the patient's situation.
3. Monitor all laboratory and diagnostic studies and report any abnormalities to the physician.
4. Administer antiemetics and analgesics based on patient assessment.
5. Identify psychosocial support systems that are available to the patient to assist with her children while she is ill in order to allay her anxieties.

Evaluation

Goals met (partially or completely) or not met (reassessment is needed).

Key Concepts

✳ Daily water requirements for the average adult are approximately 30 ml/kg (13.6 ml/lb) of body weight.

✳ The recommended dietary allowances (RDA) in kilocalories (kcal) are estimated at 33 kcal/kg (15 kcal/lb) of ideal body weight, with 46% derived from carbohydrates, 30% from fat, and 24% from protein. The body must also be supplemented with electrolytes, vitamins, minerals, and various trace elements to maintain homeostasis.

✳ Osmolality is the osmotic pull exerted by all particles per unit of water. The dissolved particles that primarily exert this pull are serum sodium, urea, and glucose.

✳ To calculate serum osmolality, the following formula is used: Multiply the serum sodium by 2; add the BUN, which has been divided by three; add the glucose, which has been divided by 18.

✳ The major indications for the initiation of intravenous infusion therapy are as follows:

   – Fluid volume maintenance

   – Fluid volume replacement

   – The provision of a vehicle to administer medications

   – The transfusion of blood and blood products

   – The provision of nutritional supplementation

✳ Infusates are categorized as follows:

   – **Crystalloids:** Solutes, which, when placed in a solvent, homogeneously mix with it, dissolve, and cannot be distinguished from the resultant solution. They are able to diffuse through membranes. Such infusions are usually electrolyte solutions that may be isotonic, hypotonic, or hypertonic.

– **Colloids:** Glutinous substances whose particles, when submerged in a solvent, cannot form a true solution because their molecules do not dissolve, but remain uniformly suspended and distributed in the fluid. Colloid infusions expand volume by raising colloid osmotic pressure.

– **Hydrating solutions:** Infusions that supplement caloric intake, supply nutrients, and provide free water for maintenance, rehydration, or to promote effective renal output.

The nurse should be able to determine the tonicity of any infusion his patient receives. He must remember that the number of ions of electrolytes equals the osmolarity of the electrolyte solution. Percentage solutions express the number of grams of solute per 100 grams (1 ml) of solvent. One gram of dextrose equals 3.4 kcal. One millimole of monohydrate dex-

trose equals 198 mg of monohydrate dextrose. One mOsm of monohydrate dextrose equals 1 mOsm of osmotic pressure, and 1 mg equals 1 ml.

Example: Monovalent normal saline = 154 mEq/L. There are 154 mEqs of sodium and 154 mEqs of chloride, making the osmolarity of the solution 308 mOsm/L.

Example: 1 L 5% dextrose in water 5×3.4 kcal = 17 kcal/100 ml or 170 kcal/L.

Example: 1 L 5% dextrose in water has 5 g of dextrose/100 ml or 50 g of dextrose/L (50,000 mg/ml). 50,000 mg dextrose/L divided by 198 mg/mOsm equals 252.52 mOsm/L.

Using the information presented in this chapter, the nurse should be able to determine which type of infusion is appropriate for his patient, and identify the assessment factors, nursing interventions, and precautions needed to provide a safe level of care.

Review Questions and Activities

1. Calculate the daily water requirements for the following:
   (a) a 24-year-old female who is 5'4" tall and weighs 126 lbs.
   (b) a 48-year-old male who is 6'2" tall and weighs 192 lbs.
2. Estimate the recommended daily allowances for the two people in question number 1.
3. Formulate the serum osmolality of patients with the following laboratory values:
   a. Na = 146 mEq/L b. Na = 137 mEq/L
   BUN = 15 mg/dl   BUN = 10 mg/dl
   Glucose = 110 mg/dl Glucose = 80 mg/dl
4. List two infusions for each category (crystalloid, colloid, and hydrating solutions) and calculate the caloric content and osmolarity of each.
5. Using the following case study, write a nursing care plan with three to five appropriate nursing diagnoses. Determine what type of IV infusion might be used for this patient. Include supporting rationales.

   Mr. Manning had an appendectomy 48 hours ago and is recuperating at home. He is 50 years old, a long-distance freight driver with a 10-year history of moderate hypertension. He is 6'1" tall and weighs 235 lbs. He has smoked one to two

packs of cigarettes per day for 32 years, drinks two to six beers per day on his days off work, and eats mainly in fast-food restaurants and truck stops.

While Mr. Manning is sitting up in bed watching television, his son observes that his dad is restless, perspiring profusely, and seems to be gasping for air. Mr. Manning says he "feels nervous" and has a "feeling of tightness" in his chest when taking a deep breath. His physician is called and advises that Mr. Manning go to the emergency department immediately.

Upon admission to the E.D., Mr. Manning's vital signs are T 100.6., BP 96/50, P 118, R 32. There is jugular vein distention (JVD) and the nurse notices that the patient's right leg is edematous, compared to the left leg. There is a right pleural friction rub. Additional assessment data reveals the following:

CBC	RBCs	=	6.1, Hgb = 18; Hct = 54
ABGs	PO_2	=	65 (indicative of hypoxemia)
	PCO_2	=	25 (indicative of hypocarbia)
	pH	=	8 (indicative of respiratory alkalosis)

Electrolytes

Na	=	134
K	=	5.2
Cl	=	92
PO_4	=	1.6

Chest x-ray   Normal

Lung scan   Abnormal ventilation and perfusion (indicative of pulmonary embolism)

Orders

O_2 with nebulization and CO_2 reservoir

Demerol 100 mg with Phenergan 25 mg IM stat and q 4 hr prn

Valium 10 mg PO stat and prn restlessness

PT and PTT stat

Transfer to intermediate care unit.

Call results of coagulation studies for heparin drip and additional orders.

Patient Preparation and Site Selection for Peripheral Intravenous Infusion Therapy

COMPETENCIES

Upon completion of this chapter, the reader should be able to:

✳ List the major advantages and disadvantages of intravenous or intravascular infusion therapy.

✳ Review the anatomy of the integumentary system and the circulatory system.

✳ Discuss the importance of psychological preparation for the patient who is about to undergo infusion therapy and for the nurse who administers it.

✳ Review the components of physical preparation for the patient about to undergo infusion therapy in terms of safety, comfort, and position.

✳ List and describe each of the sites that may be accessed by the nurse and used for peripheral intravenous infusion therapy.

✳ Assess the factors that determine the choice and selection of sites for peripheral venipuncture and infusion therapy.

KEY TERMS

arteriole	integumentary system	tunica adventitia
bioavailability	intravascular	tunica externa
capillaries	pharmacokinetics	tunica intima
cubital fossa	sebaceous	tunica media
dermis	semi-Fowler's position	varices
epidermis	subcutaneous	veins
fascia	sudoriferous	venules
Fowler's position	syncope	

There are distinct advantages and disadvantages to deliberate before instituting peripheral infusion therapy. Although the advantages usually outweigh the disadvantages, the decision must be based on the patient's situation and the pharmacokinetics and bioavailability of the products that need to be administered. **Pharmacokinetics** is the study of drug action and metabolism in the body, including the processes of absorption, distribution, duration of action, and methods of excretion. **Bioavailability** refers to the rate and concentration of drug entry into the circulatory system and its pharmacologic response at the site of action. Both of these factors must always be considered when deciding to administer fluids or medications to a patient. Table 7-1 compares and contrasts the advantages and disadvantages of peripheral IV therapy.

ANATOMY REVIEW

To facilitate vascular access the nurse must have a sound knowledge of the anatomy and physiology of the integumentary and circulatory systems. Just as the person traveling by car across unfamiliar country must know how to read and

Table 7-1 | Advantages and Disadvantages of Peripheral IV Infusion Therapy

ADVANTAGES	DISADVANTAGES
1. It provides a route for immediate availability to the systemic circulation without regard to gastrointestinal functioning or subcutaneous or intramuscular conditions.	1. There is a greater possibility of a serious allergic reaction occurring because of rapid delivery to the systemic circulation. Once administered, an IV drug cannot be retrieved.
2. Drug absorption is more predictable.	2. There is always the possibility of fluid overload.
3. Blood levels of the drug can be maintained for even distribution and titrated according to the patient's needs.	3. Should an error occur in dosage or administration, the potential for dangerous outcomes is amplified.
4. It provides a reliable route for emergency conditions.	4. There is always the possibility of infection and sepsis whenever the skin barrier is breached through percutaneous puncture.
5. It is ideal for drugs that cannot be given orally due to poor absorption and failure to reach the general circulation for systemic distribution.	5. There is pain associated with cannula insertion as well as psychological discomfort associated with the knowledge that an indwelling device is in place.
6. It provides a route for drugs that cannot be given by other routes (such as heparin, which cannot be given orally or intramuscularly).	6. There may be impaired mobility, depending on placement of the IV.
7. It is often the only available route for the unconscious or uncooperative patient.	7. The potential for nerve or vessel damage exists with improper venipuncture technique and incorrect cannula placement.
8. It is ideal for patients who are nauseated, vomiting, or have any gastrointestinal disruptions.	8. There may be pain associated with the administration of irritating drugs.
9. There is less discomfort because, once initiated, the site may be accessed for 72 hours or more.	9. Tissue damage can occur with extravasation of vesicants.
	10. There is always the potential for phlebitis, thrombophlebitis, or embolization.

follow maps and adapt to diverse terrains in order to reach his destination, so must the nurse understand the topography of the skin and the mapping of circulatory vessels in order to approach them correctly. It is imperative that she know which routes of circulatory transportation will facilitate movement of needed products to the appropriate destinations in the body. "Site selection for vascular access shall include assessment of the patient's condition, age and diagnosis, vascular condition. Infusion device history, and type and duration of therapy" (INS, 2000, Standard 43, S37).

The Integumentary System

The **integumentary system** (Figure 7-1) is composed of the outer coverings that insulate and provide the first line of defense in protecting the body from microbial invasion and injury. The **epidermis** is the outermost skin layer, composed of epithelial cells, but devoid of blood vessels. It guards against injury by its slightly acidic pH that destroys many bacteria, its varying degrees of thickness, and its dense tactile sensory supply. The epidermis also determines skin pigmentation and, to some extent, protects the body from ultraviolet damage.

The **dermis**, or corium, is often called the true skin. It is composed of connective tissue, blood and lymphatic vessels, nerves, muscles, hair follicles, and **sudoriferous** (sweat) and **sebaceous** (oil) glands. The sensory nerves that are

> ## NURSING TIP
>
> ### *Clinical Justification in Litigation*
>
> Should the nurse be involved in litigation, she must be able to assert that, at the time of insertion, the most appropriate vein for the patient was used. To ensure this, she must have a thorough understanding of the venous anatomy. She must select the most appropriate venous cannulation site and assess for any complications that might occur. The nurse must always be able to give sound clinical justification for the vein she chooses to use for infusion therapy.

sensitive to hot, cold, pain, pressure, and touch are also found in this layer—an important fact to remember when assessing patients for complications, especially pain. The sebaceous and sudoriferous glands and their duct systems are referred to as skin appendages, as are the hair and nails.

The **subcutaneous** tissue, the layer that lies below the dermis, is not part of the integumentary system but binds with it. It is made up of loose connective tissue and stored body fat, and is correctly called fascia. **Fascia**, remember, is a network of fibrous membranes that cover, bind, and support the muscular system.

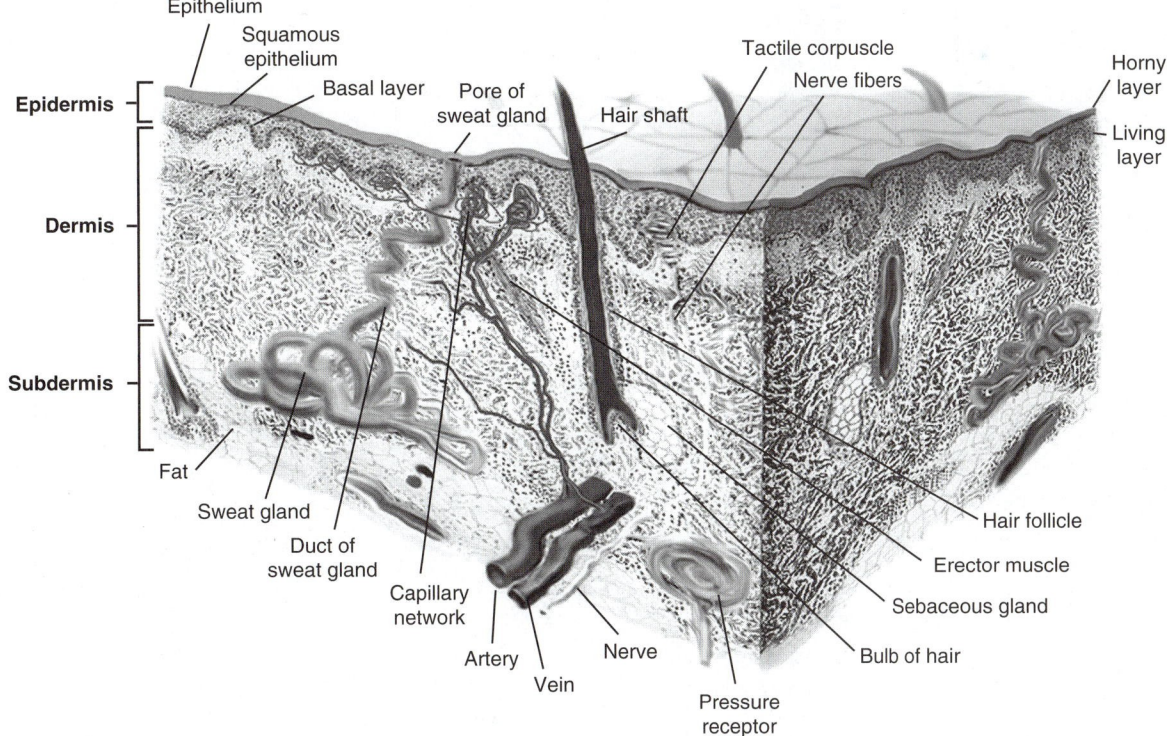

Figure 7-1 | The skin and its layers: A three-dimensional view

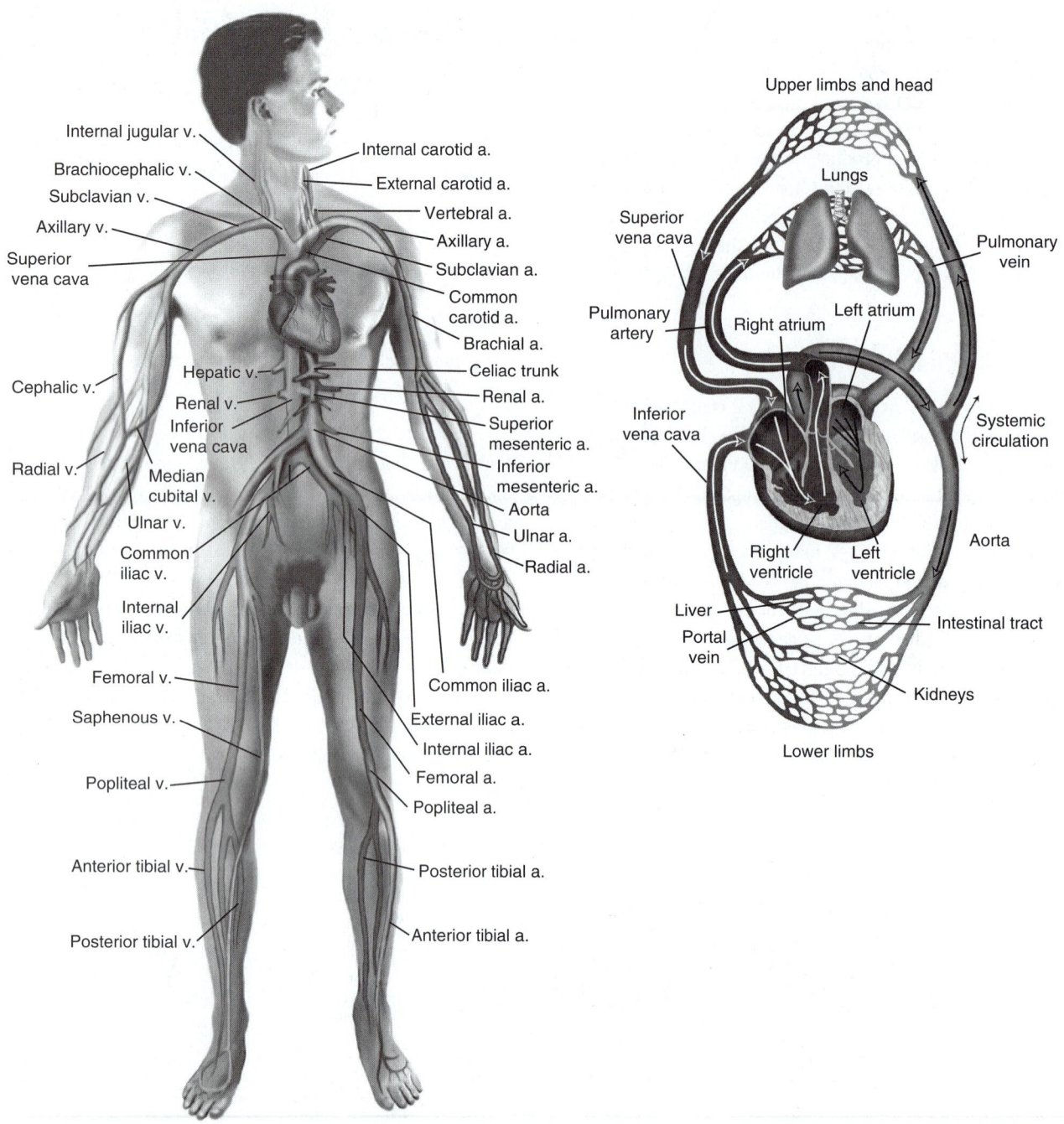

Figure 7-2 | Systemic circulation

The Circulatory System

The general, or systemic, circulation (Figure 7-2) is responsible for the transport of blood and nutrients, the elimination of waste products, temperature balance, and bacterial protection (Table 7-2). The cardiopulmonary circulation includes blood flow through the heart (Figure 7-3) and its movement through the lungs (Figure 7-4). The heart pumps the blood throughout the body via three types of blood vessels: arteries and arterioles, veins and venules, and capillaries.

Table 7-2 | Four Major Functions of Systemic Circulation

Transportation	The blood carries oxygen, water, nutrients, and secretions to all of the body systems and tissues.
Excretion	The blood picks up carbon dioxide and waste products and transports them to sites for elimination from the body.
Equalization	The blood contributes to balanced body temperature.
Preservation	The blood protects the body from bacterial invasion.

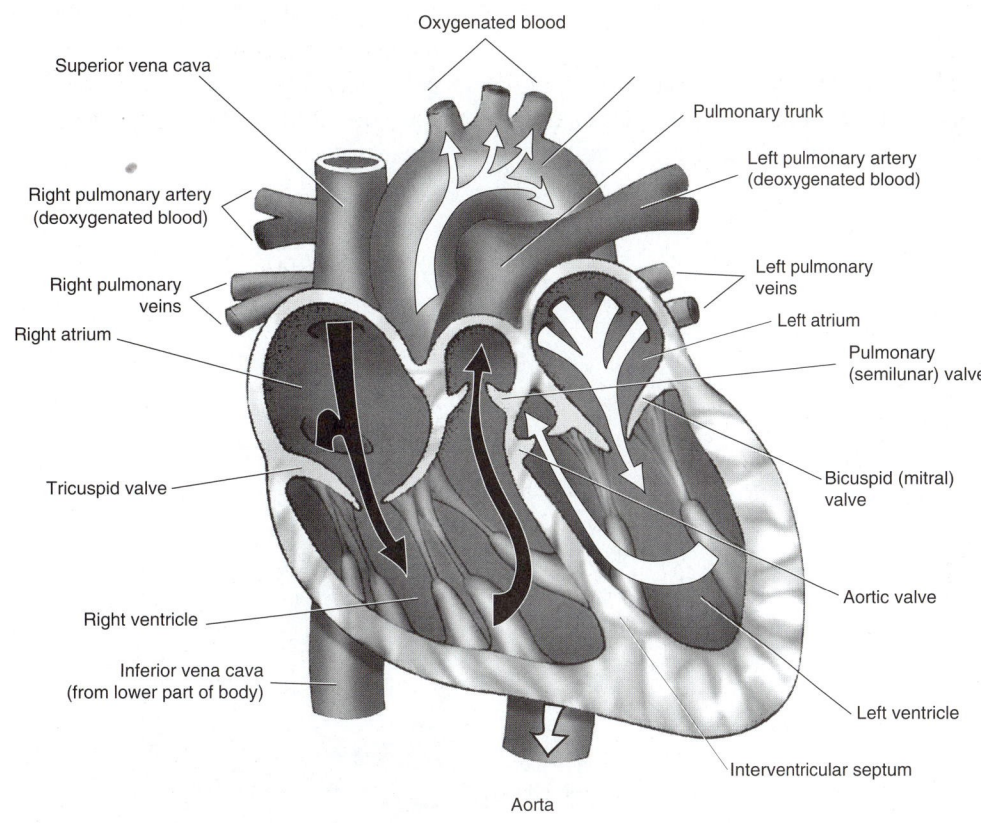

Figure 7-3 | Cardiac circulation: The structures and blood flow within the heart

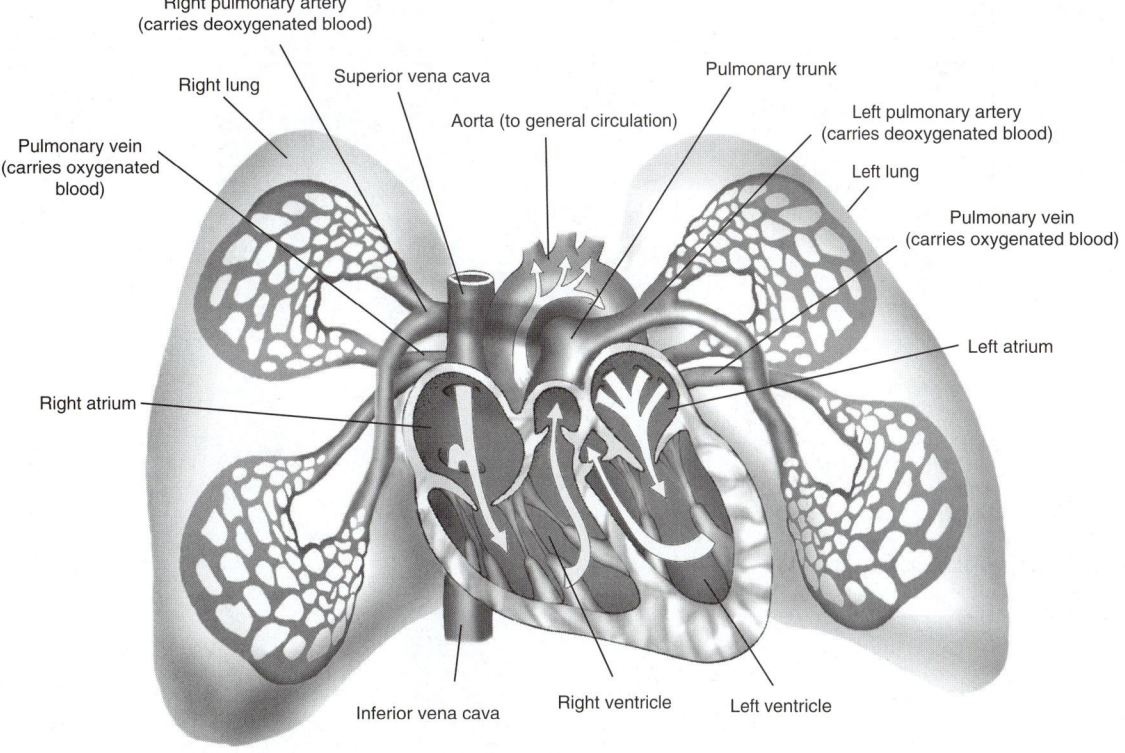

Figure 7-4 | Pulmonary circulation

Arteries and Arterioles

The arteries carry blood away from the heart via the aorta to the systemic circulation and the branches of the pulmonary artery to the lungs. They are thick-walled, highly elastic, and transport blood under potent pressure. They distribute blood throughout the body (Figure 7-5). With the exception of the pulmonary artery, which carries deoxygenated blood away from the heart to the lungs, arteries transport only oxygenated blood.

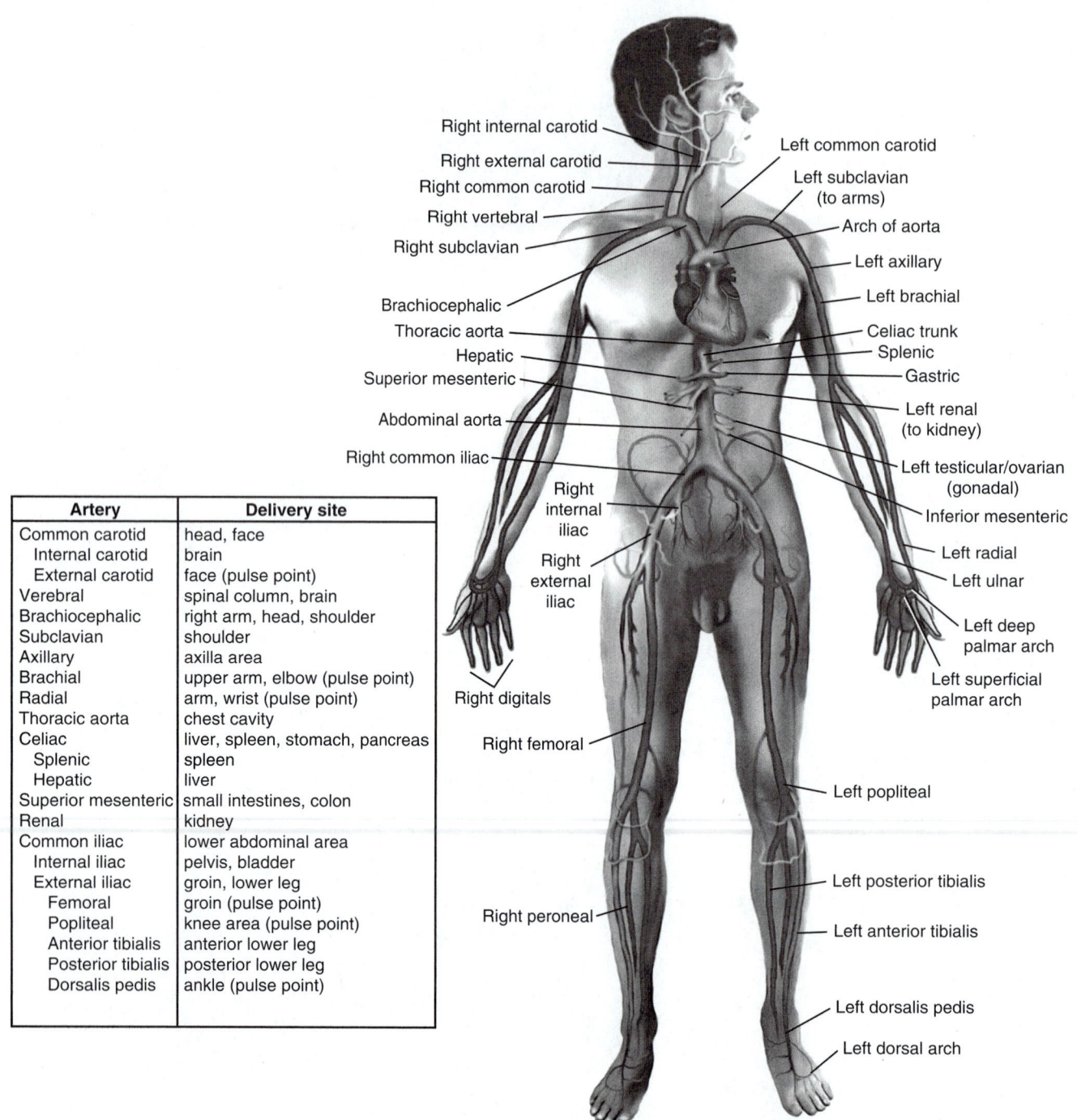

Artery	Delivery site
Common carotid	head, face
Internal carotid	brain
External carotid	face (pulse point)
Verebral	spinal column, brain
Brachiocephalic	right arm, head, shoulder
Subclavian	shoulder
Axillary	axilla area
Brachial	upper arm, elbow (pulse point)
Radial	arm, wrist (pulse point)
Thoracic aorta	chest cavity
Celiac	liver, spleen, stomach, pancreas
Splenic	spleen
Hepatic	liver
Superior mesenteric	small intestines, colon
Renal	kidney
Common iliac	lower abdominal area
Internal iliac	pelvis, bladder
External iliac	groin, lower leg
Femoral	groin (pulse point)
Popliteal	knee area (pulse point)
Anterior tibialis	anterior lower leg
Posterior tibialis	posterior lower leg
Dorsalis pedis	ankle (pulse point)

Figure 7-5 | Arterial distribution

Arteries

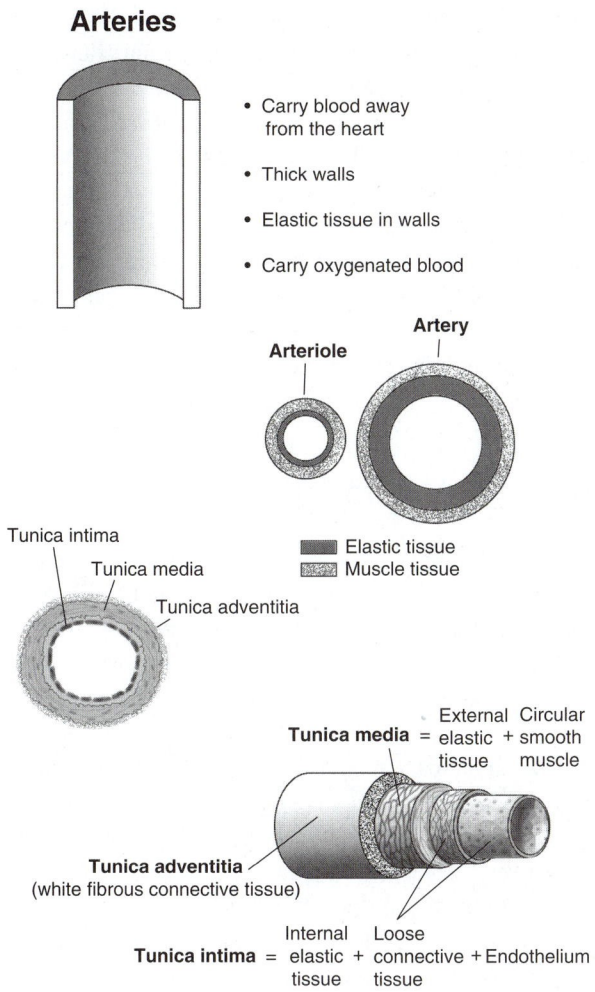

- Carry blood away from the heart
- Thick walls
- Elastic tissue in walls
- Carry oxygenated blood

Figure 7-6 | Arterial anatomy

The wall of an artery (Figure 7-6) is divided into three strata.

1. A white fibroelastic coat (**tunica adventitia** or **tunica externa**), the outermost layer, is composed of a layer of loose connective tissue that surrounds the vessel.
2. A yellow fibrous middle layer (**tunica media**) has the vital function of regulating blood flow through the artery by controlling its diameter. It is composed of some elastic fibers and smooth muscle that forms a spiral within the layer.
3. A serous layer (**tunica intima**) is the innermost coat and forms the internal lining of the artery. It is made up of endothelial cells that form a basement membrane, a subendothelial connective tissue layer, and a pliant inner lamina.

Arteries, the largest being the aorta and the pulmonary trunk, diminish in size as they branch into the organ tissues of the body until becoming **arterioles**, the very smallest of arteries. The distal portion of the arterioles branch into capillaries, the delicate tributaries of arteries, called metarterioles. Arterial (and arteriolar) communication with the venous system (via the venules) occurs in the microscopic system known as the capillary network or capillary bed (Figure 7-7).

Capillaries

The **capillaries** (Figure 7-8) are the smallest blood vessels in the body, being merely an endothelial cell layer thick. Although they are not composed of any muscle tissue, they regulate blood flow through the action of small precapillary sphincters located at the arteriolar-capillary junction. They are selectively permeable, permitting oxygen, nutrients, and plasma (or interstitial fluid, as it is classified when in the capillary bed) to pass out into the surrounding tissues, while directing carbon dioxide and waste products back into the circulation. The ISF is returned to the circulation via the lymphatics, which assist in maintaining fluid equilibrium in the interstitium. (Remember that, if it were not for the work of the lymphatics, the body would succumb to fluid volume overload within 24 hours.) Capillary selectivity is also evident in the fact that blood is transported to the tissues in proportion to the needs of individual organs.

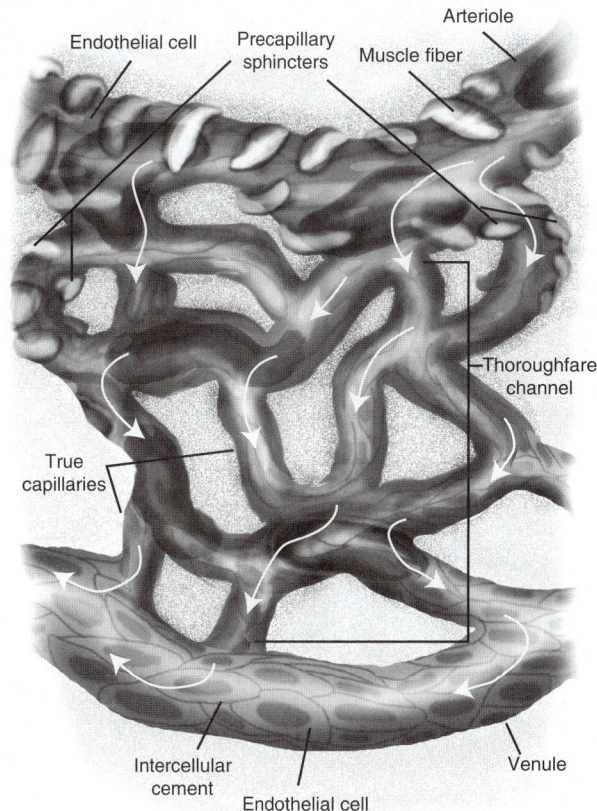

Figure 7-7 | Capillary bed connecting an arteriole with a venule

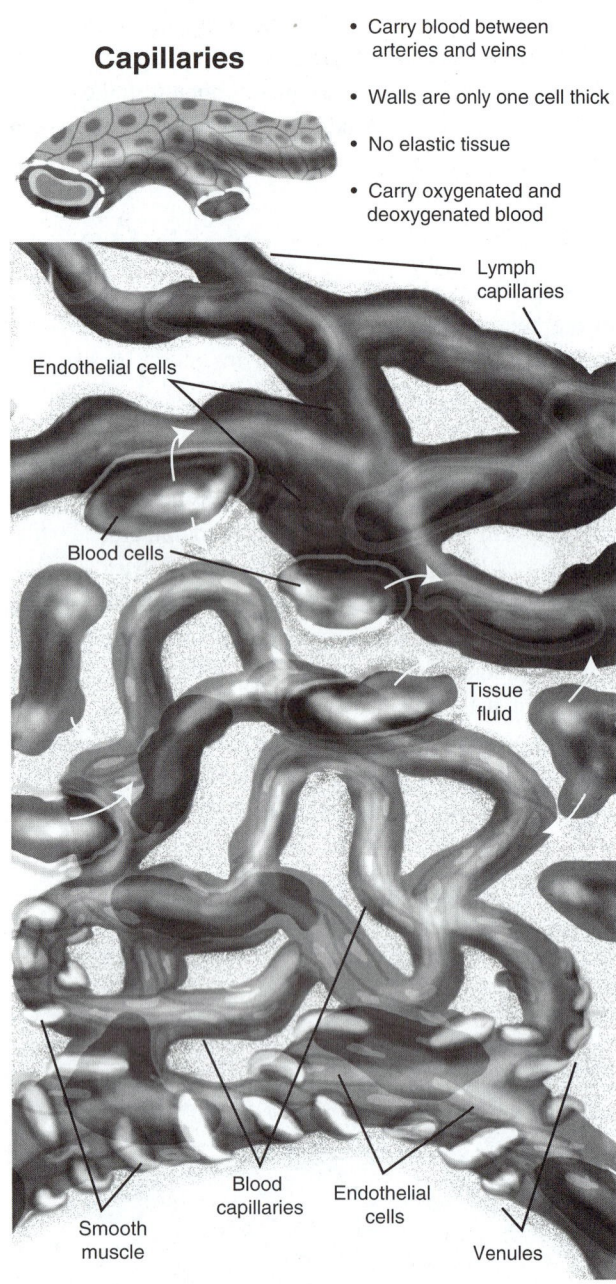

Capillaries

- Carry blood between arteries and veins
- Walls are only one cell thick
- No elastic tissue
- Carry oxygenated and deoxygenated blood

Lymph capillaries

Endothelial cells

Blood cells

Tissue fluid

Smooth muscle

Blood capillaries

Endothelial cells

Venules

Figure 7-8 | Capillary anatomy

Veins and Venules

Venules are the first circulatory vessels to receive blood containing carbon dioxide and waste products when it leaves the capillaries. Although scarcely larger in size than capillaries, they are lined with a small amount of muscle tissue, which assists the movement of blood into the **veins**. Veins are vessels that return blood to the heart and lungs and transport waste products to excretory locations (Figure 7-9). Veins are similar to arteries in appearance but differ morphologically. Venous walls are thinner in diameter, have much less elasticity, and are lined with valves, which serve to deter the

backflow of blood into the capillary bed (Figure 7-10). These valves are especially important because venous flow must overcome gravity. For this reason, the veins of the legs are more abundantly supplied with valves (but are also more susceptible to **varices**, the twisted, dilated veins that are the sequelae of distention, dilation, diminished elasticity, and incomplete valve closure). In addition to the valves, the contractions of muscles around the veins (skeletal muscles of the arms and legs, and the thoracic and abdominal muscles that rise and fall during normal respiratory movement) promote the return flow of blood to the heart.

PATIENT PREPARATION

The administration of peripheral IV therapy has become commonplace in most health care settings. In the interest of cost containment, governmental and insurance regulations are becoming more and more stringent, leaving the acute care setting available to only the sickest patients, or those in need of special procedures who cannot be accommodated safely on an outpatient basis or in the home. Ninety percent or more of the patients in some hospital units may be receiving some form of IV therapy via peripheral or central venous access lines. For those undergoing outpatient surgical procedures, peripheral infusions run throughout most of their stay. Due to the limitations dictated by Medicare and Diagnosis Related Groups (DRGs), the insurance industry, and the shift to managed care, as well as personal preferences, many patients are receiving intravenous therapies at home. There has been a dramatic conversion to IV home care for antibiotic and chemotherapy administration, hydration, pain control, hyperalimentation, as well as advanced HIV disease-related therapies, and the administration of growth hormone and immune globulins. In addition, dobutamine (for patients with severe congestive heart failure who are not candidates for heart transplantation) and tocolytic therapy (to prevent the premature onset of contractions in women who have not sustained full-term pregnancies) are being administered in the home.

Psychological Preparation

A person who is psychologically prepared for an event is better equipped to cope with the circumstances of that situation. This holds true for any new experience in life, but is even more important for the person who is ill, in an unfamiliar environment, and in need of services and procedures to which he is unaccustomed. The patient undergoing infusion therapy is usually very sick and has multiple lifestyle changes and personal crises to deal with. Any event, no mat-

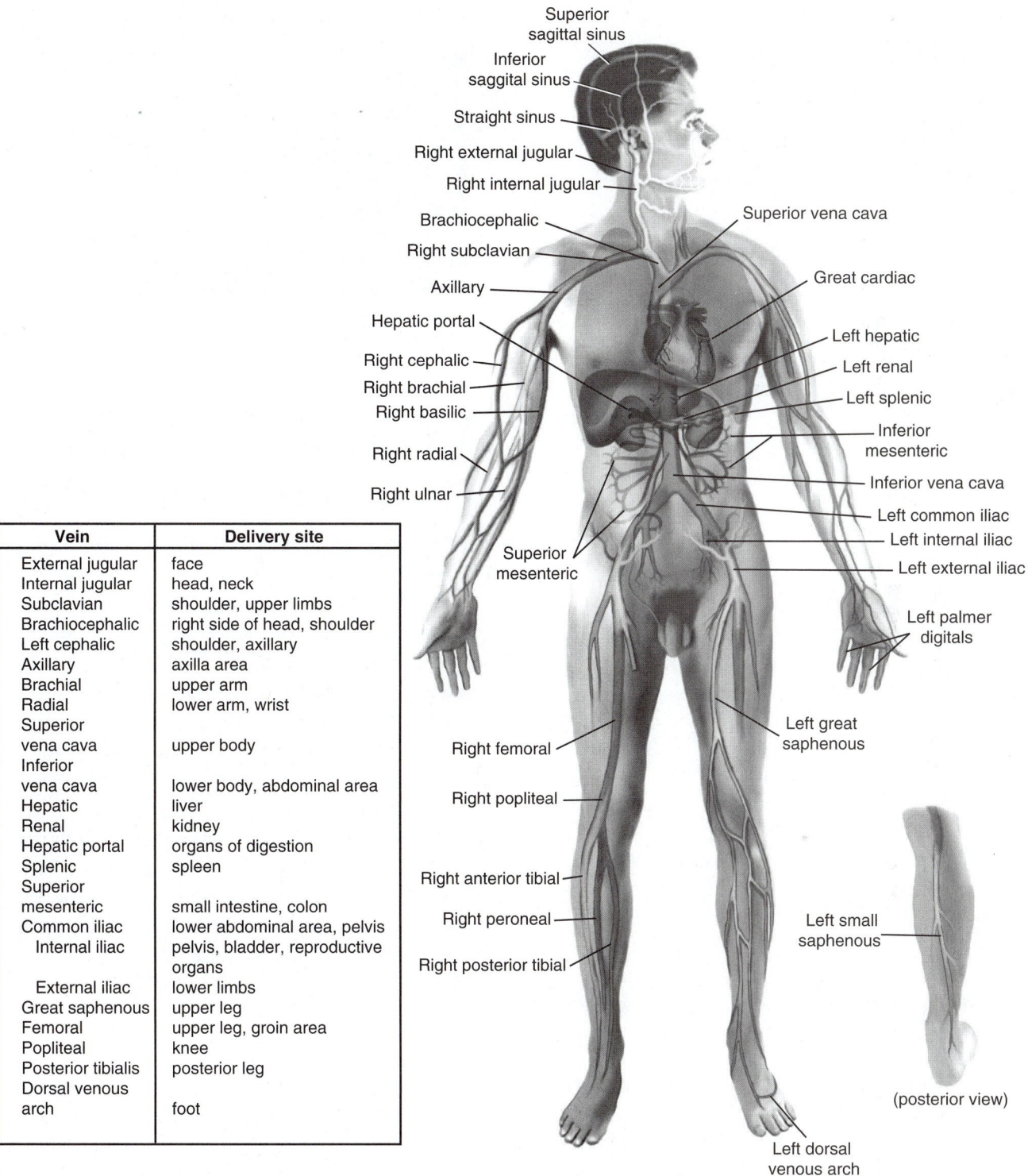

Vein	Delivery site
External jugular	face
Internal jugular	head, neck
Subclavian	shoulder, upper limbs
Brachiocephalic	right side of head, shoulder
Left cephalic	shoulder, axillary
Axillary	axilla area
Brachial	upper arm
Radial	lower arm, wrist
Superior vena cava	upper body
Inferior vena cava	lower body, abdominal area
Hepatic	liver
Renal	kidney
Hepatic portal	organs of digestion
Splenic	spleen
Superior mesenteric	small intestine, colon
Common iliac	lower abdominal area, pelvis
Internal iliac	pelvis, bladder, reproductive organs
External iliac	lower limbs
Great saphenous	upper leg
Femoral	upper leg, groin area
Popliteal	knee
Posterior tibialis	posterior leg
Dorsal venous arch	foot

Figure 7-9 | Venous distribution

ter how insignificant it may seem to someone else, can produce added stress for the patient (Figure 7-11).

When a patient is in need of IV therapy, it is imperative that he is mentally and emotionally prepared. For most people, the thought of being stuck with a needle is not pleasant.

Even though the need for treatment is inevitable, the circumstances surrounding the situation can be manipulated so that the experience is less traumatic.

The nurse must always remember that psychological preparation not only helps the patient adapt, but also

Veins

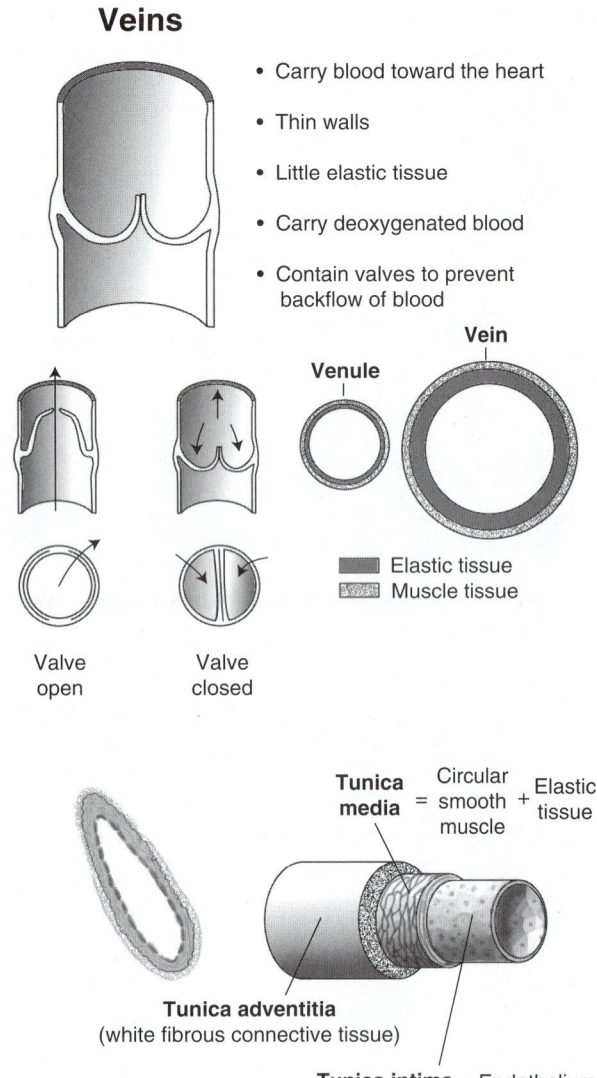

- Carry blood toward the heart
- Thin walls
- Little elastic tissue
- Carry deoxygenated blood
- Contain valves to prevent backflow of blood

Venule   Vein

■ Elastic tissue
▨ Muscle tissue

Valve open

Valve closed

Tunica media = Circular smooth muscle + Elastic tissue

Tunica adventitia (white fibrous connective tissue)

Tunica intima = Endothelium

Figure 7-10 | Venous anatomy

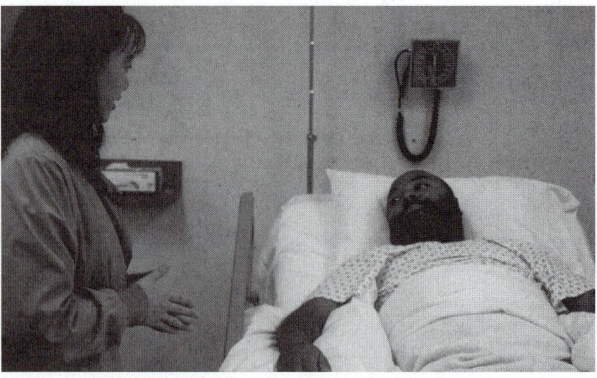

Figure 7-11 | Physical and psychological preparation for successful IV therapy

facilitates the initiation of IV therapy for the nurse. If venipuncture and the introduction of the cannula into the vein is to proceed smoothly, the patient must be relaxed. If he is not at ease, he experiences a sympathetic response, also called the fright, flight, fight, freeze reaction. When this occurs, the veins may spasm or constrict. The blood is then shunted from the peripheral circulation to the vital organs, thus making venous access very difficult, if not impossible. Extreme anxiety can cause **syncope** (fainting), the result of a vasovagal response.

Time, explanations, and honesty are the nurse's best allies when it comes to the patient's psychological preparation. When the nurse takes the time to explain the forthcoming procedure, and allows time for the patient to ask questions, caring and trust are imparted, and obstacles to communication are breached. The nurse must be honest regarding the procedure in terms of the expected time the IV will be needed, why it is needed, and the amount of discomfort, immobility, and inconvenience that will be associated with it.

If a nurse tells a patient that needlesticks or injections will not hurt, but feel just like a "little" mosquito bite, she is not being honest. A mosquito bite is not evident until after the venom has been injected and the area starts to itch; the sting itself is painless. Needlesticks, for the most part, do impart various degrees of discomfort. The patient needs to know that the pain is temporary and should diminish once the cannula is in place.

NURSING TIP

Pain Reduction

It is imperative that the nurse be honest regarding the type and severity of discomfort associated with any procedure. If pain is anticipated, the patient should be told. He should be instructed regarding any measures that might make it less distressing for him, then be reassured that the nurse will do everything possible to expedite the procedure and make it as painless for him as she can. The nurse should intervene to make any painful procedure less uncomfortable by employing appropriate (and substantiated) physical, pharmacological, and psychological measures.

It is always a good idea to explain the positive aspects of any procedure in terms of how the patient will benefit from the therapy. Sometimes, just the thought that what is being done is expected to promote health and comfort relieves much of the pain and stress associated with illness and treatment. The nurse's demeanor is also significant, making it very important that she appear confident and knowledgeable in order to elicit the patient's cooperation and decrease his anxiety.

Physical Preparation

In addition to psychological preparation, if the patient is to adapt to treatment, he must be physically prepared. Physical comfort, along with the confidence that he is in a safe environment and under the care of competent individuals, constitutes expectations that are the right of every patient. In readying a patient for venipuncture and infusion therapy, there are several prerequisites that must be addressed, primarily those of safety, comfort, and correct positioning.

Safety

The nursing assessments and interventions that promote and contribute to the patient's safety prior to the initiation of peripheral infusion therapy include, but are not limited to, the following:

1. Verification of the physician's order
2. Correct patient identification
3. Validation that the ordered infusion is appropriate for the patient
4. Confirmation that the patient is not allergic to anything that is to be administered
5. Confirmation that all supplies and equipment for venipuncture are sterile and handled aseptically, and that they have not exceeded their expiration dates
6. Documentation of significant laboratory and diagnostic reports
7. Strict asepsis in the preparation of all products to be used for venipuncture and IV infusion
8. The provision of a safe environment for the patient during infusion therapy in terms of bed rails, restraints, movement, and ambulation
9. Assessment and selection of the peripheral vessel that is appropriate for the type of infusion(s) ordered
10. Teaching measures that will instruct the patient about what he needs to report in terms of activity, discomfort, or signs and symptoms associated with any untoward reaction

Comfort

The administration of any peripheral infusion imposes some degree of restriction for the patient in terms of mobility and sustaining activities of daily living (ADLs). Although the ambulatory patient may get up and move around during IV therapy, measures must be employed to prevent dislodgment of the cannula or disconnection of any portions of the setup. Should the closed, sterile system be breached, the potential for contamination and the introduction of infection escalates.

NURSING TIP

Veins to Avoid

It is important to remember that veins in the limb located on the side of the body where a radical mastectomy with lymph node stripping and dissection has been performed are to be avoided due to altered circulation and impaired venous return. Likewise, an edematous extremity or extremity that has sustained third-degree burns should also be bypassed. If the IV is being inserted to provide access during surgery, the access site should present minimal interference with the surgical procedure or positioning during the intraoperative and postoperative periods.

Prior to the initiation of IV therapy, there are several nursing assessments and interventions that need to be employed in the interest of the patient's physical comfort. These include, but are not limited to the following:

1. Determining whether the patient is right handed or left handed (The nurse should make all efforts to access an appropriate vein in the patient's nondominant hand, so the patient can carry out ADLs without compromising the IV. The nurse should also avoid using veins in areas of flexion or in the antecubital fossa unless such areas are immobilized in a safe manner.)

2. Allowing the patient to carry out ADLs (bathing or showering, oral care, hair care, toileting) prior to the initiation of therapy, if time permits

3. Securing IV tubing that is of a length appropriate for minimally restricted movement by the patient during the infusion

4. Providing loose-fitting bed clothes that will not restrict movement or fluid flow, and allow for easy removal when they need to be changed, without interfering with the IV

5. Providing privacy

N U R S I N G   A L E R T

Hemodialysis Considerations

Never access, for peripheral intravenous therapy, an arteriovenous fistula, graft, or shunt that has been surgically placed for hemodialysis (Figure 7-12). In fact, the arm in which one of these devices is present should not be used for IV therapy, blood pressure monitoring, nor any procedure that might restrict blood flow to the dialysis access site.

Position

Prior to the initiation of IV therapy, the patient should be positioned in a manner that allows for optimum conditions for venous access. Although cannulation can be performed when the patient is in a flat, supine position, it is preferable that he be placed in the **Fowler's position**: semi-sitting with the torso and head elevated between 40 and 60 degrees (Figure 7-13). The knees may be flexed and supported by pillows (**semi-Fowler's position**). The arms should be positioned so that they are at the patient's side, with the intended site of venipuncture at a level lower than the heart, to promote venous filling.

Measures need to be taken to make the patient as comfortable as possible during infusion therapy. He should understand that he can move the extremity with the IV, rather than keep it totally immobile, so circulation is maintained. An arm board may be unnecessary if the nurse appropriately selects and cannulates the vein, allowing for natural anatomic splinting by the bones. Should immobilization of the extremity be required, the nurse must follow agency policy and procedural guidelines regarding the use of arm boards, restraints, or any stabilization devices. "Protocol for the use of restraints shall be consistent with state and federal regulations . . . shall be in accordance with the order of a physician or a prescriber authorized by the state Nurse Practice Act" (INS, 2000, Standard 37, S33). When an arm board is applied, the nurse must protect circulatory status and flow, and be able to monitor the infusion site. "An arm board should be used to facilitate infusion delivery when the catheter is placed in or around an area of extremity flexion" (INS, 2000, Standard 36, S32). The nurse must always keep in mind the potential for nerve and muscle damage that can accompany the use of restraining devices. It is important to remove any device at frequent intervals in order to adequately assess circulatory status. "The arm board should be removed and the patient's extremity circulatory status should be assessed at established intervals" (INS, 2000, Standard 36, S33). Pillows can be provided to support the extremity and to position the patient comfortably. Depending on his condition, the patient may be able to ambulate and shower, as long as the cannula and IV equipment are secured and the insertion site is protected from moisture and contamination.

INTRAVASCULAR SITE SELECTION

There are many factors that must be considered, from patient, nursing, and medical perspectives, when selecting an appropriate intravascular site. The site selected should provide the most appropriate access to the vessel for the intended therapy and accommodate administration of the prescribed infusion while minimizing any associated risks or complications. **Intravascular** access refers to entrance into arteries, veins, or capillaries. Veins, because they are so profuse and can usually be accessed easily, are most commonly used, and are predominantly focused on in this text, with this chapter addressing commonly used peripheral venous sites. (See Chapter 12, which details the central venous access sites used to administer therapy and their associated protocols, as well as other advanced fluid or medication delivery routes.)

When the nurse is responsible for initiating infusion therapy, she must take into consideration the patient's age, health status, diagnosis, condition of the site to be accessed, and the

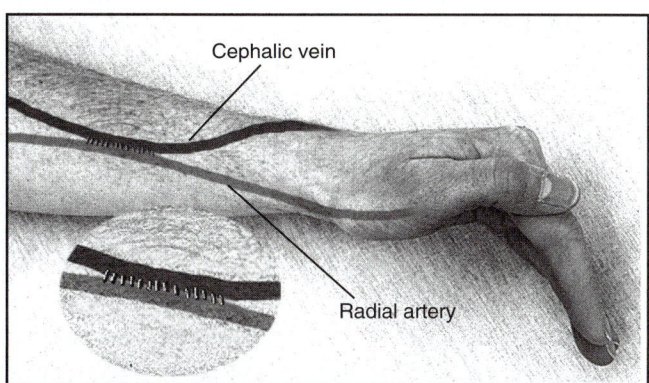

A. An arteriovenous fistula is the direct communication between an artery and a vein, in which a surgical incision is made into each vessel, after which the two are sutured together.

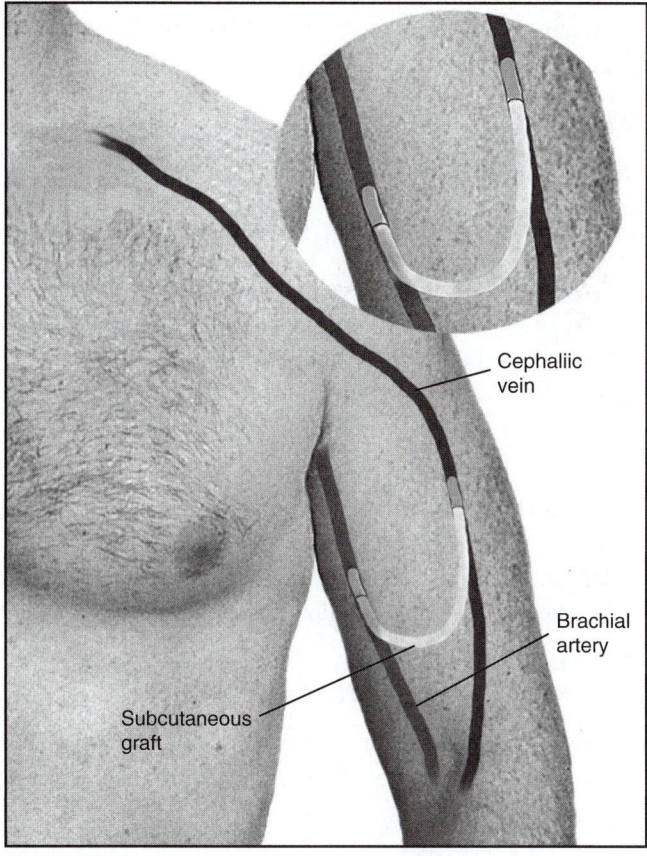

B. An arteriorvenous graft is where a natural graft (autograft or bovine graft) is tunneled under the skin and connected to the distal end of an artery and the proximal end of a vein.

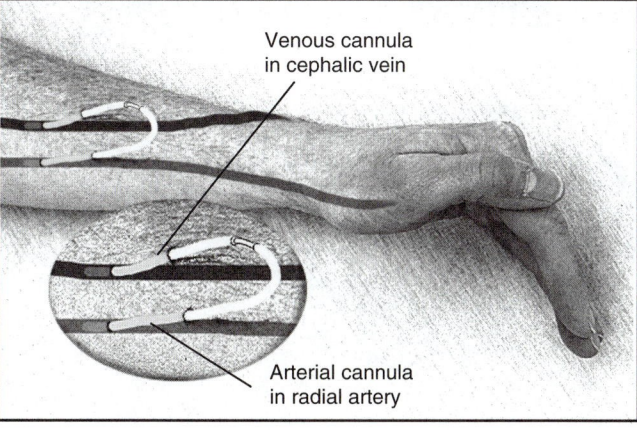

C. A shunt is an artificially constructed passage to divert blood flow from an artery to a vein, in which one transparent silicon cannula is threaded into an artery and another into a vein. The two are tunneled to the surface of the limb and connected to form a loop by joining them together with a silicon connector.

Figure 7-12 | Surgical arteriovenous communications: (A) arteriovenous fistula; (B) arteriovenous graft; (C) arteriovenous shunt

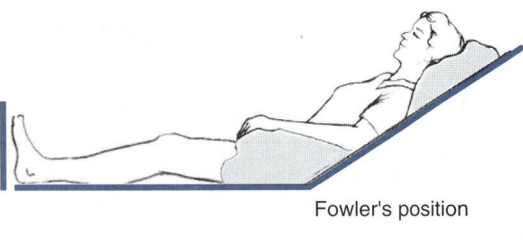

Fowler's position

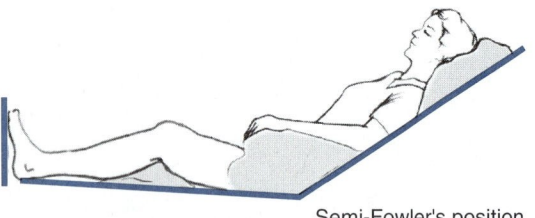

Semi-Fowler's position

Figure 7-13 | Fowler's and semi-Fowler's positions

purpose, duration, and possible side effects of therapy. The nurse is expected to have a sound understanding of the anatomy and physiology of the vascular system and the access sites that may be used whether she initiates the therapy or manages and monitors the infusion started by someone else.

Peripheral Intravenous Routes

When selecting an appropriate vein for infusion therapy, the nurse must take into consideration, based on the patient's circumstances, the purpose of therapy, the proposed duration that the IV will be needed, and the condition and location of usable veins.

Prior to setting up or bringing any IV equipment to the patient's bedside, the nurse should spend some time with the patient, explaining all components of the proposed therapy

and providing some time for the patient to ask questions. At this time the nurse can visually inspect the patient's skin and veins and palpate proposed access sites, to locate the most appropriate vessel in which to initiate therapy. She might want to apply a tourniquet, shine a flashlight over the arm, or utilize a device such as the Venoscope II Transilluminator (Figure 7-14) to detect the most suitable veins for use. When it is decided which vein will be employed, using one of these measures, the nurse might want to mark the intended vein with a surgical marking pen. During this time, she can also predict the ease or difficulty of venous access and determine the measures she might need to take to facilitate successful venipuncture. Before starting the IV, the patient's permission must be obtained.

NURSING TIP

Obtaining Permission

Before performing venipuncture and starting an infusion on an adult, the nurse must obtain his permission. Failure to do so constitutes assault and battery.

There are several issues that must be addressed and considered prior to commencing infusion therapy. These include things that the nurse should accomplish and those that she must avoid, that is, the dos and don'ts of IV site selection and therapy initiation (Table 7-3).

Upper Extremity Access Sites

Venous cannulation, for infusion therapy, should begin at the distal-most area of the upper extremity and proceed

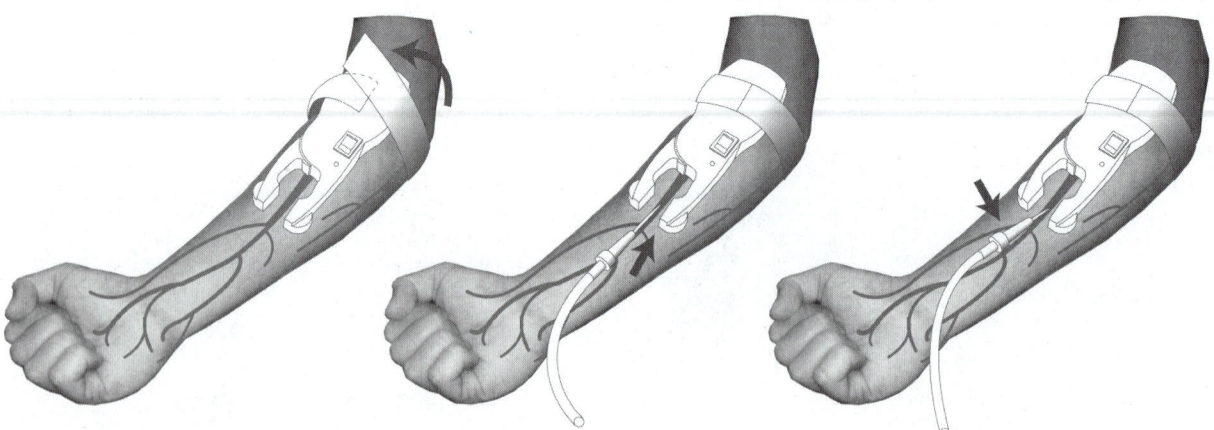

Figure 7-14 | The Venoscope II Transilluminator® (Courtesy of Venoscope, LLC, Lafayette, LA)

Table 7-3 | The Dos and Don'ts of IV Site Selection

DO	RATIONALE
Use the distal veins of the upper extremities first, with subsequent venipunctures proximal to the previous sites.	The venous network above previously used sites will not be punctured. By alternating limbs, the previously used vein can heal.
Palpate the veins prior to venipuncture.	From palpation, the nurse can determine the condition of the patient's veins, differentiate them from arteries, and locate deeper, larger veins, which are stronger and more suitable for IV therapy.
Use veins appropriate for the prescribed infusate. Larger veins should be used for irritating or hypertonic preparations.	Hypertonic or irritating infusates cause discomfort when infused into small veins where there is reduced hemodilution and the intima of the vein can be damaged.
Use veins that will most likely sustain the infusion for 48 to 72 hours.	With prolonged infusion therapy, all measures must be taken to preserve peripheral veins.
Use the smallest cannula that will deliver the prescribed infusate.	The cannula size should allow for adequate blood flow and hemodilution while delivering the infusate at the appropriate rate and causing minimal discomfort.

DON'T	RATIONALE
Do not use the veins of the lower extremities in adults and children who are walking. If an emergency exists, and they must be used, change the site as soon as the patient is stabilized.	The circulation in these veins is more sluggish than in the upper body, thereby increasing the risk of phlebitis, thrombosis, and embolism.
Do not use veins that are irritated or sclerosed from previous use.	Use of such veins produces undue discomfort for the patient and increases trauma and the possibility of phlebitis and infection.
Avoid areas of flexion, unless the joint is immobilized.	The catheter may kink and restrict the flow of fluid, or it may break. If a steel needle is used, it may puncture the vessel wall, infiltrate, or cause damage to surrounding tissues and nerves. Using these areas limits the patient's movement and independence.
Avoid veins in the antecubital fossa.	It is difficult to adequately immobilize this area and movement of the cannula can result in infiltration and mechanical phlebitis. Damage to the antecubital veins restricts use of distal veins in the extremity that feed into these vessels.
Do not use a tourniquet on fragile veins.	The pressure of the tourniquet may cause rupture of the venous wall during venipuncture, resulting in hematoma and damage to the vein.
Do not use the veins in an extremity: • On the side of the body where a radical mastectomy has been performed with lymph node dissection/stripping • That is impaired as a result of a CVA • That is partially amputated, or has undergone reconstructive or orthopedic surgery • That has sustained third degree burns	Circulation in these areas is impaired, with altered venous and lymphatic flow, which can cause or exacerbate edema.
Do not use an arteriovenous fistula, shunt, or graft for peripheral infusion therapy.	These routes, which are surgically constructed, must be preserved for hemodialysis access.

proximally, with subsequent cannulation being made proximal to the previously cannulated site. Table 7-4 profiles which veins should be used and their indications for use. As always, when electing to cannulate a particular vein for any infusion, the nurse must assess the patient and his condition, the indication(s) for therapy, the product(s) to be infused, and the projected time the therapy will be employed. "Site selection for vascular access shall include assessment of the patient's condition, infusion device history, and type and duration of therapy." (INS, 2000, Standard 43, S37).

Veins of the Hands
The digital veins of the hands are the small vessels in the dorsal and lateral sections of the digits, or fingers. They are small and communicate to form the metacarpal veins, those

Table 7-4 | Upper Extremity Venous Access Sites: Indications for Use

	VEINS								
	Digital	Metacarpal	Cephalic	Accessory Cephalic	Median Cephalic (Antecubital)	Basilic	Median Basilic (Antecubital)	Median Cubital (Antecubital)	Median Antebrachial
USAGE CHARACTERISTICS									
Ideal for short-term use	✔	✔							
Use with small-gauge cannula	✔	✔							
Use with nonirritating fluids	✔	✔							
Naturally splinted by bone			✔	✔	✔	✔			
Requires artificial splinting	✔				✔		✔	✔	✔
Accommodates large-gauge cannula			✔	✔	✔	✔	✔	✔	
Accommodates longer cannula			✔	✔		✔			
Close proximity to artery					✔			✔	
Thin-walled vein	✔	✔							
ADVANTAGES									
Best choice for early IV use		✔							
Easy access		✔	✔	✔	✔	✔	✔	✔	
Good visibility		✔	✔		✔	✔	✔		
Does not impair mobility			✔	✔		✔			
Allows for good hemodilution			✔	✔	✔	✔	✔	✔	✔
Ideal for phlebotomy						✔	✔	✔	
Ideal for blood transfusion				✔	✔	✔			
DISADVANTAGES									
Impairs mobility	✔	✔			✔		✔	✔	✔
Discomfort on insertion	✔	✔				✔	✔		✔
Infiltrates easily	✔						✔	✔	✔
Tends to roll with venipuncture				✔		✔			✔
Difficult to splint	✔				✔			✔	✔
Vessels, tissues, nerves are easily damaged					✔		✔	✔	✔
Difficult to visualize with edema or obesity	✔		✔	✔	✔				
Inflames easily		✔							

that lie on the dorsum of the hand over the metacarpal bones, and are tributaries of the dorsal venous arch. Figure 7-15 illustrates the venous circulation of the hand.

Veins of the Arms

The cephalic vein emanates from the metacarpal vein at the radial portion of the lower forearm and proceeds upward, above the radial-humeral joint, on the radial margin of the upper arm, at which point it becomes the upper cephalic vein. The accessory cephalic vein branches off from the cephalic vein and continues to run along the radial surface of the forearm, whereas the median cephalic vein branches toward the inner aspect of the forearm.

The basilic vein radiates upward from the metacarpal veins on the ulnar aspect of the forearm, past the elbow to the upper arm, with the median basilic branching on the palmar side of the forearm. In the upper arm, the basilic and cephalic veins merge with the axillary vein, which leads into

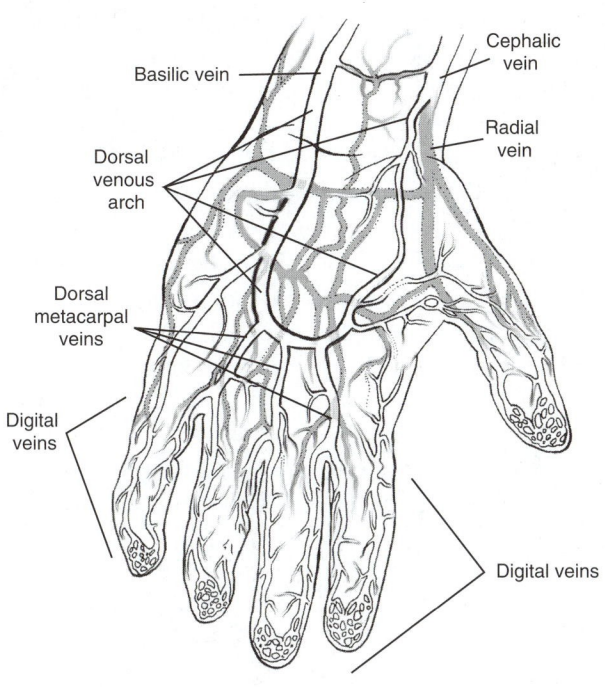

Figure 7-15 | Superficial and deep veins of the hand

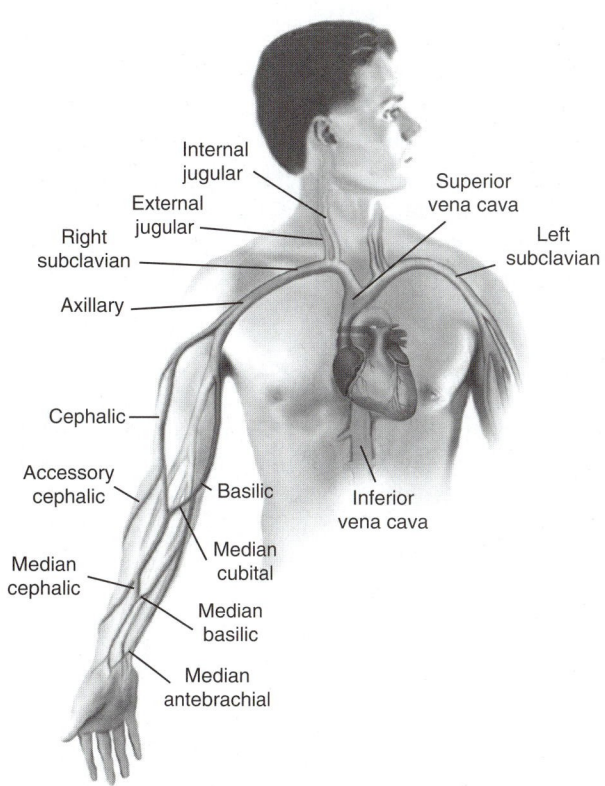

Figure 7-17 | Superficial and deep veins of the arm and upper torso

the subclavian vein. Figures 7-16 and 7-17 illustrate the venous circulation of the arms and upper body.

The antecubital veins (also called median veins because they extend centrally from the palmar region of the forearm) are three vessels that lead into the **cubital fossa**—the triangular region that lies anterior to and below the elbow. The median cephalic branches from the cephalic vein on the radial aspect of the arm, the median basilic emanates from the basilic vein on the ulnar side, and the median cubital branches from the basilic vein in front of the elbow. Table 7-4 compares and contrasts the indications and uses for peripheral access sites of the hands and arms.

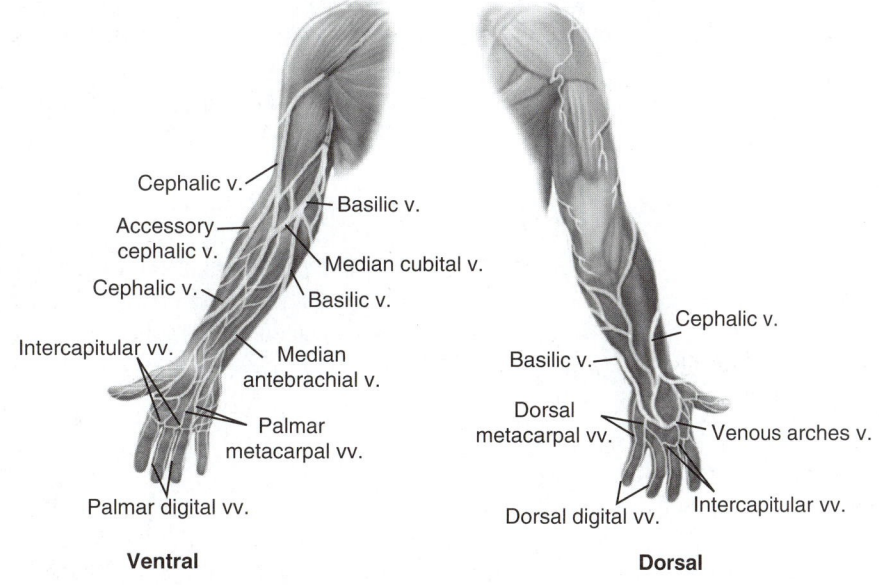

Ventral

Dorsal

Figure 7-16 | Superficial and deep veins of the arm

Veins of the Upper Body

The veins of the upper body consist of larger vessels that channel blood to the heart. The subclavian veins originate from the axillary veins where the cephalic and basilic veins merge in the upper chest and shoulder regions. The internal and external jugular veins drain blood from the head and neck regions into the superior vena cava, the large vessel that empties into the right atrium of the heart.

Lower Extremity Access Sites

"Veins of the lower extremities should not be used routinely in the adult population due to risk of embolism and thrombophlebitis" (INS, 200, Standard 43, S37). Although not recommended for use in adults or walking children because of circulatory compromise and the potential for thromboembolic disorders, the lower extremity vessels (Figure 7-18) sometimes have to be accessed in emergency situations. If used, there needs to be a written medical order, as well as agency policy to uphold this procedure. There must be full documentation to support the reason for lower extremity cannulation and the site must be changed as soon as the patient's condition warrants it. If it is absolutely necessary to use the leg veins, the best choices are usually those on the dorsum of the foot, over the metatarsal bones, or the saphenous vein, where it surfaces in the ankle area.

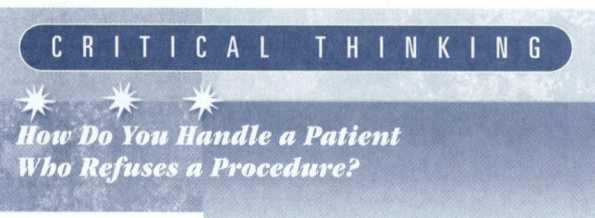

CRITICAL THINKING

How Do You Handle a Patient Who Refuses a Procedure?

Your patient, whose physician has ordered an intravenous infusion, refuses to allow you to start it. He is pale, trembling, and the palms of his hands are cool and clammy. What would you say? What would you do? What are his rights? What is your responsibility?

To begin with, always bear in mind that a patient has the right to refuse treatment, but before notifying the physician of this, you have several options:

Listen. Give him a chance to verbalize his feelings and fears.

Be nonjudgmental. Maintain eye contact and interest in what he has to say.

Reassure. Assure him that nothing will be done without his consent. Clearly state that he certainly has the right to refuse treatment and that you will abide by his wishes.

Investigate. Try and find out why he does not want the treatment—again, in a nonjudgmental manner. He may have had an unfavorable experience in the past and need clarification and explanations.

Explain. When a patient is apprehensive, he may need reinforcement as to why treatment is needed and how it can help him.

Report. If he still refuses, notify the physician.

Document. Record all assessment data, verbal and nonverbal, to substantiate the refusal.

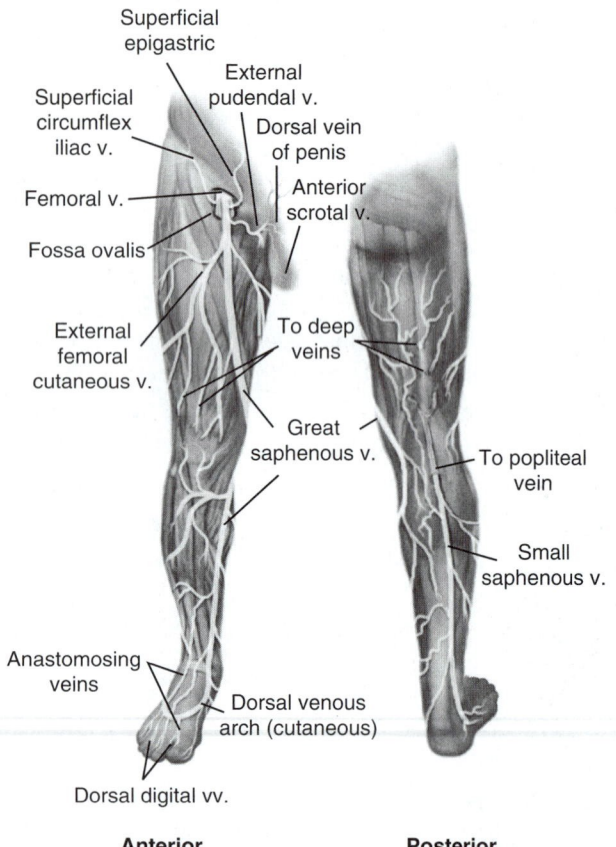

Figure 7-18 | Superficial veins of the lower limbs

Key Concepts

✳ There are distinct advantages and disadvantages that must be deliberated from the standpoint of medical judgment, nursing liability, and the patient's clinical status, safety, and comfort when the decision to institute peripheral IV infusion therapy is under consideration.

✳ To correctly and safely facilitate vascular access, the nurse must have a sound knowledge of the anatomy and physiology of the integumentary and circulatory systems.

✳ The integumentary system is composed of the outer covering that insulates and provides the first line of defense in protecting the body from microbial invasion and injury. It is made up of the epidermis (the outermost layer), which is composed of epithelial cells; and the dermis (corium), called the true skin, which is composed of connective tissue, blood and lymphatic vessels, nerves, muscles, hair follicles, and sebaceous and sudoriferous glands.

✳ Arteries, which carry blood away from the heart, are thick-walled (three layers), highly elastic, and transport under potent pressure. They merge into arterioles, which branch into capillaries (the smallest blood vessels in the body), where arterial and venous communication takes place.

✳ Once blood leaves the capillaries, it enters the venules and passes to the veins (where blood returns to the heart and the transport of waste products to areas of excretion takes place). Veins have thinner walls than arteries, have much less elasticity, and are lined with valves that serve to deter the backflow of blood into the capillary beds.

✳ Prior to the initiation of IV therapy, the patient must be prepared psychologically and physically. Psychological preparation reduces the patient's apprehension, helps him adapt, and facilitates the initiation of therapy for the nurse. Physical preparation includes measures that promote safety, comfort, and positioning.

✳ Intravascular site selection for infusion therapy is determined by the patient's condition, the purpose of therapy, and its proposed duration. Intravascular access refers to the entrance into arteries, veins, or capillaries and cannot be initiated without proper consent.

✳ The usual intravenous sites the nurse can access are the veins in the hands and arms, starting therapy at the most distal point, with subsequent punctures performed proximally. Unless it is an emergency, the lower extremity vessels should not be used on adults or children (who are walking), because of compromised blood return, making the patient more susceptible to thromboembolic disorders. If such a vein must be used, the site is to be changed as soon as the patient is stabilized and an upper extremity vein can be cannulated.

Review Questions and Activities

1. List five factors the nurse must consider when choosing an IV site.
2. Using another person's arm and hand, identify the vessels that would be appropriate for peripheral IV access when an isotonic, hypotonic, or isotonic solution is ordered.
3. In light of the physiology and mechanics of circulatory and lymphatic flow, explain why an IV infusion should not be initiated in the extremity on the side of the body where a radical mastectomy has been performed.
4. Draw a two-column chart to compare arteries, arterioles, capillaries, venules, and veins, in terms of their size, structure, anatomic location, elasticity, and blood flow.
5. Based on the following information, what measures would you take to prepare this patient physically and

psychologically for her prescribed treatment regimen? What, specifically, would you say and do regarding the IV you must start?

Miss Lucci is a 22-year-old college student, admitted to your unit for a possible ruptured ovarian cyst. Her physician has ordered several diagnostic tests and has given stat orders for her to be NPO with continuous IVs infusing at 125 cc/hr. As you begin to perform your admission assessment and explain what the doctor has prescribed, Miss Lucci begins to tremble and cry, saying, "I am so afraid of hospitals. The thought of being stuck with needles terrifies me. I feel like I am going to faint."

Chapter 8

Equipment and Supplies Employed in the Preparation and Administration of Intravenous Infusion Therapy

COMPETENCIES

Upon completion of this chapter, the reader should be able to:

✳ Analyze and identify the nurse's role and responsibility regarding the use of equipment and supplies used for infusion therapy.

✳ Identify the types of infusate containers available and indications for their use.

✳ Describe the features of the various primary and secondary infusate administration sets and the accessory devices that can be used with them.

✳ Explain how needleless systems and needlestick protection devices operate.

✳ Distinguish between the commonly used peripheral venous access devices.

✳ List the materials used to prepare and maintain the integrity of the percutaneous infusion site.

✳ Differentiate between the types of manual, gravity control, and electronic infusion devices used to regulate intravenous infusions.

(back) check valve
drop factor
extension set

filter, IV
patient-controlled analgesia (PCA)
priming volume

stopcock

The practice of intravenous infusion therapy has rapidly advanced to one of the most sophisticated specialty areas in nursing. The knowledge, skill, and expertise required to perform procedures in this highly technical realm involves the use of some traditional, but mostly innovative, state-of-the-art equipment. Such items pass through many hands and fall under the guidelines and requirements set forth by federal, state, and local authorities, as well as private, legal, and financial sectors. These groups, via their dictates, are committed to a universal cause—the well-being and safety of all health care consumers and providers.

The equipment and supplies available for use in the delivery of infusion therapy are constantly being evaluated and updated. Manufacturers strive to provide equipment that is on the cutting edge in terms of patient safety and comfort, nursing productivity, cost-effectiveness, and environmental preservation.

It is the responsibility of the nurse to develop and maintain expertise in the use and maintenance of any equipment utilized in the delivery of IV therapy. He is obligated to understand how various products function and know where to turn for information and problem solving. The nurse is often involved in clinical trials of products as well as the decision-making processes regarding what supplies will be adopted for use in his place of employment.

INFUSATE CONTAINERS

The containers used for the delivery of intravenous infusions, for the most part, are made of flexible plastic materials. Because of the chemical makeup of some infusates, however, glass containers are also used. When using any of these containers, the nurse must always do several things prior to setting up and administering the infusate, to ensure patient safety. He must read the label to ascertain that the infusate is the correct one ordered for his patient and check the expiration date. He must evaluate the container, making sure that all seals are intact and that there are no breaks in its integrity. The fluid should be checked for clarity and the absence of particulate matter. Manufacturer and additive labels are affixed to containers in an inverted position so they can easily be read when the container is hanging upside down on an IV pole.

Glass Containers

Glass containers are vacuum systems that require a vent to replace infused fluid with air. The vacuum must be released in order for the solution to flow. The venting can be accomplished with use of vented administration set tubing or through an internal system in which the bottle contains a tube that allows air to enter and collect in the space above the fluid level. In the vented administration set, the bottle is sealed with a solid rubber stopper with one hole, covered by a latex rubber disc that maintains the vacuum. Once the disc is removed and the administration set attached, filtered air enters the container through an airway that is built into the administration set spike. With the internal system, the rubber closure for the bottle has two openings, one with a filtered strawlike tube that extends into the bottle and one for the administration set (both sealed with a latex rubber disc that preserves the vacuum inside the bottle). Once the latex disc is removed and the container is spiked, air enters into the solution container through the filtered tube. In both systems the vacuum-preserving latex disc is secured with an aluminum, peel-off band. Fluid graduation marks are molded into the glass. At the bottom of the bottle is an aluminum band and bail for hanging on an IV pole when the bottle is inverted (Figure 8-1).

Once a glass solution bottle is opened by a pharmacist for the introduction of an admixture, it is sealed with a tamper-proof closure to prevent alteration of the infusate after it leaves the pharmacy. This device cannot be removed without being torn. If it is not fully intact, the infusate must not be used.

Plastic Containers

Plastic containers that house intravenous infusates are constructed of semirigid or flexible materials. Even though they can be punctured or broken, they have a greater safety factor and are more functional than glass bottles, especially in emergency and community health settings.

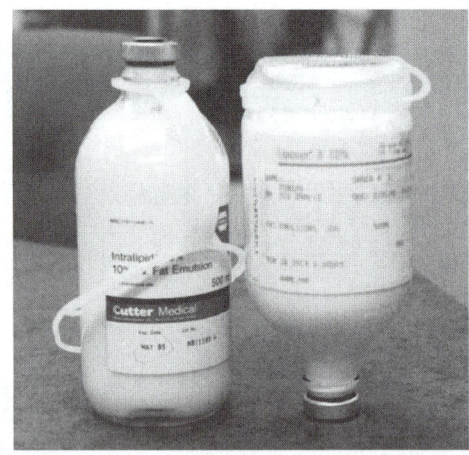

A.

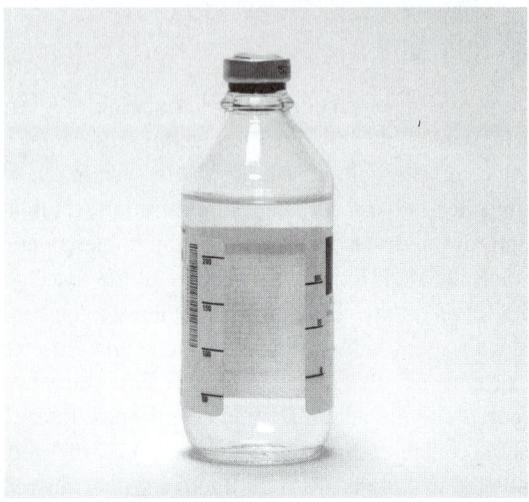

B.

Figure 8-1 | Glass IV bottles (B. Courtesy of Baxter Healthcare Corporation)

Individual plastic containers are made of the same materials, rather than a combination of glass, plastic, rubber, and metal (found in glass systems). Semirigid containers are generally made of biologically inert, non-toxic PVC (polyvinyl chloride) or polyolefin. To provide flexibility in the manufacture of pliable, collapsible bags, the phthalate plasticizer, DEHP (Di [2-ethylhexyl] phthalate) has been added to the PVC for many years. Some companies have elected not to use PVC/DEHP due to concerns regarding the safety of exposure to this chemical. The Food and Drug Administration (FDA) issued a public health notification regarding the use of the DEHP plasticizer and its ability to leach out of plastic medical devices into the solutions that come in contact with the plastic. The amount of DEHP that will leach out depends on the temperature, the lipid content of the liquid, and the duration of contact with the plastic. Exposure to DEHP has produced a range of adverse effects in laboratory animals. Of greatest concern, based on existing studies, are the effects the chemical may have on the male

reproductive system and the production of normal sperm (FDA Center for Devices and Radiological Health, 2002b). Most infusion companies are no longer making IV bags with PVC/DEHP, even though the International Agency for Research on Cancer (IARC) has reclassified DEHP as "not classifiable as to carcinogenicity to humans" (IARC, 2000). Instead, manufacturers are using polyolefin, a biologically inert, clear, flexible, non-DEHP nontoxic plastic that is ecologically favorable because it is biodegradable and will incinerate into carbon dioxide and water. Infusion containers made with polyolefin are as drug-compatible as those made of glass.

Flexible Plastic Containers

The soft, plastic containers, which are most common and widely used, are totally closed systems that do not require venting because they are not vacuum sealed (Figure 8-2). They are free of air and impervious to moisture. Because they can withstand extremes of temperature, these bags are used for additives that must be stored under refrigeration or require freezing prior to administration. These bags are available in a wider variety of sizes than other containers, ranging from 50 to 2000 ml. The major problems associated with the use of plastic IV bags is that they can be easily punctured during spiking and small breaches in the integrity of the plastic may go unnoticed, thus allowing for the entry of organisms into the system.

Unless admixtures have been added in the pharmacy, flexible plastic IV bags are contained in an opaque, outer plastic wrap that must be torn off to expose the IV container. Extending from the top of all flexible IV bags is a flat continuation of the plastic that has a hole for hanging on an IV pole. Depending on the manufacturer, there may be one or two extensions protruding from the bottom of the bag. If there are two, one is the administration set port, encased in a protective, easily removable plastic pigtail that maintains the port's sterility prior to spiking, and the other is an injection port for adding medication. Inside the administration port (about 0.5 in) is a polyvinyl diaphragm that prevents loss of infusate prior to spiking, even if the pigtail is removed. When this diaphragm is punctured with the administration set spike, infusate flows into the administration set. Once pierced, the diaphragm is not resealable. The other extension from the IV bag is covered by a latex rubber medication port that allows for introduction of additives via a syringe and needle or needleless connection plug. When there is only one extension from the bag for the administration set, the medication port, which is a resealable latex disk, is found on the lower portion of the IV bag.

Information regarding the product, expiration date, and fluid graduation marks are imprinted into the plastic by the manufacturer. Never write directly on a flexible plastic bag with a ballpoint pen or any type of indelible marker. The pen may puncture the bag and the indelible marker ink may

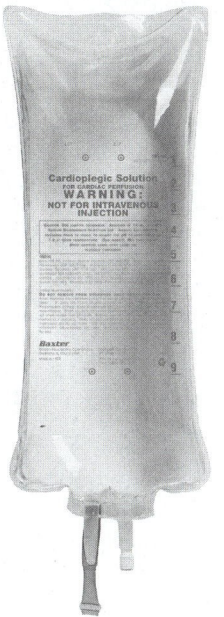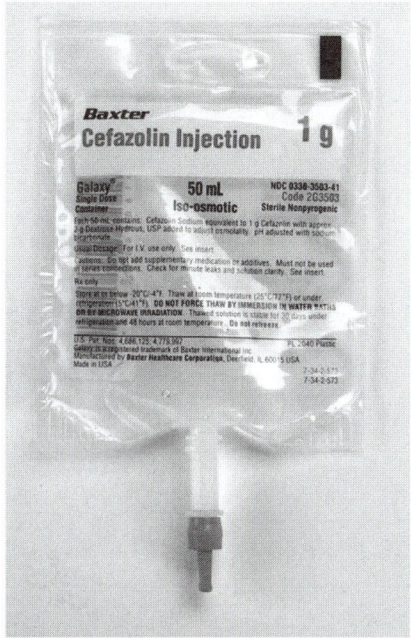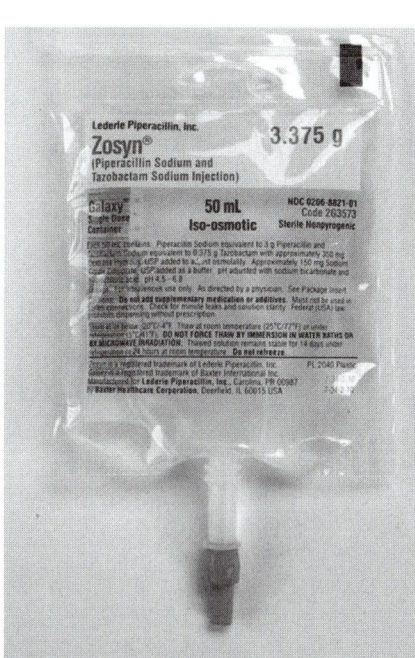

Figure 8-2 | Flexible IV Containers (Courtesy of Baxter Healthcare Corporation)

NURSING ALERT

Writing on IV Bags

Never write directly on a flexible plastic IV bag with a ballpoint pen or any type of indelible marker.

absorb into the plastic and contaminate the infusate. If additional information is to be added, it must be affixed with a label.

As with glass containers, tamperproof additive caps are available for use with flexible plastic IV bags (Figure 8-3). The cap fits over the medication port and indicates that a pharmacist has added medication to the infusate and that the admixture has not been tampered with since leaving the pharmacy.

Flexible plastic IV bags are used for reduced-volume (50 or 100 ml) piggyback containers of 5% dextrose in water and 0.9% sodium chloride (Figure 8-4). Medications are added to these bags for intermittent administration. For commonly used drugs, especially antibiotics, the plastic minibags are filled with ready-to-use medications at the time of manufacture. It is the responsibility of the nurse to know which of these need to be refrigerated or kept at room temperature prior to administration. Some minibags, such as the MiniBag Plus® system by Baxter (Figure 8-5), are manufactured with the capability of attaching a vial of medication. By manipulating the minibag and the medication vial, the medication

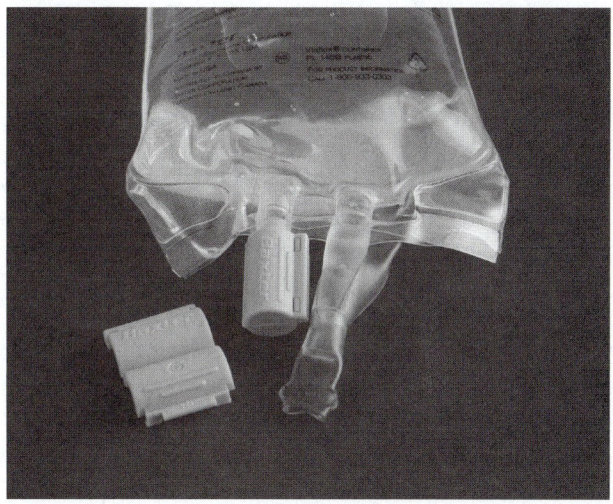

Figure 8-3 | Additive cap for VIAFLEX plastic container used to provide evidence that medication has been added to VIAFLEX containers (Courtesy of Baxter Healthcare Corporation)

and diluent can be mixed immediately prior to administration, thus eliminating the need for refrigeration.

Semirigid Plastic Containers

Semirigid containers (Figure 8-6) are made of polyolefin and do not contain plasticizers, thus preventing chemical leaching and the extraction of DEHP into the solution they enclose. They are ideal for use, too, when the additive is of a chemical nature that predisposes it to bind to the interior of

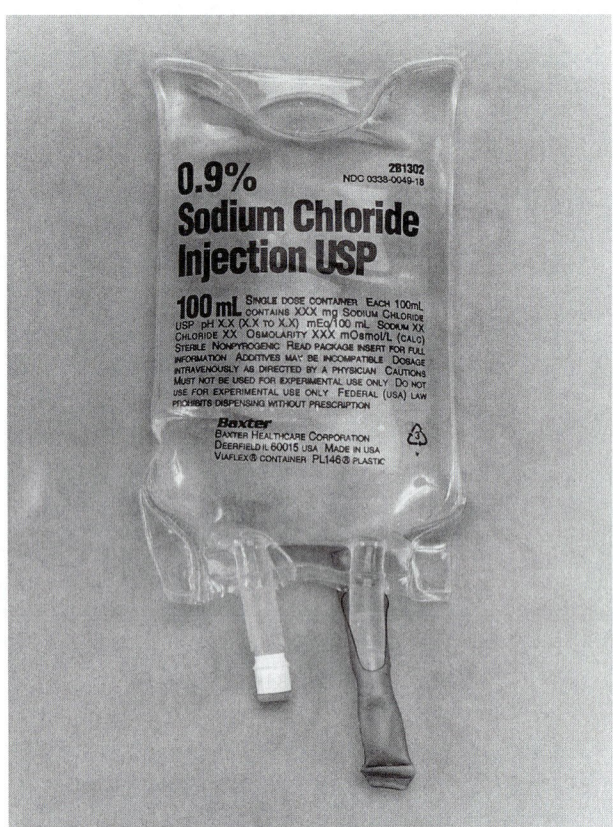

Figure 8-4 | MiniBag® Reduced-Volume Piggyback Container (Courtesy of Baxter Healthcare Corporation)

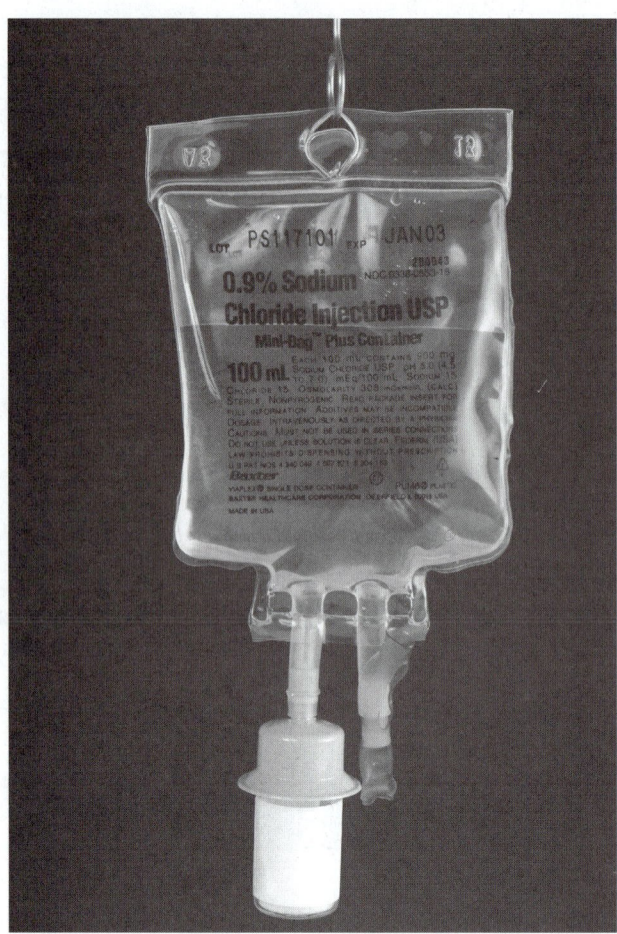

Figure 8-5 | MiniBag Plus® (Courtesy of Baxter Healthcare Corporation)

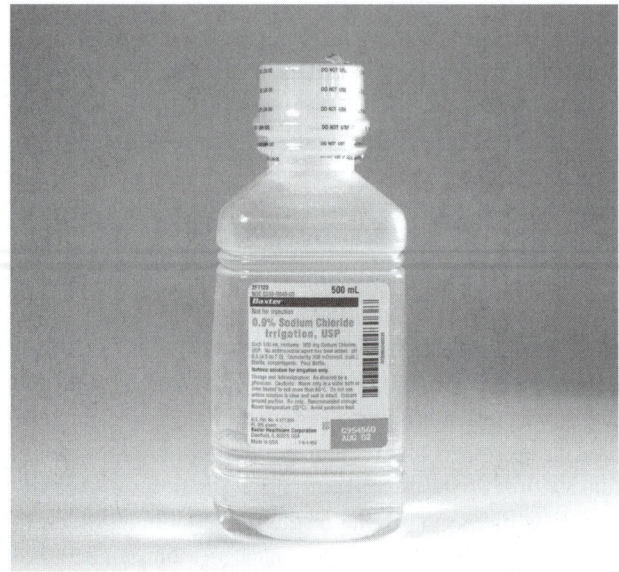

Figure 8-6 | Rigid Plastic Container (Courtesy of Baxter Healthcare Corporation)

pliable plastic bags, thus altering the proper drug delivery dosage. Some types are non-air–dependent systems and do not require venting because they collapse as they empty, while others, like glass bottles, have a vent mechanism that allows air to enter the system and replace the fluid. These containers combine the characteristics of glass bottles (form, easy-to-read calibration marks, and prevention of chemical leaching) with those of flexible bags (shatter-proof, ease of storage and transport, and reduced chance of puncture).

INFUSATE ADMINISTRATION SETS

The IV administration set is the tubing that delivers fluid or medication from the infusate container to the patient (Figure 8-7). Administration sets range in style from basic, general-purpose ones to complex, multifeature, multifunction sets. The traits they all have in common are a spike insert (usually with a finger guard for ease of insertion) at one end that fits into the administration set port of the infusate container, followed by a drip chamber, where solution flows prior to its entry into the

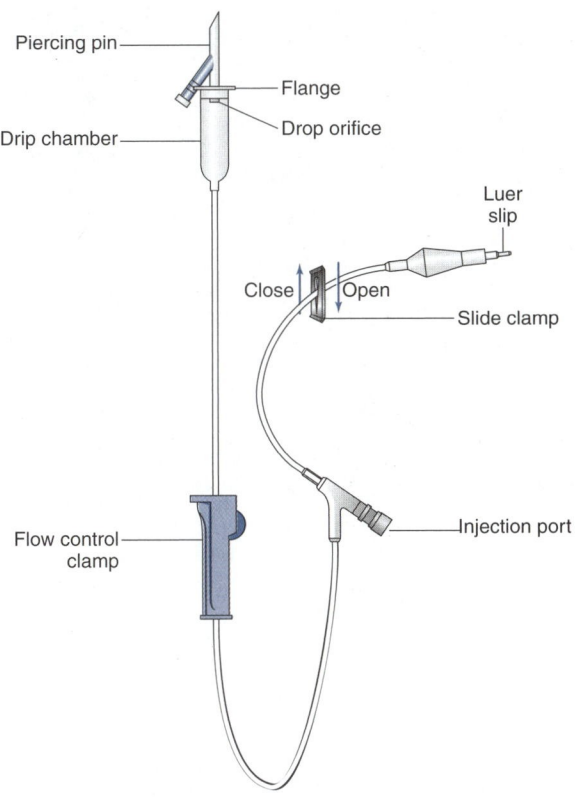

Figure 8-7 | Basic Administration Set

tubing. The tubing on all sets has a screw, roller, and slide clamp (screw and roller clamps usually also have slide clamps lower down the tubing) that provides a means for the nurse to regulate flow using one hand (Figure 8-8). (While screw and roller clamps are used to regulate the drops of the infusate flow, the slide clamp functions only as an on-off clasp.) The tubing terminates in a sterile-capped adapter to which a cannula hub can be attached. The adapter may be straight, where it fits directly into the cannula hub (with a direct push, without twisting), or manually twists and screws on to the hub of the cannula, which provides a firm attachment that cannot be pulled out (Luer-Lok®) (Figure 8-9).

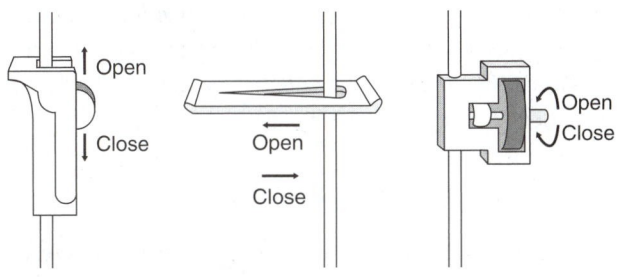

Figure 8-8 | Administration Set Tubing Clamps

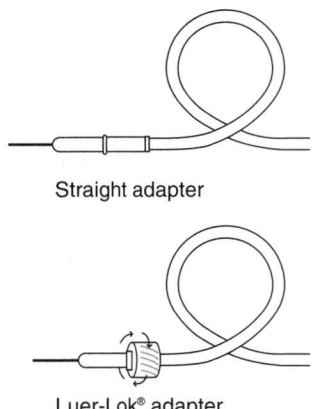

Figure 8-9 | Straight and Luer-Lok® Cannula Hub Adapters

Administration sets are available as vented systems, which are used for vacuum infusate containers that do not have their own built-in mechanisms for air displacement (glass and some semirigid bottles), or nonvented systems, for use with flexible plastic bags and other nonvacuum receptacles. They are also available for exclusive use with electronic infusion devices (EIDs), and vary according to the manufacturer.

Administration sets, based on their manufacturer-specific proportions, primarily determine the rate at which fluid can be delivered to the patient. In order for the nurse to accurately manage the delivery of infusate to a patient, he must know how much fluid the administration set he is using transports. This is determined by the drop factor.

Drop Factor

The **drop factor** is the number of drops needed to deliver 1 ml of fluid and is based on the size of the hollow, internal diameter (bore) of the administration tubing. The drop factor is clearly stated on the administration set package. Sets are made to deliver either macrodrops or microdrops. Macrodrip sets deliver 10 to 20 drops/ml while microdrip tubings dispense 60 drops/ml (minidrip) (Figure 8-10 and 8-11). The nurse calculates the rate of IV flow in drops per minute. In addition to these standard tubings, there are also specialized extra large (macrobore) and extra small (microbore) tubings that are used in specialized settings and circumstances. The former are used in emergency surgical and trauma situations when large volumes of blood or fluid must be infused rapidly. The latter are designed for the delivery of small amounts of precisely controlled fluid or medication in situations where volume restriction is critical, such as for neonatal care and for epidural infusions. (See Chapter 10 for a review of formulas and calculations.)

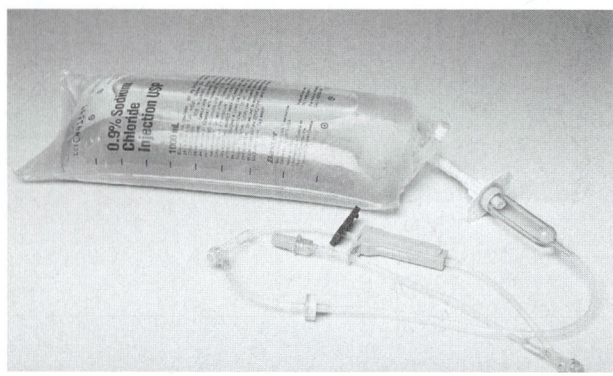

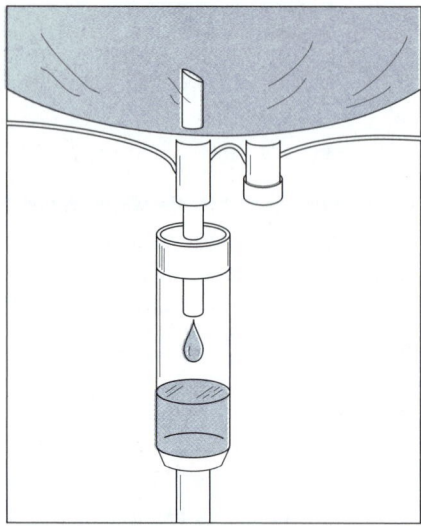

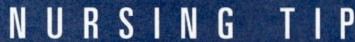

Figure 8-10 | Macrodrip Tubing

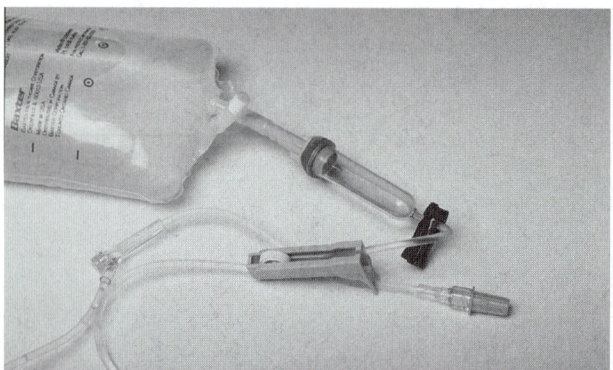

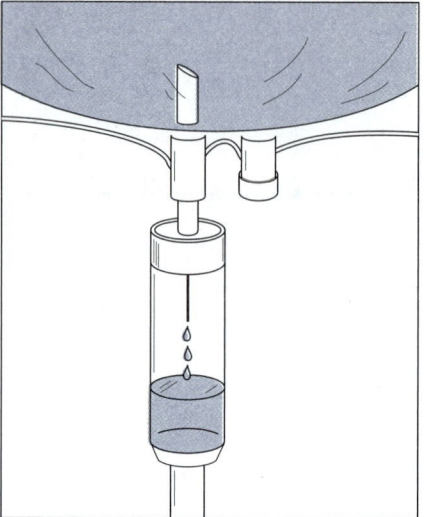

Figure 8-11 | Microdrip Tubing

NURSING TIP

Four Essentials of IV Infusions

In order to correctly deliver and manage an intravenous infusion, the nurse must know four things:

1. The prescribed volume to be infused
2. The prescribed time for the infusion
3. The drop factor
4. The mathematical formula needed to calculate the rate

Primary Administration Sets

Primary administration sets (also referred to as basic or standard sets) are those that are spiked into one (single line) or two (Y-type sets) main infusate containers and carry fluid via one tube directly to the patient. At the distal end, where they attach to the cannula, they may terminate in straight, flashtube, or Luer-Lok® male adapters. Primary tubing sets are available in macrodrop or microdrop sizes and come in varying lengths to accommodate patient needs (Figure 8-12). They are available with or without check valves, to prevent retrograde flow, and may contain one or several injection ports. It is from the primary sets that secondary administration tubings are added as well as other attachments, such as extension tubings, flow control devices, filters, and various adapters.

Single Line Primary Administration Sets

Single line primary sets have one spike that extends proximally from the drip chamber that is inserted into one main bag of infusate. The tubing distal to the drip chamber terminates in the male-adapter end that connects to the hub of the vascular access device in the patient.

Y-Type Primary Administration Sets

Y-type administration sets have two equal-length tubes (each having its own roller clamp and, sometimes, its own drip chamber) that extend above one drip chamber and are able to access two primary infusates simultaneously or alter-

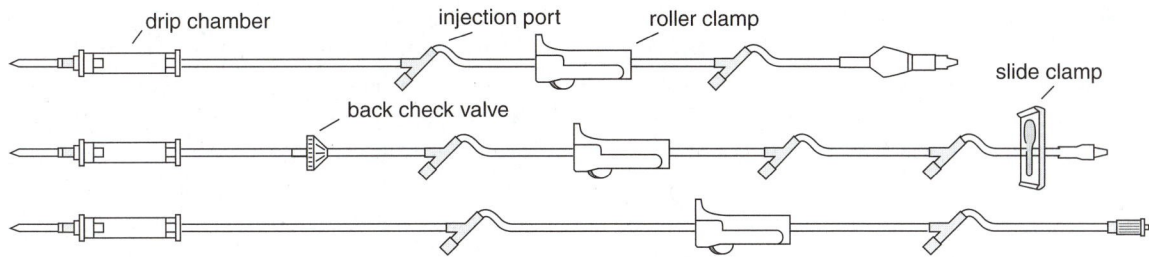

Figure 8-12 | Primary Administration Set

nately. The fluids reach the patient via one common tubing that extends distally from the common drip chamber, making it necessary for the two infusates to be compatible with each other. Such tubings are frequently used in emergency, surgical, and critical care situations and often have macrobore tubing, designed to deliver large quantities of infusate over a faster period than could be accomplished with standard macrodrop administration sets. Blood administration tubings are Y-type sets, but differ somewhat in design than standard primary Y-type sets.

It is crucial for the nurse to understand the physical principles associated with venting and the use of Y-type sets in order to prevent the possibility of air entering the circulatory system, resulting in air embolism. Y-type sets are not vented and, therefore, must be used only with collapsible infusion containers. Because flexible, plastic containers collapse, there is no air in the system. If Y-type sets are used with vented containers and one bottle infuses before the other, the empty receptacle functions as a vent (due to atmospheric pressure in the bottle and tubing exiting it, that exceeds that in the tubing distal to the control clamp). Air then enters the tubing and is siphoned into the circulation, causing a potentially fatal air embolism.

NURSING ALERT

Preventing an Air Embolism

Y-type administration sets should be used only with nonvacuum, flexible, collapsible, infusion containers where there is no air in the system and venting is unnecessary. If vented containers are used in a Y set, air can be drawn into the circulatory system and result in an air embolism, if the vented container empties before the infusate in the other container is finished infusing.

Check Valves

A **check valve** (also termed back-check or one-way valve) functions to prevent retrograde solution flow (Figure 8-13). Check valves are in-line components of many primary admin-

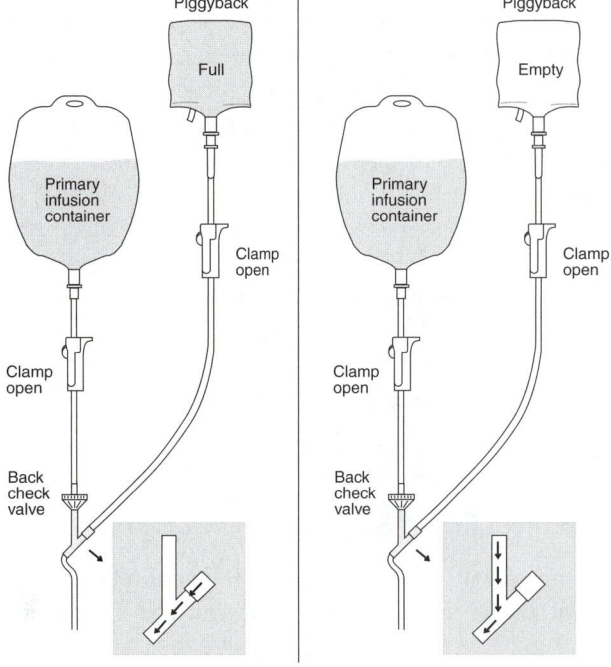

Figure 8-13 | Check Valve and Its Mechanics of Function

istration sets. They are most commonly used when secondary IV lines are in place for intermittent infusion, to inhibit the back flow of secondary infusate into the primary infusate. They also serve to constrain the backflow of blood from the cannula into the IV tubing.

The mechanism of action of the check valve is as follows.

1. The primary infusate is infusing at the prescribed rate by gravity (and is not clamped off prior to the initiation of the piggyback infusion).
2. The secondary infusate, of a lesser volume, is piggybacked into the primary line.
3. The level of the secondary infusate container is elevated above the level of the primary container.
4. The clamp on the tubing of the secondary container is opened, activating the back-check valve due to the pressure exerted by the piggyback solution. (Elevation and gravity increase pressure in the smaller secondary container, even though the primary container is larger.)

5. When the secondary infusate container empties and its fluid descends into its tubing, the decreased pressure in this line (and the greater pressure in the primary line) causes the back-check valve to release, thus activating flow in the primary line, which resumes at its previously set rate.

Secondary Administration Sets

Secondary administration sets are often referred to as piggyback or add-a-line sets and are used to deliver continuous or intermittent doses of fluid or medication (Figure 8-14). These sets are ideal, and widely used, because patients do not have to undergo additional venipunctures, nor does the primary IV have to be interrupted for administration of these therapies. They are usually connected with a needle or needleless adapter into an injection port immediately distal to the back-check valve of the primary tubing. Some primary administration sets are available with a closed-system connection to the secondary line, so that the system does not have to be breached, thus avoiding the possibility of microbial introduction into the setup.

Volume-Control Administration Sets

Volume-control administration sets are limited-volume, cylindrical solution compartments that extend from the primary

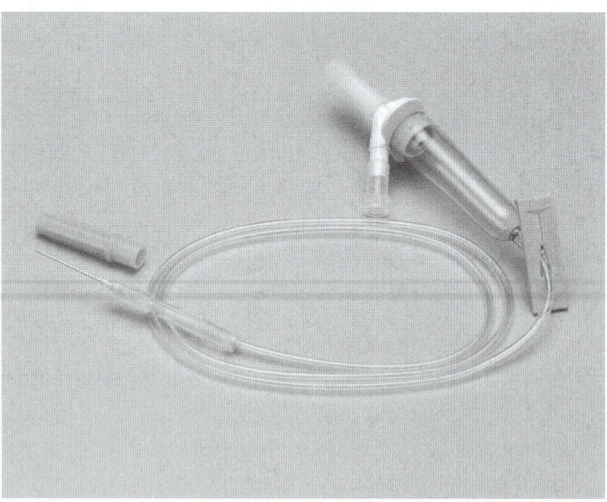

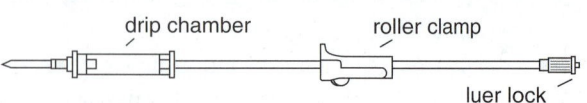

Figure 8-14 | Secondary Administration Set

infusate container and have their own tubing that joins with the patient's IV cannula (Figure 8-15). They are designed to accurately calibrate and dispense restricted quantities of fluid or medication. While these are used widely in pediatric infusion therapy, they are also used to administer small quantities of critical medications and to limit IV intake in adult patients who are severely restricted in their fluid intake. Though sometimes used for intermittent medication delivery, even though they alter the infusion schedule of the primary infusate, they have largely been replaced by secondary administration sets for this purpose.

Blood and Blood Product Administration Sets

Blood administration sets are generally Y-type tubing devices, for use with primary infusates of 0.9% sodium chloride and blood and blood products (Figure 8-16), although straight-line sets are used when blood or blood constituents are the only components to be infused. They must be used in conjunction with cannulas that are large enough for red blood cells to pass through. These sets are blood-product specific and contain in-line filters with a pore size of 170 (minimum) to 260 μm that are designed to screen out clots and other debris that accumulate during the processing, transport, and storage of blood products. The use of blood administration sets should not exceed a 4-hour time period, as bacterial contamination can develop and the filters become less effective. Specialty sets are available for the administration of platelets, cryoprecipitate, and direct IV push of small aggregates of blood component.

Blood administration sets are designed for infusion by gravity or for use with electromechanical infusion devices that have been tested and approved for blood component delivery. They are manufactured for use with special blood administration equipment, such as special filters, specifically designed external pressure infusion cuffs (that do not exceed 300 torr and are used only with large-bore cannulas), and for connection with in-line blood warming devices that do not exceed 38°C (Figure 8-17).

Lipid Administration Sets

Lipids, or fat emulsions, are supplied in glass containers and require special, vented tubing that is supplied by the pharmacy with the release of each bottle of fat emulsion. Lipid-containing infusates have been known to leach phthalates from the bags and tubings of PVC with DEHP. As a result of this concern, fat emulsions are supplied in glass containers, accompanied by nonphthalate infusion sets.

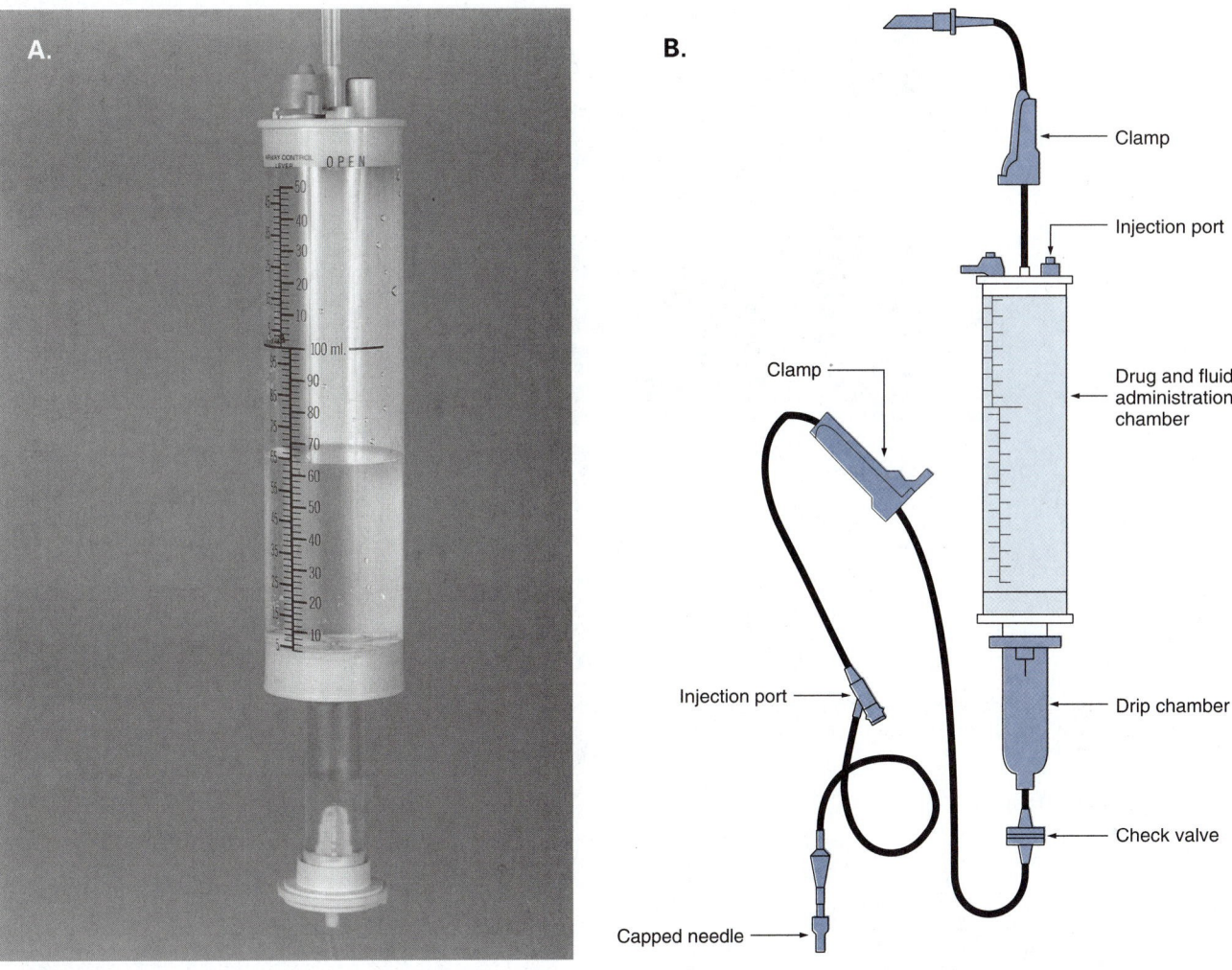

Figure 8-15 | Volume-Control Administration Set (A. Courtesy of Baxter Healthcare Corporation)

Accessory Devices for Use with IV Administration Sets

There are numerous accessory products for use with primary IV lines. Ancillary add-on devices should only be used when an integral tubing system, containing all the components needed to deliver an infusion, is not available. Whenever an infusion line is breached, in order to add nonessential components, the potentiality for inadvertent contamination occurs.

Filters

An **IV filter** is a porous medium through which impurities and particulate matter in an infusate pass, for the purpose of separating and trapping them, thus preventing them from entering the patient's circulation during infusion therapy. Filters are available as integral components of IV adminis-

tration sets (Figure 8-18) or can be added on (Figure 8-19). As a general rule, the Centers for Disease Control and Prevention (CDC) (2001a) does not recommend the use of filters for nonblood infusates. When any filter is used, it is important that the nurse follow the manufacturer's guidelines, so as not to damage the membrane.

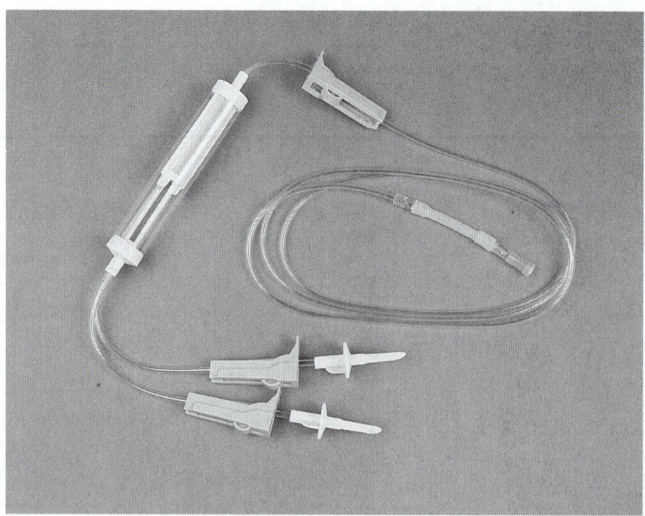

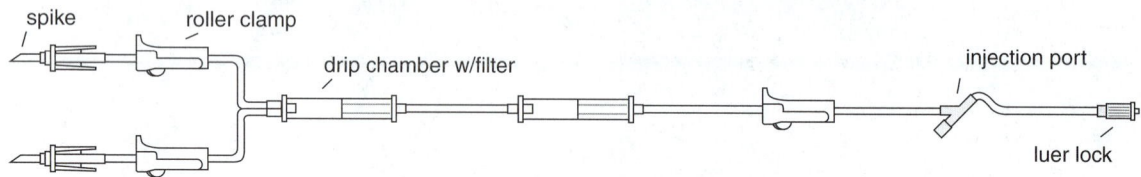

Y-type, drip chamber with (170μ) blood filter, pump chamber, three roller clamps, injection site 6" above distal end, two-piece male Luer-Lok® adapter.

Figure 8-16 │ Y-type Blood Administration Set

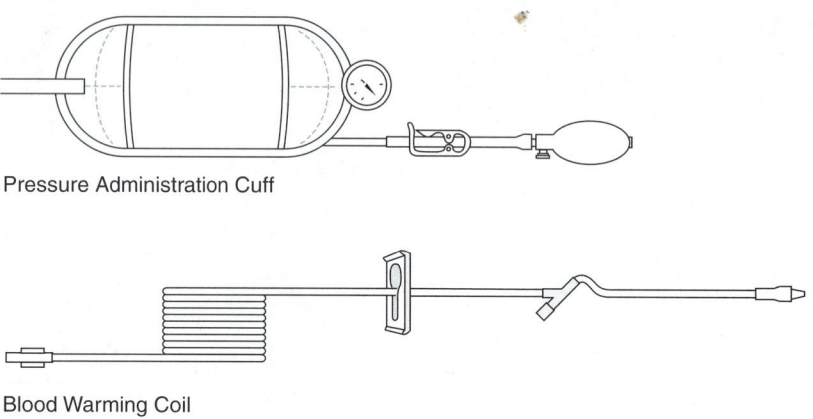

Pressure Administration Cuff

Blood Warming Coil

Figure 8-17 │ Blood Administration Accessory Equipment

Extension Sets

An **extension set** is a segment of IV tubing that is added to a primary administration line for the purpose of adding length (Figure 8-20). Extension tubings come in a variety of sizes to meet individual clinical needs, so the nurse should use only the length necessary to provide the needed elongation. If too short, the purpose is not accomplished; if too long, there is the possibility of kinking, catching on equipment, or falling on the floor and being stepped on. For purposes of safety and infection control, extension tubings should always

have Luer-Lok® adapters on both ends to avoid an inadvertent disconnection. Unless absolutely necessary, the CDC does not recommend the routine use of extra tubing (CDC, 2001).

Adapters and Connectors

Connectors attached to IV administration sets are special tubings or adapters that add versatility to the infusion line. They should be used only when they are absolutely necessary and their features are not available in integral systems (CDC,

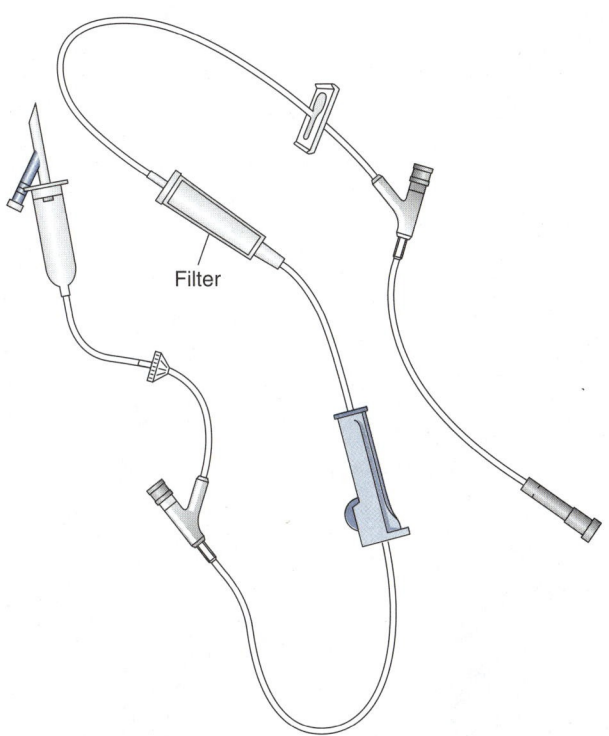

Figure 8-18 | In-line Filter

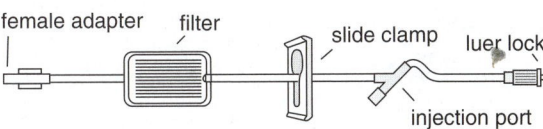

Figure 8-19 | While not normallly recommened, this is an example of a type of add-on filter that could be used.

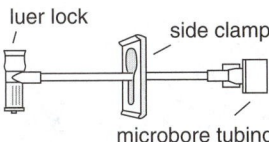

Figure 8-20 | Extension Tubings

2001). The nurse must remember that every time a closed system is breached the potential for contamination and infection increases.

When using any type of adapters or connectors, the nurse must know their priming volumes. The **priming volume** is the amount of infusate needed to replace the air in the IV adapter or connecting device. Failure to add the appropriate quantity of fluid could result in an air embolism.

Stopcocks

A **stopcock** is a device that controls the directional flow of infusate through manual manipulation of a direction-

regulating valve (Figure 8-21). IV infusion stopcocks operate as three- or four-way mechanisms. A three-way stopcock connects two lines of fluid to a patient and provides a mechanism for either one to run to the patient (like a faucet, where either the hot or the cold water can run [alone] into a container). In a four-way stopcock, the valve can be manipulated so that one or both lines can run to the patient, alone, or in combination (like a faucet, where hot water can run, cold water can run, or both can run together).

Ports and Connectors

Ports and connectors are adapters that can be added to infusion lines, serving as add-on viaducts that couple with the cannula hub or other IV lines. These are available as T ports, J loops, U connectors, or Y connectors (Figure 8-22). There are also add-ons, referred to as PRN adapters or injection caps (Figure 8-23), that affix only to the cannula hub (when there is no further use for continuous fluid administration) for intermittent use, or to keep the cannula line to the vein open. Ports are designed with integral injection sites for needleless access. A needleless system is the preferred method to access an injection/access port. Port systems are manufactured with one connection or as multiflow structures (containing one, two, or three injection ports).

The T port attaches to the cannula at the rigid portion of the device (where the top of the T has an injection port on one side and the cannula connector on the other), which extends to a 4- to 6-in. segment of tubing (the "leg" of the T), containing a slide clamp, that Luer-Loks® to the IV administration tubing. T ports are suitable for patients who are ambulatory and can be disconnected from their IV line for short periods of time for showering, ambulating, or other activities.

Serving essentially the same purpose as T ports, J loops and U connectors are rigid in form, making them more cumbersome and clumsy to handle, thus predisposing to inadvertent cannula movement during use. They do not have slide clamps, so the introduction of air or the retrograde flow of blood during connection or disconnection from the cannula hub is a possibility. Some do not have injection ports.

The Y connector is a device that provides an access route for two IV fluids to infuse at the same time. The upper

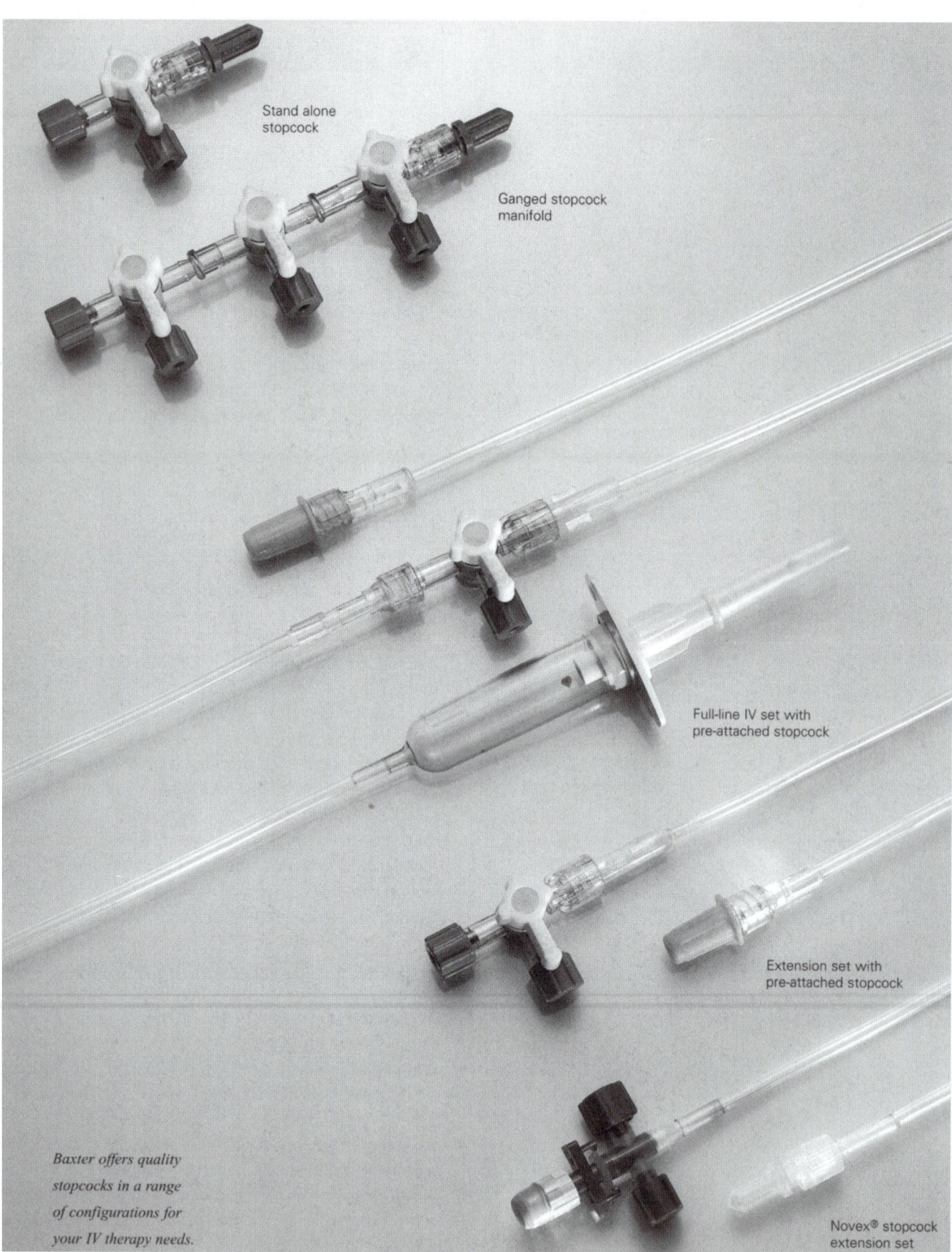

Figure 8-21 | Stopcocks (Courtesy of Baxter Healthcare Systems)

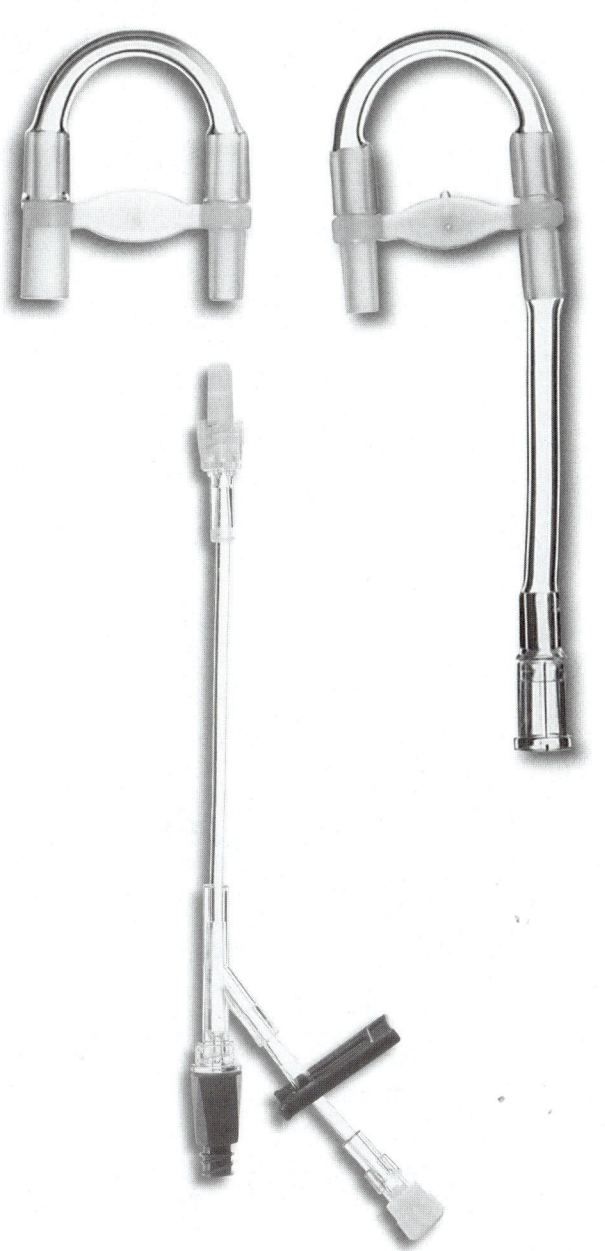

Figure 8-22 | Ports and Connectors (Courtesy of BD Medical Systems)

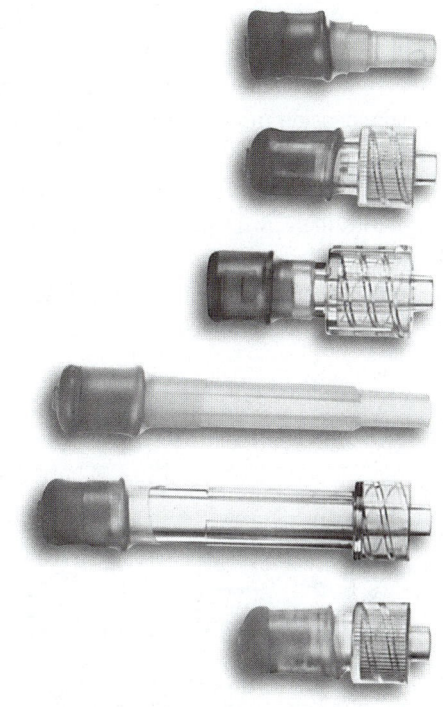

Figure 8-23 | PRN Adapters (Courtesy of BD Medical Systems)

NURSING TIP

Knowing Your Equipment

The nurse must be familiar with all types of ports and connectors available in his place of employment and choose the one most congruous with the patient's situation. There are advantages and disadvantages associated with all of the devices on the market and the nurse must keep in mind the potential outcomes associated with their use.

"arms" of the Y connect to the infusates, while the "leg" of Y attaches to the cannula hub.

NEEDLELESS SYSTEMS AND NEEDLESTICK SAFETY SYSTEMS

According to the CDC, 384,000 percutaneous injuries (needlesticks and other sharps injuries) occur annually among health care workers in U.S. hospitals. Among these injuries, 236,000 resulted from hollow-bore needles, which have the greatest potential to transmit bloodborne pathogens (General Accounting Office, 2000). Numerous studies have documented the efficacy of needleless IV-access devices in reducing the risk of IV-related injuries.

Needleless systems are state-of-the art technology in the practice of intravenous therapy. Other than the initial stick to insert the cannula into the patient's vein, there is no need for further use of needles during treatment.

Needleless systems eliminate up to 80% of needles and are used to connect IV devices, administer infusates and medications, and sample blood. Some, such as Burron Medical's SAFSITE™ System, are made in such a way that they are compatible with different manufacturers' IV administration sets and extension tubings, syringes, catheters, and medication vials. Others, such as Baxter's Interlink™ access system (Figure 8-24) offer complete needleless programs designed for use with their own equipment.

Although not needleless, other products have been developed to prevent needlestick injuries, such as self-sheathing needles and needle-locking devices, used in IV therapy as well as other parenteral routes. Figure 8-25 illustrates how the Critikon PROTECTIV™ IV catheter safety system works.

VENOUS ACCESS DEVICES

There are numerous venous access devices on the market that are available for one-time use, short-term use, or

Securing the locking cannula

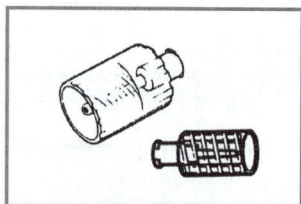

1. The InterLink™ Threaded Lock Cannula is a streamlined locking device for securing I.V. catheter connections.

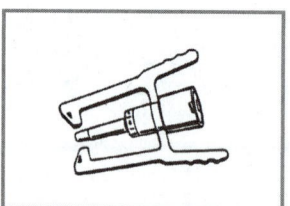

1. The InterLink™ Lever Lock Cannula is an easy-to-use device for securing I.V. connections.

Y-Site access

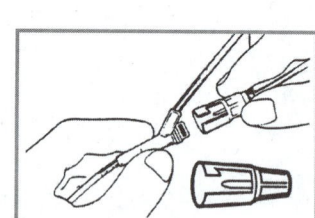

1. The InterLink™ Set allows access to the I.V. line without a needle.

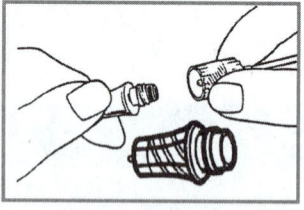

2. Insert InterLink™ Threaded Lock Cannula into InterLink™ injection site.

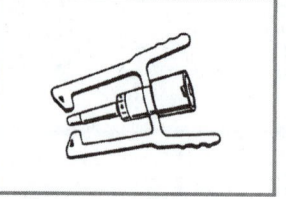

2. Grasp levers and insert the InterLink™ Lever Lock Cannula into InterLink™ injection site.

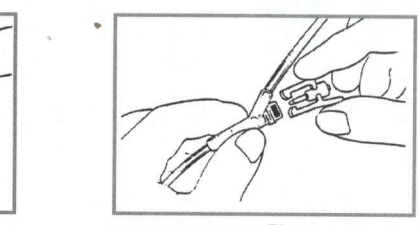

2. The InterLink™ Y-Lock inserts and twists into the InterLink™ Y-Site for a safe and secure connection.

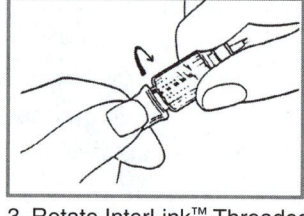

3. Rotate InterLink™ Threaded Lock Cannula clockwise until securely engaged.

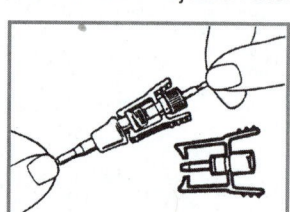

3. Release levers to lock cannula into place.

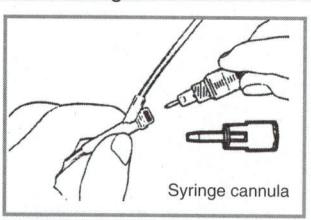

3. The InterLink™ Lever Lock Cannula is an easy-to-use device for securing I.V. connections.

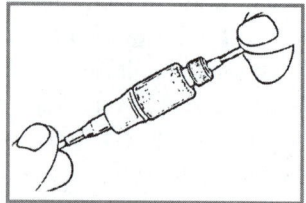

4. The Threaded Lock Cannula provides a closed system that minimizes touch contamination.

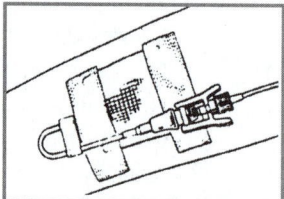

4. The Lever Lock Cannula rests comfortably against patient's skin.

Syringe cannula

4. An InterLink™ Cannula attached to a syringe is ideal for injecting bolus dose medications into the InterLink™ Y-Site.

Figure 8-24 | Interlink™ Needleless System (Courtesy of BD Medical Systems)

extended use, which are left in place and remain functional for months, even years. Most of these are inserted by nurses (some requiring nurses to have special training or certification), while others are inserted by physicians (usually anesthesiologists or surgeons) or nurse anesthetists. Once inserted, however, the responsibility for patient monitoring, management, and maintenance becomes the primary responsibility of the registered nurse in collaboration with the physician and other health care workers.

Peripheral Venous Access Devices

Peripheral venous access devices range in variety from straight steel and winged needles to catheters made of Teflon,® polyurethane, PVC, polyethylene, silicone, or other materials. They vary in length and gauge to meet the needs of a wide variety of patients, ranging from the premature neonate (with tiny, difficult-to-access veins) to the elderly (with delicate, fragile, easily broken veins). (See Chapters 9, 15, and 16 regarding their insertion and use.)

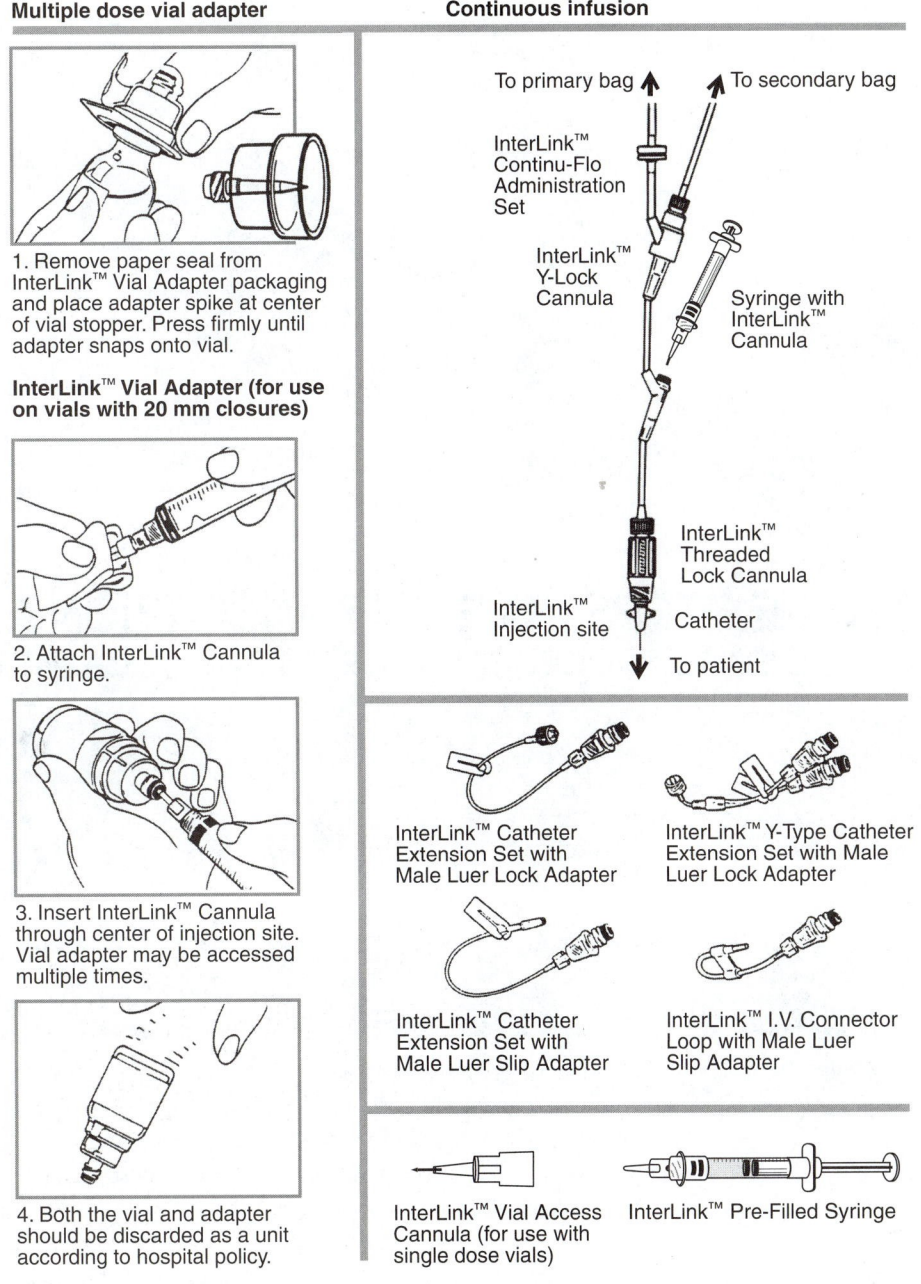

Multiple dose vial adapter

1. Remove paper seal from InterLink™ Vial Adapter packaging and place adapter spike at center of vial stopper. Press firmly until adapter snaps onto vial.

InterLink™ Vial Adapter (for use on vials with 20 mm closures)

2. Attach InterLink™ Cannula to syringe.

3. Insert InterLink™ Cannula through center of injection site. Vial adapter may be accessed multiple times.

4. Both the vial and adapter should be discarded as a unit according to hospital policy.

Continuous infusion

To primary bag / To secondary bag

InterLink™ Continu-Flo Administration Set

InterLink™ Y-Lock Cannula

Syringe with InterLink™ Cannula

InterLink™ Threaded Lock Cannula

InterLink™ Injection site / Catheter

To patient

InterLink™ Catheter Extension Set with Male Luer Lock Adapter

InterLink™ Y-Type Catheter Extension Set with Male Luer Lock Adapter

InterLink™ Catheter Extension Set with Male Luer Slip Adapter

InterLink™ I.V. Connector Loop with Male Luer Slip Adapter

InterLink™ Vial Access Cannula (for use with single dose vials)

InterLink™ Pre-Filled Syringe

Figure 8-24 | continued

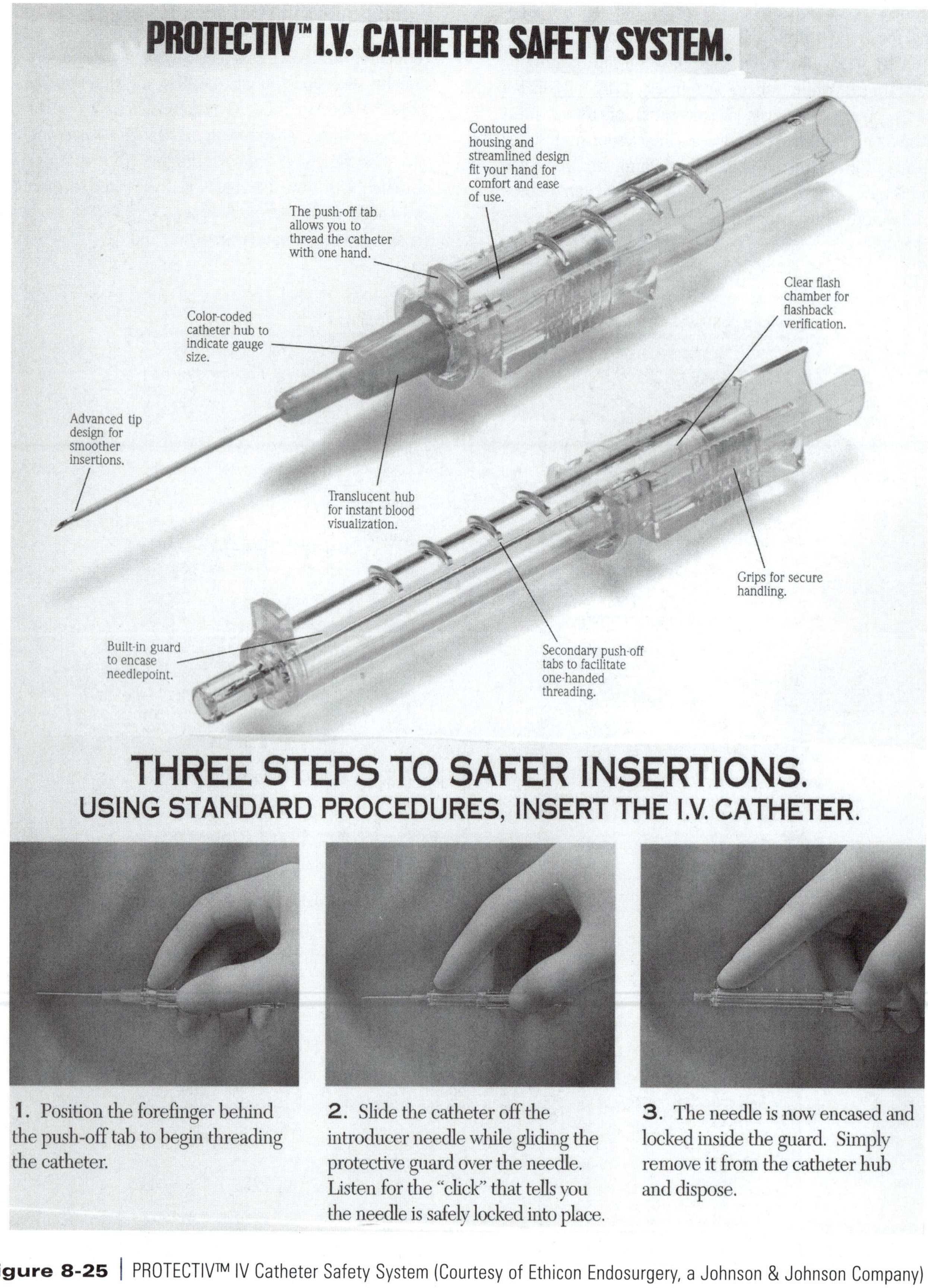

PROTECTIV™ I.V. CATHETER SAFETY SYSTEM.

Contoured housing and streamlined design fit your hand for comfort and ease of use.

The push-off tab allows you to thread the catheter with one hand.

Clear flash chamber for flashback verification.

Color-coded catheter hub to indicate gauge size.

Advanced tip design for smoother insertions.

Translucent hub for instant blood visualization.

Grips for secure handling.

Built-in guard to encase needlepoint.

Secondary push-off tabs to facilitate one-handed threading.

THREE STEPS TO SAFER INSERTIONS.
USING STANDARD PROCEDURES, INSERT THE I.V. CATHETER.

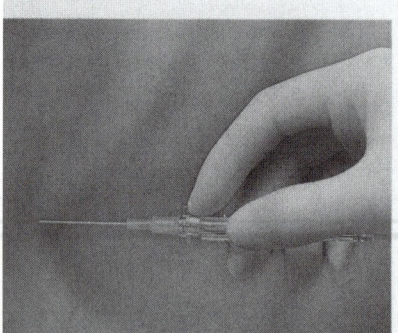

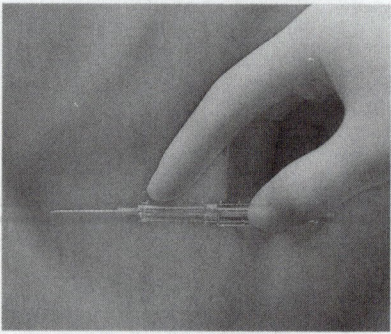

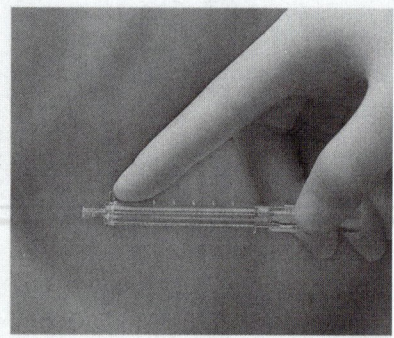

1. Position the forefinger behind the push-off tab to begin threading the catheter.

2. Slide the catheter off the introducer needle while gliding the protective guard over the needle. Listen for the "click" that tells you the needle is safely locked into place.

3. The needle is now encased and locked inside the guard. Simply remove it from the catheter hub and dispose.

Figure 8-25 │ PROTECTIV™ IV Catheter Safety System (Courtesy of Ethicon Endosurgery, a Johnson & Johnson Company)

NURSING TIP

Needlestick Injury Facts and Data*

- Number of health care workers in United States: Approximately 8 million

- Number of needlestick injuries per year: an estimated 600,000–800,000

- Incidence of needlestick injuries at a hospital in one year: an estimated 30 injuries per 100 beds

- Occupational setting for needlestick injuries: 35% in patient rooms, 22% in operating rooms, 8% in emergency departments, and 7% in intensive care units

- HIV transmission from 1985–June 1999: 55 documented cases; 44 from hollow-bore needles (data not available for hepatitis B and C)

- Items most frequently causing needlestick injuries: 1. Syringe (28% of injuries), 2. Suture needle (15%), 3. IV catheter (6%)

- Ranking of "high-risk"devices that cause needlesticks (blood-filled, large-bore needles): 1. IV Catheter, 2. Butterfly needle, 3. Syringe

*Source: EPINet, the Exposure Prevention Information Network, 2001

NURSING ALERT

What to Do Following Blood Exposure

- Wash any needlestick punctures and cuts with soap and water.

- Flush splashes to the nose, mouth, or skin with water; irrigate the eyes with clean water, 0.9% sodium chloride solution, or sterile ophthalmic irrigants.

- Report the exposure to the department responsible for managing exposures.

- Start postexposure treatment, if recommended, as soon as possible.

Straight Steel Needles

Straight steel needles come in a variety of gauges (27 ga to 14 ga) and lengths (¼ in. to 3 in.). The hub can attach to the

tip of a syringe or to infusate tubing with either a straight connector or Luer-Lok™ adapter (Figure 8-26). For IV use, needles should have a sharp, well-tapered bevel for ease of insertion and less patient discomfort.

Steel needles were commonly used for all vein cannulations prior to the introduction of IV catheters. They are rarely used today except for the direct delivery of IV medication, due to the fact that they tend to dislodge and infiltrate more frequently than catheters. "The use of stainless steel needles should be limited to short-term or single-dose administration" (INS, 2000, Standard 44, S39).

Winged Needles

Winged needles have one wing or two (referred to as butterflies) that connect with the needle on one side and a segment of infusion tubing, ending in a hub and protective cap, on the other (Figure 8-27). The wings are the portion of the device that are held in an upright position between the thumb and forefinger during needle insertion to facilitate movement into the vein. Once the needle is in the vein, the wings are placed in a flat position and taped to the skin to secure the device. Prior to insertion, the tubing, which varies in length from 3½ in. to 12 in., should be primed with normal saline to prevent the entry of air into the circulation.

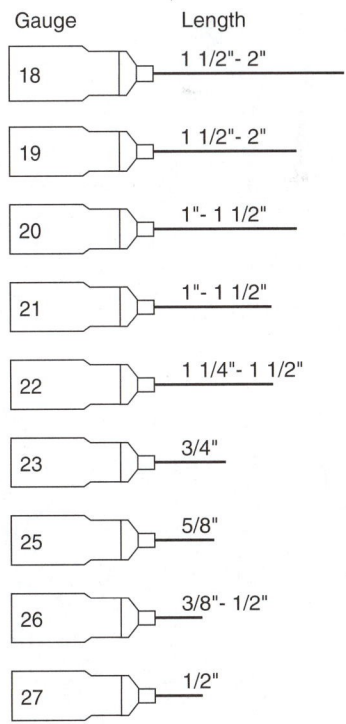

Gauge	Length
18	1 1/2"- 2"
19	1 1/2"- 2"
20	1"- 1 1/2"
21	1"- 1 1/2"
22	1 1/4"- 1 1/2"
23	3/4"
25	5/8"
26	3/8"- 1/2"
27	1/2"

Figure 8-26 | Straight Steel Needles

MINICATH™

E-Z SET™

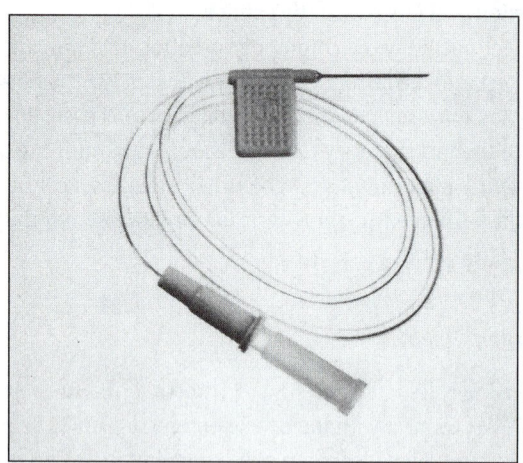

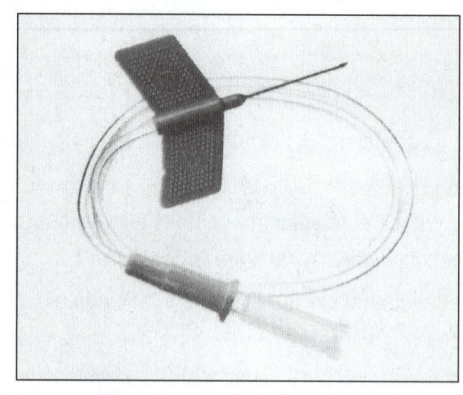

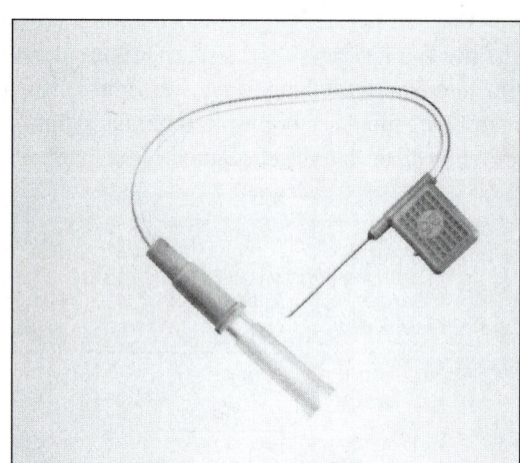

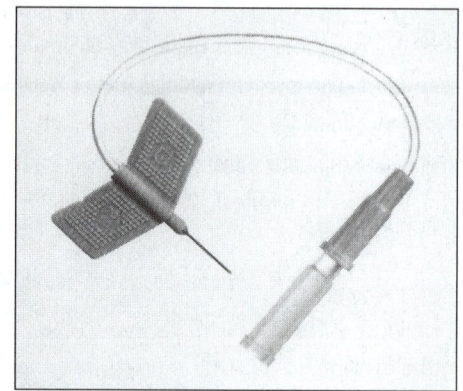

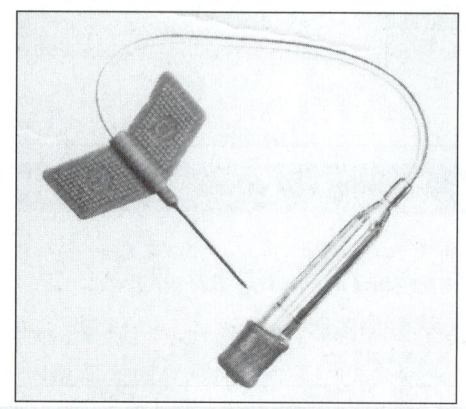

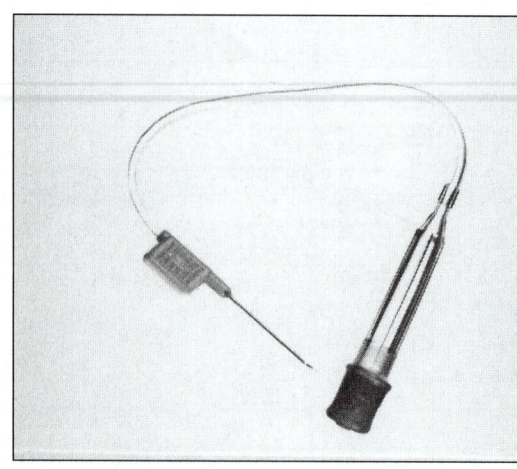

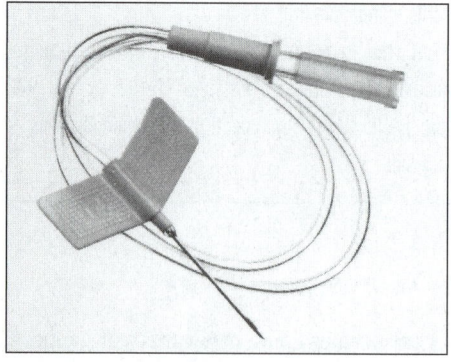

Figure 8-27 | Winged Infusion Sets (Courtesy of BD Medical Systems)

If secured properly, winged needles stay in the vein quite well and provide a good means of venous access for short-term infusions of 24 hours or less. Nonetheless, they are not frequently used for adult infusion therapy other than to deliver one-time IV medications or to draw blood. They continue to be used in pediatric services to access surface veins in the head (referred to as scalp-vein needles).

Peripheral Venous Access Catheters

A peripheral venous access catheter, the most commonly used IV device, is used to enter the superficial and deep veins of an extremity, the neck, or the head (Figure 8-28). It is a two-part flexible cannula in tandem with a rigid needle or stylet that is used as a guide to puncture and insert the catheter into the vein. The stylet connects with a clear chamber that allows for visualization of blood return indicating successful venipuncture and facilitates removal of the needle. The hub of the cannula is plastic and color-coded to indicate length and gauge. It can range in length from 1/4 in. to 12 in. (midline or midarm cannulas) and can be thin or thick-walled. Every catheter should be radiopaque so that it can be detected radiologically should it break off and embolize. There are numerous varieties and sizes of peripheral catheters available, all manufactured with safety, ease of insertion, convenience, and cost-effectiveness in mind.

The over-the-needle peripheral catheter (ONC) is a flexible cannula that encases a steel needle or stylet device and is the most commonly used peripheral IV device. Once the vein is accessed, the catheter is threaded into the vessel, and the stylet is withdrawn. Venous access can be discerned by a retrograde flow of blood from the vein into the flash chamber, a plastic compartment in back of the cannula hub, or with immediate visualization of blood in the catheter via a notched needle, such as INSYTE-N® (Figure 8-29) (see Chapter 9 for the various methods of catheter placement in the vein).

The through-the-needle catheter (TNC) is the opposite of the ONC, as the flexible cannula is encircled by the steel needle. As originally designed (and infrequently used today), the needle is withdrawn once venous access is achieved and secured in a protective shield outside the body on the skin. The TNC, mainly seen in peripherally inserted central venous access devices, has a steel or plastic encasement that can be removed after the catheter is advanced into the vein. The steel needle has a slit along the length of its shaft that can be split apart and removed, whereas the plastic type can be peeled off. Due to the risk of puncture or shearing, through-the-needle catheters are not used for routine peripheral venous access.

Catheters are made of various biocompatible materials designed for ease of insertion, while preventing vein irritation and reducing the propensity for infection. Teflon® has been used extensively in the past, but newer, state-of-the-art materials are being developed on a regular basis.

Central Venous Access Catheters

Central access catheters encompass a wide variety of devices that may be peripherally inserted or surgically implanted. The use of these products is often design-specific (see Chapter 12).

VEIN ILLUMINATION DEVICES

The use of illumination devices has facilitated the practice of intravenous access and infusion therapy for patients who are in need of IVs but have veins that can neither be seen nor palpated. The Venoscope II® Transilluminator works by directing a high-intensity cool light down into the subcutaneous tissue and creating a uniform area of orange-like reflection from the fatty tissue (Figure 8-30). The light is flush with the skin; by moving it around the extremity, a dark line can be seen between the two arms of the Venoscope II, which is the vein. The vein's deoxygenated blood absorbs the light, whereas the fatty tissue reflects the light.

After the vein is recognized, the nurse depresses both arms of the light on either side of the dark line to determine if the vein is soft and patent or hard and sclerotic. If the line disappears and then reappears when pressure is released, it is a vein that is capable of transmitting fluids and medications. If the dark line does not disappear and reappear (blanch), it is not a vein and an attempt at cannulation should not be undertaken.

INFUSION SITE PREPARATION AND MAINTENANCE MATERIALS

Prior to the insertion of a venous access device, the appropriate dressing materials must be obtained and the skin must

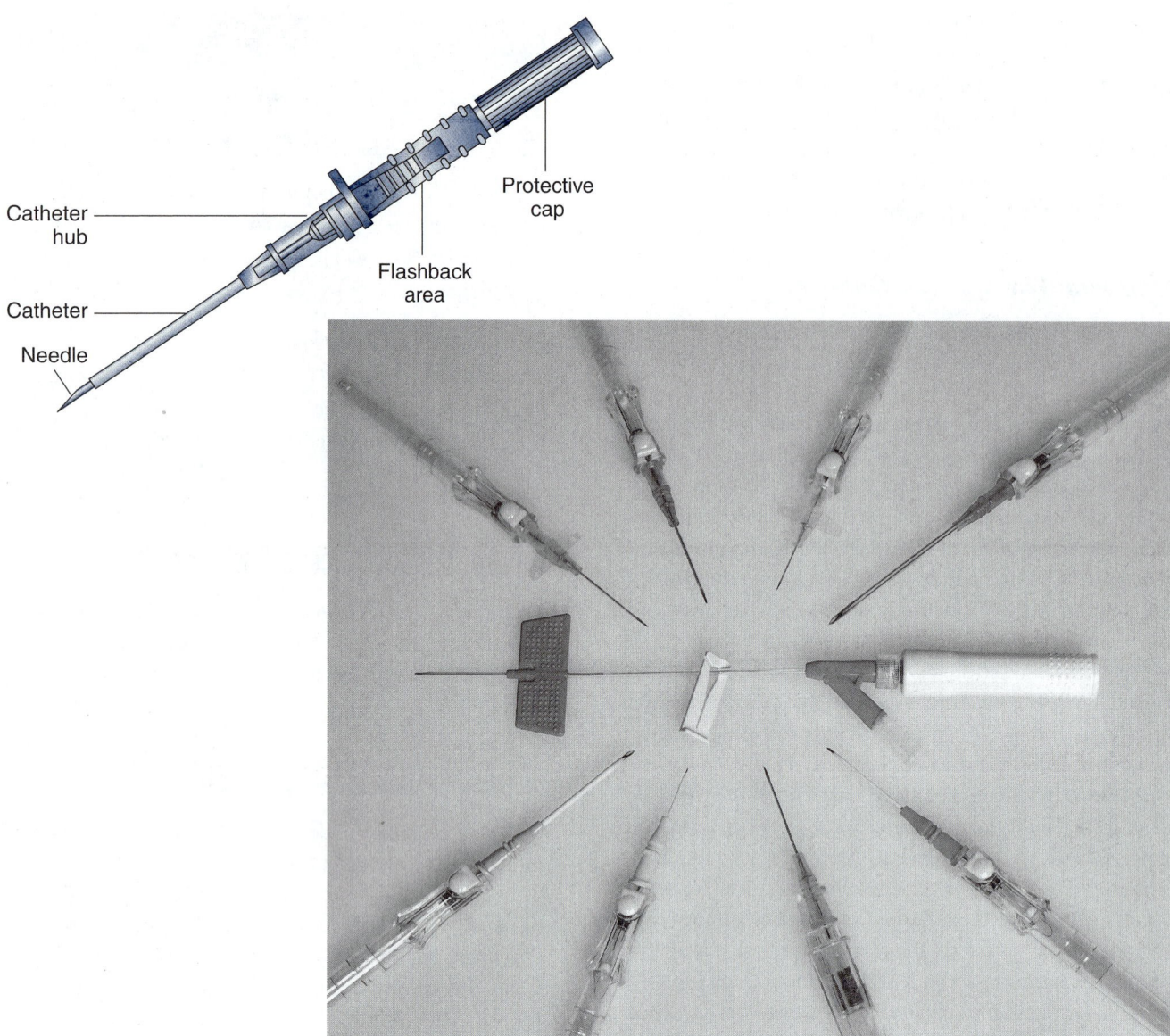

Figure 8-28 │ Over-the-needle Catheter

be properly cleansed. Once in place, the IV device must be suitably secured to allow for regular site assessment, the prevention of cannula movement or dislodgment, and to maintain asepsis and prevent catheter-related infection (CRI). This is accomplished with the use of several items, procured individually or in kits. Selection of such articles is based on individual patient situations and conditions, following the recommendations set forth by the CDC, INS standards, and agency protocols.

Skin Preparations

Prior to the insertion of a vascular access device, the client's skin must be prepared, using an antimicrobial barrier. One of the most important measures for preventing CRIs, in addition to strict attention to proper hand hygiene, is antisepsis of the insertion site. In the United States, povidone iodine has been the most commonly used antiseptic for cleansing catheter insertion sites. However, preparation of central venous and arterial sites with a 2% aqueous chlorhexidine gluconate has been shown to lower BSI rates as compared to site preparation with 10% povidone-iodine or 70% alcohol. The rate of catheter-related bloodstream infections when CHG was used was 84% lower than the rates when the two other antiseptic regimens were used (CDC, 2002a). Commercially available products containing 2% CHG were not available in the United States until July 2000, when the U.S. Food and Drug Administration (FDA) approved a 2% aqueous chlorhexidine preparation for skin antisepsis.

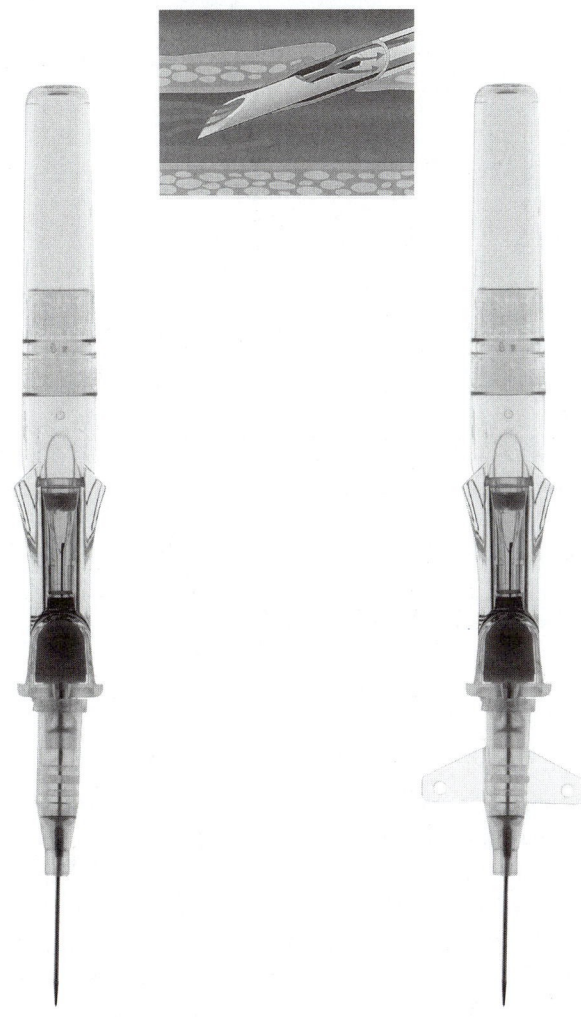

Figure 8-29 | INSYTE-N® IV Catheter with notched needle (which confirms venipuncture at the point of insertion) (Courtesy of BD Medical Systems)

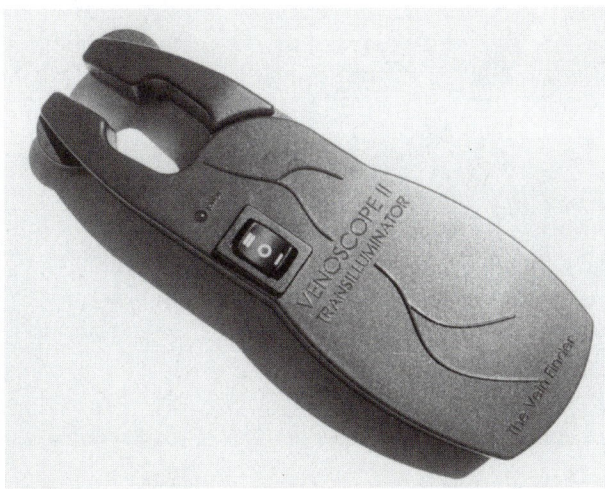

Figure 8-30 | Venoscope II Transilluminator (Courtesy of Venoscope, LLC)

The CDC, in the Guidelines For Prevention of Intravascular Device-Related Infections, 2002, suggests that the skin, prior to catheter insertion and during dressing changes, be cleansed with an appropriate antiseptic. A 2% chlorhexidine-based preparation is preferred, but an iodophor, tincture of iodine, or 70% alcohol may also be used (CDC, 2002a). The antiseptic must remain on the insertion site and be allowed to air dry before catheter insertion. Povidone iodine is to remain on the skin for at least two minutes, or longer if it is not yet dry before insertion. The use of organic solvents (e.g., acetone and ether) on the skin before insertion of catheters or during dressing changes is not recommended. When CHG or povidone iodine are used in conjunction with alcohol, the alcohol must always be used first. The alcohol must not be used to wipe off the iodophor because the iodophor exerts a prolonged antimicrobial effect. Skin preparations are available in the form of swabsticks, prep pads, or plastic (cotton-tipped) squeezable vials for one-time use (Figure 8-31).

It is not recommended that antimicrobial ointments be applied to the catheter site at the time of catheter insertion or during routine dressing changes. The use of polyantibiotic ointments that are not fungicidal may significantly increase the rate of colonization of the catheter by *Candida* species (CDC, 2002a).

Dressings

The dressing used to cover the skin surrounding a percutaneous device should be either a sterile gauze or a sterile, transparent, semipermeable dressing (CDC, 2002a). Tunneled CVC sites that are well healed might not require dressings. Transparent, semipermeable polyurethane dressings are popular among practitioners because they reliably secure the vascular access device, allow for continuous visual inspection of the catheter site, let patients bathe and shower without saturating the dressing, and require less frequent changes than do standard gauze and tape dressings; the use of these dressings saves personnel time. Data suggest that transparent dressings can be safely left on peripheral venous catheters for the duration of catheter insertion without increasing the risk for thrombophlebitis (CDC, 2002a). The choice of dressing can be a matter of preference. If blood is oozing from the catheter insertion site, a gauze dressing might be preferred.

If the patient is diaphoretic, or if the site is bleeding or oozing, a gauze dressing is preferable to a transparent, semipermeable dressing. A catheter-site dressing is to be replaced if it becomes damp, loosened, or visibly soiled. The dressing is to be changed at least weekly for the adult and adolescent patient depending on the circumstances of the individual patient. Topical antibiotic ointments or creams are not recommended for use on insertion sites (except

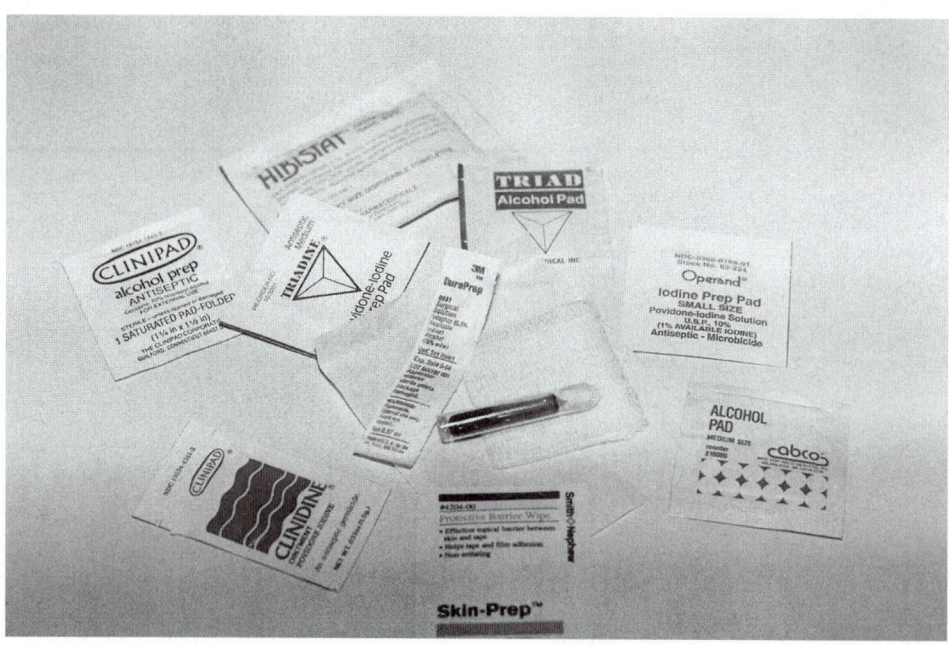

Figure 8-31 │ Antiseptic Skin Preparations

when using dialysis catheters) because of their potential to promote fungal infections and antimicrobial resistance (CDC, 2002a).

There are several types of transparent membrane dressings (TMDs) available that vary in size and thickness and are designed for one- or two-handed application (Figure 8-32). They are also referred to as transparent semipermeable membranes (TSMs). The newer gauze dressings combine the dressing and tape in one component, such as 3M™ Medipore and pad adhesive wound dressing and Smith and Nephew's Primapore.™ ConMed™'s Veni-Gard® features a transparent

membrane, a waterproof foam perimeter, and pre-cut accessory tape strips all in one (Figure 8-33).

A hydrophilic chlorhexidine-impregnated sponge (Biopatch™) is used by some agencies. It is placed over the site of short-term arterial and central venous catheters and has been shown to reduce the risk for catheter colonization and CRBSI (CDC, 2002a). Thus far, adverse systemic effects have not resulted from use of this device. When used, however, it should be according to institutional policy, after the skin has been prepped with an appropriate (agency-approved) antimicrobial barrier.

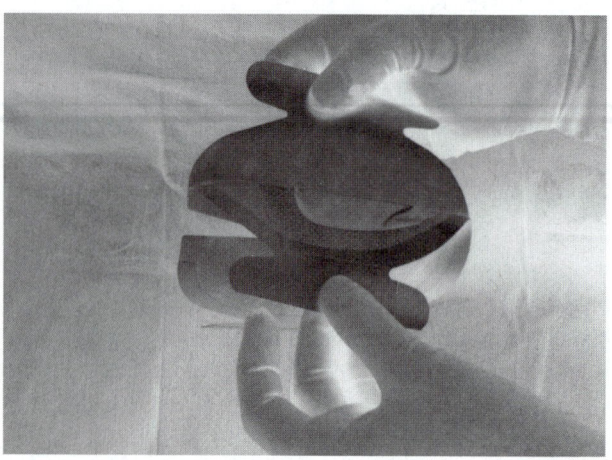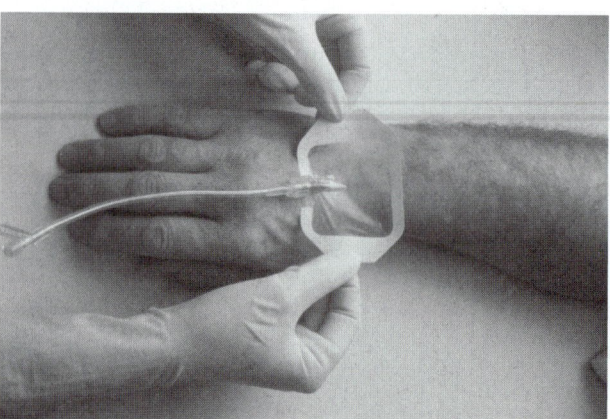

Figure 8-32 │ Transparent Semipermeable Membrane Dressings (Courtesy of 3M)

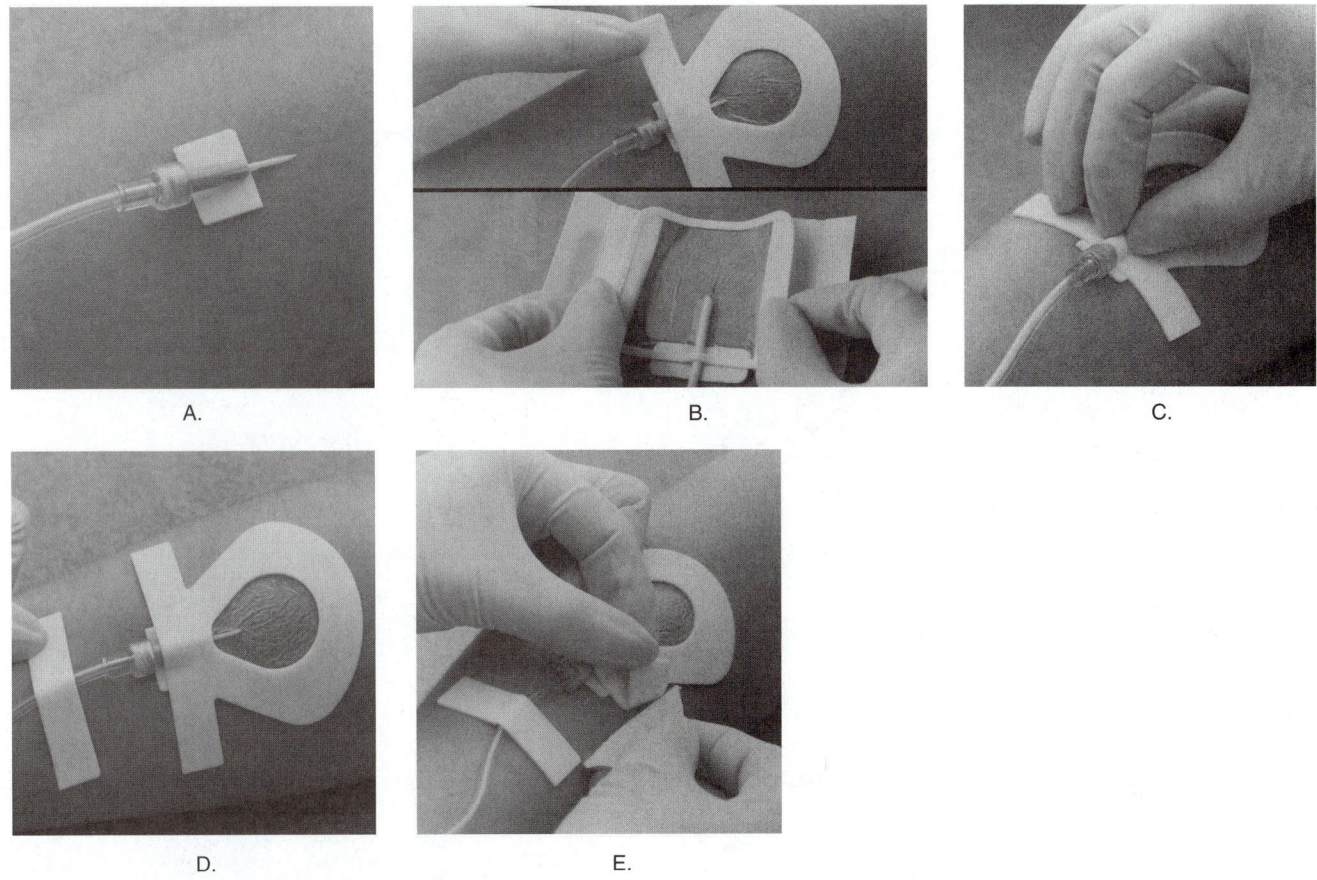

A.   B.   C.

D.   E.

Figure 8-33 | Veni-Gard® Transparent Membrane Dressing with Waterproof Foam Perimeter and Pre-cut Accessory Strips. Guidelines for use: A. Place foam pad. B. Apply dressing. C. Pinch to occlude. D. Secure with accessories. E. Remove with alcohol. (Courtesy of ConMed™ Corporation)

Kits

There are various prepackaged kits used to start IVs. They are supplied with or without peripheral venous access devices and contain all of the routinely used equipment needed to start an IV (Figure 8-34), including the tourniquet, antiseptic skin prep, gauze, tape, and a dressing.

In general, if available in an agency, the prepackaged starter kits are used only when IV therapy is initiated. If the vein is not accessed on the first attempt or when site dressings need to be reinforced or redressed, just the supplies needed are procured.

INFUSION REGULATION SYSTEMS

Traditionally, IVs infuse by gravity flow, measured in drops per minute (gtt/min), which the nurse adjusts manually with the roller or screw clamp on the administration set. Now there are numerous mechanical and electronic devices available that assist the nurse in maintaining the infusion rate.

Mechanical Gravity Control Devices

Mechanical gravity control devices such as the Baxter Control-A-Flo® infusion regulator (Figure 8-35) are flow-regulating mechanisms that attach to the primary infusion administration sets and are manually set to deliver specified volumes of fluid per hour. They are available as dials, with clocklike faces, or as barrel-shaped devices with cylindrical controls. There are flow markings, which are approximate, that must be verified by counting the drops per minute, based on the administration set drop factor.

There are several of these devices on the market, all with varying degrees of accuracy. There can be discrepancies of up to ±25% due to the patient's condition, positioning, activity level, and venous pressure. Restriction of fluid flow can occur because of kinking or obstruction of the IV tubing.

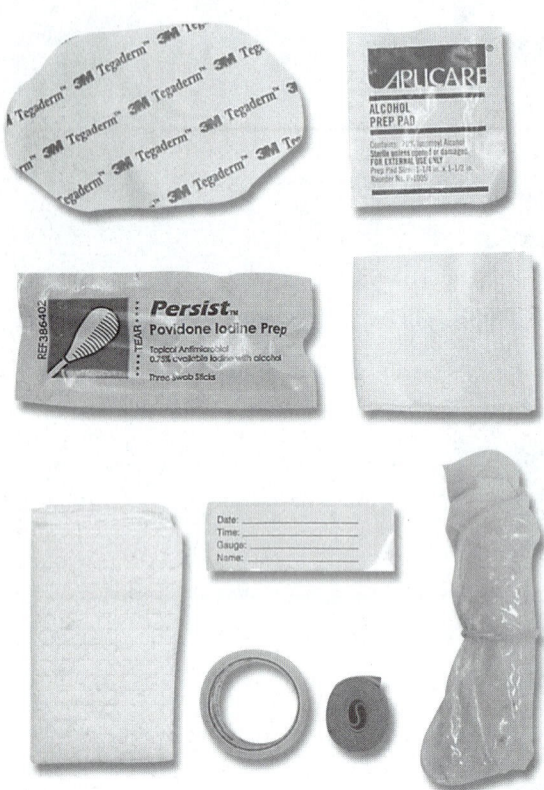

Figure 8-34 | IV Start Kit (Courtesy of BD Medical Systems)

These generally should be used only for short periods, such as for transport of patients between services, and must be checked frequently for infusion accuracy. The 3M™ IV Flow Regulator has a patented, pressure-sensitive membrane that compensates for fluctuations in pressure, providing a constant volumetric output to maintain the set flow rate within ±10%. It self-adjusts to compensate for patient movement and venous pressure changes, so it may be safely used with lipids and antibiotics, as well as for hydration.

Electronic Infusion Control Devices

Electronic infusion devices (EIDs) are regulating mechanisms that are powered by electricity, battery packs, or both. They have evolved over the past 25 years into safe, accurate, state-of-the art infusion-regulating machines that deliver fluids and medications accurately (±5%) and are capable of being programmed to infuse several infusates at different rates and volumes simultaneously. They have sensors that detect air in the line, changes in pressure, and signal when infusions have terminated. The nurse is alerted to problems

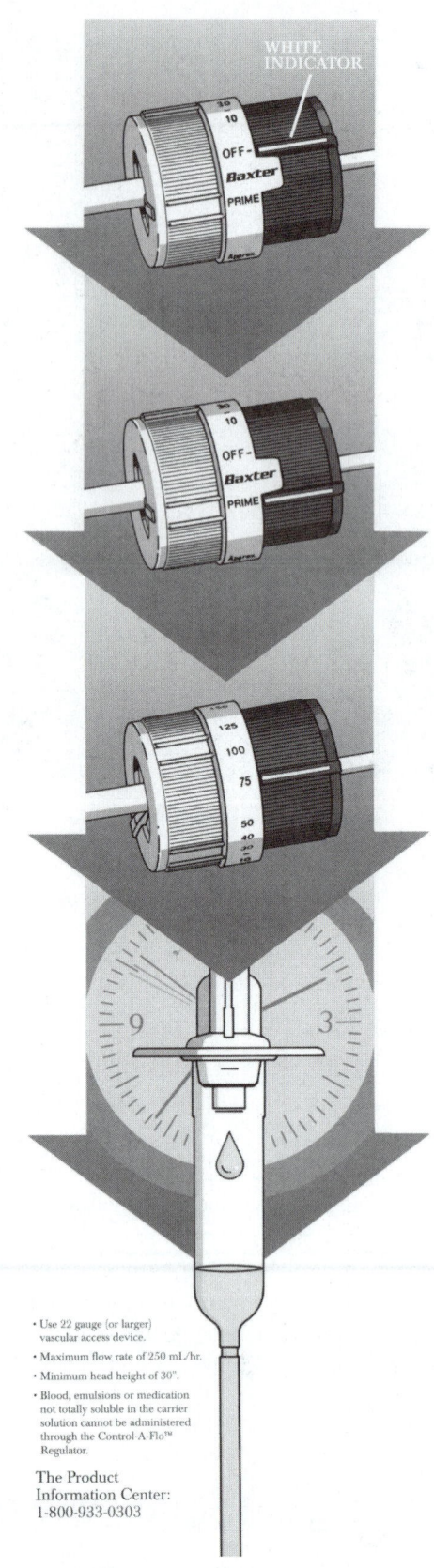

- Use 22 gauge (or larger) vascular access device.
- Maximum flow rate of 250 mL/hr.
- Minimum head height of 30″.
- Blood, emulsions or medication not totally soluble in the carrier solution cannot be administered through the Control-A-Flo™ Regulator.

The Product Information Center: 1-800-933-0303

Figure 8-35 | Control-A-Flo® (Courtesy of Baxter Healthcare Corporation)

through systems of light-emitting diode (LED) or liquid crystal display (LCD) read-outs, alarms that sound, and lights that flash. Most newer models have built-in mechanisms to prevent unintended free flow of infusate to the patient, should the administration set be removed from the machine (Figure 8-36).

It would be almost impossible for the nurse to be familiar with all of the EIDs on the market today. It is important that he learn how to use correctly the product line his agency has adopted and be able to program it safely, use its features to the fullest capacity, and know how to troubleshoot problems. An EID, no matter how sophisticated, is not a substitute for regular patient observation and evaluation.

EIDs operate through various mechanisms; the two most common are peristalsis-driven and cassette operated. In the peristaltic system, fluid is propelled through the infusion line when intermittent wavelike movement (from rotary-driven cams or fingerlike projections) exerts pressure on a portion of the administration tubing that is housed in the EID. The cassette system has a mechanism in the machine that accepts set-selective disposable administration tubing that controls the volume of infusate being delivered to the patient.

Electronic infusion devices are driven by one of two methods, the controller mode or the pump mode. Some machines are designed to function as both, such as those in the IMED® line, which offers more versatility.

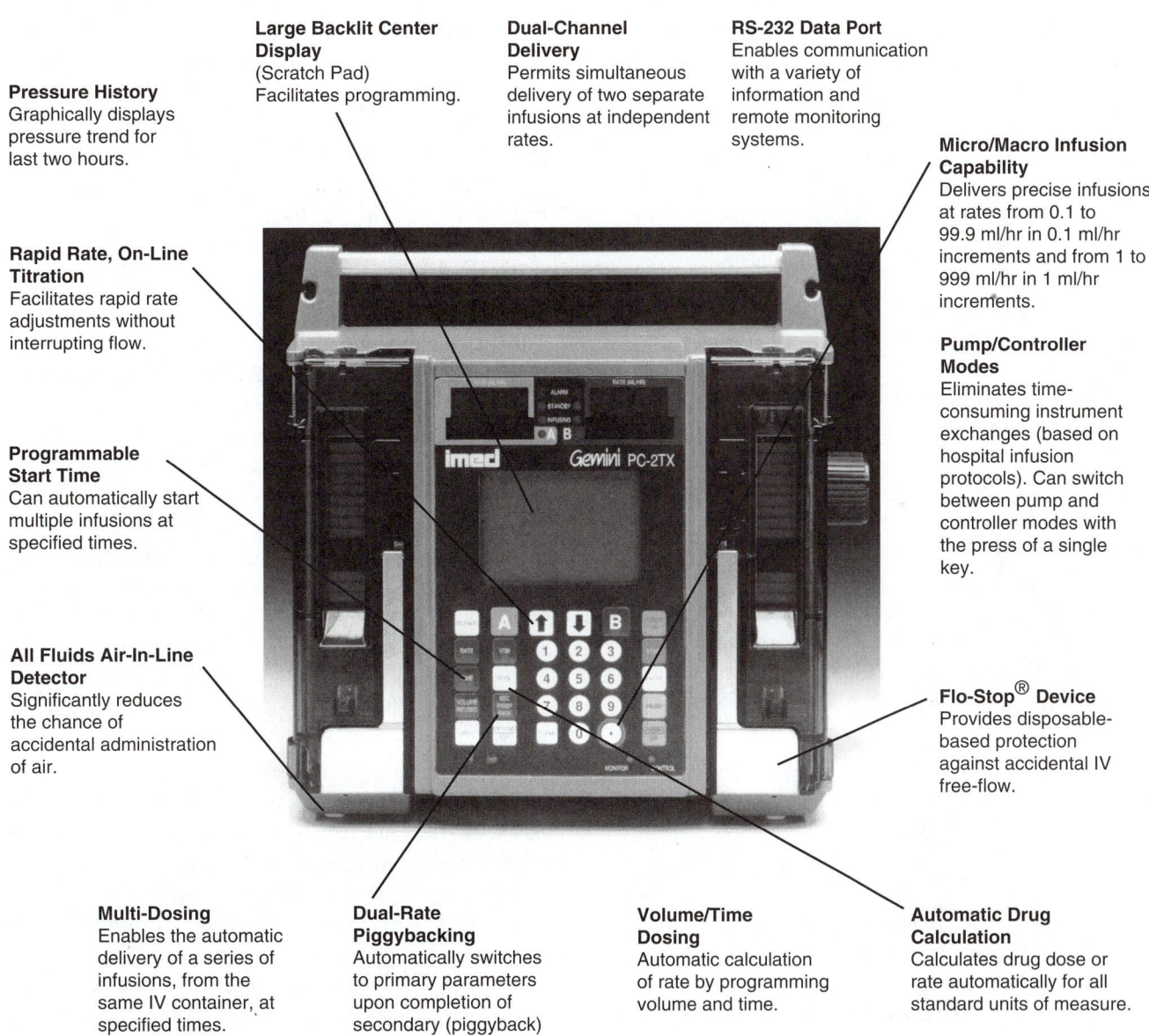

Pressure History
Graphically displays pressure trend for last two hours.

Large Backlit Center Display
(Scratch Pad)
Facilitates programming.

Dual-Channel Delivery
Permits simultaneous delivery of two separate infusions at independent rates.

RS-232 Data Port
Enables communication with a variety of information and remote monitoring systems.

Micro/Macro Infusion Capability
Delivers precise infusions at rates from 0.1 to 99.9 ml/hr in 0.1 ml/hr increments and from 1 to 999 ml/hr in 1 ml/hr increments.

Rapid Rate, On-Line Titration
Facilitates rapid rate adjustments without interrupting flow.

Pump/Controller Modes
Eliminates time-consuming instrument exchanges (based on hospital infusion protocols). Can switch between pump and controller modes with the press of a single key.

Programmable Start Time
Can automatically start multiple infusions at specified times.

All Fluids Air-In-Line Detector
Significantly reduces the chance of accidental administration of air.

Flo-Stop® Device
Provides disposable-based protection against accidental IV free-flow.

Multi-Dosing
Enables the automatic delivery of a series of infusions, from the same IV container, at specified times.

Dual-Rate Piggybacking
Automatically switches to primary parameters upon completion of secondary (piggyback) infusion.

Volume/Time Dosing
Automatic calculation of rate by programming volume and time.

Automatic Drug Calculation
Calculates drug dose or rate automatically for all standard units of measure.

Figure 8-36 | The Gemini PC-2tx™ Volumetric Pump/Controller (Courtesy of Alaris Medical Systems)

Controllers

An EID with a controller mode functions as an electronic "eye" that "watches" the drops flow, according to the pre-set rate through a drop sensor system. It generates gravitational flow. There is no force exerted by the EID, so the flow rate is influenced by the height at which the IV container is hung. When hung 36 in. above the IV site, there should be sufficient pressure for the infusate to infuse by gravitation into a peripheral vascular line. Should any resistance to flow develop, the alarm on the machine will sound.

Pumps

An EID that functions in the pump mode provides a driving force to overcome resistance to pressure in order to propel the infusate. It generates positive pressure flow. If the fluid does not flow by gravity, the pump produces the needed pressure for the infusion. There is greater delivery accuracy with a pump. A pump has pre-set pressure restrictions, so it cannot overcome forces that exceed its maximum pre-set pressure. Pressure is gauged in pounds per square inch (psi), with up to 15 psi considered a safe maximum. Pressure greater than this in the infusion line signals the alarm to sound on the pump. Pump devices that generate positive pressure flow include peristaltic, syringe, and pulsatile pumps.

"The safety features . . . should be of prime consideration . . . (and) include, but are not limited to, audible alarms, battery life and operation indicators, anti-free-flow protection, adjustable occlusion pressure levels, accuracy of delivery indicator, drug dosage calculation, in-line pressure monitoring, and antitamper mechanisms" (INS, 2000, Standard 39-II, S35). As sophisticated as an EID may be, it is never to be used as a substitute for nursing care and supervision. The nurse always maintains responsibility and accountability for monitoring the patient, the prescribed infusion, and the proper flow rate. The nurse is expected to be able to properly manage the brand of EID used by the employing agency. When using an EID, the manufacturer's guidelines should be adhered to and precautions regarding electrical safety must be followed (INS 2000, Standard 39-II, S35).

Syringe Pumps

The syringe pump is a syringe barrel with a capacity of up to 60 ml and a plunger that operates electronically. A lead, screw motor-driven system pushes the plunger to deliver fluid or medication at a rate of 0.01 to 99.9 ml/hr (Figure 8-37), depending on the model. It is a precisely accurate delivery system that can be used to administer very small volumes. Some models have program modes capable of administration in mcg/kg/min, mcg/min, and ml/hr. The syringe,

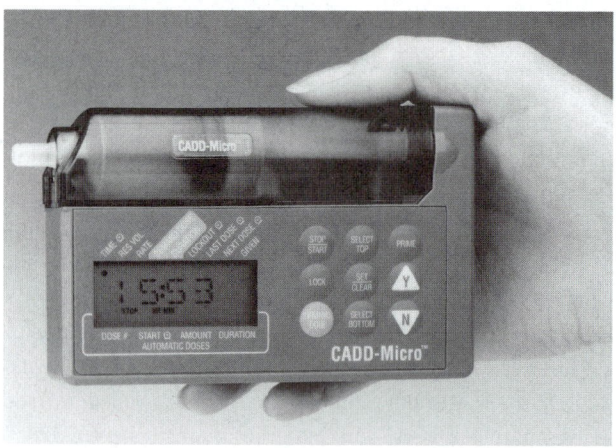

Figure 8-37 | CADD-Micro™ Ambulatory Infusion Pump. (Courtesy of Deltec, Inc.)

which is usually filled in the pharmacy, can be safely stored at room temperature or under refrigeration prior to use.

Most syringe pumps are designed to deliver continuous and bolus doses. They are frequently used in neonatal care, critical care, and anesthesia services, but are also used for patient-controlled analgesia.

Patient-Controlled Analgesia Systems

Patient-controlled analgesia (PCA) is a drug administration system that enables the patient to self-administer and regulate the delivery of medication for pain control on an as-needed (prn) basis. The candidate for this device must be mentally lucid in order to use the device correctly. The advantage of such a system is that the patient can administer a bolus of analgesic with the simple press of a button before the pain becomes too severe, thus maintaining a relatively pain-free state. When this method is used, much less medication is usually required by the patient.

PCAs are available in a variety of models, with variations in size, weight, portability, and volume delivery, depending on patient needs. Some can deliver continuous as well as bolus, intermittent, and taper-down dosages. The ones used in hospitals and other health care facilities are usually larger, heavier, and require suspension on an IV pole or table, while those designed for ambulatory patients are smaller, lightweight, and less bulky (Figure 8-38).

PCA can be used to deliver medication via IV, epidural, or subcutaneous routes. It must be programmed, according to medical orders, to regulate drug dosage, time intervals between boluses, and lock-out intervals (the period of time following drug delivery when the machine will not release any additional medication). The nurse should have knowledge of analgesic pharmacokinetics and equianalgesic dosing, contraindications, side effects, appropriate administration modalities, and anticipated outcome, and

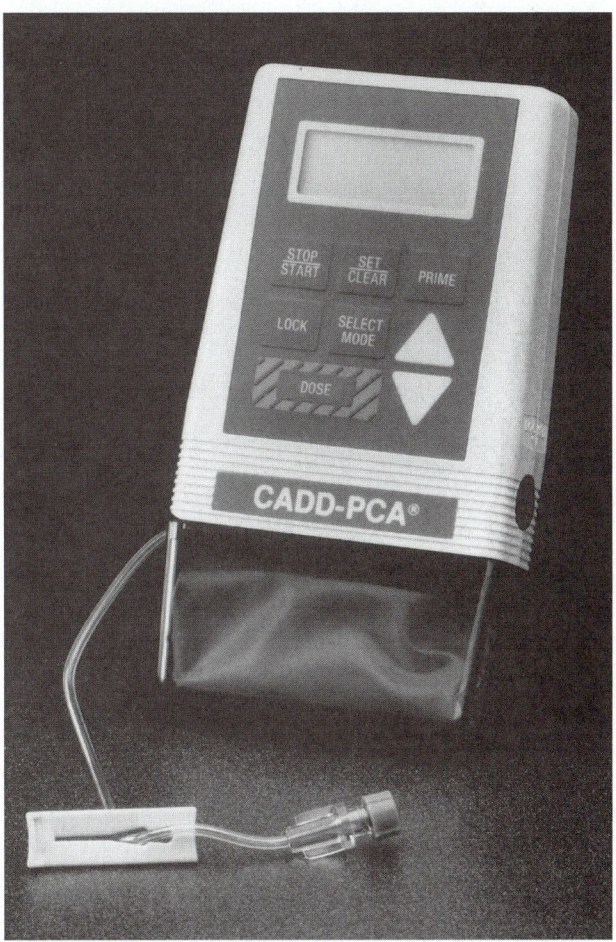

Figure 8-38 | CADD-PCA® (Courtesy of Deltec, Inc.)

should document this information in the patient's medical record (INS, 2000, Standard 72, S 68). The nurse should be educated and competent in the preparation and use of the PCA device, including programming the device to deliver prescribed therapy, administration and maintenance procedures and use of lock-out devices (INS, 2000, Standard 72, S 65).

Ambulatory and Disposable Infusion Systems

Ambulatory infusion systems are designed for patients who need parenteral medication or nutritional support, yet are able to be at home and maintain varying levels and degrees of activity. Some PCAs, as discussed previously, fall into this category, along with a large variety of others. These systems are usually lightweight, portable (with carrying cases, belt attachments, or back packs), and are powered by alkaline batteries or rechargeable NiCd batteries, but also have AC power adapters. The manufacturers of most ambulatory systems have 24-hour clinical communication centers that link the patient with the infusion service and provide clinical field nurses. They all furnish patient education information that is easy to follow, in written and audiovisual formats.

Disposable Infusion Devices

Disposable infusion devices are the newest innovations to facilitate home infusion therapy. They are closed-system mechanisms that have preattached administration tubings and air elimination filters. They are self-priming and are programmed to deliver specified volumes of infusate (50 to 250 ml) at predetermined rates. Disposable infusion structures are either elastomeric or positive-pressure systems. Although costly, patients prefer them over traditional ambulatory infusion devices because they are simple to learn, uncomplicated to use, and are completely disposable.

The framework of an elastomeric system consists of a protective outer shell, the elastomeric infusion membrane (preattached to the administration set), a 1.2 μ filter, and a volume control regulator. The driving force is the elastomeric membrane (like a balloon), which generates pressure as it collapses which, in turn, provides the thrust that delivers the infusate. The flow control device, along with the pressure in the elastomeric membrane, determines the infusion rate. The Eclipse™ (Figure 8-39) from BLOCK Medical is just one example of an elastomeric infusion structure. Other commonly used systems are the Homepump™ (BLOCK), Baxter's Intermate® (Figure 8-40), McGaw's Readymed™, and MedFlo® (Secure Medical).

A positive-pressure system, such as the SideKick® (I-Flow Corporation), has a disposable infusion system cartridge (the DISC) encased in a reusable positive-pressure infuser. The

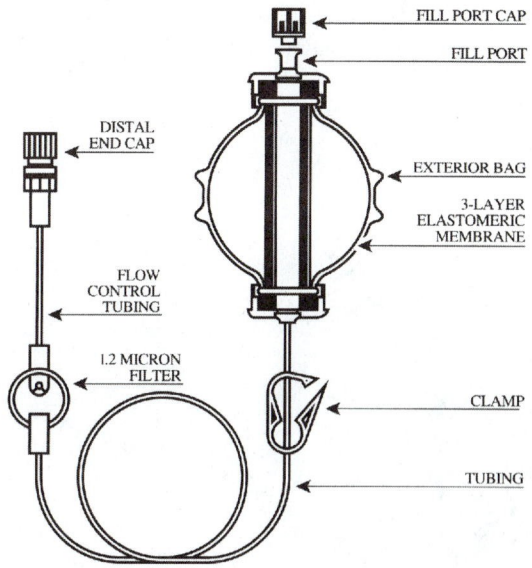

Figure 8-39 | Eclipse™ Elastometric Infusion System (Courtesy of I-FLOW Corporation)

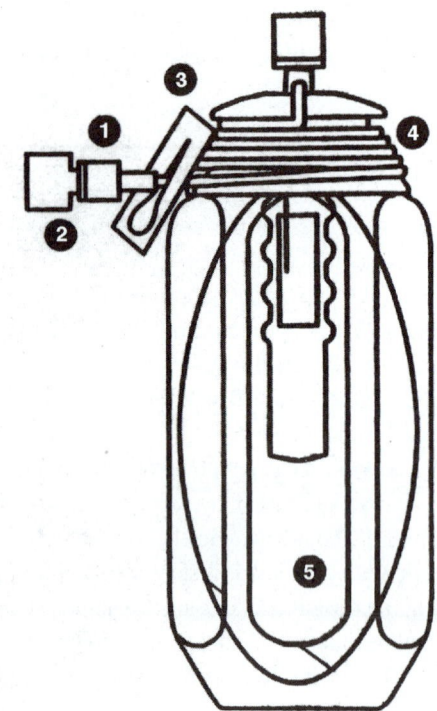

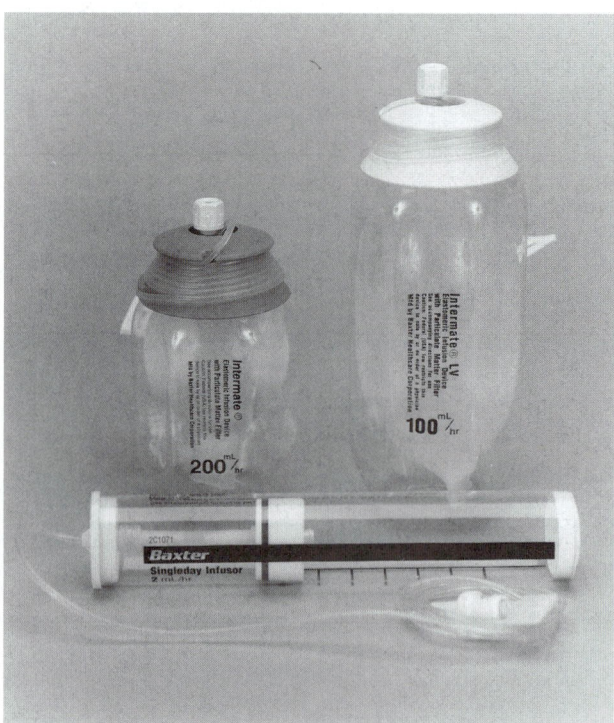

Figure 8-40 | Intermate® and Infusion Elastomeric Systems. 1. Luer-Lok connector attaches the Intermate system tubing directly to IV line. 2. Winged Luer-Lok cap protects the Luer-Lok connector. 3. Slide clamp stops fluid medication when pushed to the closed position. Medication flows when clamp is in the open position. 4. Tubing carries the fluid medication. 5. Balloon holds the fluid medication. When filled, the balloon moves medication down the delivery tubing. (Courtesy of Baxter Healthcare Corporation)

encasement has a top and bottom half, both of which are joined when screwed together. There is a spring coil in the top half of the infuser, and the DISC is loaded into the bottom half. When the two halves are screwed together, the spring exerts pressure on the DISC, and the infusate flows through the administration tubing (Figure 8-41).

LABELS

Labels are a quality assurance tool that alert all members of the health care team to the status of intravenous infusions (Figure 8-42). Legible labeling provides pertinent and easily identified information regarding the cannula, dress-

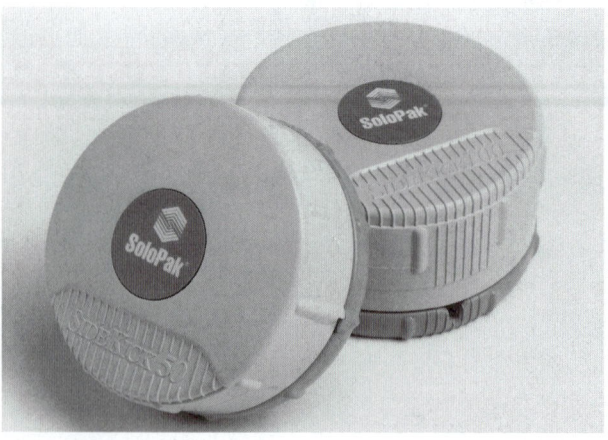

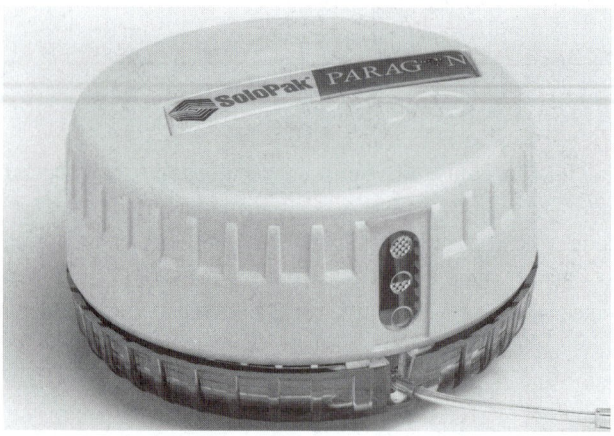

Figure 8-41 | The SideKick™ and Paragon™ Spring-Loaded Positive Pressure Drug Delivery Systems (Courtesy of I-FLOW Corporation)

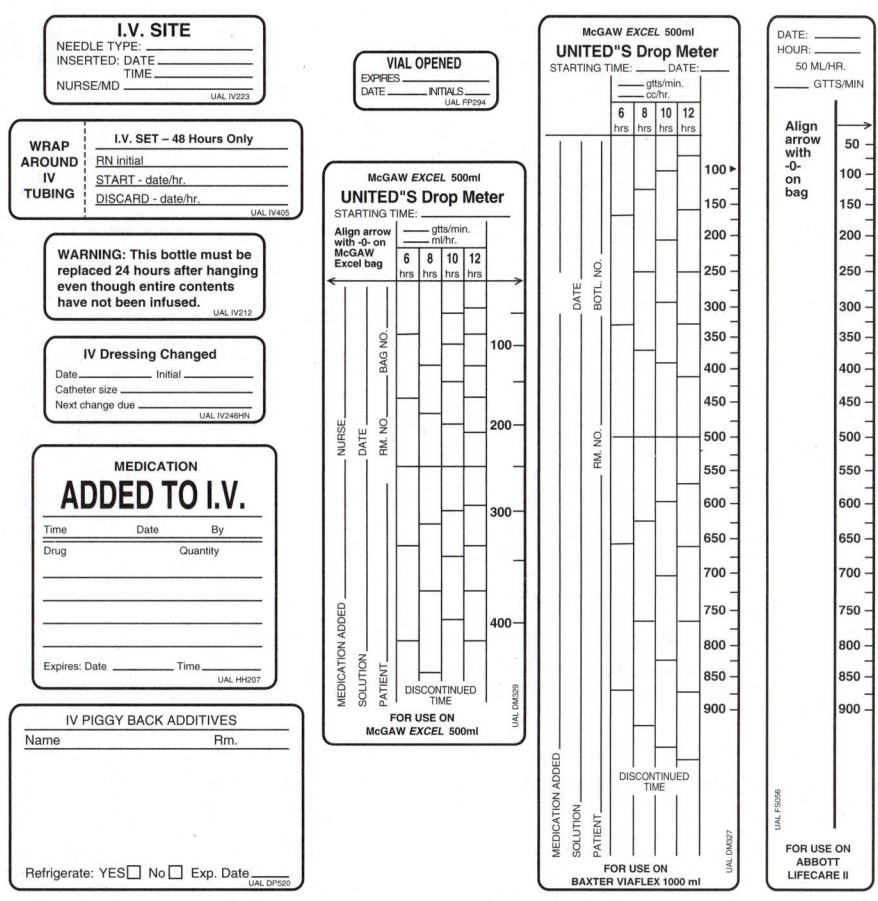

Figure 8-42 | IV Labels (Courtesy of United Ad Label Company, Inc.)

ing, infusate, medication, and administration set. Labels must be affixed to infusate containers, administration set (primary and secondary) tubings, and dressing sites. They may also be placed on the patient's bed and chart. The main purpose of labels in IV therapy is to denote start, stop, and discontinuation times (see Chapter 9, for labeling protocols).

HANGING DEVICES FOR IV EQUIPMENT

There are many hanging devices available to hold IV containers and infusion devices (Figure 8-43). They vary according to the setting in which they are used. They consist of a pole with hanging loops or projections that are usually mounted on wheels (but may also be stationary or attached to the patient's bed). Some are heavy and constructed to hold several infusate containers, machines, monitors, and other devices, while others are lightweight and portable and designed for ease of movement and ambulation.

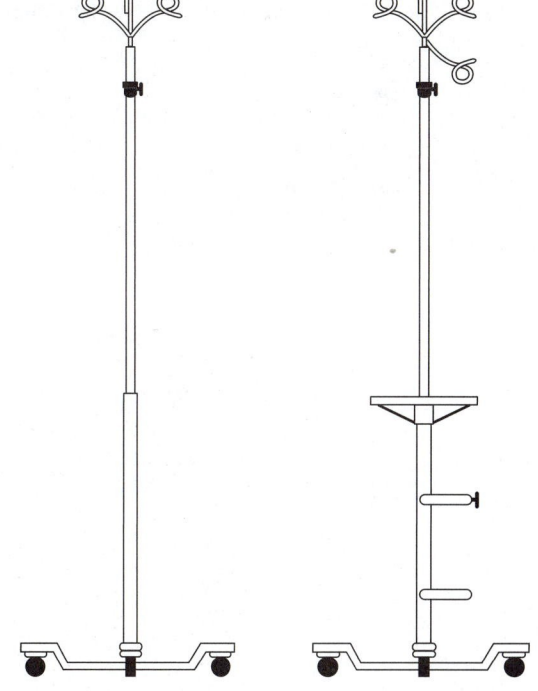

Figure 8-43 | IV Poles

Key Concepts

✳ The nurse must be familiar with the numerous equipment items and supplies needed to safely carry out intravenous infusion therapy. This includes but is not limited to the following:

- The types of infusate containers available

- The categories of administration set tubings and the devices that can be added to them

- The various types of peripheral venous access cannulas available and their indications for use

- The materials needed to prepare and maintain a percutaneous venous access site

- The categories of infusion devices available and the manner in which they operate

✳ Although the nurse cannot be familiar with every brand of every product manufactured, it is important that he know and understand how to use all of the equipment adopted for use in his place of employment.

Review Questions and Activities

1. List three nursing responsibilities and associated rationales regarding the equipment and supplies used of IV therapy.

2. Explain the difference between vented and nonvented infusate containers.

3. If you see that someone has written on a plastic IV infusate container with an indelible marker, what should you do? How would you go about ensuring that such a practice be stopped?

4. Explain and diagram the difference between straight adapters and Luer-Lok® adapters.

5. What is a drop factor? Where would you find it? What are the drop factors for the primary and secondary IV administration sets used in your agency?

6. Why must fat emulsions be contained in glass containers and delivered with special tubing?

7. Explain the concept of priming volume for IV administration sets and cannulae.

8. Why have needleless systems developed? How do they relate to OSHA guidelines regarding needlestick injuries?

9. List the three most common bloodborne pathogens that can be transmitted through needlestick injuries.

10. Differentiate between a straight steel needle and a winged (butterfly) infusion set.

11. Differentiate between an over-the-needle (ONC) and a through-the-needle (TNC) IV catheter.

12. Describe the differences of mechanical gravity control devices, electronic infusion controllers and pumps, and syringe pumps.

13. Describe the use of labels in the delivery of IV therapy.

Chapter 9

The Delivery, Care, Maintenance, and Discontinuation of Intravenous Infusion Therapy

COMPETENCIES

Upon completion of this chapter, the reader should be able to:

✳ Evaluate the dual importance of psychological and physical preparation for the patient in need of infusion therapy.

✳ Identify the anatomical areas and vessels where vascular cannulation is contraindicated for routine IV use.

✳ Explain how training devices and simulated veins help the nurse develop the experience and the dexterity needed for successful vascular access.

✳ Review the components of the medical order for IV infusion therapy.

✳ State the correct use of a tourniquet for peripheral venous access in terms of indications, application, and duration.

✳ Compare the general procedures and sequencing used to enhance venous identification and access with those procedures needed for patients with compromised circulatory conditions.

✳ Evaluate the nurse's role in identifying allergies to tape, iodine, and latex products.

✳ Assemble the items required to initiate a primary peripheral IV infusion.

✳ Demonstrate the following:

– How to set up a primary IV infusion

– How to antiseptically prepare the skin prior to infusion therapy

– Two methods of accessing a peripheral vein using an over-the-needle catheter

– How to access a vein with a winged infusion set

- Two methods of dressing a peripheral IV site

- The correct method to piggyback a secondary infusion to a primary IV line

- The correct method to connect and maintain an intermittent infusion line

- The correct method to discontinue an infusion line

- The correct method to administer medications by direct intravenous delivery with a syringe connected to a straight needle and a winged infusion set

✳ Analyze the components of labeling, reporting, and documentation, and their importance, in the practice of peripheral infusion therapy.

✳ Write a nursing care plan for a perioperative patient requiring peripheral infusion therapy.

KEY TERMS

compartment syndrome	hooding	tourniquet
floating	laminar air flow	

In the preceding chapters all of the important parameters that provide the infrastructure for IV therapy have been covered. In this chapter, the steps and procedures involved in the initiation, maintenance, supervision, and discontinuation of IV therapy will be detailed. It is important that the reader refer back to the information presented in the supporting chapters whenever necessary.

PREPARATION GUIDELINES FOR INFUSION THERAPY

In addition to the principles and concepts previously discussed, the nurse must bear in mind that several important prerequisites must be taken into consideration before the initiation of infusion therapy. The safety and comfort of the patient are paramount and are achieved by following the policies and procedures mandated by regulatory agencies and the nurse's employer.

Before initiating IV therapy, a full assessment is mandatory. Vascular access devices for routine IV use must not be introduced into the following areas:

1. An extremity with an arteriovenous fistula or graft (which is usually intended for hemodialysis cannula-

tion). "AV fistulas and hemodialysis catheters should not be used for routine administration of parenteral medications and/or solutions, except upon the order of a physician or authorized prescriber" (INS, 2000, Standard 52, S46).

2. An arm on the side of a mastectomy with axillary dissection, or orthopedic or plastic surgery subject to lymphedema and inadequate venous return. With surgical innovations, less radical procedures are performed and lymphedema or impaired vascular venous return may not be a problem following surgery for breast cancer.

3. An extremity on the side of the body affected by a CVA, because of diminished sensation and movement.

4. An extremity that has been burned, because of skin or vessel damage, diminished sensation, and decreased venous return.

5. Veins that are sclerotic or phlebitic.

6. Areas of recent infiltration.

Training Devices

Prior to the initiation of infusion therapy it is important for the nurse to have developed a level of proficiency that allows for successful venipuncture and vein access. Expertise, of course, is developed only through practice. For the student (and the nurse who has been away from

NURSING TIP

Principles of Safe Practice

It is important to remember that, while procedures and protocols may vary from state to state or agency to agency, the underlying principles regarding safe practice in the delivery of IV therapy do not change.

NURSING ALERT

Staying Abreast of Changes in the Field

With the rapid ongoing changes in IV therapy in recent years, the nurse must be fully cognizant of the responsibilities and liability associated with this practice specialty. It is critical to know and understand the following:

1. Established standards of the nurse practice act in the state in which licensure is held
2. Centers for Disease Control and Prevention (CDC) guidelines
3. Occupational Safety and Health Administration (OSHA) mandates
4. Standards set forth by the Infusion Nurses Society (INS)
5. Policies and procedures set forth by the employing agency

These are the five parameters against which the nurse will be judged should she be sued for malpractice in an IV therapy-related situation.

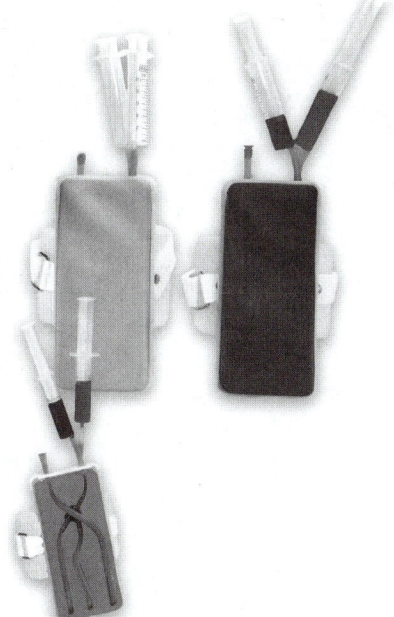

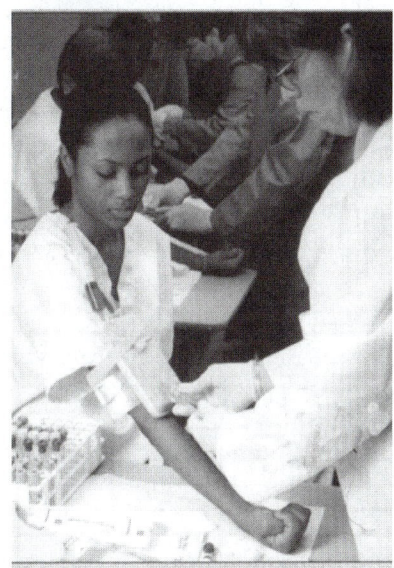

Figure 9-1 | The Venatech IV Trainer

IV practice for a period of time), it is advisable that preparation in a learning laboratory or practice setting precede clinical application. This can be accomplished using simulation mannequins, fabricated veins, and with supervised practice on peers.

There are various training devices (mechanical and computer-simulated) that allow phlebotomy practice on adult (Figure 9-1), pediatric, and geriatric "veins" as well as nephrology fistulas and grafts and various venous access devices. They provide wide variances in the sensations and feelings the nurse experiences with actual venipuncture on a living person, and have modes for practicing the maneuvers and dexterity skills used in clinical practice. It is important to inspect and palpate veins on a variety of persons—peers, family members, and patients of different ages and body types—to develop a feel for distinctions in skin texture and the elasticity and turgor of peripheral veins.

Another recommended method of practice is simulated veins. These are commercially available, but can also be easily made. To make a practice "vein," place a 6- to 8-in. segment of flexible plastic tubing (about the diameter of an administration set line) on a table and tape both ends down. Cannulation can be practiced while allowing for visualization of the actual entry, advancement, and placement of the cannula into the "vein" (Figure 9-2). This method also demonstrates how a vein can roll during venipuncture.

A similar but more realistic method of simulating the tactile sensation and cannulation of a real vein was developed

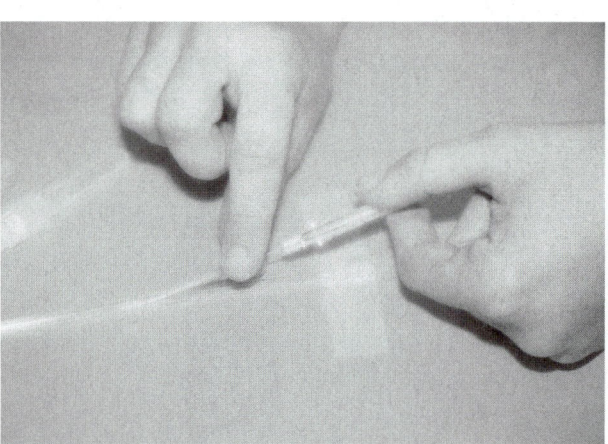

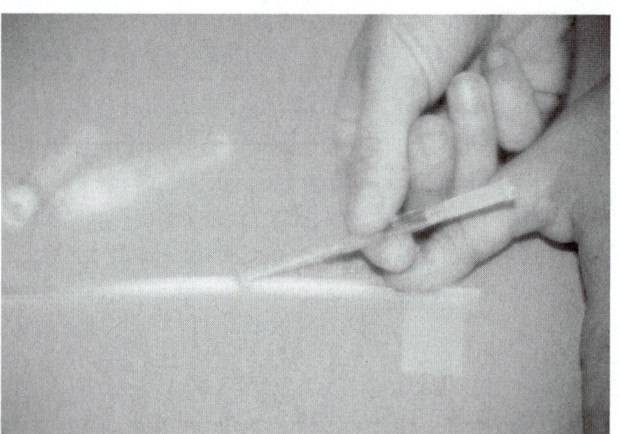

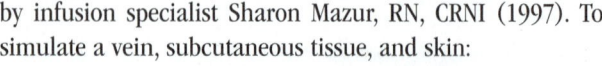

Figure 9-2 │ Vein simulation using a segment of plastic tubing

by infusion specialist Sharon Mazur, RN, CRNI (1997). To simulate a vein, subcutaneous tissue, and skin:

- Fill, without expanding, a long (4-inch to 6-inch), thin party balloon (the kind used to make animals and hats) with tomato juice and knot the end securely. Mexican-made balloons, if available, work best.
- Place the juice-filled balloon over a damp household sponge (approximately 4 inch wide × 6 inch long × 1 inch thick), which serves as the subcutaneous tissue.
- Encase the "vein"-covered sponge in "skin" by wrapping a thin, waterproof covering, such as a strip of vinyl shower curtain, around it. The covering should be opaque so that the vein cannot be seen, only palpated. Tape the covering in place on the underside of the sponge.

Medical Order

Infusion therapy is a collaborative function that integrates medicine, nursing, and pharmacology. It cannot be initiated without the order of a physician or legally authorized prescriber. The order must be appropriate for the patient and properly written in the medical record. "Verbal orders should be signed by the physician within an appropriate time frame in accordance with state and federal regulations and organizational policies and procedures" (INS, 2000, Standard 10, S18). (Figure 9-3). The essentials of any prescription include the patient's name and location; the date (and preferably the time); the name of the medication or infusate, including the dose, quantity, frequency, route, and necessary directions or precautions regarding administration; and the physician's signature. Generic or brand names may be used.

Legibility, which depends on the handwriting of the physician and the experience of the nurses and pharmacists reading medical orders, must also be considered. Whenever there

is any doubt regarding legibility or the intention of the physician, it must be questioned. Never make assumptions! An order for initiation of therapy should be written and signed by the prescriber and must be "clear, concise, legible, and complete before the nurse may initiate therapy" (INS, 2000, Standard 10, S18). If the order is not clear, the nurse must contact the prescriber for clarification.

NURSING TIP

Physician's Orders

The physician's order for any infusion must include all of the following, written on the patient's medical record:

1. Date and time of day
2. Infusate name
3. Route of administration
4. Dosage of infusate
5. Volume to be infused
6. Rate of infusion
7. Duration of infusion
8. Physician's signature

Although abbreviations are not recommended because of possible misinterpretations that may result in errors, they are widely used. It is very important that the physician, nurse, and pharmacist comprehend, and are in accord with, the commonly used abbreviations in the setting in which they practice. Doubts must always be clarified. Appendix A lists many of the abbreviations related to medications, in terms of their names, dosages, and scheduling.

There are many different brands of drugs available within the same category. They may be identical to each other in terms of their chemical makeup or pharmacologic proper-

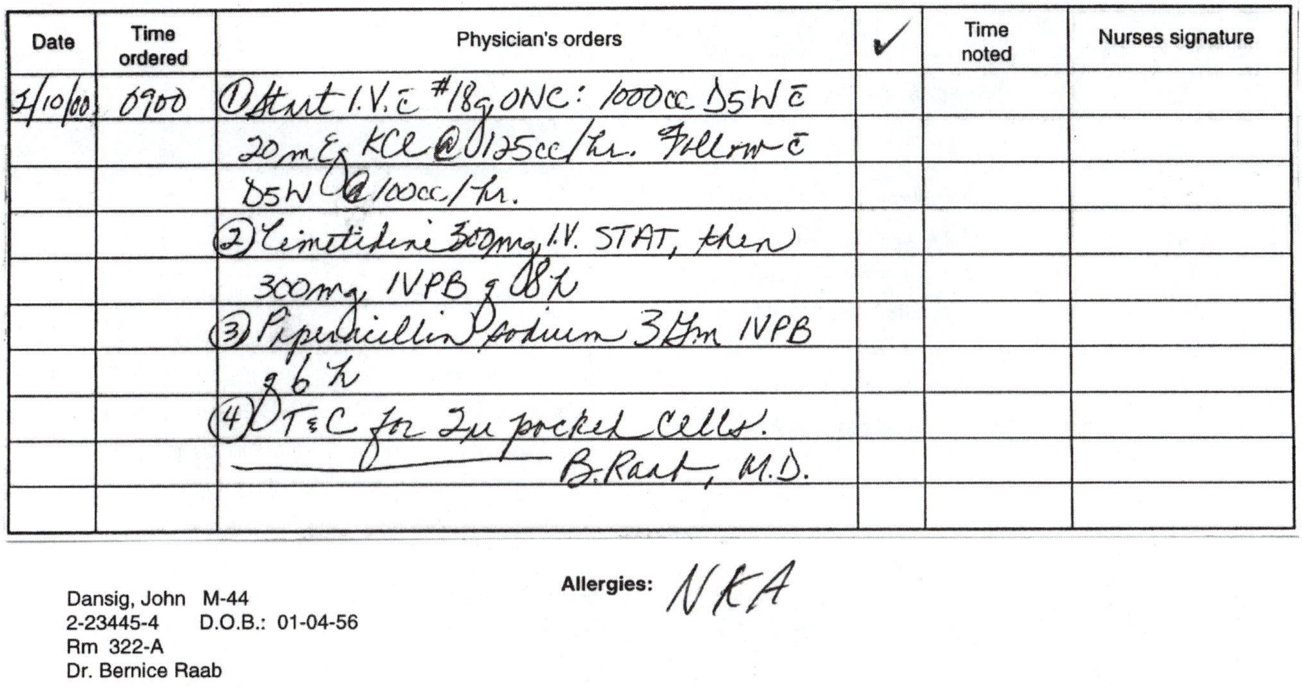

Date	Time ordered	Physician's orders	✓	Time noted	Nurses signature
1/10/00	0900	① Start I.V. c̄ #18g ONC: 1000cc D5W c̄			
		20 mEq KCl @ 125cc/hr. Follow c̄			
		D5W @ 100cc/hr.			
		② Cimetidine 300mg I.V. STAT, then			
		300mg IVPB q 08 h			
		③ Piperacillin sodium 3 Gm IVPB			
		q 6 h			
		④ T & C for 2u packed cells.			
		———— B. Raab, M.D.			

Allergies: *NKA*

Dansig, John M-44
2-23445-4 D.O.B.: 01-04-56
Rm 322-A
Dr. Bernice Raab

Figure 9-3 | Infusion orders

ties. This is often the case with antibiotic classifications, such as the ampicillins and the cephalosporins. In order to minimize duplication, most institutions have instituted the formulary system, a program in which only one drug (a generic equivalent) from a particular category is selected for use, rather than stocking every one on the market. The nurse should be aware of the formulary system so as not to be confused when the medical order is written for a brand name drug, but the pharmacy dispenses a generic equivalent.

Formulary drugs are decided upon by Pharmacy and Therapeutics (P & T) Committees within institutions (made up of pharmacists, nurses, physicians from various services, infection control personnel, and others) with selection criteria usually including safety, therapeutic effect, and cost. These panels authorize the pharmacy to stock and dispense the generic equivalents of the various brands of drugs ordered by physicians.

Hand Hygiene

It cannot be stressed often enough that proper hand hygiene is the single most important means of preventing the spread of infection. The nurse must clean her hands by washing or use of an alcohol-based rub or gel before gathering and setting up equipment and before using it on a patient. Hand hygiene must be carried out immediately after contact with a patient or his belongings and before touching other patients or items. Hands are to be sanitized before donning gloves and immediately upon removal. Since touch contamination is a common source

for the transmission of pathogens, proper hand hygiene reduces the risk of cross-contamination. Hands are to be cleansed by washing or with the use of alcohol-based rubs or gels (CDC, 2002d).

Patient Preparation and Vein Evaluation

Once the nurse has verified an IV order, but before preparing the necessary equipment and transporting it to the patient's room, it is important to take a few minutes to apprise the patient of the situation. This prepares him psychologically, allows for questions and explanations, and gives the nurse an opportunity to evaluate venous accessibility. This not only gives the nurse a better idea of what she will be dealing with but also provides the opportunity to reassure the patient and establish rapport.

During this short period that precedes the initiation of infusion therapy, when the nurse has the opportunity to assess and evaluate the patient's veins, she should have a tourniquet available in order to examine one or several areas for the best possible venipuncture site. If the nurse foresees that finding a suitable vein may be difficult, there are measures that can be taken to enhance venous access.

Tourniquet Application

A **tourniquet** is an encircling device consisting of a segment of rubber tubing or a strip of Velcro® strapping that temporarily arrests blood flow to or from a distal vessel. A blood pressure cuff is sometimes used as a tourniquet by inflating it to a reading midway between the patient's systolic and diastolic pressures or just below his diastolic pressure. Unless disposable tourniquets are available, reusable ones should be disinfected between use or covered with a throwaway plastic sheath during use to avoid cross-contamination between patients. Remember: Tourniquets may be a source of latex exposure.

The most important thing to remember when utilizing a tourniquet is to apply it so that only venous, and not arterial, blood flow is suppressed. To ensure this, the nurse must always be able to palpate or auscultate a pulse distal to the tourniquet. See Skill 9–1 for the proper method of applying a tourniquet.

Methods to Enhance Venous Access

If after assessing the patient's veins the nurse finds an appropriate site for venipuncture, she then prepares the necessary equipment for infusion therapy. Should she find that venous access may be difficult, there are steps that should be taken to facilitate cannulation and insertion.

The following procedures, used alone or in conjunction with the others, are commonly employed, in the ensuing order, to expedite venous access. Be sure to explain to the patient what will be done before each procedure is initiated.

1. *Gravity.* Place the extremity intended for venipuncture below the level of the patient's heart for several minutes. If the veins do not distend, do this with a tourniquet in place.
2. *Fist clenching.* Ask the patient to open and close his fist or squeeze and release his hand around a rolled wash cloth or the lowered bed rail. If the veins do not distend, do this with a tourniquet in place.
3. *Friction.* Gently stroke the skin over the veins intended for venipuncture. Doing this with an alcohol pledget creates heat, which enhances venous distention. If the veins do not engorge, do this with a tourniquet in place.
4. *Percussion.* Gently tap the area of skin over a vein using the thumb and index (or third) finger, or pat the area using light to moderate force (to engorge the vein with blood). If veins do not engorge, do these maneuvers with a tourniquet in place.
5. *Compresses.* With the extremity placed below the level of the patient's heart, apply warm compresses for 10 to 15 minutes prior to venipuncture. Immediately before the intended IV site is to be prepped with an antiseptic, fresh, warm compresses may be applied for a few additional minutes, with a tourniquet in place, to further enhance vein distention.

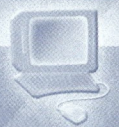

SKILL 9-1

Tourniquet Application

Equipment Needed:

Tourniquet

Implementation/Action	Rationale
1. Check the physician's order.	A physician's order is a legal requirement for infusion therapy.
2. Introduce yourself to the patient.	By introducing yourself, you convey courtesy, establish/promote the nurse-patient relationship, instill patient trust, and thus alleviate anxiety.
3. Identify the patient by checking the wrist band against the doctor's order and asking the patient, if conscious, to state his/her name.	Proper identification ensures that the procedure is being performed on the correct patient.
4. Verify the allergy status of the patient.	This is a patient safety measure.
5. Explain the proposed procedure in terms the patient can understand.	The patient has the right to know what is being done and the right to refuse care.
6. Carry out proper hand hygiene.	Good hand hygiene is the single most important means of preventing the spread of infection.
7. Gather equipment.	This serves to economize time and reduce patient anxiety.
8. Provide for privacy.	Privacy allows the patient to maintain dignity.
9. To correctly apply the tourniquet, hold one end in the dominant hand and the other end in the nondominant hand (Figure 9-4).	

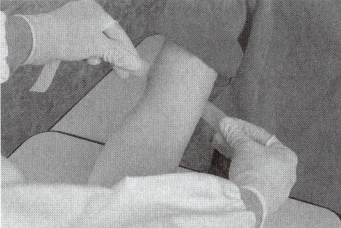

Figure 9-4 | A tourniquet positioned 3 to 4 inches above the intended venipuncture site

10. Encircle the extremity 3 to 4 inches above the venipuncture site. Lay one length over the other, close to the skin, as if tying a knot (Figure 9-5). The end of the tubing in the nurse's dominant hand is not brought through completely (as it would be if tying a knot) but tucked under the other segment (Figure 9-6).

This ensures one-handed release of the tourniquet by pulling on the end of the tucked-under segment.

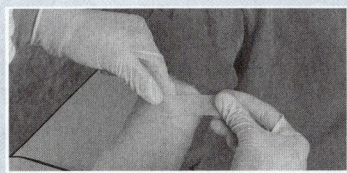

Figure 9-5 | Stretch the tourniquet tight and cross the ends.

(continues)

Tourniquet Application (continued)

Implementation/Action	Rationale

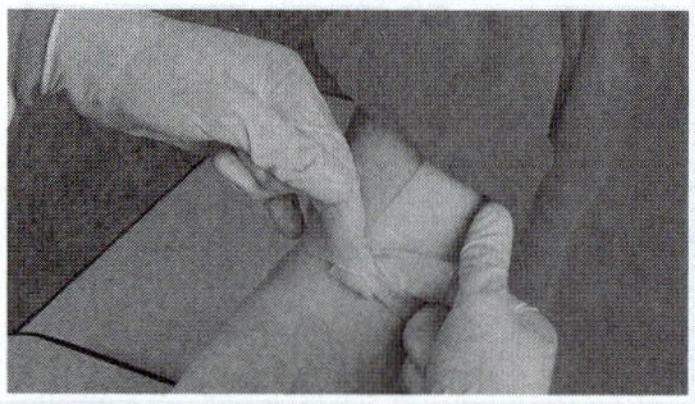

Figure 9-6A | Tuck one portion of the tourniquet under the other.

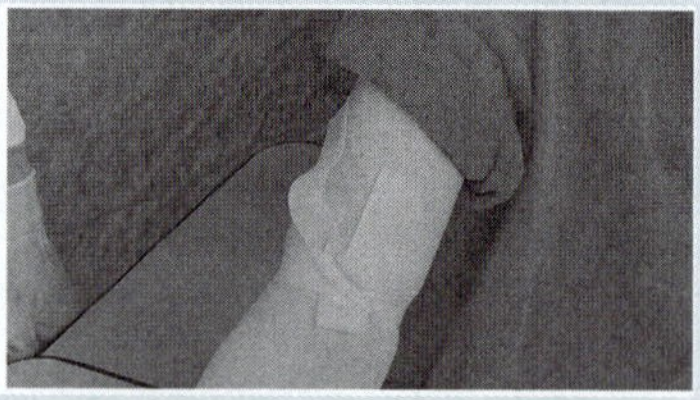

11. Assess for a pulse distal to the application site.
12. To remove the tourniquet, pull the end of the tucked portion.

Figure 9-6B | The ends of the tourniquet should be pointing upward and not hanging in the venipuncture site.

Palpation or auscultation of a pulse ensures that arterial blood flow is not hindered.

6. *Multiple tourniquets.* This process increases tissue oncotic pressure and forces blood into collateral veins to distend them. It is employed when the usual veins accessed for IV therapy are not viable and collateral vessels must be used. The process is as follows:

(a) Apply one tourniquet to the upper arm (about 2 to 3 inches above the antecubital fossa) for two minutes while applying pressure with downward stroking movements from the tourniquet to the hand. Check for arterial pulses distal to this tourniquet.

(b) After two minutes, apply a second tourniquet to the forearm about 2 to 3 inches below the antecubital fossa and continue with the downward stroking movements. At this point, collateral veins usually become visible.

(c) If collateral veins do not appear after two minutes, place a third tourniquet above the wrist and release the tourniquet on the upper arm. Continue to stroke the hands to locate collaterals in the hands and fingers.

(d) Remove all tourniquets before six minutes have passed.

(e) Should a venous access site still not present itself, the physician should be notified.

7. *Transillumination.* Darken the room so that the lighting is dim and hold the VENOSCOPE® II Transilluminater so that the arms are flush against the patient's skin. Gradually slide the device along the extremity until a dark shadowy line appears between the fiberoptic

arms, indicating that a vein is present. Apply downward pressure over the two arms to check for blanching.

Veins in the lower extremity should not be used. If they must be accessed, there should be a medical order. They are used only for a short period of time until other upper body sites can be found or placement of a central line can be instituted. When lower extremity veins are used, there must be frequent circulatory assessments and range-of-motion exercises (active, passive, or both) must be instituted to maintain adequate venous return.

NURSING TIP

Checking for Blanching

Remember, for a vein to be viable, it must be able to be blanched. To check for blanching, apply downward pressure over or on each side of a vein. If the vein disappears with the pressure, then reappears when the pressure is removed, the vein is viable. A sclerotic vein will not blanch.

Hair Removal

If necessary, prior to initiating IV therapy, hair may need to be removed. This should be done only if there is enough hair to impede vein visualization, site disinfection, cannula insertion, or dressing adherence. Hair is to be removed by gently clipping it close to the skin, without scratching the skin. Shaving, because of the potential for microabrasion and the introduction of contaminants, should not be used, nor should depilatories be applied because of the possibility for skin irritation or allergic reactions (INS, 2000, Standard 45, S40). An electric shaver may be used, depending on institutional policy, if it belongs to the patient or if the shaving heads can be changed or disinfected between patient use. An electric shaver should not be used if breaches in skin integrity result from its use.

Special Considerations Regarding Venous Access

In addition to the previously discussed problems, other circumstances and conditions may impede venous access. In these situations there are special techniques the nurse may need to utilize to facilitate cannulation.

Patients Receiving Anticoagulation Therapy

Patients receiving anticoagulants are prone to bleeding that can range from local ecchymoses to major hemorrhagic complications. A primary nursing consideration for such patients is to monitor them closely and avoid any procedures that might enhance bleeding during IV therapy.

Precautions are especially necessary when IV therapy is being initiated. If possible, tourniquets should be avoided to prevent subcutaneous bleeding and bruising. If they must be used, they should be applied as loosely as possible. Venous distention may be accomplished using gentle constriction with towels, cotton batting, or even the hands of another person encircling the extremity and applying gentle pressure during cannulation.

During the application of the antimicrobial preparation, care must be taken to avoid excess pressure. The smallest cannula that will accommodate the vein and deliver the ordered infusate should be selected to prevent unnecessary traction against the skin during cannulation. Dressings must be removed gently, using alcohol or an adhesive solvent, to avoid any tearing movement that might result in superficial bruising. If cannulation is not successful after the vein has been entered, measures must be taken to diminish bleeding into the surrounding tissues and reduce bruising.

Patients with Altered Skin and Vessels

Special precautions must be taken if patients have irritated, burned, or diseased skin. Alternate measures, in accord with institutional policies, may need to be taken during skin antisepsis to prevent further irritation and discomfort. Since photoexposure may cause discomfort, special, indirect lighting is usually employed when locating a vein and during

cannulation. Venous distention may be achieved using measures similar to those required for patients receiving anticoagulants.

For patients with fragile, delicate veins, the use of tourniquets is discouraged. These fine vessels may break ("blow") when they distend with tourniquet application or when accessed during venipuncture. Such veins are usually seen in frail, elderly patients and patients receiving corticosteroid therapy. (See access maneuvers in Chapter 16.)

Some patients develop sclerosed veins from frequent IV therapy, collagen-related disease processes, or illicit intravenous drug use. These veins are hard and often cordlike, nonelastic, and do not blanch when pressure is applied over or around them. Sclerotic veins cannot be accessed, so transillumination may be needed to locate deeper veins. The multiple tourniquet technique, to find collateral vessels, may also be used.

CRITICAL THINKING

Respecting a Patient's Privacy While Maintaining IV Care Priorities

Sometimes the nurse is faced with a situation in which there are no viable peripheral veins for infusion therapy because the patient has a history of illicit IV drug use. The physician may need to put an IV line in a central vein in the neck area. In such a circumstance, when the patient's family members come to visit, they may ask you why the IV is in such an unusual place. A parent might say to you, "When I needed one, the nurse put it in a vein in my forearm. Why does my son need it in his neck?" How would you handle this situation? What are your patient's rights regarding confidentiality in this case?

Patients with Peripheral Edema

Venous access in patients with peripheral edema is very difficult and not without risk. Because of increased oncotic pressure in the tissues that surround the vessels, venous access is complicated. If cannulation is successful, the vessel may collapse from the oncotic pressure created by the edema. When venous access is achieved and maintained, another potential problem, infiltration (because of the edema) is hard to identify. Should infiltration occur, **compartment syndrome**, in which the function and viability of nerves and vessels are threatened when they are confined and constricted by fluid pressure, can result.

Because veins cannot be visualized, the nurse must locate veins based on anatomical landmarks. Venous access is best accomplished by applying digital pressure with the heel of the hand (for 15 to 20 seconds over the proposed vein) to displace tissue pressure. When the pressure is removed, the edema is temporarily gone (displaced) and the vein can be seen. Cannulation must follow quickly or the edema will shift back and obliterate the vein again. For the purpose of asepsis, and since the nurse must work quickly, it is a good idea to have prepped the intended venipuncture area first and apply digital pressure with a sterile glove prior to cannulation. Some nurses apply the pressure using a 70% alcohol pledget.

Obese Patients

Obese patients may have easy-to-visualize surface veins or deeply imbedded vessels, depending on how the adipose tissue displaces them. If they migrate toward the surface of the extremity, cannulation is accomplished as it would be for an average-sized person. For deep vessels, anatomical landmarks must be used in conjunction with a longer cannula that can gain access to them. Multiple tourniquets and vein illumination may also be necessary.

Allergies

It cannot be stressed often enough that the nurse must take advantage of every possible situation to determine whether or not a patient has allergies. These include medications, foods, animal and insect matter, latex, and environmental substances. The patient and family should be questioned during the initial assessment and the nursing history, but also throughout the course of care. Questions regarding allergies should always be asked prior to giving medications, especially those administered parenterally. The nurse must know where emergency drugs used to counteract allergic reactions are located. When administering care to a patient in the home, the nurse must have access to emergency drugs and any equipment needed to counteract allergic reactions. Once it is determined that a patient has allergies, such information must be placed in the medical record and clearly labeled on his identification bracelet, chart, bed, MAR, and on all communication media with the pharmacy, x-ray, and laboratory departments, and all other services used by the patient (Figure 9-7).

Iodine Allergy

With infusion therapy it is important to determine whether a patient is allergic to iodine and its derivatives, since such products are often used in skin antisepsis. If a patient does not know whether or not he is allergic to iodine, he should

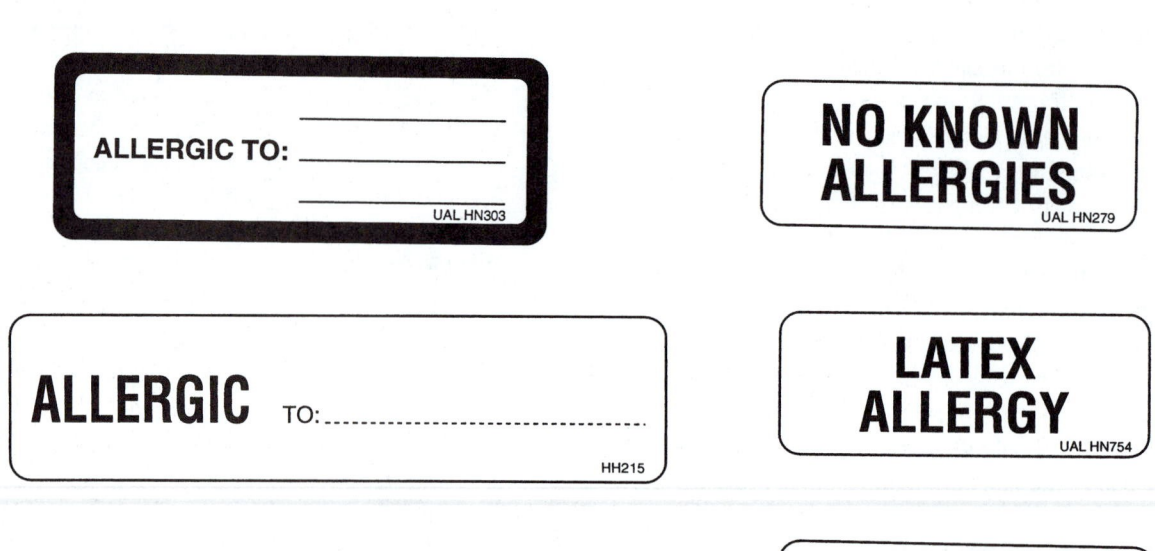

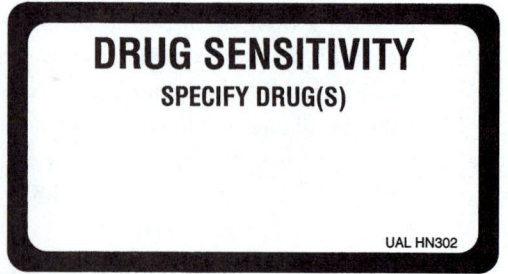

Figure 9-7 | Allergy labels *Courtesy of United Ad Label, Inc., Brea, CA*

be questioned regarding allergies to fish, especially shellfish. If there is any doubt, iodine preparations should not be used. If a patient has a known allergy to iodine, the prepping solution of choice is 70% isopropyl alcohol. The alcohol is to be applied with friction for a minimum of 30 seconds or until the final applicator is visually clean. CHG, if institutionally-approved, may also be used.

Tape Allergy

Another consideration regarding allergies concerns tape. Many people who have not had problems with tape or dressings in the past develop sensitivities to it over time. It is important to assess for any problems with tape that may develop during the course of nursing care and be alert to redness, rashes, or patient complaints of itching when tape is used. The problem with tape may be associated with the adhesive used on it or the fact that it is made of latex.

Latex Allergy

Latex refers to the natural rubber product manufactured from a milky fluid that is primarily obtained from the rubber tree (*Hevea brasiliensis*). Latex has become a major health concern with patients and health care personnel having developed, or become aware of, an allergy to latex. Increasing numbers of people in the workplace have been affected due to the extensive use of the product as a component of many medical and consumer devices. Some synthetic rubber materials may be referred to as "latex" even though they do not contain the protein that produces latex allergy.

It is estimated that 10–17% of health care workers have already become sensitized to latex, and over 2% have occupational-induced asthma as a result of latex exposure. The Food and Drug Administration (FDA) has received more than 1,000 reports of adverse health effects from exposure to latex, including 15 deaths due to such exposure (OSHA, 2002). Documented reactions to latex

> ### NURSING ALERT
>
> #### Powdered Gloves and Hand Creams
>
> The starch powder used to coat and lubricate some latex gloves becomes coated with latex protein and is inhaled during glove application and removal. It is better to use powder-free gloves. Oil-based hand creams and lotions should not be used with gloves because they cause latex deterioration, which increases exposure to latex proteins (Petsonk, 1997).

> ### NURSING TIP
>
> #### Latex Reactions
>
> Patients at risk for latex-related reactions include the following:
>
> 1. Women (who account for 75% of all reported cases)
> 2. Asthmatics
> 3. Persons with histories of allergies
> 4. Persons with occupational latex exposure, such as health care workers, artists and painters, rubber industry workers
> 5. Persons with allergies to fruits and vegetables, especially avocados, bananas, chestnuts, kiwis, and other tropical fruits (due to reciprocal reaction of these foods and latex allergens)
> 6. Persons who undergo intermittent catheterization
> 7. Persons with long histories of genitourinary or intra-abdominal surgeries

> ### NURSING TIP
>
> #### Latex Balloons
>
> Remember, latex balloons, which are often brought to patients in the home or hospital setting, are a source of latex allergy exposure. Mylar balloons should be used instead of latex to protect latex-sensitive individuals.

include mild contact dermatitis, rhinitis, conjunctivitis, urticaria, bronchospasm, and severe systemic anaphylaxis.

The FDA and OSHA advise health care professionals to identify latex-sensitive patients and be prepared to treat them. Many common household items contain latex or its by-products. Home-bound patients who perform self-catheterization or undergo intermittent catheterization are at risk for latex-related allergic reactions. Allergic individuals must avoid latex products and use appropriate substitutes that meet federal safety guidelines. Synthetic rubbers, polyethylene, silicone, or vinyl can be used effectively as alternatives to natural rubber latex. Latex materials labeled hypoallergenic are not necessarily latex-free and may not prevent adverse reactions because they may contain the latex proteins and chemicals responsible for sensitization.

The FDA recommendations to health professionals include the following:

1. Questioning for latex sensitivity during the taking of general histories on all patients
2. Using devices made with alternative materials, such as plastic
3. Being alert to the fact that an allergic reaction may occur whenever latex-containing devices are used, especially when the latex comes in contact with mucous membranes
4. Alerting patients with suspected allergic reactions to latex to possible latex sensitivity and advising them to consider immunologic evaluation
5. Advising patients to tell health professionals and emergency personnel about their latex sensitivity and consider advising them to wear a medical identification bracelet

INITIATION OF INFUSION THERAPY

After all of the preparatory steps have been taken, the nurse is ready to gather and set up the appropriate equipment and start the infusion. She must check the order, identify that it is for the right patient, and verify infusate compatibility. The infusate container should be compared directly with the physician's order to be sure it is correct, and pharmacy admixtures must be verified. If the IV order is for blood or blood products, anticoagulants, or chemotherapy, institutional protocols usually require verification checks by two licensed nurses. It is very important for the nurse to know what is required by the agency that employs her.

Equipment Preparation and Setup

The equipment needed for the infusion should be set up away from the patient's room in an environment that minimizes the chance for contamination. If possible, a separate room or area that has good lighting is preferable. Noise and traffic should be kept to a minimum so there is no unnecessary distraction for the nurse and the least amount of air movement. All nonsterile supplies must be clean, such as any outer packaging, IV poles, or electronic infusion devices.

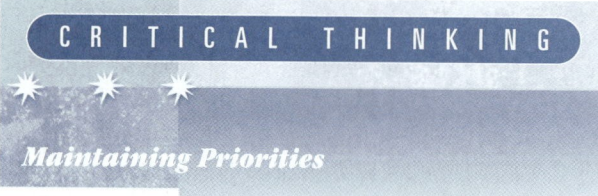

CRITICAL   THINKING

Maintaining Priorities

You are preparing to set up an IV infusion that is ordered stat. The only IV pole on your unit was just used by another patient and is contaminated with splatters of blood. What would you do in this situation?

Primary Infusion Setup

Prior to starting an intravenous infusion, the correct infusate needs to be set up with a primary administration set (Figure 9-8). If piggyback medications or secondary infusions are ordered or anticipated, procure a set that has a check valve and injection ports. The interior of the tubing, both ends, as well as the IV fluid, need to be kept sterile to avoid contamination. Gravity flow tubing, or tubing that is not pump specific, is available in macrodrip (usually 15 drops per ml) and microdrip (usually 60 drops per ml).

Many tubings are specifically used for certain types of IV pumps. Although the principles for setting up the infusion remain the same, directions should be checked for any specific tubing as the manufacturer may have slight variations for setting up their particular brand of tubing.

To set up a primary infusion, the nurse must strictly adhere to established step-by-step protocols, as illustrated in Skill 9-2.

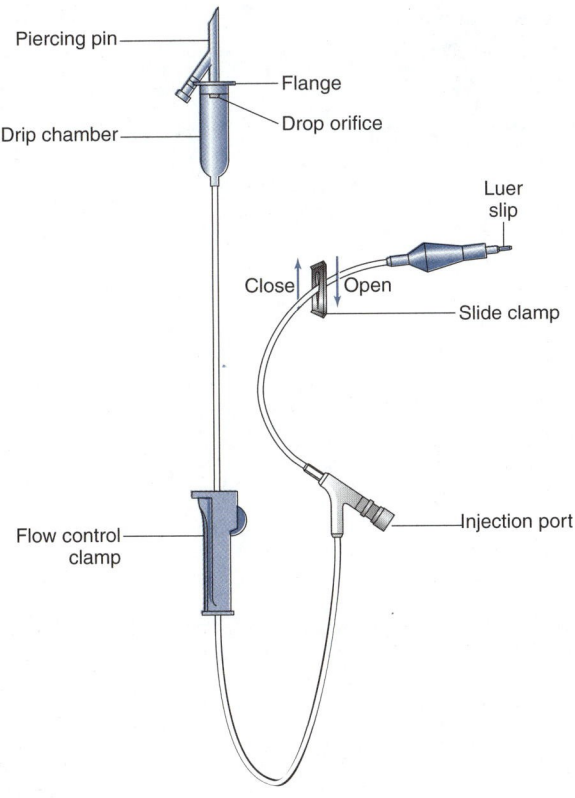

Figure 9-8 | Proper setup of a primary infusion line

Administration Guidelines for Peripheral Infusion Therapy

With all of the proper equipment ready and the correct infusion prepared, the nurse can proceed to the bedside. As discussed earlier, the ideal situation is one in which the nurse has had the opportunity to establish rapport, give thorough explanations regarding the prescribed therapy, assess the patient and his venous status, and allow for questions and answers. Even if time is of the essence, shortcuts cannot be taken when it comes to safety, comfort, and communication. (A brief review of the risks and complications [Chapter 5] and patient preparation and site selection [Chapter 6] are very important here.) Patient identity must be verified, and asepsis must be a major concern. Allergies and fluid or medication compatibilities need to be double-checked. The room should be equipped to accommodate both the patient and the nurse, and it should have good lighting and a comfortable temperature. If time and the patient's condition permits, he should be given the opportunity to use the bathroom prior to starting the IV. If possible, site selection should be in the patient's nondominant hand or arm so he can carry out routine activities of daily living during infusion therapy. If the extremity to be used for the IV is

---

SKILL 9-2

Primary Infusion Setup

Equipment Needed:	Implementation/Action	Rationale
Intravenous infusate	1. Check the physician's order.	A physician's order is a legal requirement for infusion therapy.
Primary IV administration set	2. Introduce yourself to the patient.	By introducing yourself, you convey courtesy, establish/promote the nurse-patient relationship, instill patient trust, and thus alleviate anxiety.
IV pole	3. Identify the patient by checking the wrist band against the doctor's order and asking the patient, if conscious, to state his/her name.	Proper identification ensures that the procedure is being performed on the correct patient.
Label for the IV bag		
Label for the tubing	4. Verify the allergy status of the patient.	This is a patient safety measure.
Implementation	5. Explain the proposed procedure in terms the patient can understand.	The patient has the right to know what is being done and the right to refuse care.
IV start kit	6. Carry out proper hand hygiene.	Good hand hygiene is the single most important means of preventing the spread of infection.
cannula	7. Gather the ordered IV fluids, appropriate tubing, and a clean IV pole	This serves to economize time and avoid undue anxiety for the patient.

(continues)

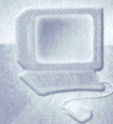

SKILL 9-2

Primary Infusion Setup (continued)

Implementation/Action	**Rationale**
for set up in an uncontaminated area away from the patient's room. If a pole-mounted EID (electronic infusion device) is needed, check that it is in proper working order and that the batteries are charged.	
8. Check the IV fluid for type and amount, expiration date, clarity, and leaks in the bag or bottle. For plastic infusate containers, remove the outer tear-off wrap, following the manufacturer's directions. (This will have been removed in the pharmacy if an admixture has been ordered.)	**This ensures the fluid is appropriate, safe to use, and sterile, in order to prevent complications, including infection.**
9. Check for the expiration date on the IV tubing container and open it. Ensure that the sterile cover is over the infusate spike and the distal end where the IV cannula connects are intact. (If the cannula end has a "breathable" attachment, it will not have a cover over it.) Once the set is removed from its package, keep it coiled and contained above waist level (Figure 9-9).	**This may prevent the tubing from falling on the floor and becoming contaminated.**

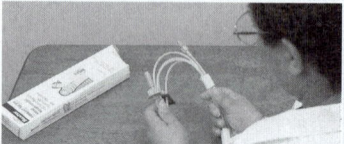

Figure 9-9 | Remove the tubing from the packaging and keep it coiled.

10. Close the roller clamp on the administration set tubing (but not the slide clamps, if there are any).	**Prevents the fluid from spilling when the tubing is primed.**
11. Hang the IV fluids that are in plastic bags on an IV pole. Place glass containers on a clean counter.	**This will prevent unnecessary air from entering the tubing.**
12. To spike a plastic bag:	
a. Secure the neck of the bag with the thumb and index finger of the nondominant hand and remove the sterile cover on the administration set port with the dominant hand (Figure 9-10).	

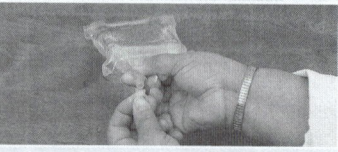

Figure 9-10 | Open the plastic tab covering the IV port, taking care to maintain its sterility.

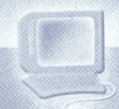

SKILL 9-2

Primary Infusion Setup

Implementation/Action	**Rationale**
b. Remove the sterile cover from the tubing administration set spike. Do not touch the spike itself.	This will prevent the spike from becoming contaminated. If it is touched, it will need to be replaced.
c. To spike the bag, grasp the middle of the outside surface of the administration port, holding it vertically between the thumb and index and third finger of the nondominant hand. Holding the fingerguard area below the spiked portion of the administration set, insert the spike into the administration port, using a straight, twisting motion (see Figure 9-11).	This ensures free flow of the infusate into the tubing, preventing leakage and precluding contamination.

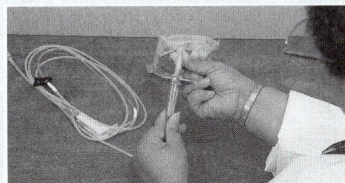

Figure 9-11 | Spike the IV bag.

To spike a glass bottle...

a. Be sure to use the appropriate administration set. A vented set must be used if there is no internal venting system in the bottle.	To prevent air from entering the line while the infusion is running.
b. With the bottle standing upright on a level surface, hold it in place with the nondominant hand and peel off the outer aluminum band from the top of the bottle with the dominant hand.	
c. Remove the rubber disk stopper, which seals the vacuum and sterile lid of the bottle where the administration port sits. If an admixture has been instilled, the aluminum cap and rubber stopper will already have been removed in the pharmacy and sealed with a tamperproof closure, which must be torn off before spiking. Do not touch the top of the bottle where the administration port or vent outlet sits. If it is touched, the top must be thoroughly wiped with a 70% alcohol solution prior to spiking.	To prevent contamination of the infusate.
d. Remove the sterile cap from the spike and push it into the port with a straight (not twisting) movement.	

(continues)

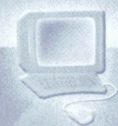

SKILL 9-2

Primary Infusion Setup (continued)

Implementation/Action	**Rationale**
e. Suspend the bottle on the IV pole by the aluminum bale at the bottom of the container.	
13. Squeeze the drip chamber to allow it to fill $\frac{1}{3}$ to $\frac{1}{2}$ full (Figure 9-12) or to the level of the manufacturer's imprinted marking on the chamber.	**This allows for observation of the drip rate.**

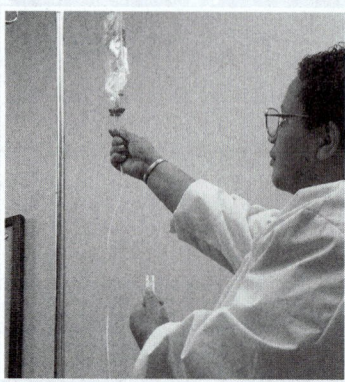

Figure 9-12 | Allow the drip chamber to fill half way.

14. Remove the sterile cap from the distal end of the administration set. Make sure to maintain the sterility of the cap. Prime the administration tubing by holding the distal end of the administration set over (but not touching) a basin, paper towel, or sink. Slowly open the roller clamp to purge air from the set (Figure 9-13). As the fluid approaches the check valve or any injection ports, invert those sites and tap on them to remove any trapped air.	**Purges air from the line while maintaining sterility.**

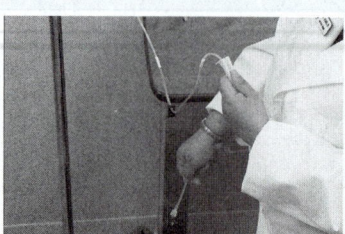

Figure 9-13 | Allow the infusate to run through the tubing and then clamp the tubing to remove all air from the line.

SKILL 9-2

Primary Infusion Setup

Implementation/Action	Rationale
15. Once the infusate reaches the distal end of the administration set and there are no visible air pockets, the tubing can be clamped, recapped (if appropriate), and hung over the top of the IV pole for transport to the patient's room.	**Prevents fluid from leaking and maintains sterility of the set.**
16. Connectors and add-on devices may be added before or after priming, depending on the manufacturer's guidelines. The priming volume is stated on the packaging.	**It is important for the nurse to remember to purge air from any add-on device to prevent air embolism.**
17. Label the infusate container and the administration set with date and time per institutional policy (Figure 9-14).	**This will indicate when the infusate and/or tubing replacement is necessary.**

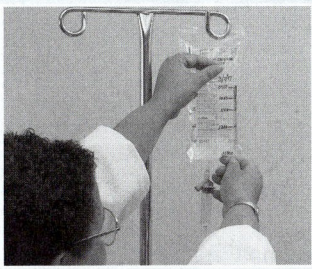

Figure 9-14 | Label the IV bag.

18. Adjust the height of the infusate container to approximately 36 inches above the intended IV insertion site.

not clean, it should be washed with soap and water, rinsed, and dried prior to precannulation antisepsis. The bed should be elevated so the nurse can comfortably assess the patient, prepare the IV site, and initiate the infusion. For the patient's safety and convenience, the bed should be returned to its low position after the infusion is started.

Starting an Infusion

The ensuing guidelines and protocols should be closely followed for the safe administration of any infusion.

1. Ask the patient to state his full name, if he is able to do so. Verify identity with the chart and the identification bracelet.
2. Introduce yourself to the patient.
3. Provide privacy.
4. Explain the proposed procedures in terms the patient can understand. Remember, the patient has the right to know what is being done and the right to refuse treatment.
5. Elevate the bed to a level conducive to starting the IV to prevent straining the nurse's back.
6. Place the patient in a semi-Fowler's or Fowler's position.
7. Protect the patient's clothing and bedding with an underpad or towel.
8. Carry out proper hand hygiene.
9. Set up all of the necessary supplies on the bedside stand or overbed table in the order they will be used, and tear or cut tape strips into the needed lengths. A few strips of paper tape should be available in addition to the start-kit tape. Because paper tape is easy to handle while wearing gloves and is easily removable, it is good to use it to stabilize the IV tubing, once it has been connected

to the cannula, while the IV site dressing is being applied. Without this, it is easy for the weight of the tubing to pull the cannula out of the vein before the site dressing and regular tape are applied.

10. Gloves are worn to protect the nurse from exposure to blood and do not need to be sterile. For the convenience of the nurse, it is suggested that, before donning them, all of the supplies needed to perform venipuncture and dressing of the IV site be arranged, the vein selected, and the site prepped. The gloves can be applied while the final antiseptic is drying.

11. Select a vein based on the type of infusion therapy and the anticipated duration.

12. Apply a tourniquet 2 to 3 inches below the antecubital fossa for venous access in the lower arm or hand. For veins that are not readily visible, as with the obese person, position the tourniquet 2 to 3 inches above the intended venipuncture site. Depending on the nurse's experience

and the time needed for cannulation, the tourniquet may be left on during site preparation or removed. If it is anticipated that more than four to six minutes will be needed from the time of tourniquet placement to venous cannulation, the tourniquet should be applied, the vein located, the tourniquet removed, the site prepped, and the tourniquet reapplied before cannulation.

Preparing the Site

Correct infusion site preparation is necessary to prevent injury and the introduction of microorganisms that can predispose an individual to infection. Skin preparation can be done using 70% isopropyl alcohol and 2% aqueous chlorhexiden gluconate, povidone-iodine, or 70% tincture of iodine. Institutional policy should be followed; in general, the procedure for preparing the site is outlined in Skill 9-3.

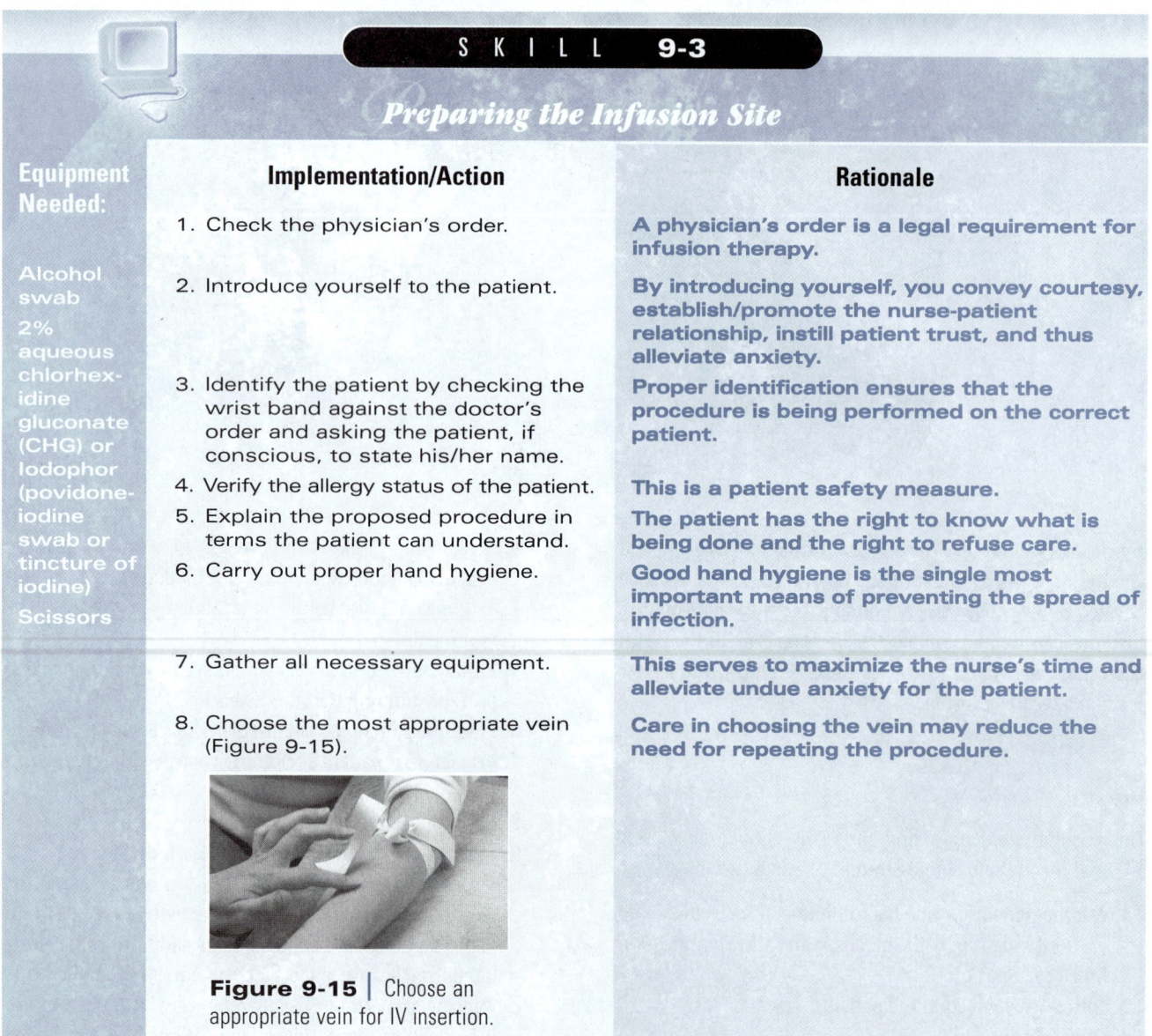

SKILL 9-3

Preparing the Infusion Site

Equipment Needed:	Implementation/Action	Rationale
Alcohol swab	1. Check the physician's order.	A physician's order is a legal requirement for infusion therapy.
2% aqueous chlorhex-idine gluconate (CHG) or Iodophor (povidone-iodine swab or tincture of iodine)	2. Introduce yourself to the patient.	By introducing yourself, you convey courtesy, establish/promote the nurse-patient relationship, instill patient trust, and thus alleviate anxiety.
	3. Identify the patient by checking the wrist band against the doctor's order and asking the patient, if conscious, to state his/her name.	Proper identification ensures that the procedure is being performed on the correct patient.
	4. Verify the allergy status of the patient.	This is a patient safety measure.
	5. Explain the proposed procedure in terms the patient can understand.	The patient has the right to know what is being done and the right to refuse care.
Scissors	6. Carry out proper hand hygiene.	Good hand hygiene is the single most important means of preventing the spread of infection.
	7. Gather all necessary equipment.	This serves to maximize the nurse's time and alleviate undue anxiety for the patient.
	8. Choose the most appropriate vein (Figure 9-15).	Care in choosing the vein may reduce the need for repeating the procedure.

Figure 9-15 | Choose an appropriate vein for IV insertion.

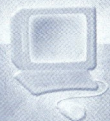

SKILL 9-3

Preparing the Infusion Site

Implementation/Action	Rationale
9. Assess for intact, non-bruised skin.	Undamaged skin prevents skin damage and lessens the chance for microbial introduction into the body.
10. If excessive hair is present, clip short with scissors.	Removal of excess hair enhances visualization and palpation of the vein, enhances adherence of the dressing, and eliminates undue discomfort when the dressing is removed.
11. Assess the patient for allergies.	Determination of allergies will prevent a sensitivity reaction.
12. Cleanse the site with 70% isopropyl alcohol. Using friction, begin at the intended cannulation site and work outward 2 to 3 inches, in a concentric circle, for 20 to 30 seconds. Do not backtrack over a previously cleaned area. Allow the alcohol to air-dry. Do not blow on or fan the skin and do not wipe the alcohol off the area.	This removes surface microorganisms.
13. Using the same directional movement, cleanse the site thoroughly with 2% aqueous chlorhexidine gluconate, povidone-iodine, or tincture of iodine (Figure 9-16). If tincture of iodine is used, the site should be wiped gently with a sterile gauze.	This product is irritating to the skin of some individuals.

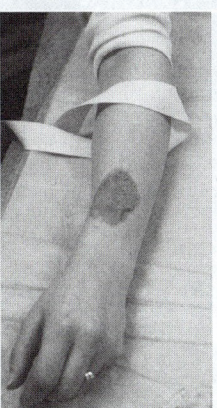

Figure 9-16 | Cleanse the site with alcohol and then iodophor.

14. Proceed with venipuncture.

Preparing the Local Anesthesia

The use of local anesthetics for peripheral cannulation is dictated by institutional policy. The most common products used are lidocaine, normal saline, and EMLA® cream.

Lidocaine

The routine use of lidocaine is generally not recommended. Most nurses agree that the risks of allergic reaction, inadvertent injection into a vessel, the need for an additional needle stick, and vein obliteration (due to tunica media relaxation) outweigh the benefits of reduced anxiety and increased comfort. They believe that one stick for cannulation done expeditiously is safer and causes the patient the least amount of distress. However, when used, 0.05 to 0.2 ml of 1% lidocaine (Xylocaine) without epinephrine is injected with a 27- to 25-ga., ¼- to ½-inch needle into the tissue below or to the side of the intended cannulation site. When a superficial wheal forms, it is massaged with an alcohol pledget to speed absorption and prevent obliteration of the vein. The anesthetic effect usually occurs within ten seconds. Always follow institutional policy regarding this practice.

Normal Saline

Normal saline (NS), or 0.9% bacteriostatic sodium chloride, produces essentially the same anesthetic effect as lidocaine. The ethyl alcohol used as the preservative causes the numbing sensation. The NS does not cause smooth muscle relaxation of the vein wall, nor does it sting (as lidocaine does). A larger volume of NS can be injected, making the anesthetic more powerful. To make the procedure virtually painless, the needle (27- to 25-ga., ¼- to ½-inch) should be introduced bevel down. Before inserting the needle, apply pressure with the needle bevel down for a few seconds, then pass the needle under the skin. Inject the NS over the vein, then on each side of the vein. Most nurses who routinely use local anesthesia injections prior to cannulation prefer normal saline to

lidocaine since it does not have the potential to cause an untoward effect.

EMLA® Cream

EMLA® cream is a eutectic mixture of 2.5% lidocaine and 2.5% prilocaine as an oil in water emulsion. It is applied to intact skin under an occlusive dressing. It provides dermal analgesia by releasing lidocaine and prilocaine from the cream into the epidermal and dermal layers of the skin in the vicinity of dermal pain receptors and nerve endings. EMLA® works well when time is not a major consideration. The onset, depth, and duration of dermal analgesia depends on the duration of application. For IV therapy, it should be in place for at least one hour prior to venipuncture and cannula placement. It is used frequently for peripherally inserted central lines and in pediatric settings. Because it causes relaxation of the tunica media, the vein may be obliterated and difficult to access.

Astrazeneca, Inc. recommends the following steps for the application of EMLA® cream:

1. Remove the backing from an EMLA® patch (Figure 9-17A).
2. Peel the paper liner from the paper framed dressing.
3. Apply the EMLA® patch, being careful not to spread out the cream. Smooth down the dressing edges carefully and be sure the dressing is secure to avoid leakage. (This is especially important when the patient is a child.) (Figure 9-17B)
4. Remove the paper frame. The time of application can be marked directly on the occlusive dressing (Figure 9-17C). EMLA® cream must be applied at least one hour before the start of a routine procedure and two hours before the start of a painful procedure.
5. Remove the occlusive dressing, wipe off the EMLA® cream, clean the entire area with an antiseptic solution,

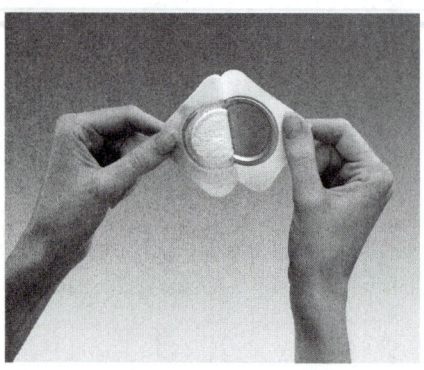 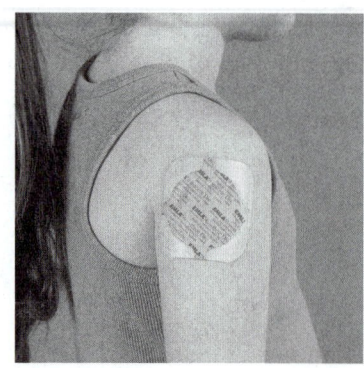 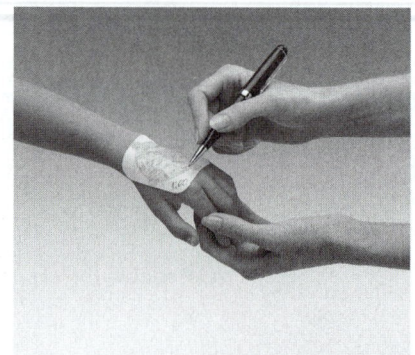

Figure 9-17 | (A) Peel the backing from the EMLA® patch. (B) Apply the patch to the skin. (C) Label the dressing around the patch. *Courtesy of AstraZeneca, LP, Wayne, PA*

and prepare the patient for the procedure. The skin anesthesia will be effective for at least one hour after removal of the occlusive dressing.

(Reproduced with permission of Astrazeneca, Wilmington, DE)

Iontophoresis

The skin can be desensitized using iontophoresis of lidocaine (Numby Stuff by Iomed), an alternative to EMLA®, when time is of the essence. Whereas EMLA® takes about an hour to exert the effect of numbness, iontophoresis takes about ten minutes. It is a fast, noninvasive system that utilizes a mild electrical current to deliver local anesthetic to the skin without causing tissue distortion (such as the wheal that occurs with injection). The system consists of a set of electrode pads. One pad, which contains Iontocaine (2% lidocaine and epinephrine 1:100,000 topical solution), is placed over the intended venipuncture site. The other electrode is placed on the skin about 4 to 6 inches (10–15 cm) away from the drug-delivery site. A handheld device controls a steady, low electrical flow of current that initiates the delivery of ion salts into the skin layers to provide local anesthesia to a depth of up to 10 mm.

Vein Cannulation

Prior to cannulation, take the distal end of the IV administration tubing that is hanging over the IV pole and position it in close proximity to the IV insertion site. Gently loosen the cap, but do not remove it. Sterility must be maintained until it is connected to the cannula hub.

Over-the-Needle Catheter (ONC) Insertion

The most commonly used angiocatheter to start an infusion is the over-the-needle catheter (ONC). An ONC is a flexible catheter, encased with a metal stylet, that is used to pierce the skin and vein, and which attaches to the infusion tubing (once the stylet has been removed). The ONC has essentially replaced straight, steel needles that were, at one time, the main delivery device for fluids into the vein.

An ONC can be inserted using a one-handed or two-handed technique (Figure 9-18). It can be threaded into the vein or "floated" in. The nurse's experience and the manufacturer's guidelines determine what method should be used. See Skill 9-4 for the general procedure for ONC insertion.

> ### NURSING TIP
>
> **Cannulating ONCs**
>
> The two methods used to cannulate ONCs are:
>
> 1. **One-handed technique.** Using one hand (while the other anchors the vein), the skin is entered, the vein cannulated, and (with the index finger or thumb) the cannula is advanced off the needle/stylet and into the vein, and the needle is discarded or retracted into its protective shield.
> 2. **Two-handed method.** The cannula is inserted into the vein, using one hand, while the other anchors the vein. Once a backflash of blood occurs, one hand (that anchored) is used to stabilize the cannula hub while the other removes the needle/stylet.

Figure 9-24 illustrates cannulation with a Y-type catheter. In this type of system, the stylet is removed from an accessory port rather than through the insertion route. With this method, the administration set tubing can be connected prior to cannulation, providing a bloodless IV start.

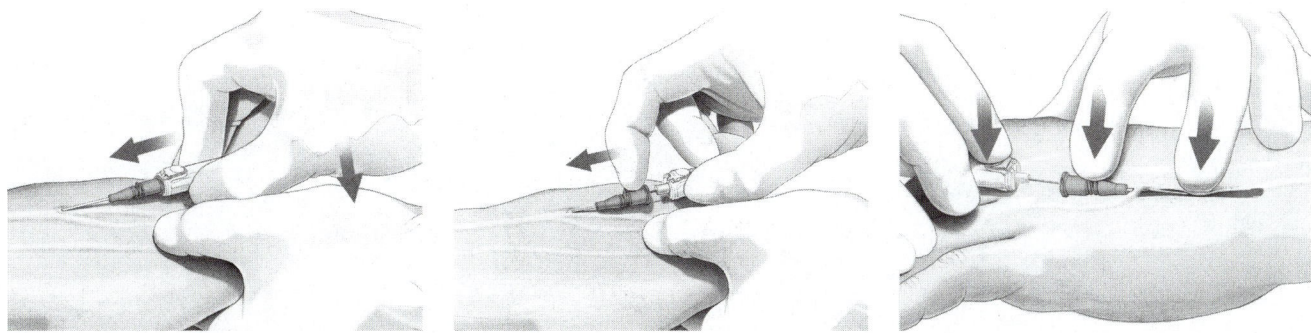

Figure 9-18 | Over-the-needle catheters can be inserted using a one-handed technique in which the catheter is inserted into the vein (A) and the index finger is used to slide the catheter into the vein while the needle is being retracted (B) or by using a two-handed technique in which one hand anchors the vein and holds the catheter while the other retracts the needle (C). *Courtesy of BD Medical Systems, Franklin Lakes, NJ*

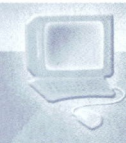

SKILL 9-4

Starting an IV: Over-the-Needle Catheter

Equipment Needed:

Properly set-up primary infusion line

Appropriate ONC

IV start kit

Paper tape

Scissors

Protective underpad

Disposable gloves

Sharps container

Implementation/Action	Rationale
1. Check the physician's order.	A physician's order is a legal requirement for infusion therapy.
2. Introduce yourself to the patient.	By introducing yourself, you convey courtesy, establish/promote the nurse-patient relationship, instill patient trust, and thus alleviate anxiety.
3. Identify the patient by checking the wrist band against the doctor's order and asking the patient, if conscious, to state his/her name.	Proper identification ensures that the procedure is being performed on the correct patient.
4. Verify the allergy status of the patient.	This is a patient safety measure.
5. Explain the proposed procedure in terms the patient can understand.	The patient has the right to know what is being done and the right to refuse care.
6. Carry out proper hand hygiene.	Good hand hygiene is the single most important means of preventing the spread of infection.
7. Set up all the necessary supplies on the bedside stand or overbed table in the order in which they will be used. Cut any tape that will be needed. Inspect the ONC to be sure that the needle bevel is sharp and smooth. Read the manufacturer's directions regarding inspection and manipulation of the ONC.	Maintains order, lessens the chance for contamination, and conserves time.
8. Provide privacy.	To maintain patient dignity.
9. Elevate the bed level.	Conducive to a successful procedure and alleviates back strain for the nurse.
10. Place the patient in a Fowler's or semi-Fowler's position with extremity intended for cannulation below the level of the patient's heart.	Enhances venous access and ensures successful cannulation.
11. Protect the patient's clothing and bedding with protective underpad or towel.	To prevent contamination with blood, alleviate the need to change clothing/linen, and to save time.
12. Apply the tourniquet and identify the most appropriate vein for cannulation, preferably in the nondominant hand (Figure 9-19).	

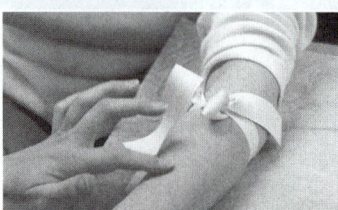

Figure 9-19 | Choose an appropriate vein for IV insertion.

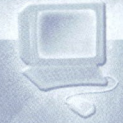

S K I L L   9-4

Starting an IV: Over-the-Needle Catheter

Implementation/Action	Rationale
a. Select a vein, using the most distal vein first.	If the vein is later damaged, the proximal segment can be used.
b. Avoid bony prominences.	To decrease discomfort and prevent inadvertent infiltration from venous puncture.
c. Use the nondominant hand.	Allows for freedom of movement.
d. Avoid areas of rash or broken skin.	To decrease risk of infection.
13. Remove the tourniquet, leaving it under the extremity.	So it is ready for use after the site has been antiseptically cleansed.
14. If there is an excessive amount of hair at the venipuncture site, clip the hair at the site. Do not shave the area.	Clip the hair to ensure adhesion of the dressing and reduce the discomfort when the dressing is removed. Shaving can cause microabrasions that may provide a site for microbial growth.
15. Antiseptically prepare the site according to policy (Figure 9-20).	Prevents infection.

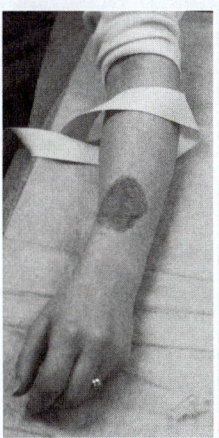

Figure 9-20 | Cleanse the site with alcohol and iodophor.

Implementation/Action	Rationale
16. Don gloves.	For protection of nurse from contamination with blood.
17. Apply tourniquet to occlude venous flow.	For venous distention and enhanced venipuncture and cannulation.
18. Palpate for and ensure presence of a pulse distal to the tourniquet.	To ensure that arterial blood flow is intact. Occlusion of arterial flow can cause damage to the extremity.
19. Remove the needle cover and tell the patient that the needle is going to enter the vein.	The patient has the right to know when the stick will occur.
20. Anchor the vein below the intended insertion site with gentle skin traction. Using the thumb of the nondominant hand, pull the skin taut.	Anchoring the vein properly is the key to successful cannulation.
21. Hold the ONC by the needle hub flash chamber, *not* the color-coded hub of the catheter unit, with the bevel up.	To prevent separation of the needle and catheter.

(continues)

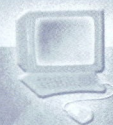

SKILL 9-4

Starting an IV: Over-the-Needle Catheter (continued)

Implementation/Action	Rationale
22. Entry of the over-the-needle catheter can be either via a direct or indirect method. For the direct-entry method, position the needle over the vein with the needle in the bevel-up position and pointing in the direction of the blood flow. In this method, the needle passes through the skin, over and directly into the vein in one maneuver. For the indirect entry method, position the needle in the bevel-up position and alongside the vein, pointing in the direction of the blood flow. In this method, the needle enters the skin, is maneuvered alongside the vein, and then enters the vein.	**The ONC must be inserted in the direction of venous return (toward the head) to prevent damage to the venous valves. This method is generally used for veins that are well developed and that have good elasticity.** **This method is used for veins that roll or may "blow" with the direct approach.**
23. Use a 15-degree angle for insertion into superficial veins and a 25- to 30-degree angle for insertion into deeper veins (Figure 9-21).	**Use of the proper angle of insertion will help to prevent too shallow or too deep penetration. Care must be taken not to immediately lower the cannula angle once in the vein, so as not to pierce the opposite vein wall.**

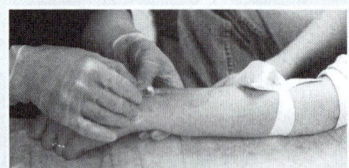

Figure 9-21 | Insert the ONC with the bevel up at a 20- to 30-degree angle to the skin.

Implementation/Action	Rationale
24. Observe for flashback of blood in the flash chamber. *Note:* Upon entry into the tunica adventitia (outermost) layer of the vein, the nurse may feel a slight "pop" (or sensation of release of pressure), depending on the brand of catheter used. Some of the newer types, such as those made with Vialon®, provide such a sharp, smooth insertion that there is little or no characteristic "pop" upon vein access	**Flashback confirms vein entry.**
25. Once the over-the-needle catheter is in the vein, lower the needle until it is almost flush with the skin to avoid puncturing the opposite vein wall, then advance the needle and catheter unit so that the catheter tip is in the center of the vein lumen.	**To maintain the integrity of the vein.**
26. Advance the catheter, using one of the following techniques: • Advance the whole unit—needle and catheter—into the vein, then retract the needle.	

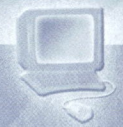

S K I L L   9-4

Starting an IV: Over-the-Needle Catheter

Implementation/Action	**Action/Rationale**
• Stabilize the needle-flash chamber and gradually advance the catheter off the needle, threading it into the vein lumen, until the desired length has been inserted (Figure 9-22). If the catheter does not thread smoothly or blood flow ceases, remove the catheter and needle together, apply pressure to the site, and attempt venipuncture in another site, using a new device.	

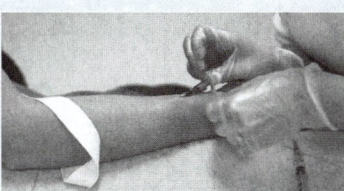

Figure 9-22 | Loosen the stylet and advance the catheter into the vein.

Implementation/Action	**Action/Rationale**
• To use the **hooding** method, hold the catheter unit stationary and advance the catheter off the needle no more than a $1/4$ inch, *hooding* the tip of the needle inside the catheter. If preferred, pull the needle back no more than a $1/4$ inch to achieve the same result. Grasp the color-coded catheter hub and advance the hooded needle or catheter as a unit into the vein. When it is in place, remove the needle.	
• To use the **floating** method, the needle and catheter are advanced about halfway into the vein (verified by flashback), at which point the tourniquet and needle are removed. The cannula hub is then attached to the infusion tubing, the flow control clamp is slowly opened, and the infusion is started. The catheter is then *floated* into the vein with the infusate. *Note:* For this method to work well, the skin and vein must remain anchored with one hand. If anchoring is not maintained, the catheter may meet resistance from skin traction at the insertion site.	
27. Release the tourniquet. Do not touch the end of the catheter hub or the IV insertion site. A sterile 2 × 2-inch gauze pad may be placed under the catheter hub.	**To avoid contamination and to provide an aseptic field when removing the needle and connecting the administration set.**

(continues)

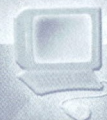

SKILL 9-4

Starting an IV: Over-the-Needle Catheter (continued)

Implementation/Action	Rationale
28. Remove the needle and dispose of it in the sharps container (Figure 9-23).	**To prevent needlestick injury.**

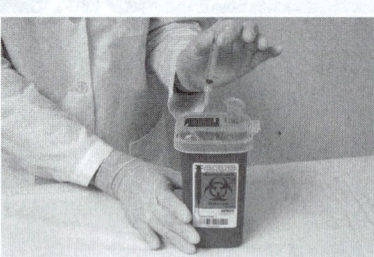

Figure 9-23 | Dispose of the needle in the sharps container.

Implementation/Action	Rationale
29. Connect the infusion tubing with a gentle push-and-twist motion.	**To secure the junction and prevent leakage and contamination.**
30. Place a strip of paper tape over the tubing.	**To stabilize it and prevent inadvertent dislodgement of the cannula from the vein.**
31. Open the flow clamp and observe the insertion site and vessel pathway as the infusate freely enters the vessel. Adjust the flow rate.	**To ascertain that the vein is intact and that there is no infiltration of infusate.**
32. Remove the strip of paper tape. Dress the site per agency policy.	**It is important to follow the policy designated by your agency.**
33. Remove gloves and carry out proper hand hygiene.	**To prevent cross-contamination.**
34. Label the site at the side of the dressing with the date, time, IV device used, and your initials.	**Legal protection of the patient and nurse.**
35. Label the infusion container and all administration sets that are used.	**Legal protection of the patient and nurse.**
36. Return the bed to the lowest position, lower the head of the bed (if appropriate for the patient), and raise the bedrails.	**Safety, in terms of fall prevention, is enhanced when the bed is in the low position and the rails are up.**

If cannulation is unsuccessful, the entire procedure must be repeated at another site. It is not recommended that cannulation be attempted by the same nurse more than two times (INS, 2000, Standard 48 S43), as this may put undue stress on the patient and the nurse, both tending to lose confidence. If possible, another person should attempt to perform the procedure. The nurse should not allow herself to become distressed over this or let it diminish her self-confidence. As proficient as she may be at venipuncture and cannulation, there are times when the procedure does not progress as planned. It is better to be forthright about this (in her own regard and for the patient's sake) and let someone else attempt cannulation.

NURSING ALERT

Flashback

Flashback may occur when the needle (only), and not the catheter tip, has entered the vein. Do not use flashback as a signal to withdraw the needle.

Straight Needle

Straight needles are seldom used anymore for infusion therapy, but are still used for blood sampling and blood donation. When they are used to deliver infusates, it is best to

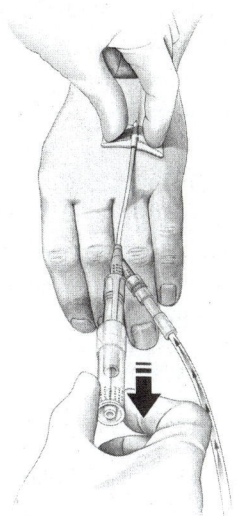

Figure 9-24 | Y-style catheter allows bloodless insertion of an IV because the infusate can begin flowing before removing the stylet. *Courtesy of BD Medical Systems, Franklin Lakes, NJ*

NURSING TIP

To prevent blood leakage while removing the needle and connecting the administration set tubing, apply digital pressure to the vein just above the catheter tip, using the fourth or fifth finger of the nondominant hand, while holding the cannula hub securely with the thumb and index finger

For patients with thin, fragile veins, this practice is not recommended, as the pressure, especially if it is inadvertently applied over the tip of the catheter, could bruise the vein wall. In this situation, work quickly to connect the cannula hub with the administration set tubing. This is why it is important to shield the area under the extremity with a protective cover.

NURSING ALERT

Maximum Cannula Use

Never stick a patient more than one time with the same cannula. If venipuncture is unsuccessful, the cannula must be properly disposed of and a new one inserted.

NURSING ALERT

Avoiding a Catheter Embolus

Do not, under any circumstances, reinsert the needle into the catheter at any time. The needle could sever the catheter, resulting in a catheter embolus.

CRITICAL THINKING

Handling a Coworker Situation

As you enter your patient's room to care for him, you see a nurse trying to start an IV on the patient in the other bed. You notice that she has reused the same ONC three times for different unsuccessful sticks. You offer to go and get her some new catheters, but she says, "I've already gone through four and must have stuck him eight times." You offer to try to start the IV for her but she replies, "I'm determined to get this IV started if it takes all day." You see that the patient is very apprehensive, flushed, and diaphoretic. What would you do in this situation?

NURSING TIP

Advancing the Catheter

It is suggested that the catheter not be advanced completely up to the hub, but that approximately ⅛ in. of catheter remain visible outside of the body. In the rare, unforeseen event that the catheter and hub should separate, the catheter could be retrieved with forceps.

NURSING ALERT

Checking for a Needle in the Patient's Bedding

Do not leave the needle or stylet in the patient's bed. Check before completing the procedure.

use veins that are naturally splinted by bone to hinder movement of the needle within the vein. Steel needles must never be used to deliver fluids or medications that may cause tissue necrosis should extravasation occur. The correct method follows.

1. Select the smallest needle that will accommodate the vein yet deliver the ordered infusate. The needle can be inserted using one of two methods, depending on the nurse's preference and the condition of the patient's vein:
   (a) Connect the needle to the end of the administration set tubing, remove the needle cap while maintaining its sterility, and slowly open the tubing clamp to purge the needle of any air. Reclamp the tubing and recap the needle.
   (b) Prepare the site and don gloves.
   (c) Enter the vein, bevel up, and advance the needle into the vein. Once in the vein, there may be a small back-flash of blood into the IV tubing, depending on venous pressure, to verify placement. If this does not occur, slowly open the tubing clamp and slowly run the infusate, watching the site and palpating around it. A cool sensation and skin-tightening would indicate infiltration. If the site looks and feels normal, loosely tape the IV tubing with paper tape to the patient's arm. Lower the IV container below the IV site with the clamp fully open. A retrograde flow of blood into the tubing indicates placement in the vein. Hang the IV and

regulate it. The site should be dressed and secured in the same manner as an ONC.

2. The other method used to insert a steel needle is to connect it to a syringe containing 3 cc to 5 cc of normal saline.
   (a) Prime the needle and enter the vein, bevel up. To verify placement, pull back on the syringe plunger to visualize a backflow of blood.
   (b) Secure the needle, remove the syringe, connect the cannula hub to the administration set, and regulate the infusion. Secure and dress the site.

IV therapy can be administered through a winged infusion set, also known as a butterfly needle. This is a short metal needle that lies within the vein during infusion therapy. The needle extends from soft plastic wings and is connected to a short, permanently attached, extension tubing. The wings provide a means to stabilize the cannula when secured with tape. The wings are flexible and can be bent upward to act as a handle when inserting the needle. Since this is a metal needle, there is an increased chance of the needle becoming dislodged during therapy. Winged metal needles are usually used to provide IV therapy to infants or for very short-term drug or fluid administration, such as a one-time order. It is generally a nursing judgment, based on accurate assessment, as to which type of device is most appropriate for a particular client. The most common site for insertion of a winged needle is the dorsal surface of the hand and the smaller veins in the forearm. See Skill 9-5 for the procedure for inserting a winged infusion set.

SKILL 9-5

Starting an IV: Insertion of a Winged Infusion Set

Equipment Needed:	Implementation/Action	Rationale
	1. Check the physician's order.	A physician's order is a legal requirement for infusion therapy.
Winged infusion needle Gloves Tourniquet	2. Introduce yourself to the patient.	By introducing yourself, you convey courtesy, establish/promote the nurse-patient relationship, instill patient trust, and thus alleviate anxiety.
Alcohol swab 2% aqueous chlorhexi-drine gluconate (CHG) or Iodophor swab	3. Identify the patient by checking the wrist band against the doctor's order and asking the patient, if conscious, to state his/her name.	Proper identification ensures that the procedure is being performed on the correct patient.
	4. Verify the allergy status of the patient.	This is a patient safety measure.
	5. Explain the proposed procedure in terms the patient can understand.	The patient has the right to know what is being done and the right to refuse care.
	6. Carry out proper hand hygiene.	Good hand hygiene is the single most important means of preventing the spread of infection.

(continues)

SKILL 9-5

Starting an IV: Insertion of a Winged Infusion Set (continued)

Equipment Needed (*continued*):	Implementation/Action	Rationale
	7. Gather equipment.	Having all equipment at hand will save time and lessen patient anxiety.
Tape	8. Provide for privacy.	Preserves patient dignity.
5 ml syringe	9. Assess for an appropriate vein in the nondominant hand/arm (Figure 9-25). A vein should be chosen at the most distal site, working upward in a proximal direction.	This allows the patient freedom of movement to carry out basic activities of daily living while the IV is in place.
Agency-Approved dressing		

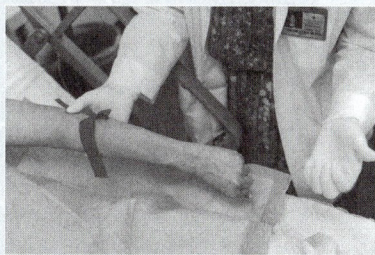

Figure 9-25 | Choose an appropriate vein for IV insertion.

	Implementation/Action	Rationale
	10. Apply the tourniquet; this should be 2 to 3 inches above the intended venipuncture site for most patients.	Allows for the dilation of veins.
	11. Cleanse the skin with alcohol starting at the insertion site and working outward in a circular motion. Once the site is cleansed, do not retouch the site, unless with a sterile gloved finger or a gloved finger that has been prepped with 70% isopropyl alcohol.	Prevents the spread of infection.
	12. Cleanse the skin with 2% aqueous chlorhexidine gluconate, povidone-iodine, or agency-approved iodophor if the patient is not allergic (Figure 9-26).	Prevents the spread of infection.

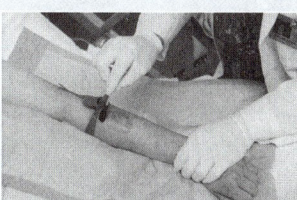

Figure 9-26 | Cleanse the site with alcohol and iodophor.

	Implementation/Action	Rationale
	13. Don gloves while the iodophor is drying.	Protects the nurse and prevents cross contamination.
	The following method works well for patients who have well-developed, elastic veins, with good venous pressure.	
	14. Hold the skin below the insertion site taut.	Holds the vein in place during the venipuncture.

(continues)

SKILL 9-5

Starting an IV: Insertion of a Winged Infusion Set (continued)

Implementation/Action	Rationale
15. Pick up the winged needle, holding it by the plastic wings, bevel up.	Holding the needle properly allows for easier insertion.
16. Insert the needle with the bevel up at a 20- to 30-degree angle (Figure 9-27).	Decreases the chance of puncturing both sides of the vein.

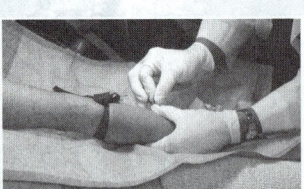

Figure 9-27 | Insert the winged needle with the bevel up at a 20- to 30-degree angle to the skin.

Implementation/Action	Rationale
17. Assess for retrograde blood flow into the tubing of the set.	To assure that the needle is in the vein.
18. Apply a strip of paper tape across the wings.	To prevent dislodgement of the needle while needed attachments are made and the dressing is applied. Paper tape is nonirritating and is easily removed when the dressing is ready for application.
19. Allow retrograde blood flow to purge the tubing of air, then connect the medication syringe and administration set tubing for the infusion, or apply a male-adapter plug as appropriate and instill a saline lock.	To achieve required infusion therapy.
20. Apply the appropriate dressing.	To secure the IV and preclude the entry of microbes at the site.
21. Remove the tourniquet.	Prevents tissue and nerve damage.
22. Write (to the side of the dressing or on a piece of tape or labeling) the date, time, needle size (length and gauge), and your initials.	Provides information for other nurses and prevents complications.
23. Provide patient teaching.	Decreases patient anxiety, allows the patient to participate in care.
24. Make the patient comfortable.	Decreases patient anxiety.
25. Document the procedure in the medical record in the nurse's notes and appropriate infusion flow sheets. If medications are administered, document in the MAR.	Provides for continuity of care.

A variation in technique can be used when it is anticipated that backflow of blood into the winged set tubing will be sluggish.

Implementation/Action	Rationale
1. Attach a syringe containing 3 to 5 ml of normal saline to the winged infusion set and prime the tubing and the needle.	To verify placement within the vein and purge the line of air.

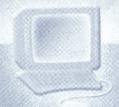

S K I L L   9-5

Starting an IV: Insertion of a Winged Infusion Set

Implementation/Action	Rationale
2. Perform venipuncture.	**To access the circulatory system.**
3. Once the needle is in the vein, the plunger is retracted to elicit a blood return and withdraw air from the tubing.	**This is to verify cannulation of the vein and prevent the introduction of air into the system.**
4. Inject an amount of saline to clear the tubing of blood.	**To ascertain that the vein is functional and to remove blood from the tubing.**
5. Once the tubing is purged of air with the blood, connect the medication syringe and administration set tubing for the infusion, or apply a male-adapter plug as appropriate and instill a saline lock.	**To achieve required infusion therapy.**
6. Apply the appropriate dressing.	**To secure the IV and preclude the entry of microbes at the site.**

Securing the IV Site with Dressings and Tape

As discussed earlier, the IV site can be dressed with a transparent membrane dressing or a gauze-and-tape covering, depending on the patient's clinical situation and institutional policy. The most important factor, regardless of the type of dressing used, is that the site must be able to be assessed frequently in order to troubleshoot problems. The dressing should be secured around the catheter hub to protect the IV site and to prevent the dressing from coming off (Figure 9-19). Additional tape is only to be used to secure the administration set tubing. In an oriented, noncombative adult, the IV site dressing and two to three additional strips of tape are generally all that are required to maintain an IV. Additional adhesion is superfluous in that it adds unnecessary bulk, is a potential skin irritant, and provides a medium for contamination. To avoid circulatory impairment, tape must never encircle an extremity.

Two major considerations must be kept in mind when using any IV site dressing:

1. The dressing should mold to the catheter insertion site and surrounding area so that there are no gaps or openings where contaminants can enter.
2. The dressing must be placed so that it covers only the IV site and extends up to the top margin of the cannula hub. No tape or dressing should cover the connection between the IV device and the administration set tubing. When this connection site is secured with the dressing, there is manipulation of the cannula and IV site should the administration set need to be changed, have extensions or

N U R S I N G   A L E R T

Applying Tape to an IV Site

When applying tape to an IV site or when taping an immobilizing device in place, never encircle the entire extremity with tape. This could cause circulatory impairment, especially if edema sets in or if infiltration occurs.

N U R S I N G   T I P

Tape or Dressing Removal

To prevent a skin tear when removing tape or a transparent dressing, remember the following rule: "Don't remove the tape from the skin; remove the skin from the tape."

connectors added to it, or if the infusion is disconnected and converted to an intermittent administration system.

Transparent Dressings

The transparent semipermeable dressing (TSD) (Figure 9-28) or transparent membrane dressing (TMD) is often preferred because the IV insertion site can be easily assessed. Manufacturer instructions must be followed when using TSDs. Instructions for the application of a TSD follow.

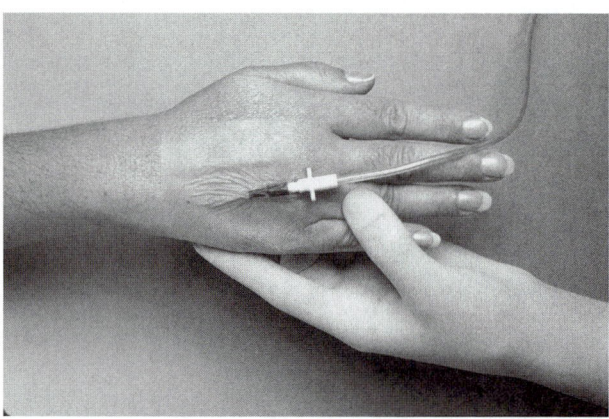

Figure 9-28 | Transparent semipermeable membrane dressing

1. Apply to dry skin.
2. Remove backing papers according to directions.
3. Gently lift the catheter, and carefully mold the transparent film around the sides of the catheter hub to form a seal.
4. Remove any additional backings or paper frames around dressing, as directed.
5. Apply additional tapes, as needed, to secure IV tubing, but do not obliterate the IV insertion site.
6. Do not apply tape over a transparent dressing.

To remove a transparent dressing, gently move the skin away from the dressing using either the stretch technique or the alcohol technique. With the stretch technique, the dressing is stretched parallel to the patient's skin in small increments until the dressing has been removed. With the alcohol (or adhesive remover) technique, the dressing is lifted around the edges and the solvent is used to break down the adhesive seal and remove the dressing.

Gauze and Tape Dressings

If an all-in-one gauze-tape dressing (Figure 9-29) is used, follow the manufacturer's directions for application and removal. If a ready-made dressing is not available, the IV site must be covered with a sterile (preferably, nonadherent) gauze that covers the prepped area. It should be taped so that there are no openings for contaminants to enter. When gauze-tape dressings are used, established institutional protocols must be followed regarding scheduled removal for changing and to assess the IV site.

Catheter Stabilization and Taping

"Cannulas shall be stabilized in a manner that does not interfere with assessment and monitoring of the infusion site or impede delivery of the prescribed therapy" (INS, 2000, Standard 49, S43). In the past, it was recommended that the needle or catheter be stabilized by taping over or around its hub in a chevron, H, or U formation before applying the

dressing. Since it is now encouraged that nothing that is not sterile come in contact with the IV site once it is prepped and cannulated other than the sterile dressing, this practice is not recommended. Some agencies recommend pre-dressing taping regimens for certain patient populations, such as pediatrics and geriatrics. Unless institutional policy dictates otherwise, there should be nothing placed between the catheter and the dressing.

In general, if an IV site requires additional protection, as for a pediatric or combative patient, the better alternative is to use a self-adherent wrap over the basic IV dressing, one which does not require adhesive, pins, or clips (Figure 9-30). The wrap

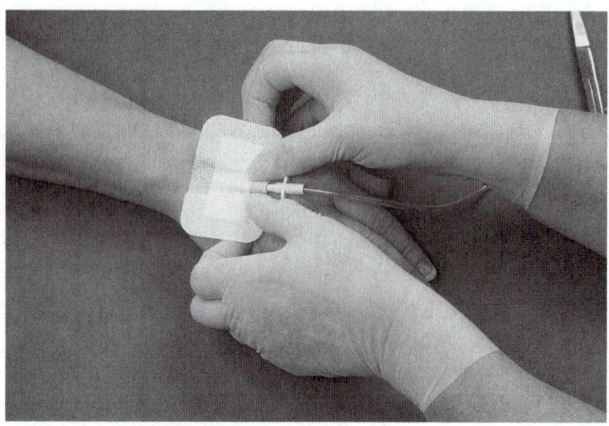

Figure 9-29 | All-in-one gauze-tape dressing

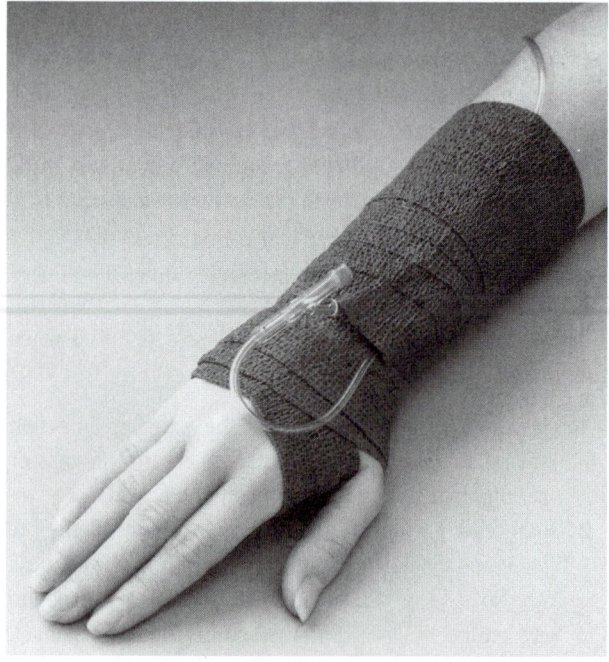

Figure 9-30 | 3M™ Coban™ Self-Adherent Wrap to secure and protect an IV over the basic site dressing
Courtesy of 3M Health Care, St. Paul. MN

stays in place to protect the IV, can be removed easily for site assessment, and can be reapplied. The use of roller bandages is not advised because they may impede circulatory flow and do not allow for visual inspection of the cannula site. "Site protection material shall allow visual inspection of the site and shall be placed so as not to impede circulation or impede infusion through the access device" (INS, 2000, Standard 49, S43).

Completing the Procedure

Lower the bed and document the procedure.

Documentation

Once the infusion is initiated, the nurse must document the following information in the nurse's notes (Figure 9-31) of the medical record.

1. Date and time started
2. Insertion site and its appearance
3. Size and type of cannulation device
4. Name of the infusate and the rate
5. Type of dressing applied
6. Number and locations of attempted cannulations and the condition of the sites (and any remedial procedures needed)
7. Patient's response to the procedure

Armboards

Unless absolutely necessary (and then only when an IV device is in an area of flexion), it is better not to restrict the patient's extremity on an armboard (INS, 2000, Standard 36, S32). If an IV device is positional in a vein, a rolled washcloth or gauze roll can often be used to support and better position it and reestablish infusate flow.

If an armboard is indispensable for the maintenance of an IV, extreme care must be taken to ensure that the area it is applied to has optimum circulation and remains functional. Measures are to be instituted to prevent restriction, discomfort, or injury while allowing for infusion site monitoring. The armboard must be removed at established intervals in order to assess circulation and movement. Federal and state mandates must be followed regarding the use of armboards and restraints and the issue must be addressed, in writing, in agency policy. If extremity restraints are ordered, care must be taken to position them away from the IV site and cannula.

PERIPHERAL INFUSION THERAPY: MAINTENANCE AND MONITORING

Once IV therapy has been initiated, it is vitally important to observe and assess the patient, monitor the IV site, and maintain the equipment. Strict adherence to safety protocols and the detection of problems, should they arise, are the most important mechanisms in preventing the complications associated with infusion therapy.

> ### NURSING TIP
>
> #### Patient-Family Teaching for Home-Bound Patients
>
> For home-bound patients, where frequent nursing assessment is not feasible, the patient and family should be instructed regarding IV therapy. It is important that they understand what to look for and what situations require reporting.

Observation and Assessment

The patient undergoing any type of infusion therapy should be monitored every hour at a minimum. If the individual's condition warrants it, more frequent checks may be necessary. He must be observed as well as questioned regarding his status. Any change in his color, skin turgor, level of consciousness, or

Nurse's Notes

DATE	TIME	ASSESSMENT DATA	NURSING INTERVENTIONS	EVALUATION
6-2-99	0840	Pt. c/o "burning and stinging" when ONC inserted. 6 mm raised, circular ecchymotic area around insertion site after ONC removal.	Venipuncture attempted in Rt. dorsal metacarpal vein over 3rd finger with 20 g 1" Jelco ONC. 2" × 2" pressure dressing applied following removal.	Pt. said it is "sore, but feels OK."
	0855		20 g 1¼" Jelco ONC inserted above Lt. dorsal venous arch into cephalic vein. 1000 cc D₅W @ 125 cc/hr per IMED (controlled mode). Op Site TSM to site.	Pt. says site and arm "feels fine."

Figure 9-31 | Documentation in the nurse's notes

Nurse's Notes

DATE	TIME	ASSESSMENT DATA	NURSING INTERVENTIONS	EVALUATION
8-7-98	0430	Pt. states, "I have such terrible pain in my whole arm that it woke me up. It feels like it is on fire where the needle is." Cannula insertion site (Lt. dorsal metacarpal area) is reddened, warm to the touch, and tender. Lower arm and hand are edematous. T: 101.2, P: 94, R: 26, BP: 136/90.	IV d.c. 'd, Lt. hand and forearm wrapped in moist, warm compresses and elevated on 2 pillows. Dr. Gand called (per Exchange Operator #22) regarding fever.	Pt. says Lt. arm "feels better, but the hand still hurts."
	0455		Acetaminophen gr × "p.o." IV restarted in Rt. cephalic vein (above the wrist) with 20 g 1" Insyte ONC at 100 cc/hr per IVAC pump. Tegaderm TSM to site.	Pt. says he feels better and wants to go back to sleep.
	0550	Pt. asleep. T: 99.1, P: 82, R: 18, BP: 128/90.		

Figure 9-32 | Documentation in the nurse's notes regarding a change in the patient's status and reporting

vital signs must be investigated, documented, and reported (Figure 9-32). Observation includes not only the patient but any IV equipment used. There must be thorough and accurate verbal and written communication among all personnel caring for him.

Monitoring is especially important during the period following the initiation of infusion therapy and the introduction of new medications. It is very important that the nurse stay with the patient for a short period whenever anything new is delivered. Even though a patient may not have experienced problems with something in the past, especially if taken orally, that cannot be taken for granted. Time is of the essence when problems arise with parenteral fluids or drugs, and measures must be instituted swiftly to counteract any untoward events. Monitoring is an integral part of quality improvement and risk management and it ensures patient safety.

Documentation and Reporting

It has been stressed repeatedly that the nurse must document and report all pertinent information regarding the patient's status. The saying, "not documented, not done" has become a legal standard. The patient's chart (the medical record) is where all pertinent communications regarding a patient's care and status must be documented, in addition to other forms required by the institution. Remember, documentation includes labeling.

Documentation entails recording infusion-related information in the following areas:

1. MAR
2. Nurse's notes
3. Infusion flow sheets
4. Nursing care plan
5. Intake and output records
6. General or equipment flow sheets
7. Laboratory, radiology, and other ancillary department requisitions
8. Labels:
   (a) ALLERGIC: place on and in the patient's chart, room, and bed, and all communication channels with other personnel and departments, regarding allergies and drug reactions, and attach the appropriate identification bracelet to the patient
   (b) IV site, next to the dressing, with the date and time of the cannulation; the type of device, including length and gauge; and the nurse's initials
   (c) Administration set tubing (date and time of initiation or change)
   (d) Infusate containers (date and time of start, flow level strips, medications added)

Documentation and reporting go hand-in-hand. One without the other is insufficient.

Reporting includes verbal communication to the physician supported by written notes to nursing personnel, to pharmacy, to the family, and to ancillary departments regarding any pertinent occurrences and changes regarding the patient's status. Even though information is written in the patient's chart, failure to report it to the appropriate individuals means communication is incomplete and may be invalidated in a court of law.

Infusion Site Maintenance

The proper maintenance of the IV site is essential to preventing complications. Since the site provides accessibility to the circulatory system, measures must be taken to avoid microbial contamination and chemical or mechanical trauma. The policies and procedures of the institution regarding the frequency of site monitoring and maintenance should be followed. In addition, monitoring must be dictated by the patient's condition and age, the type of infusion device, the kind of therapy he is receiving, and the setting in which care is delivered.

The most recent CDC Guidelines regarding IV site care (CDC, 2001c) recommend the following:

1. The IV insertion site is to be visually inspected and manually palpated, through the intact dressing, on a daily basis. If the dressing prevents palpation and visualization because it is large or bulky, it must be removed for assessment and a new one reapplied.
2. Hands are to be washed, using an antiseptic-containing product, before palpating, inserting, changing, or dressing any intravascular device.
3. Wear (sterile or nonsterile) vinyl or latex gloves during insertion of intravascular catheters and during dressing changes (per OSHA Standards).
4. Dressings are to be left in place until the catheter is removed or changed, or the dressing becomes damp, loosened, or soiled. Dressings need to be changed more frequently for patients who are diaphoretic.

Equipment Protocols

The equipment used for infusion therapy must be used correctly, regularly monitored, and properly maintained for the safety of the patient and the personnel using it. The CDC guidelines regarding IV equipment (CDC, 2002a) include the following:

1. Select the catheter, insertion technique, and insertion site with the lowest risk for complications (infectious and noninfectious) for the anticipated type and duration of IV therapy.
2. Allow the antiseptic (2% aqueous chlorhexidine gluconate [CHG], 10% povidone-iodine, 2% tincture of iodine, or 70% alcohol) to remain on the insertion site and to air dry before catheter insertion. Allow the povidone-iodine to remain on the skin for at least two minutes, or longer if it is not yet dry before insertion. Do not apply organic solvents (e.g., acetone and ether) to the skin before insertion of catheters or during dressing changes.
3. Once an intravascular device is inserted, the date and time of insertion must be recorded in an obvious location near the insertion site (e.g., on [and to the side of] the dressing or on the bed).
4. In adults, replace short, peripheral venous catheters at least every 72–96 hours to reduce the risk for phlebitis. If sites for venous access are limited and no evidence of phlebitis or infection is present, peripheral venous catheters can be left in place for longer periods, although the patient and the insertion sites should be closely monitored. Do not routinely replace midline catheters to

reduce the risk for infection. In pediatric patients, leave peripheral venous catheters in place until IV therapy is completed, unless a complication (e.g., phlebitis and infiltration) occurs.

5. When adherence to aseptic technique cannot be ensured (i.e., when catheters are inserted during a medical emergency), replace all catheters as soon as possible and after no longer than 48 hours.

6. Use clinical judgment to determine when to replace a catheter that could be a source of infection. Replace any short-term CVC if purulence is observed at the insertion site, which indicates infection.

7. Promptly remove any intravascular catheter that is no longer essential.

8. Replace administration sets, including secondary sets and add-on devices, no more frequently than at 72-hour intervals, unless catheter-related infection is suspected or documented. Replace tubing used to administer blood, blood products, or lipid emulsions (those combined with amino acids and glucose in a 3-in-1 admixture or infused separately) within 24 hours of initiating the infusion. If the solution contains only dextrose and amino acids, the administration set does not need to be replaced more frequently than every 72 hours. Replace tubing used to administer propofol infusions every 6 or 12 hours, depending on its use, per the manufacturer's recommendation.

9. Complete the infusion of lipid-containing solutions (e.g., 3-in-1 solutions) within 24 hours of hanging the solution. Complete the infusion of lipid emulsions alone within 12 hours of hanging the emulsion. If volume considerations require more time, the infusion should be completed within 24 hours. Complete infusions of blood or other blood products within 4 hours of hanging the blood. No recommendation can be made for the hang time of other parenteral fluids but most agencies do not recommend leaving any infusate hanging for more than 24 hours.

10. Change the needleless components at least as frequently as the administration set. Change caps no more frequently than every 72 hours or according to manufacturers' recommendations. Ensure that all components of the system are compatible to minimize leaks and breaks in the system. Minimize contamination risk by wiping the access port with an appropriate antiseptic and accessing the port only with sterile devices.

11. Do not use filters routinely for infection-control purposes.

IV Medication Administration During Infusion Therapy

When IV medications are ordered while an infusion is running, there are several administration options. They may be added to the primary infusate container, given via a secondary administration set, added through an injection port in the primary administration tubing, or given by direct injection into another vein that is not concurrently receiving any infusates. If the first three options are used, it is critical that the nurse check for chemical, physical, and therapeutic compatibility between the medications and the delivery systems.

Adding Medications to the Infusion Container

In general, admixtures are dispensed directly into infusate containers in the pharmacy by pharmacists who use strict asepsis. Admixing is done under laminar air flow hoods, where air is constantly filtered of contaminants. **Laminar air flow** refers to air that moves along separate but parallel flow paths into filters where contaminants are removed. It was common practice in the not-too-distant past for nurses to prepare their own admixtures for primary infusions. The CDC now recommends that all parenteral admixtures be aseptically prepared in the pharmacy under laminar-flow hoods (CDC, 2002a).

In some circumstances the nurse may have to add newly ordered medications to an already hanging infusion. Prior to doing this, several areas need to be addressed:

1. *Compatibility.* The nurse must verify that the drug can be mixed with the existing infusate.

2. *Concentration.* Depending on the amount of infusate remaining in the primary container, would the addition of the medication render a safe dilution? (An example here would involve adding potassium chloride to a primary container. Unless there is enough infusate to dilute the drug, the concentration of KCl might be too great, which could result in a cardiac dysrhythmia.)

3. *Stability.* How long will the drug be stable once it is added to the infusion?

If after all precautions are taken and the nurse does add medication to a primary container, she must prepare the admixture using strict asepsis. If taken from a glass ampule, a depth-filter needle must be used to draw up the medication to remove any glass fragments that may have fallen into the solution when the ampule was broken. It must be replaced with a standard needle or appropriate needleless device before expelling the drug from the syringe into the IV container.

The administration set tubing must be clamped and the infusion container must be removed from the IV pole prior to injecting the drug. The injection port must be swabbed with 70% alcohol, the medication injected, and then the bag or bottle must be gently rocked back and forth to thoroughly mix the added drug with the fluid. It can then be rehung, the clamp opened, and the rate adjusted. The container must be labeled to indicate what drug and dose was added, the date and time, the amount of infusate in the container when the admixture was prepared, the name of the person who prepared and added it, and the expiration time. See Skill 9-6 for the step-by-step procedure used to add medication to an infusion container.

Secondary Medication Administration Piggybacked into the Primary Infusion Line

The secondary infusion is initiated after the primary infusion is in progress. It is the most common method to administer IV medications concurrently with the primary infusion. It is

coupled to the primary infusion line at the first injection port below the check valve.

The piggyback is able to function concurrently with a primary infusion only when it is suspended higher than the primary line (which must have a back-check valve). By opening the clamp on the secondary line, the primary infusion temporarily stops flowing. When the piggyback infusion is complete and the infusate in its tubing falls below the level of the primary line drip chamber, the back-check valve opens and the primary infusion

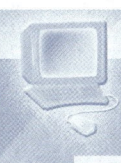

SKILL 9-6

Adding Medication to an Infusion Container

Equipment Needed:	Implementation/Action	Rationale
Vial or ampule of appropriate medication	1. Check the physician's order.	A physician's order is a legal requirement for infusion therapy.
	2. Introduce yourself to the patient.	By introducing yourself, you convey courtesy, establish/promote the nurse-patient relationship, instill patient trust, and thus alleviate anxiety.
Syringe and appropriate needle to draw up and deliver the medication into the infusate container	3. Identify the patient by checking the wrist band against the doctor's order and asking the patient, if conscious, to state his/her name.	Proper identification ensures that the procedure is being performed on the correct patient.
	4. Verify the allergy status of the patient.	This is a patient safety measure.
	5. Explain the proposed procedure in terms the patient can understand.	The patient has the right to know what is being done and the right to refuse care.
	6. Carry out proper hand hygiene.	Good hand hygiene is the single most important means of preventing the spread of infection.
Filter needle (if medication is contained in a glass ampule)	7. Gather equipment.	Saves time, prevents interruptions during procedure.
	8. Check the medication for the name, dosage, expiration date, appropriate appearance, and the integrity of the container.	To ensure that it is appropriate and safe to use, and to ensure sterility.
70% isopropyl alcohol swabs	9. Draw up the medication dose as prescribed.	
	10. Clamp the tubing on the infusate administration tubing.	To allow for proper admixing of the drug and prevent bolus administration.
	11. Remove the infusion container from the IV pole.	
	12. Swab the injection port on the infusate container with the alcohol.	To prevent entry of microorganisms into the infusate during injection of the medication.
	13. Inject the medication into the injection port.	

(continues)

SKILL 9-6

Adding Medication to an Infusion Container (continued)

Implementation/Action	Rationale
14. Gently rock the infusion container back and forth.	To thoroughly mix the medication into the infusate and prevent the formation of bubbles.
15. Hang the container on the IV pole.	
16. Discard the used syringe into the sharps container.	To prevent needlestick injury.
17. Open the clamp on the IV tubing and regulate the rate.	To resume flow of the infusate and administer medication delivery.
18. Stay with the patient for five minutes.	To assess for any untoward effects of the drug.
19. Affix a label to the infusate container to indicate the addition of the drug. The label should contain the following: a. Name of drug b. Dose of drug c. Date d. Time the drug was added e. Amount of infusate in container when drug was added. f. Expiration time g. Nurse's name	
20. Carry out proper hand hygiene.	To prevent cross-contamination.
21. Document in the MAR.	Legally documents the drug and dose given and method of delivery.

resumes. Skill 9-7 summarizes the steps in initiating a secondary infusion.

Adding Medications Through the Infusion Line

Some IV medications that would normally be delivered directly into the vein by bolus injection can be administered through an injection port in the primary administration set if the patient already has an IV running.

When administering any IV push medication it is very important to check for compatibility between the infusing product and the drug. Failure to do so could cause a precipitate to form, which could obstruct the infusion line or, if it entered the patient, could damage the vein or embolize. It is also critical that any required nursing interventions that accompany the drug's administration be verified. These often

NURSING TIP

Adding Medication to an Existing Infusion Container

When adding a medication to an existing infusion container, *never* inject it into the bag or bottle while it is hanging and infusing. This would deliver the drug to the base of the container, where it would infuse as a bolus dose to the patient. There are documented cases where this practice has resulted in serious complications and death.

NURSING TIP

Bolus Injection

The term *bolus injection* actually refers to the slow injection of a drug directly into a vein. Contrary to what some nurses believe, it does not mean to administer the drug via an existing infusion line.

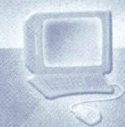

SKILL 9-7

IV Piggyback

Equipment Needed:	Implementation/Action	Rationale
Disposable gloves	1. Check the physician's order.	A physician's order is a legal requirement for infusion therapy.
Medication prepared in a labeled infusion container	2. Introduce yourself to the patient.	By introducing yourself, you convey courtesy, establish/promote the nurse-patient relationship, instill patient trust, and thus alleviate anxiety.
Secondary IV tubing with appropriate needle and hanging device, or needleless system, as appropriate	3. Identify the patient by checking the wrist band against the doctor's order and asking the patient, if conscious, to state his/her name.	Proper identification ensures that the procedure is being performed on the correct patient.
	4. Verify the allergy status of the patient.	This is a patient safety measure.
	5. Explain the proposed procedure in terms the patient can understand.	The patient has the right to know what is being done and the right to refuse care.
70% isopropyl alcohol swab	6. Carry out proper hand hygiene.	Good hand hygiene is the single most important means of preventing the spread of infection.
	7. Provide privacy.	To maintain patient dignity.
Tape or manufacturer-specific coupling device	8. Obtain the medication and verify that it is correct and compatible with the current infusate, and check the expiration date. If the medication is refrigerated, it should be removed from the refrigerator 20 to 30 minutes before administration. If the medication is stored at room temperature, it should be opened immediately before administration. Set up all the necessary supplies.	Maintains order and conserves time.
MAR		
Primary infusion delivery tubing with backcheck valve	9. Don gloves.	Protects nurse from contamination should hands come in contact with blood.
	10. Open the sterile container with the secondary medication administration set.	
	11. Clamp the secondary medication administration set and spike the medication container without contaminating it.	
	12. Do not fill the drip chamber and do not prime the tubing in the conventional manner.	To maintain a closed system and prevent retrograde microbial entry into the line.
	13. Swab the injection port directly below the check valve on the primary tubing with alcohol.	To promote asepsis and preclude microbial entry into the system.
	14. Attach the secondary tubing to the cleansed injection port with the appropriate needle or needleless adapter.	To prepare for the administration of the medication.
	15. Lower the secondary bag below the level of the port it is tethered into while the primary infusate is still running.	To ready the secondary line for priming.

(continues)

SKILL　9-7

IV Piggyback (continued)

Implementation/Action	Rationale
16. Slowly open the clamp on the secondary administration set and let the infusate from the primary line purge the secondary tubing of air (via retrograde fluid flow). When the drip chamber is one-half to two-thirds full, close the roller clamp on the secondary set.	To complete priming the secondary line.
17. Attach the hanger, included in the secondary set, and attach it to the primary infusate container (making the primary container hang lower than the secondary container).	To promote gravitational flow.
18. Open the roller clamp on the secondary tubing and infuse the piggybacked infusate at the prescribed rate. Do not close the clamp on the primary infusion.	When the piggyback has infused, the negative pressure will activate the check valve and the primary infusion will resume dripping.
19. Tape or affix a manufactured coupling device to secure the connection between the primary and secondary line.	To prevent inadvertent disconnection.
20. Assess the patient's response.	
21. Document the procedure.	

include vital signs (which may be required before, during, and after administration), patient teaching regarding sensations he may experience during or following administration, the amount of time needed to safely inject the drug, side effects associated with too-rapid infusion, and patient safety precautions.

DISCONTINUATION OF PERIPHERAL INFUSIONS WHILE RETAINING VENOUS PATENCY

Once the need for a primary infusion is no longer needed, the bag or bottle and administration set tubings can be removed, and an intermittent infusion plug can be attached to the hub of the cannula. This is usually done in order to keep the IV line available in case it is needed later or to keep it for administering intermittent medications.

After verifying the order, the nurse obtains an intermittent infusion plug, also called a male adapter plug (formerly called a heparin lock) and a 2 cc syringe of 0.9% NaCl. The appropriate needleless connectors are used for access to the intermittent infusion plug. The infusion is turned off, gloves are applied, and the administration set tubing is disconnected from the cannula. The sterile cap on the intermittent plug is removed and the adapter is attached to the cannula hub. The rubber stopper is swabbed with 70% alcohol and 2 cc of normal saline is injected to flush the cannula (See Skill 9-9).

In the past, the saline flush was followed by 1 ml of heparin (10 units per ml). The CDC (CDC, 2001) recommends that heparin be used only when intermittent infusion devices are used for blood sampling. Normal (0.9%) saline is just as effective as heparin in maintaining catheter patency and reducing phlebitis among peripheral catheters. In addition, recent in vitro studies have suggested that the growth of coagulase-negative staphylococci (CoNS) on catheters may be intensified in the presence of heparin. CoNS growth is inhibited by edetic acid (EDTA), making it the subject of clinical trials and testing to judge its efficacy for use in catheter flushing. Until further clinical trials substantiate otherwise, heparin is no longer routinely recommended for intermittent flushing.

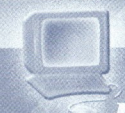

SKILL 9-8

IV Drug Administration into an Existing Infusion Line

Equipment Needed:	Implementation/Action	Rationale

Equipment Needed:

Watch with second hand

Disposable gloves

Medication in vial or ampule

Filter needle to draw up medication (if in glass ampule)

Sterile syringe, appropriate for the volume of medication to be injected. (Once drawn into the syringe, the syringe must be labeled.)

Sterile needles or needleless adapter, appropriate to access the injection port of the infusion line

Sterile needles appropriate to access the vein and deliver the prescribed medication

Two syringes containing NS (labeled)

70% isopropyl alcohol swabs

Sharps container

Implementation/Action

1. Check the physician's order.

2. Introduce yourself to the patient.

3. Identify the patient by checking the wrist band against the doctor's order and asking the patient, if conscious, to state his/her name.

4. Verify the allergy status of the patient.

5. Explain the proposed procedure in terms the patient can understand.

6. Carry out proper hand hygiene.

7. Provide privacy.

8. Elevate the bed level.

9. Assess vital signs and LOC and record.

10. Set up all the necessary supplies on the bedside stand or overbed table in the order in which they will be used.

11. Ascertain that the medication to be injected is compatible with the existing infusion. (If it is not compatible, the injection must be preceeded and followed with normal saline [or manufacturer-provided diluent] while the tubing above the injection site is stopped of infusate flow either by pinching off or with the inherent slide clamp on the tubing set.)

12. Don gloves.

13. Swab the injection port nearest to the client with the alcohol.

14. Insert the needle or needless adapter into the port.

15. Stop the primary infusion by pinching the administration set tubing closed just behind the injection port (or, if the administration set has one, close the slide clamp).

16. Inject the medication according to directions.

Rationale

A physician's order is a legal requirement for infusion therapy.

By introducing yourself, you convey courtesy, establish/promote the nurse-patient relationship, instill patient trust, and thus alleviate anxiety.

Proper identification ensures that the procedure is being performed on the correct patient.

This is a patient safety measure.

The patient has the right to know what is being done and the right to refuse care.

Good hand hygiene is the single most important means of preventing the spread of infection.

To maintain patient dignity.

Conducive to a successful procedure and alleviates back strain for the nurse.

To provide baseline physical and mental status.

Maintains order, lessens the chance for contamination, and conserves time.

To prevent any medication reactions.

Protects nurse from contamination should hands come in contact with blood.

Asepsis.

To deliver the medication IV.

(continues)

SKILL 9-8

IV Drug Administration into an Existing Infusion Line (continued)

Implementation/Action	Rationale
17. Remove the syringe or needle and dispose of it properly in the sharps container.	**To prevent needlestick injury or contamination to others.**
18. Check to be sure the infusion is running at the appropriate rate and adjust as required to maintain the schedule.	**Ensure effective treatment.**
19. Return bed to normal position.	**Patient safety.**

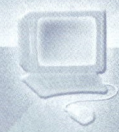

SKILL 9-9

Using a Peripheral Intermittent Infusion Device

Equipment Needed:

Intermittent infusion plug (sterile), with integral extension tubing and slide clamp. Disposable gloves 3 ml syringe filled with sterile normal (0.9%) saline, with appropriate connector to accommodate needle or needleless system. If a needle is used, it must be small (27 to 25 gauge) and short (1/2 to 5/8 inch in length).

Implementation/Action	Rationale
1. Check the physician's order.	**A physician's order is a legal requirement for infusion therapy.**
2. Introduce yourself to the patient.	**By introducing yourself, you convey courtesy, establish/promote the nurse-patient relationship, instill patient trust, and thus alleviate anxiety.**
3. Identify the patient by checking the wrist band against the doctor's order and asking the patient, if conscious, to state his/her name.	**Proper identification ensures that the procedure is being performed on the correct patient.**
4. Verify the allergy status of the patient.	**This is a patient safety measure.**
5. Explain the proposed procedure in terms the patient can understand.	**The patient has the right to know what is being done and the right to refuse care.**
6. Carry out proper hand hygiene.	**Good hand hygiene is the single most important means of preventing the spread of infection.**
7. Provide privacy.	**To maintain patient dignity.**
8. Elevate the bed level.	**Conducive to a successful procedure and alleviates back strain for the nurse.**
9. Set up all the necessary supplies on the bedside stand or overbed table in the order in which they will be used.	**Maintains order, lessens the chance for contamination, and conserves time.**
10. Don gloves.	**Protects nurse from contamination should hands come in contact with blood.**
11. Open the sterile container with the intermittent injection plug, remove the sterile cap, attach the syringe of normal saline, prime the plug, and leave the syringe attached.	**To maintain sterility and prevent air entry into the circulatory system.**

(continues)

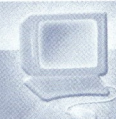

SKILL 9-9

Using a Peripheral Intermittent Infusion Device

Equipment Needed (*continued*):	Implementation/Action	Rationale
	12. Stop the infusion.	To stop the flow of infusate into the vein.
Antiseptic swab (normally 70% isopropyl alcohol)	13. Loosen the existing infusion tubing, remove the tubing, remove the sterile cap (if present) on the Luer-Lok®, and insert the intermittent infusion plug, screwing it securely onto the cannula hub (Figure 9-33).	To insert the plug in exchange for the infusion and maintain sterility and patency of the line.

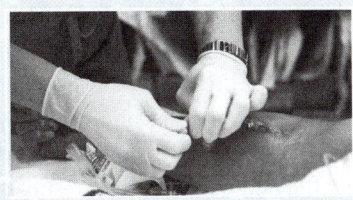

Figure 9-33 | Screw the intermittent infusion device onto the cannula hub.

Trans-parent semi-permiable membrane (TSM), if required

14. Open the slide clamp on the set, aspirate, and slowly inject the saline. Stop injecting when the last 0.5 ml of saline remains and immediately close the slide clamp on the set (Figure 9-34).

To saline-lock the plug and maintain positive pressure in the line.

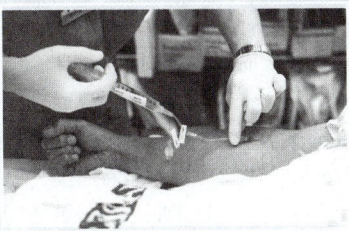

Figure 9-34 | Inject saline into the device to maintain pressure and patency in the line.

15. Dispose of the syringe in the sharps container.

To prevent needlestick injury or contamination.

16. Properly dispose of the infusate and tubing.

To dispose of contaminated, expired materials.

17. Remove gloves and carry out proper hand hygiene.

Prevent the cross-contamination of microorganisms from the nurse to other patients.

18. Document the procedure.

When an intermittent line is inserted but no IV medications are ordered, the usual maintenance routine is to assess the site, check for cannula patency, and instill 2 cc of 0.9% saline every 8 to 12 hours. To check for patency, the syringe is attached to the intermittent plug and the plunger is pulled back to elicit a blood return. There may or may not be a return because a fibrin shield forms at the tip of most cannulas (a homeostatic defense mechanism that occurs when the skin barrier is broken) that prevents retrograde blood flow, yet allows infusates to pass into the system. If there is no blood return the nurse should gently inject the saline while palpating the infusion site and observing. If the cannula is out of the vein, the saline will infiltrate the surrounding tissue, raising it, and giving it a cool feeling. Otherwise, the saline will enter the cannula and vein to maintain patency.

When any medication is administered into an intermittent infusion device, the protocol to be followed is the S-A-S method:

1. Carry out proper hand hygiene.
2. Assess the site.
3. Don gloves.
4. Disinfect the cannula port.
5. Verify cannula and venous patency. If resistance is met, do not exert pressure on the syringe plunger to restore patency.
6. Slowly instill 2 ml of normal saline (0.9% NaCl) to clear the lock—**S**.
7. Administer the prescribed medication—**A**.
8. Flush with normal saline to clear the lock—**S**.
9. Maintain positive pressure during and after flushes to prevent reflux of blood. (See *Nursing Tip*.)
10. Remove gloves and carry out proper hand hygiene.
11. Document according to agency policy.

If multiple IV medications are ordered at one time, the normal saline is to be instilled between the administration of each one. The normal saline must always be given after any medications are injected to clear the cannula of the drug and maintain patency. Positive pressure must be maintained within the cannula lumen during and following a flush to prevent reflux of blood into the lumen.

In the event that heparin is ordered, the traditional S-A-S-H sequence protocol would be used:

1. Carry out proper hand hygiene.
2. Assess the site.
3. Don gloves.
4. Disinfect the cannula port.
5. Verify cannula and venous patency. If resistance is met, do not exert pressure on the syringe plunger to restore patency.
6. Slowly instill 2 ml of normal saline (0.9% NaCl) to clear the lock—**S**.
7. Administer the prescribed medication—**A**.
8. Flush with normal saline to clear the lock—**S**.
9. Connect the heparin-filled syringe (usually 1 ml of 10 units/ml) to the cannula port and flush—**H**.
10. Maintain positive pressure during and after flushes to prevent reflux of blood. (See *Nursing Tip*.)
11. Remove gloves and carry out proper hand hygiene.
12. Document according to agency policy.

Do not use the S-A-S-H method for peripheral IV lines unless it is backed by institutional policy or specifically ordered by the physician.

Turbulent flushing may assist in minimizing fibrin collection and clot formation on peripheral catheters, just as it does with central lines This type of flushing is accomplished by exerting a driving motion on the syringe plunger with a pulsatile, push-pause technique. This introduces turbulence into the cannula of the IV device, which creates a swirling (true flushing motion). The result is a vigorous movement that can remove blood cells, fibrin, or protein buildup on the walls of the cannula.

N U R S I N G   A L E R T

Maintaining Positive Pressure in Cannula Lumen

It is imperative that positive pressure be maintained within the lumen of the catheter during and following the administration of a flush solution to prevent reflux of blood into the cannula lumen. A positive displacement device helps to eliminate fluid backflow by generating a positive pulse of fluid directed toward the catheter tip as the male Luer-Lok adapter is removed from the device. When flushing a positive displacement device, remove the syringe *before* clamping.

N U R S I N G   T I P

Positive Pressure Technique

- When using a blunt cannula or needle, withdraw the blunt cannula or needle as the last 0.5 ml is flushed inward.
- When using a Luer activated device:
  - As the last 0.5 ml is flushed inward, clamp the extension tubing.
    or
  - Maintain pressure on the plunger and clamp the extension set at either end.

DISCONTINUATION OF PERIPHERAL INFUSION LINES

An IV is discontinued when ordered by the physician, when the infusion line is no longer needed, or if it must be terminated because of complications. Skill 9-10 summarizes the steps for discontinuing peripheral infusion lines.

MEDICATION ADMINISTRATION BY DIRECT INTRAVENOUS BOLUS DELIVERY

When the patient does not have an infusion line in place but requires intravenous medications, the medication must be injected directly into the vein. Either a straight needle or a winged tip administration set connected to a syringe can be used.

Straight Needle and Syringe

For medications that can be injected over a short time period (usually less than 60 seconds), a straight needle attached to a syringe is generally used (see Skill 9-11).

Winged Administration Set and Syringe

A winged administration set is generally used when the medication to be administered takes more than a minute to inject (such as IV phenytoin, where the rate is not to exceed 50 mg/min). Using this method, the nurse can comfortably position herself next to the patient without straining her back. If any interventions need to be taken during administration of the medication (such as blood pressure or pulse monitoring), the syringe can be set down next to the patient's extremity or taped to it without the needle becoming dislodged from the vein (see Skill 9-12).

NURSING ALERT

Time Parameters

The term *IV bolus* or *IV push* does not indicate an appropriate injection rate. If the prescriber does not order time parameters, it is the nurse's responsibility to consult with the phyiscan as well as a reliable drug reference source, or confer with a pharmacist to obtain a protocol for the length of time needed to administer the ordered dose. Certain drugs, such as digoxin, when administered too rapidly can cause severe bradycardia or death from cardiac arrest.

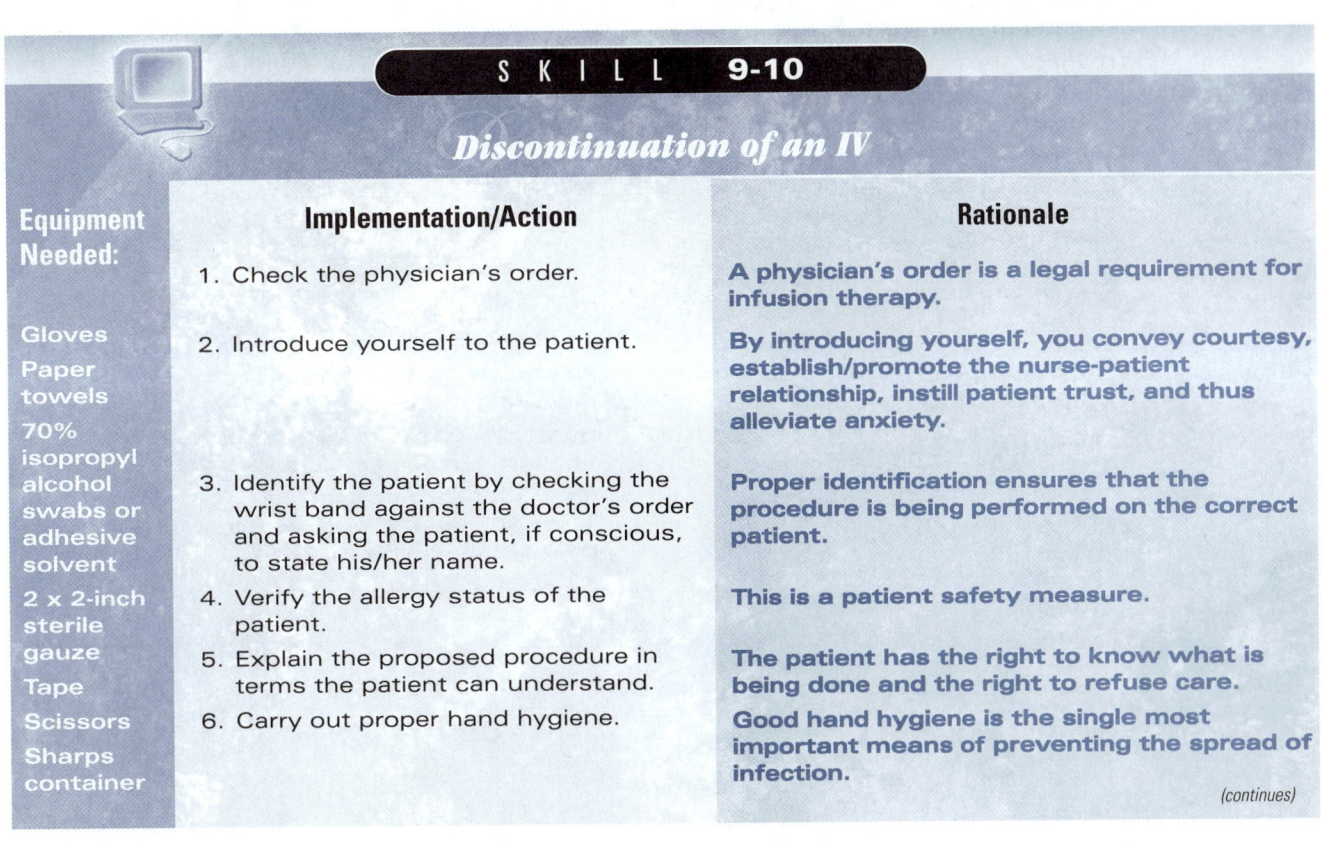

SKILL 9-10

Discontinuation of an IV

Equipment Needed:	Implementation/Action	Rationale
Gloves	1. Check the physician's order.	A physician's order is a legal requirement for infusion therapy.
Paper towels	2. Introduce yourself to the patient.	By introducing yourself, you convey courtesy, establish/promote the nurse-patient relationship, instill patient trust, and thus alleviate anxiety.
70% isopropyl alcohol swabs or adhesive solvent	3. Identify the patient by checking the wrist band against the doctor's order and asking the patient, if conscious, to state his/her name.	Proper identification ensures that the procedure is being performed on the correct patient.
2 x 2-inch sterile gauze	4. Verify the allergy status of the patient.	This is a patient safety measure.
Tape	5. Explain the proposed procedure in terms the patient can understand.	The patient has the right to know what is being done and the right to refuse care.
Scissors	6. Carry out proper hand hygiene.	Good hand hygiene is the single most important means of preventing the spread of infection.
Sharps container		

(continues)

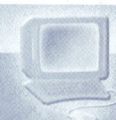

SKILL 9-10

Discontinuation of an IV (continued)

Implementation/Action	Rationale
7. Gather supplies.	To complete the skill in a timely manner.
8. Provide privacy.	To maintain patient dignity.
9. Elevate the bed.	Conducive to successful procedure and alleviates back strain for the nurse.
10. Clamp infusion tubing and turn off electronic infusion device (if appropriate).	The infusion must cease prior to removal of the IV device.
11. Cut or tear off a few strips of tape.	To apply to dressing to arrest bleeding and enclose site.
12. Don gloves.	To prevent contamination of the nurse's hands.
13. Remove all tape and loosen the skin from the edges of the dressing over the IV site very carefully, using the stretch method or alcohol (or adhesive remover) method. Be careful not to pull on the cannula.	To prevent undue trauma to the insertion site or catheter dislodgement.
14. While stabilizing the cannula hub, remove the entire IV dressing, moving in the direction of the IV device, not away from it.	To completely remove the dressing and prevent undue trauma to the insertion site.
15. Place a 2 x 2-inch sterile gauze (not alcohol) over the IV insertion site and apply gentle pressure while grasping the cannula hub and removing the catheter with one smooth movement.	To lessen pain and tissue damage as a result of catheter removal. Alcohol creates heat, increased blood flow, and can enhance post-removal bleeding.
16. Place the catheter on the paper towel.	The catheter will need to be examined.
17. Elevate the extremity and apply firm, gentle pressure to the IV site for 60 seconds, or until there is no bleeding.	Pressure prevents bleeding from the site.
18. Assess the site and apply tape firmly over the gauze. If the patient is undergoing anticoagulation therapy or has a bleeding disorder, a larger pressure dressing may be needed.	Bleeding from the site is to be prevented/arrested.
19. Examine the removed catheter.	To be sure it is intact.
20. Dispose of the IV device in the sharps container.	To prevent needlestick injury or contamination.
21. Return the bed to the lowest position and raise the bedrails.	Safety, in terms of fall prevention, is enhanced when the bed is in the low position and the rails are up.
22. Recheck the IV site.	To be sure there is no bleeding or other problem(s).
23. Document the procedure.	

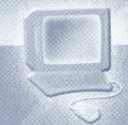

SKILL 9-11

Medication Administration by Bolus Delivery

Equipment Needed:

Gloves
Tourniquet
Two 70% alcohol pledgets or prep recommended by the institution
Sterile 2 × 2-inch gauze dressing
Paper tape

Implementation/Action	Rationale
1. Check the physician's order.	A physician's order is a legal requirement for infusion therapy.
2. Introduce yourself to the patient.	By introducing yourself, you convey courtesy, establish/promote the nurse-patient relationship, instill patient trust, and thus alleviate anxiety.
3. Identify the patient by checking the wrist band against the doctor's order and asking the patient, if conscious, to state his/her name.	Proper identification ensures that the procedure is being performed on the correct patient.
4. Verify the allergy status of the patient.	This is a patient safety measure.
5. Explain the proposed procedure in terms the patient can understand.	The patient has the right to know what is being done and the right to refuse care.
6. Carry out proper hand hygiene.	Good hand hygiene is the single most important means of preventing the spread of infection.
7. Draw the medication up in a syringe.	This is the method of accessing the drug.
8. Change the needle, attaching the smallest one that will deliver the ordered medication yet accommodate the patient's vein.	The needle needs to be changed because a larger needle is generally used to facilitate drawing up the medication. In addition, the outer surface of the needle has medication on it once it exits the medication container. The delivery needle used must protect the integrity of the skin and vein and cause little or no trauma to the patient.
9. Perform any preadministration nursing interventions, such as taking vital signs or performing neurologic or cardiovascular assessments.	Ensure the patient's safety and allow for follow-up assessment and evaluation of the patient's response to the drug.
10. Cut or tear one 4-inch strip of tape and open the 2 × 2-inch gauze without contaminating it.	
11. Apply the tourniquet and engorge the vein.	The tourniquet restricts venous blood flow; engorging facilitates venous access.
12. Prep the site using appropriate antiseptics. Work in a circular motion from the intended venipuncture site outward, extending to 2 inches. Do not backtrack. Allow the site to dry.	Proper asepsis of the site prevents antimicrobial contamination. The site must be dry before the needle is inserted so that the antiseptic will exert its effect and will not be tracked into the circulation during venous cannulation.
13. Don gloves.	Gloves are used to protect the nurse from exposure to the patient's blood.
14. Access the vein and pull back on the plunger to verify placement in the vein.	The medication must be delivered by the proper route.
15. Remove the tourniquet.	This reestablishes venous blood flow and facilitates IV medication delivery.

(continues)

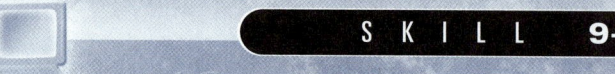

S K I L L 9-11

Medication Administration by Bolus Delivery (continued)

Implementation/Action	Rationale
16. Inject the medication.	
17. Place the 2 × 2-inch gauze over the injection site and remove the needle.	This prevents retrograde flow of blood and medication out of the vein and promotes hemostasis.
18. Elevate the extremity until bleeding stops and apply tape over the gauze.	This promotes hemostasis.
19. Dispose of the syringe properly in the sharps container to prevent needle-stick injury and adhere to safety guidelines.	
20. Remove gloves and carry out proper hand hygiene.	This prevents the spread of infection.
21. Stay with the patient and assess his response to the medication.	This provides for patient safety.
22. Perform any postadministration nursing interventions associated with the medication.	This upholds the steps of the nursing process.

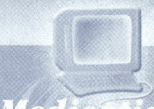

S K I L L 9-12

Medication Administration by Bolus Using a Winged Administration Set

Equipment Needed:	Implementation/Action	Rationale
Gloves	1. Check the physician's order.	A physician's order is a legal requirement for infusion therapy.
Tourniquet		
Two 70% alcohol pledgets or the antiseptic recommended by the institution	2. Introduce yourself to the patient.	By introducing yourself, you convey courtesy, establish/promote the nurse-patient relationship, instill patient trust, and thus alleviate anxiety.
	3. Identify the patient by checking the wrist band against the doctor's order and asking the patient, if conscious, to state his/her name.	Proper identification ensures that the procedure is being performed on the correct patient.
	4. Verify the allergy status of the patient.	This is a patient safety measure.
Sterile 2 × 2-inch gauze dressing	5. Explain the proposed procedure in terms the patient can understand.	The patient has the right to know what is being done and the right to refuse care.
Tape	6. Carry out proper hand hygiene.	Good hand hygiene is the single most important means of preventing the spread of infection.
	7. Draw the medication up into a syringe and cap the needle.	Capping maintains the sterility of the medication.

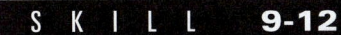

S K I L L   9-12

Medication Administration by Bolus Using a Winged Administration Set

Implementation/Action	Rationale
8. Draw up 2 to 3 ml of normal saline (0.9%) in each of two separate syringes and cap the needles.	
9. Attach a winged administration set with the smallest needle that will deliver the drug and be appropriate for the patient's vein to one of the syringes containing 0.9% saline and prime the tubing and needle on the set.	**The delivery needle used must protect the integrity of the skin and vein and cause little or no trauma to the patient. Priming prevents the entry of air into the patient's circulation.**
10. Perform any preadministration nursing interventions, such as taking vital signs or performing neurologic or cardiovascular assessments.	**This ensures patient safety and allows for follow-up assessment and evaluation of the patient's response to the drug.**
11. Cut or tear two 4-inch strips of tape and open the sterile 2 × 2-inch gauze without contaminating it.	
12. Apply the tourniquet to restrict venous blood flow and engorge the vein so venous access is facilitated.	
13. Prep the site using a circular motion extending 2 inches outward from the intended venipuncture site. Do not backtrack. Allow the site to dry.	**Proper asepsis of the site prevents antimicrobial contamination. The site must be dry before needle insertion so that the antiseptic will exert its effect and will not be tracked into the circulation during venous cannulation.**
14. Don gloves.	**Gloves are used to protect the nurse from exposure to the patient's blood.**
15. Remove the tourniquet to reestablish venous blood flow and facilitate IV medication delivery.	
16. Using the syringe attached to the 0.9% saline, insert the winged needle. Verify placement by retracting the plunger. If it's in the vein, flatten the administration set wings and place a strip of tape over them, securing the set to the patient's extremity. Slowly inject the 0.9% saline.	**The needle must be in the vein to administer an intravenous medication. By retracting the plunger, a blood return may or may not be present. Slow administration of normal saline verifies placement in the absence of a blood return. By placing a strip of tape over the wings, the needle is stabilized.**
17. Disconnect the empty syringe and attach the syringe containing the medication to the administration tubing.	
18. Inject the medication over the prescribed time.	
19. When the medication has been administered, disconnect the empty syringe and attach the second syringe of 0.9% saline to the administration set tubing. Inject the normal saline.	**The last injection of normal saline clears the tubing and needle of medication and maintains venous patency.**
20. Remove the strip of tape and place the 2 × 2-inch gauze on the injection site and remove the needle.	**This prevents retrograde flow of blood and medication out of the vein and promotes hemostasis.**

(continues)

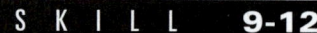

SKILL 9-12

Medication Administration by Bolus Using a Winged Administration Set

Implementation/Action	Rationale
21. Elevate the extremity and apply pressure to the injection site until bleeding stops. Apply the clean strip of tape over the gauze.	**Applying tape over the gauze promotes hemostasis.**
22. Dispose of the syringes and the winged administration set properly in the sharps container to prevent needlestick injury and adhere to safety guidelines.	
23. Remove gloves and carry out proper hand hygiene to prevent the spread of infection.	
24. Stay with the patient and assess his response to the medication.	**This provides for patient safety.**
25. Perform any postadministration nursing interventions.	**This upholds the steps of the nursing process.**

Key Concepts

* Physical and psychological preparation go hand-in-hand when administering infusion therapy to a patient.

* By using simulation mannequins and training devices, the nurse develops the confidence and dexterity necessary to successfully perform venous cannulation on patients.

* To be legally complete, the medical order for any infusion must include the following:

  – Date and preferably the time of day

  – Name of the infusate to be administered

  – Route of administration

  – Dosage of the infusate

  – Volume to be infused

  – Rate of the infusion

  – Duration of the infusion

  – Physician's signature

* The nurse must be familiar with the general procedures required to facilitate venous access in the general adult population as well as for patients with compromised circulatory conditions.

* It is critical that the nurse investigate the allergy status of every patient prior to the initiation of infusion therapy.

* In order to practice nursing in today's health care environment, the nurse must be able to know what equipment is indicated for the various types of infusion therapy, to prepare the equipment, and to use it correctly.

* It is essential that the nurse adhere to the most recent guidelines set forth by the CDC and the policies and procedural protocols of her employer when dealing with vascular access issues and administering infusion therapy.

* Prior to administering infusion therapy to a patient, the nurse must understand the principles and procedures required to safely perform the infusion.

* The nurse must understand the parameters of reporting and documentation regarding infusion therapy, and use them appropriately.

Review Questions and Activities

1. Write a nursing care plan for the patient in the following case study, focusing on his potential infusion-related needs.

> Mr. Beaupré is a 59-year-old certified public accountant. He has a wife, who does not work outside of the home, and three children (a daughter in law school, a son in college, another daughter in high school). He has a medical history of hypertension, hypercholesterolemia, and gastritis. He smokes 15 to 20 cigarettes a day. He takes Prilosec 20 mg daily, Pravachol 20 mg daily, and Zestril 10 mg daily.
>
> On April 10, after working late at the office, he stops for a pizza and a couple of beers. During the night he is awakened with severe midepigastric burning and nausea. He takes an over-the-counter antacid, which doesn't help, so he takes some more.
>
> The next day Mr. Beaupré's stomach continues to burn, but he attributes it to the long hours he has been working, since it is tax time. For lunch he has a hot dog and a cola and works late again, missing supper. When he gets home, he is too tired to eat, and goes to bed.
>
> At 0130 hours on April 12, Mr. Beaupré is awakened with severe abdominal pain, nausea, and vomiting blood. His physician is called and he is taken to the hospital. Initial assessment data reveals the following:

- Restless and agitated
- T: 97.8; P: 98; R: 28; BP: 110/78
- Hgb: 12.8; Hct: 37.2
- Stool is Hemoccult positive
- Nasogastric tube aspirate is Hemoccult positive

The initial medical orders for Mr. Beaupré include:

- NPO and ice chips prn
- Insert 18 ga. ONC
- D_5LR @ 125 cc/hr
- Type & crossmatch for 2 units packed cells
- Hourly H & H (hematocrit and hemoglobin)
- Consult with gastroenterologist for upper and lower endoscopy ASAP

2. Describe three of the conditions a patient may have that would compromise successful venous cannulation. What nursing interventions can be taken to overcome each condition?

3. Make a chart that would be useful to health care workers and patients, alerting them to sources of latex-based substances that might pose a threat to a person allergic to latex products.

4. List how each of the following five sources provide the nurse with the tools needed for protection should she be involved in IV therapy-related litigation.
   (a) State nurse practice acts
   (b) Centers for Disease Control and Prevention guidelines
   (c) Occupational Safety and Health Administration mandates
   (d) Infusion Nurses Society standards
   (e) Employer policy and procedure manuals

Mathematical Calculations for the Administration, Regulation, and Maintenance of Intravenous Infusion Therapy

C O M P E T E N C I E S

Upon completion of this chapter, the reader should be able to:

- Review common fractions, decimal fractions, percentages, and proportions.

- Differentiate among the metric, apothecaries', and household systems of weights and measurements and their relationship to infusion calculations.

- Convert commonly used measurements between the metric, apothecaries', and household systems.

- Describe the unit and milliequivalent systems and their use in intravenous infusions.

- Explain how percentages, ratio and proportion, and alligation are used in calculating infusion dosages.

- Solve infusion dosage calculations using the multistep formulas.

- Calculate infusion dosages using dimensional analysis or the factor labeling method.

KEY TERMS

alligation	factor	proportion
denominator	numerator	ratio
dimensional analysis	percent	

When the physician orders an infusion, it is the responsibility of the nurse to verify that it is correct and appropriate for the patient, and that it is properly delivered. The nurse must know how to calculate accurately the dosage of every oral and parenteral medication he administers. He must be able to regulate and maintain every infusion at the prescribed rate whether it is sustained by simple gravity flow in drops per minute or by an infusion device that is manually operated or managed electronically.

In order to calculate dosages and solutions, the nurse must have a working knowledge of the basic mathematical processes of addition, subtraction, multiplication, and division. These operations must be exercised with whole numbers, fractions, and decimals. Problems need to be calculated using percentages, ratios, and proportions. The nurse must also be able to recognize Roman numerals and Arabic numbers.

BASIC MATHEMATICAL REVIEW

Mathematical calculations for infusion therapy include common fractions, decimal fractions, percentages, ratios, and proportions. If the nurse is not comfortable working with any of these processes, it is advisable that he review the information, using a basic dosage calculation text, as this is requisite knowledge for infusion calculations. The following provides a synopsis and serves only to refresh the nurse's memory regarding the elementary steps used in these processes.

Common Fractions

A common fraction is the quotient portion of a unit quantity or a whole number. It is an expression of division, with the **numerator** (top number) divided by the **denominator** (bottom number). The denominator signifies the total number of parts into which the whole is divided, and the numerator indicates the number of those parts to be considered. Proper fractions (e.g., $\frac{5}{8}$) have a numerator that is of lesser value than the denominator, while improper fractions (e.g., $\frac{8}{5}$) have a numerator that has an equal or greater value than the denominator (making the total value greater than or equal to 1). Mixed fractions combine a whole number with a proper fraction (e.g., $1\frac{5}{8}$). In complex fractions, the numerator or the denominator may be a proper fraction, mixed fraction, or a whole number.

In order to calculate infusions, the nurse must be able to make conversions between different types of fractions, to reduce and enlarge fractions, and to add, subtract, multiply, and divide them.

Fraction Conversions

By converting fractions, the nurse can solve calculation problems easily. Solutions to the problems can be expressed in the simplest terms, thereby reducing the possibility of error.

To convert a mixed fraction to an improper fraction, multiply the denominator by the whole number and add the numerator (e.g., $1\frac{1}{2} = 2 \times 1 + 1 = \frac{3}{2}$). To convert an improper fraction to a mixed fraction or a whole number, divide the numerator by the denominator (e.g., $\frac{5}{2} = 5 \div 2 = 2\frac{1}{2}$).

Fraction Equivalents

The value of any fraction may be expressed in different ways without changing the value (equivalents) by changing the form. This can be done through reduction or enlargement. The numerator and the denominator can be multiplied or divided by the same number without changing the value of the fraction. Numbers cannot, however, be added or subtracted from the numerator and denominator without changing the value of the fraction.

To reduce a fraction to its lowest terms, divide the numerator and the denominator by the largest multiple that will go evenly into both (e.g., for $\frac{4}{8}$, 4 is the largest number that can be divided evenly into 4 and 8, reducing the fraction to $\frac{1}{2}$). If there is no common number that both can be divided by, the fraction is already in its lowest terms and cannot be reduced any further.

To raise a fraction to higher terms, multiply the numerator and the denominator by the same number (e.g., for $\frac{5}{8}$, multiply both the 5 and the 8 by 2, enlarging the original fraction to $\frac{10}{16}$).

Addition and Subtraction of Fractions

In order to add or subtract fractions, they must have the same denominator. The same, or common, denominator is the lowest number into which all denominators can be divided an even number of times. For example, to add $\frac{1}{2}$ and $\frac{3}{5}$, the lowest common denominator into which both 2 and 5 can be evenly divided is 10. Therefore, $\frac{5}{10} + \frac{6}{10} = \frac{11}{10}$ (an improper fraction) or $1\frac{1}{10}$ (a mixed fraction). To subtract, the same process applies. For example, to subtract $\frac{1}{2}$ from $\frac{2}{3}$, the lowest common denominator into which both 2 and 3 can be divided is 6. Therefore, $\frac{4}{6} - \frac{3}{6} = \frac{1}{6}$.

Multiplication of Fractions

To multiply fractions, the numerators must be multiplied and the denominators must be multiplied (e.g., $\frac{1}{3} \times \frac{1}{2} = [1 \times 1]/[3 \times 2] = \frac{1}{6}$). If necessary, to simplify the process, each should be reduced to its lowest term, through the process of cancellation, and then multiplied ($\frac{125}{250} \times \frac{5}{10}$ cancels to $\frac{1}{2} \times \frac{1}{2}$ and equals $\frac{1}{4}$). Once multiplied, if applicable, the product (answer) should be reduced to its lowest terms.

Division of Fractions

To divide fractions, the divisor is inverted, then the process of multiplication of fractions is applied (e.g., $\frac{1}{2} \div \frac{2}{3} = \frac{1}{2} \times \frac{3}{2} = \frac{3}{4}$). If necessary, cancel terms prior to multiplication (e.g., $\frac{125}{250} \div \frac{125}{375} = \frac{1}{2} \div \frac{1}{3} = \frac{1}{2} \times \frac{3}{1} = \frac{3}{2}$). Reduce the product to its lowest terms ($\frac{3}{2} = 1\frac{1}{2}$).

When dividing mixed fractions, they must first be converted into improper fractions. For example, $2\frac{5}{8} \div 1\frac{1}{3}$ is converted to the improper fractions $\frac{21}{8} \div \frac{4}{3}$ then the divisor inverted $\frac{21}{8} \times \frac{3}{4}$ and multiplied $\frac{21}{8} \times \frac{3}{4} = \frac{63}{32}$ $1\frac{31}{32}$.

Decimal Fractions

Decimal fractions are fractions that have been converted to decimals. This is done by dividing the numerator by the denominator (e.g., $\frac{1}{2} = 1 \div 2 = 0.5$). Decimal fractions have a denominator of any multiple power of 10. Zeros added after the last digit do not change the value, but those added between the decimal point and the first number in a decimal fraction do change the value. For example, $0.125 = 0.1250$ or 0.12500, but $0.125 \neq 0.0125$, or 0.00125. Always place a zero to the left of the decimal point to emphasize that it is a decimal fraction.

To convert a decimal to a fraction, the decimal number becomes the whole number in the numerator and the number 1, followed by as many zeros as there are digits to the right of the decimal point, becomes the denominator. For example, 0.5 becomes $\frac{5}{10}$, 0.50 becomes $\frac{50}{100}$, and 0.500 becomes $\frac{500}{1000}$. Always reduce the final fraction to its lowest terms ($\frac{5}{10} = \frac{1}{2}$, $\frac{50}{100} = \frac{1}{2}$, and $\frac{500}{1000} = \frac{1}{2}$).

Addition and Subtraction of Decimals

Decimal fractions can be added and subtracted by aligning the decimal points and continuing as with whole numbers. The decimal point in the total is aligned with those in the numbers to be added or subtracted. A zero is placed before the decimal point if the number is less than 1. For example, $1.50 + 2.75 = 4.25$:

$$\begin{array}{r} 1.50 \\ + \ 2.75 \\ \hline 4.25 \end{array}$$

Multiplication of Decimals

To multiply decimals, the process is the same as with whole numbers, but the placement of the decimal point depends on the number of digits to the right of the decimal point in each of the numbers being multiplied. For example, 1.45 (two places to the right of the decimal point) $\times$ 1.725 (three places to the right of the decimal point) $= 2.50125$ (five places to the right of the decimal point):

$$\begin{array}{r} 1.725 \\ \times \ 1.45 \\ \hline 8625 \\ 6900 \\ 1725 \\ \hline 2.50125 \end{array}$$

If there are fewer digits in the answer than places to the right of the decimal point in the numbers multiplied, zeros are added to the extreme left of the answer to provide the proper number of digits. For example, to multiply 0.15×0.25 ($15 \times 25 = 375$) add a zero to the left (0.0375) to allow for four places to the right of the decimal point in the answer:

$$\begin{array}{r} 0.15 \\ \times \ 0.25 \\ \hline 075 \\ 030 \\ + \ 000 \\ \hline 0.0375 \end{array}$$

To multiply decimals by a power of ten, the decimal point is moved as many places to the right as there are zeros in the multiplier. For example $2.25 \times 10 = 22.5$, $22.5 \times 10 = 225$, and $0.225 \times 100 = 22.5$.

Division of Decimals

To divide decimal fractions, move the decimal point of both the divisor (number divided by) and the dividend (number divided into) to the same number of places to the right until the divisor is a whole number. For the problem $3.75 \div 2$, the decimal point in the dividend must be moved two places to the right to make it a whole number. (The decimal fraction 3.75 is essentially multiplied by 100.) Therefore, two zeros must be added to the divisor. The problem becomes $375.000 \div 200 = 1.875$. The decimal point in the quotient (answer) is placed above the moved decimal point in the dividend. Remember, that adding zeros after a decimal point, does not alter its value ($375 = 375.000$):

$$
\begin{array}{r}
1.875 \\
200{\overline{\smash{\big)}\,375.000}} \\
-\ 200 \\
\hline
1750 \\
-\ 1600 \\
\hline
1500 \\
-\ 1400 \\
\hline
1000 \\
-\ 1000 \\
\hline
0000
\end{array}
$$

To divide a decimal by a power of 10, the decimal point is moved to the left as many places as there are zeros in the divisor. For example, $2.50 \div 10$ (1 zero) $= 0.25$ (decimal point moved one place to the left), or $1.25 \div 100$ (2 zeros) $= 0.0125$ (decimal point moved two places to the left):

$$
\begin{array}{r}
0.25 \\
10{\overline{\smash{\big)}\,2.50}} \\
2\,0 \\
\hline
50 \\
50 \\
\hline
00
\end{array}
\qquad
\begin{array}{r}
0.0125 \\
100{\overline{\smash{\big)}\,1.2500}} \\
1\,00 \\
\hline
250 \\
200 \\
\hline
500 \\
500 \\
\hline
000
\end{array}
$$

Percentages

The term **percent** means one part in a hundred ($1\% = 1$ part per hundred, $10\% = 10$ parts per hundred). The whole of anything is 100%. A percentage can be expressed either as a decimal or as a fraction.

To convert a decimal to a percentage, multiply the decimal by 100 (moving the decimal point two places to the right) and add the percent symbol (e.g., $0.45 \times 100 = 45\%$):

$$
\begin{array}{r}
0.45 \\
\times\ 100 \\
\hline
45.00
\end{array}
$$

To convert a fraction to a percentage, it is first converted to a decimal. For example, the fraction $\frac{4}{5}$ is converted ($4 \div 5$) to 0.80, then is multiplied by 100, making it 80% ($0.80 \times 100\% = 80\%$).

To find the percentage of any whole number, the percentage number must be converted to a decimal. This is done by dividing the percentage number by 100. For example, to find 5% of 50, the 5 is divided by 100 to get 0.05. The 0.05 is then multiplied by the 50 to get 2.5. Five percent of 50 is 2.5.

Ratio and Proportions

A **ratio** is a quantitative relationship of one thing to another. In mathematical expressions, a ratio is the same thing as a fraction. For infusion therapy, the ratio identifies a specific amount of medication and solution. A percentage is a fraction or ratio with a denominator of 100 (e.g., $1\% = 1$ part per 100 or $\frac{1}{100}$). When quantitative comparisons are made using ratios, the two items being compared are separated by a colon, as in 1:100.

A **proportion** is two equal ratios or an equation (mathematical association) between them. It is a method of expressing a fraction in a different form without changing its value. It is written as two ratios separated by the identical sign ($::$) or the equal sign ($=$). For example, if $\frac{1}{5}$ is to be converted to hundredths (how many $\frac{1}{100}$s equal $\frac{1}{5}$), a proportion can be determined. If x represents an unknown quantity, two methods are used to solve for x. Either the numerator of one fraction is multiplied by the denominator of the other fraction, or the means (5 and x) and extremes (1 and 100) of each fraction, set up as a ratio, are divided. The means are the second and third (or inside) terms and the extremes are the first and fourth (or outside) terms in a proportion. For converting $\frac{1}{5}$ to hundredths, the following methods can be used:

$$
\frac{1}{5} = \frac{x}{100}
$$

$$
\begin{array}{ll}
5 \times x = 1 \times 100 & \\
5x = 100 & \text{or} \quad \begin{array}{l} 1{:}5 \ ::\ x{:}100 \\ 5x = 100 \end{array} \\
x = 20 & \qquad\quad\ x = 20
\end{array}
$$

Ratios and proportions are used extensively in the dosage calculation and preparation of infusions by nurses and pharmacists.

Alligation

Alligation is the process of determining the proportion of components used in the preparation of an infusate of a specifically required strength that is not available commercially. This is done by combining a stronger infusate with a weaker one to provide the ordered dosage. Once the proportional parts are determined, the actual quantities of

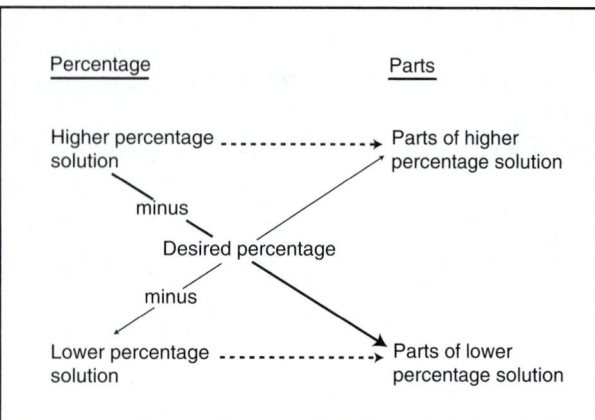

Figure 10-1 | Alligation

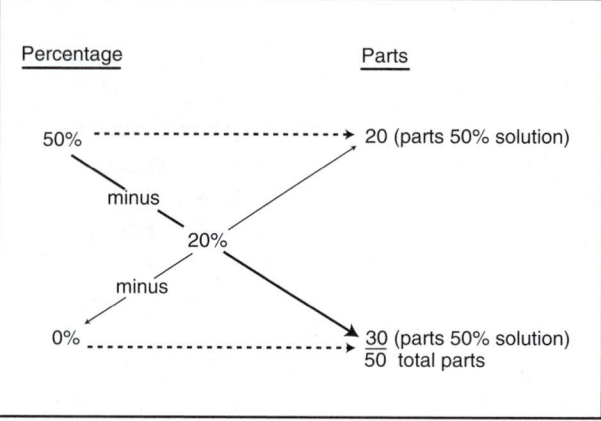

Figure 10-2 | The use of alligation to make an ordered preparation

each component needed for the total quantity can be calculated by using ratio and proportion. This is generally the pharmacist's responsibility, but in some instances it may be the nurse's duty to prepare the product.

Alligation (Figure 10-1) is set up as follows:

- The percentages of the components available to be used in mixing the solution are written on the left corners of the rectangle.
- The final percentage desired is written in the center.
- The relative parts required are calculated and written on the right corners of the rectangle.
- The desired percentage is subtracted from the higher percentage to give the proportional parts of the lower percentage solution needed (written in the lower right corner).
- The lower percentage is subtracted from the desired percentage to give the proportional parts of the higher percentage solution (written in the upper right corner).
- Once the proportional parts have been determined, the quantities of each component needed for a certain total quantity can be determined by proportion.

To clarify the preceding explanation of alligation, an example of a standard prescription may be helpful. The order calls for 1,000 ml of a parenteral nutrition solution containing 20% dextrose. The most concentrated preparation of dextrose available is a 50% solution. It now must be determined what volume of 50% dextrose must be used to prepare a 20% dextrose solution (Figure 10-2).

The problem is set up as follows:

Twenty parts of $D_{50}W$ mixed with an amino acid and sterile water (0% dextrose) solution yield a 20% dextrose concentration:

$$\frac{\text{parts of 50\% dextrose solution}}{\text{total parts}} = \frac{\text{volume of 50\% dextrose solution}}{\text{total volume}}$$

All quantities are known, except the volume of 50% dextrose needed in the final volume.

$$20 \text{ parts}/50 \text{ parts} = x/1{,}000 \text{ ml}$$
$$50 \text{ parts} \times x = 20 \text{ parts} \times 1{,}000 \text{ ml}$$
$$50x \text{ parts} = 20{,}000 \text{ ml parts}$$
$$50x = 20{,}000 \text{ ml}$$
$$x = 20{,}000 \text{ ml}/50$$
$$= 400 \text{ ml}$$

$$\begin{array}{r} 400 \text{ ml of } 50\% \text{ dextrose solution} \\ +\quad 600 \text{ ml of } 0\% \text{ dextrose solution} \\ \hline = 1{,}000 \text{ ml of } 20\% \text{ dextrose solution} \end{array}$$

(400 ml of the final volume is 50% dextrose solution, making the final volume of 0%, 600 ml)

SYSTEMS OF WEIGHTS AND MEASURES

The most commonly used weights and measures employed in the preparation and calculation of drug dosages are the metric system, the apothecaries' system, and the household system. Although the metric system is the universal standard, the English system, of which avoirdupois, apothecaries', and troy are part, continues to be used. For this reason, the nurse needs to be familiar with both.

The Metric System of Weight and Measurement

The metric system is recognized by the International System of Units (SI) as the standard units of measure and is the most widely used and accepted system employed in the prescription and dosage calculation of medications. Its basic units

Table 10-1 | Units of the Metric System

UNIT	EQUIVALENT
Length	
meter (m)	1 m = 100 cm = 1,000 mm
centimeter (cm)	1 cm = 0.01 m = 10 mm
millimeter (mm)	1 mm = 0.001 m = 0.1 cm
Volume	
liter (L)	1 L = 1,000 ml
milliliter (ml)	1 ml = 0.001 L = 1 cc
cubic centimeter (cc)	1 cc = 1 ml = 0.001 L
Weight	
gram (g)	1 g = 1,000 mg
milligram (mg)	1 mg = 0.001 g = 1,000 mcg
microgram (mcg or μg)	1 mcg = 0.001 mg = 0.000001 g
kilogram (kg)	1 kg = 1,000 g

are the gram, liter, and meter (Table 10-1). The system uses decimals (based on units of ten), so calculations are performed by multiplying or dividing by a power of ten. To use the metric system correctly, the nurse must recognize and understand the prefixes that designate the unit of measurement to be used (e.g., micro-, milli-, centi-, kilo-).

Decimals signify fractional metric units (e.g., $\frac{1}{2}$ is written as 0.5), and a zero always precedes the decimal point for any unit smaller than 1 (e.g., one half is noted as 0.5, rather than .5) to avoid errors in dosing. In this system, the metric abbreviation always follows the numerical measurement (e.g., 1.2 L).

The English System of Weight and Measurement

The English system (so called because it was brought to America by the English colonists) measures length in inches, feet, yards, and miles; weight in ounces, pounds, and tons; and volume in pints, quarts, and gallons for liquid volumes or bushels and pecks for dry volumes. Apothecaries' and household quantities have additional terms. (There is some duplication of unit terminology between the apothecaries' and household systems). Much of this system is used in everyday life and crosses over into health care. There are situations, although infrequent, in which the nurse may be required to convert between the metric, apothecaries', and household systems of measurement.

The Apothecaries' System

The apothecaries' system is an incongruent organization of units for measuring. The name of this system comes from the apothecaries (meaning pharmacists) who determined which plants had medicinal properties, then extracted the smallest amount needed to produce a therapeutic effect. The quantities of herbs and drug products were based on comparisons with common objects and terms: dram, meaning a small amount of anything; grain, meaning the size of a grain of wheat; minim, the smallest amount of anything; and scruple, meaning a small, sharp stone. Volume is measured in minims, fluid drams, fluid ounces, pints, and gallons, whereas weight is measured in grains, drams, scruples, ounces, and pounds (Table 10-2).

The apothecaries' system is unsystematic, is confusing, and requires memorization to define its components. Lower case Roman numerals represent whole numbers from 1 to 10 (i, ii, iii) and the numbers 20 and 30 (xx and xxx); Arabic numbers are used for all others. For numbers less than one, fractions are used, except $\frac{1}{2}$, which is ss). The unit abbreviation precedes the numerical measurement (e.g., gr. $\frac{1}{4}$ or gr. ii).

The Household System

The household system of weights and measurements, like the apothecaries' system, is inconsistent and requires memorization of its components. It is commonly used among the general population for recipes and measuring products within the home. Conversions are difficult because the standard measuring devices available with household measurements increments have limited ranges. Arabic numbers are used with the abbreviation, which follow the numerical measurement (e.g.,

Table 10-2 | Units of the Apothecaries' System

UNIT	EQUIVALENT
Liquid Volume	
minim (♏)	60 minims = 1 fluidram (inaccurate for measurement; referenced for the purpose of recognition)
fluidram (ʒ)	8 fluidrams = 1 fluidounce
fluidounce (℥)	16 fluidounces = 1 pint
pint (pt.)	2 pints = 1 quart
quart (qt.)	4 quarts = 1 gallon
gallon (gal.)	1 gallon = 4 quarts = 128 ounces
Weight	
grain (gr.)	60 grains = 1 dram
dram (dr.)	8 drams = 1 ounce

1 tsp.). The main benefit of this system in nursing care is to use terms patients understand and use in the home (Table 10-3). It is the least accurate of the measurement systems and is not used for intravenous calculations. The drop, which is a unit of household measurement, is used in infusion therapy. Its size, however, cannot be standardized because it is dependent on the diameter of the line from which it is dispensed.

Occasionally the nurse may encounter situations in which conversions between the metric, apothecaries', or household systems are necessary. Table 10-4 lists the commonly used equivalents between these systems.

Other Systems of Weight and Measurement

The nurse will encounter two other systems in calculating infusions: the unit and milliequivalent systems. These are frequently used to prescribe specific amounts of infusion admixtures.

The Unit System of Measurement

Synthetically made medications are manufactured under strictly controlled conditions and are very pure. Their

Table 10-3 | Units of the Household Measurement System

UNIT	EQUIVALENT
Length	
inch (in.)	12 inches = 1 foot
foot (ft.)	3 feet = 1 yard
yard (yd.)	
Volume	
drop (gtt.)	60 to 75 gtts. = 1 tsp. (inaccurate for measurement; referenced for the purpose of recognition)
teaspoon (tsp.)	3 tsp. = 1 tbsp. = ½ fl. oz.
tablespoon (tbsp. or T.)	2 tbsp. = 1 fl. oz.
ounce (oz.)	8 fl. oz. = 1 C.
cup (C.); glass (gl.)	2 C./gl. = 1 pt. = 16 fl. oz.
pint (pt.)	2 pt. = 1 qt. = 32 fl. oz.
quart (qt.)	4 qt. = 1 gal. = 128 fl. oz.
gallon (gal.)	1 gal. = 128 fl. oz.
Weight	
ounce (oz.)	16 oz. = 1 lb.
pound (lb.)	

Table 10-4 | Commonly Used Equivalents Among the Metric, Apothecaries', and Household Systems of Weights and Measurements

METRIC	APOTHECARIES'	HOUSEHOLD
Dry Weight		
60 mg to 65 mg	gr. i	
1 g	gr. xv	
15 g	drams iv (½ oz.)	½ oz.
30 g	drams viii (1 oz.)	1 oz.
	16 oz.	1 lb.
1 kg		2.2 lb.
Liquid Volume		
	1 minim*	1 gtt.*
1 ml	15–16 minims*	15–16 gtts.*
4 ml to 5 ml	fluidram i	¾ tsp.
5 ml	75 minims*	1 tsp.
30 ml	1 fluidounce (8 fluidrams)	1 fl. oz. (2 T.)
500** ml	16 fluidounces (1 pint)	16 fl. oz. (1 pt., 2 C.)
1,000*** ml	32 fluidounces (1 quart)	32 fl. oz. (1 qt.)
Length		
2.5 cm		1 in.
1 m		39.4 in.

*Minims and drops are inaccurate for measurement; referenced here for the purpose of recognition

**Rounded up from 473 ml

***Rounded up from 946 ml

potency can be accurately regulated and they are measured by weight.

Medications that are derived from biologic sources vary in potency and purity, depending on the source. Because of this variation, they are measured in units of activity instead of units of weight. They are expressed in United States Pharmacopeia or USP units, or international units (IU). A unit is a standard that represents a quantity equivalent to a particular weight of pure drug. Medications customarily quantified in units are heparin, insulin, penicillin, and some vitamins.

The Milliequivalent System of Measurement

The milliequivalent (mEq) measurement is used to express the concentration of electrolytes in a specified volume of solution. It is represented as milliequivalents per liter (mEq/L). By representing electrolytes in milliequivalents, the number of ions and their electrical charges (which measures their chemical combining ability) is expressed. One mEq of any cation (positively charged particle) is chemically equivalent to one mEq of any anion (negatively charged particle). The weight of a chemical has no relation to its chemical activity (e.g., 1 mEq of Na^+ [23 mg] combined with 1 mEq of Cl^- [35 mg] equals 1 mEq of NaCl.) For this reason, electrolytes are expressed in milliequivalents instead of weight in milligrams.

INTRAVENOUS INFUSION CALCULATIONS

When calculating intravenous infusion dosages and rates, the nurse may use multistep formulas or dimensional analysis. The method used is not important as long as the problem is set up correctly and the final calculation is accurate. If there is any doubt regarding the accuracy of a dosage or rate, the nurse must verify it with a pharmacist or another nurse.

When an infusion is ordered, it is written so that the prescribed volume of fluid will be administered over a determined time period. When calculating the rate for gravity flow, it is essential to know what the drop factor is, as the final delivery rate will be stated in drops per minute. Remember, the drop factor, which is specific to the administration set tubing, determines how much infusate is delivered in each drop. When an electronic infusion device (EID) is used, the volume (in milliliters per hour) is calculated and the machine is set to control the flow rate. Even though an infusion regulator is used, the nurse is still responsible for establishing the correct rate and maintaining it.

When calculating infusion rates, milliliters per hour, milliliters per minute, and drops per minute must all be considered. When using the multistep procedure, separate formulas are set up for each phase. When using dimensional analysis, a one-step formula is used for the entire process.

Multistep Calculation Formulas

When using the multistep method, a separate mathematical process is used to calculate the hourly rate (if appropriate), the rate per minute, and the drops per minute. When gravitational flow is calculated, rounding off is necessary.

Rounding Off

To accurately set up a problem, the hourly and minute rates are carried three places to the right of the decimal point and rounded off to two places. For drops per minute, since a portion of a drop cannot be measured, the number is rounded off to the nearest whole. The rule for rounding off to a whole number is as follows:

1. When the amount following the decimal point is less than 5, the whole number stays the same. For example, 1.49 (or less) rounds off to 1.

2. When the amount following the decimal point is 5 or more, it is necessary to round off (up) to the next whole number. For example, 1.51 rounds off to the next whole number, which is 2.

The rule for rounding off the places to the right of the decimal point, when calculating gravity flow infusion rates, is as follows:

1. Work the problem to three places to the right of the decimal point, and round off to two places.

2. When the third number to the right of the decimal point is less than 5, the second number stays the same. For example, 1.333 rounds off to 1.33.

3. When the third number to the right of the decimal point is 5 or more, the second number increases by one increment. For example, 1.666 rounds off to 1.67.

Milliliters Per Hour

To determine an infusion rate in milliliters per hour (ml/hr), it is necessary to divide the total volume (V) by the total time

(T). The formula is $V \div T = R$, where R is the rate:

$$\frac{V\,(ml)}{T\,(ml)} = R\,(ml/hr)$$

Examples:

1. Infuse 3,000 ml of D₅W IV over the next 24 hours.
   3,000 ml ÷ 24 hr = 125 ml/hr
2. Infuse 1,000 ml of D₅$\frac{1}{2}$NS IV in 10 hours.
   1,000 ml ÷ 10 hr = 100 ml/hr
3. Infuse 1,000 ml NS IV in 6 hours.
   1,000 ml ÷ 6 hr = (166.666) 166.67 ml/hr

If an infusion is ordered for a period of less than one hour, this first step is omitted. Such would be the case with the intermittent administration of an infusate (such as an antibiotic, mixed in 50 to 100 ml of normal saline that is given every 6 hr) ordered to infuse over a 30-minute period.

Milliliters Per Minute

To determine milliliters per minute (ml/min) it is necessary to multiply the number of hours of an ordered infusion by the number of minutes in an hour (60) and divide that number into the total volume. The formula is $V \div T$ (hr × 60 min) = R, milliliters per minute:

$$\frac{V\,(in\ ml)}{T\,(hr \times 60\ min)} = R\,(ml/min)$$

Examples:

1. Infuse 3,000 ml of D₅W over the next 24 hours.
   3,000 ml ÷ (24 hr × 60 min) = 3,000 ml ÷ 1,440 min
   = (2.083) 2.08 ml/min
2. Infuse 1,000 ml D₅$\frac{1}{2}$NS over the next 10 hours.
   1,000 ml ÷ (10 hr × 60 min) = 1,000 ml ÷ 600 min =
   (1.666) 1.67 ml/min
3. Infuse 1,000 ml NS in 6 hours.
   1,000 ml ÷ (6 hr × 60 min) = 1,000 ml ÷ 360 min =
   (2.777) 2.78 ml/min
4. Cefotetan 1 g q 12 hr IV per heparin lock.
   The drug is mixed with 0.9% NaCl in a 50-ml, single-use bag. (The nurse knows that this medication is usually infused over a 20- to 30-minute period.)
   50 ml ÷ 20 min = 2.5 ml/min
   50 ml ÷ 30 min = (1.666) 1.67 ml/min

Flow Rate in Drops Per Minute

To determine the drops per minute (gtts./min) of any infusion, it is necessary to know the drop factor, which is stated on the administration set package. The rate in drops per

minute is found by dividing the total volume by the total time, in minutes, and multiplying that number by the drop factor. The formula is $V \div T$ (min) × C (C = drop factor calibration) = R:

$$\frac{V\,(ml)}{T\,(min)} \times C = R\,(gtts./min)$$

Examples:

1. Infuse 3,000 ml D₅W IV over the next 24 hours.
   Drop factor (C) = 10.
   1,000 ml ÷ 24 hr = 125 ml/hr
   1,000 ml ÷ (24 hr × 60 min) = 2.08 ml/min
   2.08 ml/min × 10 gtts./ml = (20.8) 21 gtts./min
2. Infuse 1,000 ml D₅$\frac{1}{2}$NS IV over the next 10 hours.
   Drop factor = 15.
   1,000 ml ÷ 10 hr = 100 ml/hr
   1,000 ml ÷ (10 hr × 60 min) = 1.67 ml/min
   1.67 ml/min × 15 gtts./ml = (25.05) 25 gtts./min
3. Infuse 1,000 ml NS IV over the next 6 hours.
   Drop factor = 15.
   1,000 ml ÷ 6 hr = 166.67 ml/hr
   1,000 ml ÷ (6 hr × 60 min) = 2.78 ml/min
   2.78 ml/min × 15 gtts./ml = (41.7) 42 gtts./min
4. Cefotetan 1 g q 12 hr IV per heparin lock. (The drug comes mixed in 0.9% NaCl in a 50-ml, single-use bag. It is normally administered over a 20-minute period.)
   Drop factor = 10.
   50 ml ÷ 20 min = 2.5 ml/min
   2.5 ml/min × 10 gtts./ml = 25 gtts./min

Shortening the Three-Step Method

There is a shorter way to determine the rate of an infusion, by incorporating the first two steps (time in hours and minutes) and adding the drop factor to the formula. This is done by calculating the total infusion time in minutes before a formula is set up. For example, if an IV order is for 1,000 ml of fluid to infuse in 8 hr, the minutes are calculated as (8 hr × 60 min) 480, and the formula is set up as $V \div T \times C$, with C = 10. The single formula would read, 1,000 ml ÷ 480 min × 10 gtts./ml = (20.83) 21 gtts./min:

$$\frac{\overset{25}{\cancel{1,000}}\ ml}{\underset{12}{\cancel{480}}\ min} \times 10\ gtts./ml = (20.83)\ 21\ gtts./min$$

Examples:

1. 1,000 ml D₅W IV to infuse over the next 4 hours.
   Drop factor = 10.

1,000 ml ÷ 240 min × 10 gtts./ml = (41.67)
42 gtts./min

2. 2,000 ml LR IV to infuse over the next 24 hours.
Drop factor = 15.
2,000 ml ÷ 1,440 min × 15 gtts./ml = (20.83)
21 gtts./min

3. 3,000 ml $D_5\frac{1}{2}NS$ IV to infuse over the next 20 hours.
Drop factor = 15.
3,000 ml ÷ 1,200 min × 15 gtts./ml = (37.5)
38 gtts./min

4. Infuse 2 units (250 ml each) packed RBCs over the next 4 hours.
Drop factor = 20.
500 ml ÷ 240 min × 20 gtts./ml = (41.67)
42 gtts./min

Regulating the Infusion

Once the rate in drops per minute is established and rounded off, the nurse must then regulate the IV. The best way to do this is to divide the number of drops per minute by four, to roughly initiate the rate for a quarter of a minute (15 sec). For example, if the rate of infusion is 42 gtts./min, the 15-second rate would be (42 ÷ 4) 10.5, or approximately 11 drops per 15 seconds. The nurse should then place a watch with a second hand close to the drip chamber and roughly regulate the rate over a 15-second period (Figure 10-3). Once the preliminary rate is established, the nurse can fine-tune the rate over a period of 30 to 60 seconds. The nurse must recheck the rate periodically to ascertain that it is infusing as scheduled.

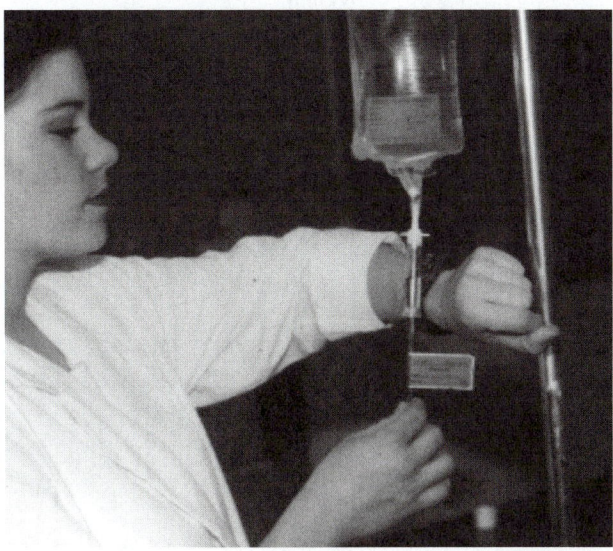

Figure 10-3 | The nurse regulates a gravity flow infusion with the second hand of a watch held adjacent to the drip chamber.

The Dimensional Analysis Method of Calculation

Dimensional analysis, also known as the factor labeling method, is a logical, systematic approach to problem-solving that does not require the memorization of terms or the learning of formulas. It is schematically organized on the basis of the ratio proportion system, but is set up so that one equation rather than several can be used to solve nearly any kind of problem. The unit measurement labels of the ratios are referred to as factors. Equations are set up starting with the unit of the answer so there is little confusion encountered in solving problems.

Dimensional analysis is based on the **factor**, which is a quantity or number that has a related unit of measurement. An example of a factor is 60 seconds equals 1 minute, with the number of seconds being the quantity and the unit of measurement being the minute. In this system, the factors are set up as a series of ratios systematically sequenced into a fractional equation. Conversion factors, which are the "knowns," are always equal to each other (e.g., 60 sec = 1 min, 12 in. = 1 ft., 30 ml = 1 oz., etc.) and are conversions that must be committed to memory.

Within the system of dimensional analysis the equation factors are also related. For each factor in a problem there is a corresponding factor, usually set up adjacent to it, that uses the same unit of measurement. Factors are usually separated from one another by a multiplication sign (×). If there is a quantity and measurement unit in an equation without a related counterpart, that factor is placed as a numerator, with a denominator of 1.

When using the dimensional analysis approach to problem solving, start with the unit of the answer (e.g., drops per minute) and then work backward, using all of the conversion factors ("knowns"). Remember that the factors must always be set up as fractions. Three steps are then used to find the answer: (1) multiplication of the numerator and (2) multiplication of the denominator, followed by (3) division of the numerator by the denominator.

Flow Rate Calculations

To calculate the flow rate of any infusion, the nurse must know the total volume to be infused, the total time for administration, and the drop factor. When using the dimensional analysis approach, he must also have committed to memory the necessary conversion factors. The following sample problems illustrate how to calculate flow rates using the factor labeling process in milliliters per hour, in milliliters per minute, and in drops per minute.

Milliliters Per Hour

When calculating the hourly rate, the unit of the answer is milliliters per hour. The framework for the equation, therefore, is ml/hr. The factors are volume in ml and time in hours. The equation is as follows:

$$\text{ml/hr} = \frac{\text{total volume in milliliters}}{\text{total time in hours}}$$

Examples:

1. Order: 1,000 ml D$_5$W IV q 8 hours.
   Calculate the hourly rate.

$$\frac{\text{ml}}{\text{hr}} = \frac{\overset{125}{\cancel{1,000}} \text{ ml}}{\underset{1}{\cancel{8}} \text{ hr}} = \frac{125 \text{ ml}}{1 \text{ hr}} = 125 \text{ ml/hr}$$

2. Order: 2,000 ml D$_{5}\frac{1}{2}$NS over the next 24 hours.
   Calculate the hourly rate.

$$\frac{\text{ml}}{\text{hr}} = \frac{\overset{\mathbf{250}}{\cancel{2,000}} \text{ ml}}{\underset{\mathbf{3}}{\cancel{24}} \text{ hr}} = (83.33) \; 83 \text{ ml/hr}$$

Milliliters Per Minute

To calculate the rate of an infusion in minutes, the unit of the answer is milliliters per minute. The framework for the equation is ml/min. The factors are the volume in ml and the time in minutes. In this case, conversion factors must be used to convert hours to minutes:

$$\frac{\text{ml}}{\text{min}} = \frac{\text{ml}}{\text{hr}} \times \frac{1 \text{ hr}}{60 \text{ min}}$$

Examples:

1. Order: 1,000 ml D$_5$W IV q 8 hr.
   Calculate the rate in minutes.

$$\frac{\text{ml}}{\text{min}} = \frac{\overset{\overset{25}{125}}{\cancel{1,000}} \text{ ml}}{\underset{1}{\cancel{8}} \text{ hr}} \times \frac{1 \text{ hr}}{\underset{12}{\cancel{60}} \text{ min}} = 2.08 \text{ ml/min}$$

2. Order: 500 ml LR IV over the next 6 hours.
   Calculate the rate in minutes.

$$\frac{\text{ml}}{\text{min}} = \frac{\overset{\overset{25}{250}}{\cancel{500}} \text{ ml}}{\underset{3}{\cancel{6}} \text{ hr}} \times \frac{1 \text{ hr}}{\underset{6}{\cancel{60}} \text{ min}} = \frac{25 \text{ ml}}{18 \text{ min}} = 1.39 \text{ ml/min}$$

Drops Per Minute

To calculate the flow rate of an infusion, the unit of the answer is in drops per minute (gtts./min). The factors are the volume in ml, the time in minutes, the drop factor, and the hour-to-minute conversion factor.

Sample Calculations:

Calculate the flow rate in drops per minute for the following infusion orders.

Infuse 1,000 ml D$_5$W IV over the next 8 hours.
Drop factor = 10.

$$\frac{\overset{1}{\cancel{10}} \text{ gtts.}}{\cancel{1} \text{ ml}} \times \frac{\overset{125}{\cancel{1,000}} \text{ ml}}{\cancel{8} \text{ hr}} \times \frac{\cancel{1} \text{ hr}}{\underset{6}{\cancel{60}} \text{ min}} = (20.83) \; 21 \text{ gtts./min}$$

Infuse 800 ml D$_5$W 0.45 NaCl IV for 10 hours.
Drop factor = 15.

$$\frac{\overset{1}{\cancel{15}} \text{ gtts.}}{\cancel{1} \text{ ml}} \times \frac{\overset{\overset{20}{\cancel{80}}}{\cancel{800}} \text{ ml}}{\underset{1}{\cancel{10}} \text{ hr}} \times \frac{\cancel{1} \text{ hr}}{\underset{\underset{1}{4}}{\cancel{60}} \text{ min}} = 20 \text{ gtts./min}$$

Infuse 250 ml D$_5$LR IV over the next 2 hours.
Drop factor = 20.

$$\frac{\overset{1}{\cancel{20}} \text{ gtts.}}{\cancel{1} \text{ ml}} \times \frac{\overset{125}{\cancel{250}} \text{ ml}}{\cancel{2} \text{ hr}} \times \frac{\cancel{1} \text{ hr}}{\underset{3}{\cancel{60}} \text{ min}} = (41.67) \; 42 \text{ gtts./min}$$

Infuse 1,200 ml 0.9% NaCl IV over the next 8 hours.
Drop factor = 20.

$$\frac{\overset{1}{\cancel{20}} \text{ gtts.}}{\cancel{1} \text{ ml}} \times \frac{\overset{\overset{50}{\cancel{150}}}{\cancel{1,200}} \text{ ml}}{\underset{1}{\cancel{8}} \text{ hr}} \times \frac{\cancel{1} \text{ hr}}{\underset{\underset{1}{3}}{\cancel{60}} \text{ min}} = 50 \text{ gtts./min}$$

Infuse 100 ml 0.45% NaCl IV over the next 8 hours.
Drop factor = 60.

$$\frac{\cancel{60} \text{ gtts.}}{\cancel{1} \text{ ml}} \times \frac{\overset{25}{\cancel{100}} \text{ ml}}{\underset{2}{\cancel{8}} \text{ hr}} \times \frac{1 \text{ hr}}{\cancel{60} \text{ min}} = (12.5) \; 13 \text{ gtts./min}$$

Give Zantac 50 mg IV stat in 50 ml 0.9% NaCl over 15 minutes.
Drop factor = 10.

$$\frac{10 \text{ gtts.}}{1 \text{ ml}} \times \frac{\overset{10}{\cancel{50}} \text{ ml}}{\underset{3}{\cancel{15}} \text{ min}} = \frac{100}{3} = (33.33) \ 33 \text{ gtts./min}$$

Give 4 mEq KCl IV diluted in 50 ml 0.9% NaCl over 30 minutes q 6 hr today.
Drop factor = 15.

$$\frac{\overset{1}{\cancel{15}} \text{ gtts.}}{1 \text{ ml}} \times \frac{\overset{25}{\cancel{50}} \text{ ml}}{\underset{\underset{1}{2}}{\cancel{30}} \text{ min}} = 25 \text{ gtts./min}$$

Ampicillin sodium 2 g plus gentamycin, 1.5 mg/kg, in 100 ml 0.9% NaCl, IV over 30 minutes on call to the O.R.
Drop factor = 15.

$$\frac{\overset{1}{\cancel{15}} \text{ gtts.}}{1 \text{ ml}} \times \frac{\overset{50}{\cancel{100}} \text{ ml}}{\underset{\underset{1}{2}}{\cancel{30}} \text{ min}} = 50 \text{ gtts./min}$$

ADJUSTMENT AND RECALCULATION OF FLOW RATES

Various factors can affect the rate of an infusion, especially when it is flowing by gravity alone. It is a major nursing responsibility to ensure that the infusion is delivered and maintained as scheduled, in spite of any obstacles. This can be done only through continuous observation and assessment of the patient, the IV site, the equipment, and the infusion. As is always the case, prevention of erratic flow rates, through meticulous nursing care, is better than having to make up for problems later.

When an infusion inadvertently gets off schedule, it is the responsibility of the nurse to use good judgment and follow established protocols to readjust the flow rate appropriately. Any modification in rate is determined by the patient's condition and diagnosis, the type of infusate being delivered and medications that may be added to it, and institutional policy. The nurse does not arbitrarily speed up or slow down an erratic rate. In general, if the patient's condition warrants it, an infusion may be adjusted to within ±25% of the original rate to put it back on schedule as closely as possible.

When adjusting an infusion, the nurse must recalculate the flow rate, staying within the ±25% limit, so that the remaining volume of infusate is calibrated to infuse within the original time frame. If the original infusion schedule is altered to such a degree that this cannot be done, the physician should be notified for further orders.

The following examples illustrate the steps that are taken to recalculate an infusion.

EXAMPLE 1

Original infusion order: 1,000 ml D_5W IV to infuse over the next 10 hours.

Infusion start time: 1,300 hours

Drop factor	= 10	
Hourly rate	= 100 ml/hr	(1,000 ml ÷ 10 = 100)
Minute rate	= 1.67 ml/min	(100 ml ÷ 60 min = 1.666)
Flow rate	= 17 gtts./min	(1.67 ml × 10 = 16.70)

At 1430 hours, the infusate level is at the 900 ml level. 150 ml should have already infused, leaving 850 ml remaining to infuse over the next 8½ hours. The nurse recalculates the IV as follows:

Hourly rate	= 105.88 ml/hr	(900 ml ÷ 8.5 hr = 105.882)
Minute rate	= 1.77 ml/min	(105.88 ml ÷ 60 min = 1.764)
Flow rate	= 18 gtts./min	(1.77 ml × 10 = 17.70)

This is a safe adjustment based on the fact that 25% of 100 ml = 25 ml, allowing for an increase in hourly volume up to 125 ml/hr (with an adjusted rate of 105.88 ml/hr).

EXAMPLE 2

Original infusion order: 1,000 ml $D_5\frac{1}{2}NS$ IV to infuse over the next 8 hours.

Infusion start time: 0900 hours

Drop factor	= 15	
Hourly rate	= 125 ml/hr	(1,000 ml ÷ 8 hr = 125)
Minute rate	= 2.08 ml/min	(125 ml ÷ 60 min = 2.08)
Flow rate	= 31 gtts./min	(2.08 ml × 15 = 31.20)

At 1200 hours, when the patient returns from x-ray, the nurse notices that the infusion he started 3 hours ago is only at the 850 ml level. By this time, 375 ml should have infused, leaving 625 ml of infusate in the IV bag to infuse over the next 5 hours. He recalculates the IV as follows:

Hourly rate	= 170 ml/hr	(850 ml ÷ 5 hr = 170)
Minute rate	= 2.83 ml/min	(170 ml ÷ 60 sec = 2.83)
Flow rate	= 42 gtts./min	(2.83 ml × 15 = 42.45)

The nurse realizes that this is an unsafe infusion volume, as it exceeds 25% over the originally ordered rate. He makes this decision based on the following calculations:

25% of 125 ml/hr (original hourly rate) = 31.25 ml/hr, allows an increase up to 156.25 ml/hr. The 170 ml/hr rate is, therefore, a 36% increase.

He notifies the physician for further orders.

CALCULATING WITH ACCURACY

In order to deliver the ordered volume of any infusion correctly, the nurse must be able to calculate the rate accurately. He must develop a sound understanding of the measurement systems, conversion factors, and the mathematical processes needed to carry out the required steps. It is important to develop a comfort level with equations, whether using multistep formulas or the dimensional analysis (factor labeling) method. This can be achieved only with practice and memorization of the necessary facts and concepts related to the dosing and delivery of medications and infusions.

There has been controversy in recent years regarding the practicality of using calculators in solving drug dosage problems. Students are now allowed to use them in some nursing programs during clinical practicum rotations or for written classroom examinations. Calculators have not been approved as yet for use during the National Council Licensure Examination for Registered Nurses (NCLEX-RN).

NURSING ALERT

Adjusting an Erratic Flow Rate

The nurse must never arbitrarily speed up or slow down an erratic infusion flow rate. In general, and only if the patient's condition warrants it, an infusion may be adjusted ±25% of the original rate to return it, as closely as possible, to its original schedule. An arbitrary adjustment that is not based on the individual patient's clinical situation may cause harm to the patient.

NURSING TIP

Using a Calculator

It is important to remember that a calculator is only as good as the skill of the person using it. If equations are set up incorrectly on paper, or if data is improperly entered, a calculator is useless. As a general rule, calculators should be used only for checking mathematical formulas. It is also necessary for them to be in good working condition and maintained according to manufacturer's specifications.

Key Concepts

* In order to administer and manage intravenous therapy, the nurse must be able to calculate and regulate infusions correctly.

* The mathematical processes required for infusion calculations include the use of common fractions, decimal fractions, percentages, ratios, and proportions.

* It is necessary for the nurse to differentiate and make conversions between the metric, apothecaries', and household systems of weights and measurements.

* The drop factor is the number of drops needed to deliver 1 ml of fluid and is determined by the diameter of the tubing through which it flows. The drop factor is listed on the administration set package. The nurse cannot calculate the rate of an infusion in drops per minute if the drop factor is unknown.

* Infusion calculations can be performed using multistep formulas or with the dimensional analysis (label factoring) method.

* In the practice of infusion therapy, it is important for the nurse to understand the concepts related to the dosing and delivery of medications and infusates and to develop expertise in using them.

Review Questions and Activities

1. Convert the following units of length, volume, and weight into the listed equivalents:

   gr i   = _____ mg

   1 g   = _____ gr

   1 g   = _____ mg

   1 mg = _____ mcg

   1 kg = _____ g

   1 kg = _____ lb.

   1 ml = _____ cc

   1 tsp. = _____ ml

   1 T   = _____ ml

   1 oz. = _____ ml

   30 ml = _____ oz.

   1 in. = _____ cm

   1 m   = _____ in.

   1 C. = _____ oz.

   1 pt. = _____ oz.

   1 qt. = _____ oz.

   1 gal. = _____ oz.

   1 lb. = _____ oz.

2. Explain the unit system of measurement. Look up the drug insulin in a nurse's drug handbook and list the protocols and precautions for administering it intravenously.

3. Explain the milliequivalent system of measurement. Look up the electrolyte supplement potassium in a nurse's drug handbook and list the protocols and precautions for administering it intravenously.

   Calculate the rates of administration for the following orders, illustrating how you arrive at your answer:

4. 1,000 ml NS IV to infuse over 12 hours.

   Drop factor: 10.

   Give: _____ ml/hr

   _____ ml/min

   _____ gtts./min

5. 500 ml D_5W IV over 6 hours.

   Drop factor: 15.

   Give: _____ ml/hr

   Give: _____ ml/min

   Give: _____ gtts./min

6. 1,200 ml 0.9% NaCl IV over 8 hours.

   Drop factor: 20.

   Give: _____ gtts./min

7. 50 ml Serum Albumin IV stat over 1 hour.

   Drop factor: 10.

   Give: _____ ml/hr

   Give: _____ gtts./min

8. 1,000 ml NS IV over 16 hours.

   Give: _____ ml/hr

   Give: _____ ml/min

   Give: _____ gtts./min (Be careful.)

Recalculate the following:

9. 1,000 ml D_5LR IV over 8 hours.

   Drop factor: 15.

   Give the initial rate in

   _____ ml/hr

   _____ gtts./min

   After 4 hours, 600 ml remain. Recalculate the rate, in

   _____ ml/hr

   _____ gtts./min

   Is this a safe readjustment (using the ±25% guideline)? Show how you determine this.

10. 2,000 ml $D_5\frac{1}{2}NS$ IV over the next 16 hours.

    After 8 hours, 1,400 ml remain. Recalculate the rate, in

    _____ ml/hr

    _____ gtts./min

    Is this a safe readjustment? Show how you determine this.

11. What parameters must the nurse take into consideration when recalculating the rate of an intravenous infusion?

12. At 0600 hours the nurse on the night shift started an IV infusion of D_5LR with 20 mEq KCl added. It was ordered to infuse at 100 ml/hr. The patient was admitted with a diagnosis of pneumonia and influenza. When you go to assess the patient at 0730, after change-of-shift report, you notice that there is only 400 ml left in the IV bag. List, in the appropriate sequence, the measures you would institute in terms of assessment, nursing interventions, reporting, and documentation.

Pharmacologic Principles Related to the Preparation and Administration of Intravenous Medications

COMPETENCIES

Upon completion of this chapter, the reader should be able to:

* Define pharmacokinetics and the processes of drug absorption, bioavailability, distribution, and biotransformation.

* Explain the mechanisms of drug action.

* Review the concepts of plasma concentration times and plasma half-lives.

* Identify how drugs are named and listed.

* Interpret the nurse's role in handling controlled substances.

* List each of the IV medication classifications.

* Differentiate among the mechanisms of action of the antimicrobial agents.

* Review how microbes develop resistance to antimicrobial preparations.

* Examine the precautions associated with intravenous administration of anticonvulsant agents.

* Categorize the cardiovascular agents in terms of their actions, side effects, and the nursing precautions associated with administering them intravenously.

* Relate how the benzodiazepine agents are categorized within several of the medication classifications.

* Interpret the use of compatibility charts for intravenous medication administration.

* Analyze the nurse's roles and responsibilities regarding the intravenous delivery of the agents included in this chapter.

Medications administered intravenously are absorbed directly into the bloodstream without having to pass through other systems or cross tissue membranes. Because the barriers that impede absorption are avoided, blood levels are reached immediately, and absorption is most efficient. Such drugs are administered not only for the treatment of disease processes and to correct homeostatic imbalances, but also are given for palliative and prophylactic purposes.

NURSING TIP

Patient-Family Teaching

It is important to remember that when medications are administered to a person for any reason—prevention, cure, or palliation—it is vital to include patient-family education regarding the drugs as an integral component of treatment. This provides a safety mechanism, fosters patient compliance, and promotes a therapeutic nurse-patient relationship, three factors that are vital to a beneficial outcome.

PHARMACOKINETICS AND MECHANISMS OF DRUG ACTION

Pharmacokinetics is the study of drug action and metabolism and relates to the disposition of drugs in the body. It deals with the mechanisms and processes of uptake and absorption, biotransformation, local and systemic distribution, duration of action, and excretion (Figure 11-1).

Drug **absorption** is the passage of a drug through a body surface into the tissues and the bloodstream. **Distribution** is the process whereby the drug is transported to its intended site. **Bioavailability** refers to the actual amount of the drug (as distinct from the amount administered) that enters the general circulation available for use. With the intravenous route of administration, the bioavailability of a drug is most comparable to its original potency and the dose administered. Bioavailability varies considerably with other routes of administration.

Drug Action

Drug action refers to the interaction of any therapeutic agent within the body and its physiochemical alteration (effects) of existing bodily processes to bring about a therapeutic effect. The most common method of drug action is through chemical bonding via target cell–receptor site interaction. Other processes, such as enzymatic interaction, cellular process alteration, chemical composition change, or metabolic pathway blockade, also relate to drug action modalities.

Drug Action through Target Cell–Receptor Site Interaction

The site of action where a drug exerts its effect is called a **target cell**. The target cell has a specific location called a receptor site where the drug interacts by forming a chemical bond in a lock-and-key type union (Figure 11-2). When the molecules of a drug fit exactly into (have an affinity for) the receptor site, a predictable therapeutic response results. If the fit is not precise, the response may be weak or ineffective (Figure 11-3).

A drug that fits and interacts with a receptor site to produce a response, thus imitating the body's own regulatory function, is called an **agonist**. To be categorized as an agonist, a drug must have two main qualities: affinity and

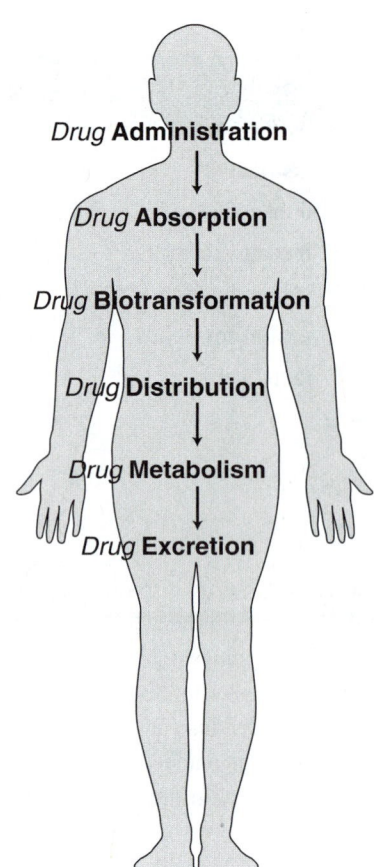

Figure 11-1 │ Pharmacokinetic processes in the body

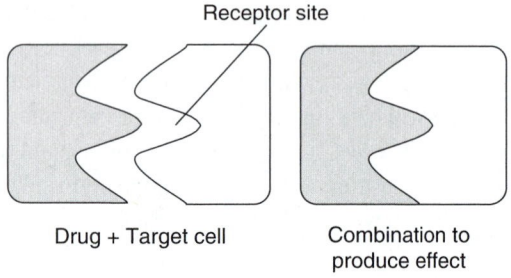

Figure 11-2 │ Lock-and-key union of drug and receptor

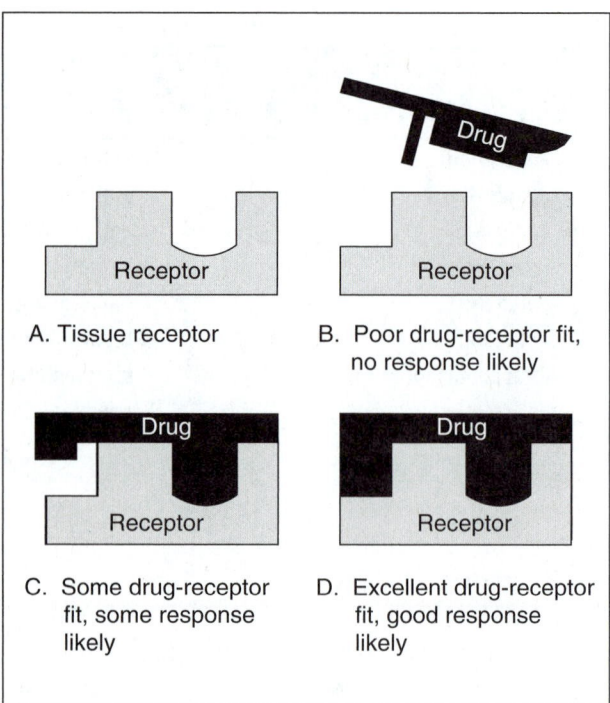

Figure 11-3 │ Drug-receptor interaction

is an **antagonist** (a receptor blocker). It may have an affinity for the site but lacks the efficacy to elicit a response (much like a key that fits into a lock, but does not open the door).

An agonist-antagonist is a drug that expends agonistic and antagonistic properties by associating with the target receptor site to invoke some pharmacologic response, while at the same time antagonizing other agonists that combine with the same receptor. There is competition between the two drugs for receptor sites. The agonist-antagonist relationship can in some instances be overcome by increasing the agonist dose.

Drug Action through Enzymatic Interaction

An enzyme, remember, is an action-specific catalyst that induces cellular biochemical changes by acting on a substrate (without being changed itself). An enzyme's catalytic energy can be inhibited by the action of certain drugs that are chemically designed to mimic the enzyme's substrate, thus blocking the enzyme's normal function. The enzyme, then, combines with the drug (called an antimetabolite) instead of its substrate. An example of such a drug is neostigmine (Prostigmin Injection).

In the neuromuscular disease myasthenia gravis, nerve impulses fail to activate muscular contraction owing to a deficiency of the neurotransmitter acetylcholine (substrate) or an excess of cholinesterase, the enzyme that catalyzes

efficacy. *Affinity* is the characteristic whereby the agonist molecule is able to attach to, interact with, or occupy a particular receptor site. *Efficacy* refers to the agonist's capability to elicit a response once it encounters the site. There are many endogenous, or naturally occurring, agonists within the body that, under normal circumstances, control various functions. These include, but are not limited to, autocoids (local modulators, such as histamine and prostaglandins), hormones, and neurotransmitters.

Any drug that interacts with the receptor site but does not cause a response or hinders or averts the action of an agonist

acetylcholinesterase (the enzyme that breaks down acetylcholine). Neostigmine, an enzyme-blocking agent, works by combining with (and thus inhibiting) the enzyme acetylcholinesterase to prevent it from inactivating acetylcholine at the myoneural junction.

Drug Action through Cellular Process Alteration

Some drugs can pass through the pores in the cellular membrane while others act by infiltration of the cell membrane or permeation of the cell itself. Because of the lipoprotein composition of the cell membrane, drugs with structural similarities, such as lipid-soluble compounds, are able to alter cellular membrane properties and gain entrance. Many of the intravenous barbiturates and anesthetic agents fall into this category. They are high water-oil soluble emulsions that are able to reach equilibrium between the blood and the brain. Their duration of action, however, is short, because they are easily redistributed into fat deposits within the body. The amount of body fat is inversely proportional to the duration of drug action, so the greater amount of adipose tissue, the shorter the duration of sedation and vice versa.

Drug Action through Physiochemical Composition Changes

Some drugs exert their effect by chemically altering the composition of body fluids. These may alter the pH by raising or lowering acidity or alkalinity levels. Examples would be ammonium chloride to treat metabolic alkalosis and sodium bicarbonate or lactate to treat acidosis.

Other drugs act by physically increasing or decreasing osmotic pressure. The osmotic diuretic mannitol, for example, increases urine production by increasing the osmolarity of the glomerular filtrate (which, in turn, decreases the reabsorption of water while increasing the excretion of sodium and chloride ions) and the plasma (which enhances the movement of water from the tissues into the intestines).

Drug Action through Metabolic Pathway Alteration

Some drugs act by altering the metabolic processes of certain cells. Such is the case with many antibiotics, which act on bacterial cells and destroy them. The antineoplastic drugs modify cellular processes by blocking genetic pathways. Others block the metabolic pathways, the release, or the re-uptake of certain neurotransmitters or autocoids. By doing this, they interfere with or obstruct the usual action of these substances on certain tissues and body systems.

Biotransformation

Biotransformation, or biodegradation, refers to the metabolism of a drug within the body. It involves the chemical alterations in pharmacologic activity that the drug undergoes once it enters the body in order to be chemically transformed or broken down. The process of metabolism limits the duration of a drug's action by inactivating it and converting it into a form that allows it to be excreted from the body. The most common site of drug biotransformation is the liver, but other organs are also involved. The kidneys, lungs, intestines, and blood plasma all collaborate to metabolize a drug so that it can be excreted.

Drug components are predominately eliminated from the body via the kidneys. The molecules may be inactivated, modified, or unchanged (from their original form) prior to excretion. If there is any metabolic delay or malfunction, drug cumulation may occur. This can result in an excessive or sustained drug response.

Intravenous Time-Response Reactions

When describing the action of drugs in the body, two expressions are used. One is the plasma concentration time and the other is the plasma half-life. Both are measured in hourly intervals.

With any method of medication administration, the quantity of a given drug rises, reaches a peak plasma level (time of maximum effect), and then begins to steadily decline. The time interval between the onset of action and the peak action varies, depending on the route used. The plasma concentration time is a graphic depiction of the time it takes for a drug to reach its peak plasma level following administration (Figure 11-4). With intravenous administration, the maximum effect is achieved immediately, whereas the time varies considerably when other routes are used.

When a drug is given over a period of time and at constant intervals, the plasma concentration reaches a uniform level and does not deviate until the drug is discontinued or changes are made in the administration schedule. If the drug is given at scheduled intervals, the peak plasma concentration occurs immediately following administration and the minimum level (trough) occurs just before the next dose is administered. It is very important for the nurse to understand this concept, because peak and trough blood levels are often ordered for patients receiving antibiotic therapy. The nurse must be sure that blood is drawn immediately following the administration of one dose and then again immediately preceding the administration of the next dose, so that accurate results are obtained.

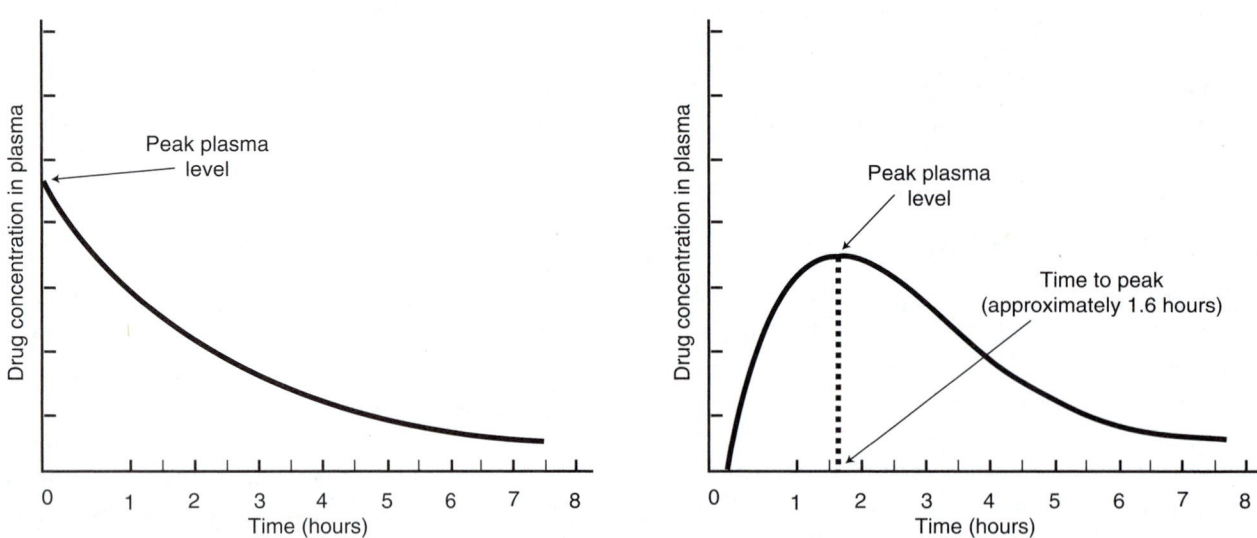

Figure 11-4 | Comparison of drug concentrations in plasma following single oral and intravenous bolus administration

---

NURSING TIP

Applying the Peak and Trough Blood Level Concept

It is very important for the nurse to understand this concept because peak and trough blood levels are often ordered for patients, especially those receiving antibiotic therapy. If accurate results are to be obtained, the nurse must ensure that the peak blood sample is drawn immediately following the administration of one dose and that the trough specimen is drawn immediately before the next dose is given.

The half-life refers to the time it takes for the body to metabolize and eliminate one half of the original concentration of an administered drug. It is abbreviated $t_{1/2}$. This is a very important consideration in determining safe adminis-

tration doses. After the first dose of a drug is administered, the subsequent doses are scheduled in accord with the half-life. For example, if the half-life of an antibiotic is 4 hours, the rate at which the concentration of the drug diminishes in the body is as follows:

Initial bolus	100 %
After 4 hours	50 %
After 8 hours	25 %
After 12 hours	12.5 %
After 16 hours	6.25 %
After 20 hours	3.125 %
After 24 hours	1.56 %

DRUG NAMES

Drug names are categorized by their chemical, generic, and brand names (Table 11-1). The chemical name of a drug

---

Table 11-1 | Drug Names

CHEMICAL NAME	NONPROPRIETARY NAME (GENERIC NAME)	PROPRIETARY NAME (BRAND OR TRADE NAME)
2,6-diisopropylphenol	propofol	Diprivan®
p-amino-N-[2-(diethylamino)ethyl]benzamide monohydrochloride	procainamide hydrochloride	Pronestyl®

delineates its molecular and chemical structure in terms of the names, numbers, and proportions of its elements. It is mainly of value to pharmaceutical chemists and is rarely used by nurses and clinical pharmacists. The generic name, more appropriately called the nonproprietary name, is the singular identification term assigned to every commercially produced pharmacologic product. The nonproprietary listing is the universal nomenclature for distinguishing one drug from another. The brand, or trade, name is the proprietary name of a drug. It is the trademarked name given to every product made by a specific manufacturer. There may be many different trade names for the same nonproprietary drug (e.g., the anti-infective vancomycin hydrochloride [nonproprietary/generic name], may be labeled with the brand names Lyphocin, Vancocin, or Vancoled). The brand name usually has the sign ® or ™, indicating that it is registered for use or trademarked by a particular pharmaceutical company.

When two drugs are combined, the resulting product is called a **combination drug**. The combination drug has a brand name, but usually no generic name, even though it is made up of two nonproprietary drugs.

INTRAVENOUS DRUG CLASSIFICATIONS

Every drug is categorized by one of two means. It may be classified according to its indication for use and therapeutic action or classified according to the body system(s) on which it exerts its effect. Intravenous drugs are most appropriately classified using the first method. Table 11-2 lists the most commonly used classifications of medications administered intravenously.

Adrenergic Agents

The term *adrenergic* pertains to the effects of sympathetic nervous system stimulation resulting from the release of epinephrine (from the adrenal medulla) and norepinephrine (liberated from postganglionic adrenergic nerve fibers). There are sites in the autonomic nerve pathways known as alpha(α)-adrenergic receptors, where excitatory reactions occur in response to adrenergic agents. Those sites where inhibitory responses to these agents occur are the beta(β)-adrenergic receptors.

Adrenergic drugs, also called sympathomimetics, imitate the action of the hormonal neurotransmitters epinephrine and norepinephrine, thus bringing about sympathetic nervous system activation. They may exert their action,

depending on their degree of selectivity for specific adrenergic receptors, through the following:

1. Central nervous system stimulation
2. Increased glycogenolysis and lipolysis
3. Increased cardiac contractility (positive inotropic effect)
4. Increased cardiac rate (positive chronotropic effect)
5. Increased cardiac conduction (positive dromotropic effect)
6. Increased cardiac electrical impulse generation (automaticity)
7. Increased renin secretion
8. Vasoconstriction of peripheral blood vessels
9. Vasodilation of skeletal muscle blood vessels

NURSING ALERT

Adrenergic Drug Metabolism

It is extremely important for the nurse to understand how adrenergic drugs are metabolized and distributed, and how they affect the body as a whole. The nurse must always keep in mind that they are associated with multisystem side effects and interactions with other drugs that can be serious or life-threatening.

Analgesic Agents

Analgesic drugs are given to relieve pain, usually without altering consciousness, and are administered intravenously for perioperative patients or those who cannot tolerate other routes of administration. The analgesics given IV are usually the opioid and some potent, nonopioid analgesics used in the treatment of moderate to severe pain that is generally visceral in origin.

The opioids, most of which are now synthetically produced copies of opium compounds, work by binding with opioid receptors in the CNS, thus inhibiting the transmission of pain impulses. Five receptors have been identified, the mu (μ), kappa (κ), sigma (σ), delta (δ), and epsilon (ϵ), with the drug action of the opioid analgesics concentrated in the first three:

1. Mu (μ) receptor:
   controls morphinelike effects of analgesia, euphoria, and respiratory depression.
2. Kappa (κ) receptor:
   controls spinal analgesia, sedation, and miosis.

Table 11-2 │ Intravenous Medications Classified According to their Indications for Use and Therapeutic Actions

CLASSIFICATION	CATEGORIES	CLASSIFICATION	CATEGORIES
Adrenergic Agents (sympathomimetic agents)	Catecholamines	Diuretics	Proximal tubule diuretics Diluting segment diuretics Loop diuretics Distal tubule diuretics Osmotic diuretics
Analgesic Agents	Opioid analgesics Nonopioid analgesics	Electrolytes	
Anesthetic Agents	Nonbarbiturates Short-acting barbiturates	Hematologic Agents	Anticoagulants Hemorheologic agents Hemostatic agents Thrombolytic agents (fibrinolytic agents) Tissue plasminogen activator
Anticoagulation Agents			
Anticonvulsant Agents	Barbiturates Benzodiazepines Hydantoins Magnesium sulfate	Histamine H-2 Antagonists	
		Hormones	Pituitary Thyroid Parathyroid Adrenal Pancreas Ovarian Testicular Pineal
Antiemetic-Antinauseant Agents			
Antimicrobials and Anti-infectives	Aminoglycosides Antifungal agents Antiparasitic agents Antiprotozoal agents Antiretrovirals Antiviral agents Beta-Lactams Carbapenems Cephalosporins Fluorquinolones (quinolones) Macrolides Monobactams Penicillins (and penicillin-related antibiotics) Sulfonamides Tetracyclines Miscellaneous	Hypnotics and Sedatives	Barbiturates Benzodiazepines
		Immunobiologic Regulators	Biologic response modifiers Immunostimulants Immunosuppressants
		Muscle Relaxants	Centrally acting skeletal muscle relaxants Neuromuscular blockers

		Nutritional Agents	Carbohydrates
			Fats
			Proteins
			Minerals
			Organic salts
			Trace elements
			   aluminum fluorine nickel
			   bromine iodine silicon
			   chromium iron zinc
			   copper manganese
			Vitamins

Anti-Inflammatory Agents	Steroidal Nonsteroidal		
Antihistamines			
Antineoplastic Agents	Alkylating agents Antibiotics Antimetabolites Hormones Plant alkaloids Miscellaneous		A (carotene) C (ascorbic acid) B_1 (thiamine) D B_2 (riboflavin) E (alpha tocopherol) B_6 (pyridoxine) folacin B_{12} (cyanocobalamin) niacin
Anxiolytic Agents	Barbiturates Benzodiazepines		
Cardiovascular Agents	Antidysrhythmic agents Antihypertensives Cardiac glycosides Cardiac stimulants	Respiratory Agents	Antitussives Bronchodilators (adrenergic agents and theophylline derivatives) Decongestants Expectorants Mucolytics
Cholinergic Agents (parasympathomimetic agents)	Direct-acting Indirect-acting		
Diagnostic Agents	Biologic in vivo agents Nonbiologic in vivo agents In vitro diagnostic agents Radiographic contrasts	Volume Expanders	Dextran Hetastarch

3. Sigma (σ) receptor:
controls hallucinatory activity, respiratory stimulation, and vasomotor excitement.

N U R S I N G   A L E R T

Opioid Side Effects

The main side effect—a potentially serious one—associated with the use of opioids is respiratory depression. The nurse must carefully assess the breathing status of any patient receiving these agents. Should any problems develop, the opioid antagonist naloxone (Narcan) must be administered intravenously. Opioids also are associated with problems of tolerance and dependence.

Drugs similar chemically and pharmacologically to the opioids but with fewer problems associated with dependence and abuse are the nonopioid analgesics. (They are not free of dependence-related problems, however, and so still must be used with caution.) Those nonopioids commonly administered intravenously are buprenorphine HCl, butorphanol tartrate, dezocine, and nalbuphine HCl. In general, to exert their effect they should be administered before pain becomes severe.

Controlled Substances

Because of the identified potential for physical and psychologic dependence and abuse, certain drugs are controlled, that is, regulated by law with regard to possession and use. These drugs are categorized under the governmental Controlled Substances Act of 1970.

N U R S I N G   T I P

Legal and Ethical Guidelines for Controlled Substances

Scheduled substances are manufactured, prescribed, dispensed, and administered under carefully controlled regulations. There are many legal and ethical guidelines the nurse must adhere to in terms of storage, handling, disposal, and documentation. Many drugs administered intravenously for purposes of analgesia, anesthesia, anxiety, hypnosis, and sedation fall under the Controlled Substances Act.

Anesthetic Agents

Anesthetics are agents that produce loss of sensation, with or without loss of consciousness, through interference with nerve conduction of painful impulses. They are categorized as general, regional, or local.

Anesthesiologists and nurse anesthetists generally administer anesthetic agents for childbirth and surgical procedures. Nurses often administer various forms of these drugs during the immediate pre- and postoperative phases of surgery and for purposes of conscious sedation or monitored anesthesia care (MAC) in the intubated patient or in patients undergoing certain diagnostic procedures. These may be given by bolus or intermittent injection. Some injectable anesthetic agents, while good for inducing and maintaining anesthesia, do not have analgesic properties. They, therefore, must be administered in conjunction with appropriate analgesia.

N U R S I N G   T I P

IV Nurse's Responsibility of Knowledge

It is very important that the nurse read and understand the protocols and compatibilities involved in preparing and administering anesthetic agents as well as the expected effects exerted in the patient. Even though the nurse may not always actually administer such agents, it is still vital that she know how they affect the patient in order to be able to assess and intervene appropriately should any untoward reactions occur.

Anticonvulsant Agents

Anticonvulsants are agents used to prevent or control seizure activity or the involuntary muscle spasms associated with certain neurological disorders. They are prescribed based on patient-specific seizure disorders and are thought to act by interfering with excessive electrical discharges of the seizure locus and surrounding cells in the CNS. There are several categories of drugs that are used to treat convulsive disorders: barbiturates, benzodiazepines, hydantoins, and magnesium sulfate.

Barbiturates

Barbiturates are nonspecific CNS depressants that control seizures by interfering with the transmission of cerebral cortex impulses. Phenobarbital sodium is a member of this class

NURSING ALERT

Anticonvulsant Precautions

Important precautions must be considered when administering intravenous anticonvulsants because of their propensity to induce respiratory depression or cardiovascular collapse. It is especially important for the nurse to check the time frames for their administration and the many drug incompatibilities associated with them. This is extremely important to remember when giving phenytoin (Dilantin), a commonly used product to treat convulsive disorders. It is given orally or intravenously, never intramuscularly. The intramuscular route is not recommended for the treatment of status epilepticus since blood levels of phenytoin in the therapeutic range cannot be readily achieved.

   IMPORTANT NOTE: This drug must be administered slowly. In adults, do not exceed 50 mg per minute intravenously. In neonates, the drug should be administered at a rate not exceeding 1-3 mg/kg/min. Severe cardiotoxic reactions and fatalities have been reported with atrial and ventricular conduction depression and ventricular fibrillation. Phenytoin should be used with caution in patients with hypotension and severe myocardial insufficiency. Hypotension usually occurs when the drug is administered rapidly by the intravenous route. The margin between therapeutic and toxic doses is very small.

and is often used alone or combined with other anticonvulsants, to manage partial and generalized seizure activity. It is given IV for acute convulsive episodes and status epilepticus and must be given slowly, at a rate not to exceed 50 mg/min. Even with slow injection, overdosage and respiratory depression can easily occur.

NURSING ALERT

Phenobarbital Sodium Dangers

Even with slow intravenous administration (not exceeding 50 mg/min) of phenobarbital sodium, overdosage and respiratory depression can occur.

Benzodiazepines

The benzodiazepines are a group of psychotropic drugs that restrict the spread of seizure-related electrical discharges from their origination point. The IV administration of the benzodiazepine diazepam (Valium) is the drug of

choice for treating status epilepticus and severe recurrent seizures.

NURSING ALERT

Cautions Regarding the IV Administration of Diazepam (Valium)

1. Carefully monitor vital signs and have emergency equipment available, as bradycardia, respiratory depression or arrest, and cardiac arrest can occur during or following injection.
2. Administer slowly (not exceeding 5 mg/min) and directly into large veins, as it is very irritating.
3. Never mix diazepam with other drugs or infusates, as it is very unstable and a precipitate may form in the vein during administration. Conventional diazepam is insoluble in any solution. Emulsified diazepam may be diluted with an emulsion base but may be destabilized (which is not always visually apparent), and is incompatible with PVC infusion sets.
4. Administer diazepam from a glass syringe, as plastic decreases drug availability, thus altering the ordered dose.

Hydantoins

The hydantoins are a group of drugs used to treat generalized tonic-clonic (grand mal) seizures as well as the convulsions that may occur following neurosurgery. Phenytoin (Dilantin) is a nonsedating drug that exerts its effect on the cerebral motor cortex by reducing the spread of spontaneous electrical discharges from rapidly firing epileptic centers in this area. It also suppresses the activity of centers in the brain stem that are responsible for the tonic phase of grand mal seizures.

NURSING ALERT

Rapid Administration of Phenytoin

Rapid IV administration (not exceeding 50 mg/min) of phenytoin (Dilantin) can result in life-threatening cardiovascular events, which include dangerous dysrhythmias/arrhythmias, CNS depression, CV collapse, heart block, and severe hypotension.

   Phenytoin administered IV must be delivered very slowly (not exceeding 50 mg/min). Rapid injection can result in life-threatening cardiovascular events, including dysrhythmias/arrhythmias, CNS depression, cardiovascular collapse, heart block, and hypotension. There have been incidences of choreoathetosis associated with rapid administration, muscle tone fluctuations that vary from hypotonic to hypertonic with extreme ranges of motion, sometimes with resultant deformities such as subluxation of shoulder and finger joints.

The hydantoin fosphenytoin (Cerebyx) may be considered safer, and a preferred choice over phenytoin (Dilantin). Cerebyx is a water-soluble prodrug, meaning that once it is injected or infused into the body, fosphenytoin is converted to active phenytoin following injection or infusion. The Cerebyx dosage is expressed in phenytoin sodium equivalents (PE). By using phenytoin sodium equivalents (PE), physicians will not have to make dosing adjustments when converting from phenytoin sodium to Cerebyx or vice versa. Fosphenytoin or Cerebyx has fewer local side effects than phenytoin injection and can safely be administered over a shorter period of time.

Magnesium Sulfate

Magnesium sulfate is a CNS depressant that also reduces contractility in cardiac, skeletal, and smooth muscle, and induces a mild diuretic and vasodilating effect. It is used to control seizures, especially those of severe preeclampsia and eclampsia as well as those induced by plasma hypomagnesemia. When convulsions are occurring, magnesium is administered undiluted and slowly (at a rate not exceeding 1.5 ml of a 10% solution/min). For IV infusion, 4 g are diluted in 250 ml of 5%D in normal saline and administered slowly (not exceeding 3 ml/min).

Antiemetic and Antinauseant Agents

Antiemetics are agents that prevent or arrest vomiting, and **antinauseants** are agents that prevent the occurrence of nausea. These are the same medications that are administered for the treatment of motion sickness, vertigo, and the gastrointestinal upset associated with antineoplastic and radiation therapy.

Nausea and vomiting are reflex symptoms that occur secondary to other conditions, diseases, medications, or toxins that stimulate the vomiting center in the medulla. Since they are symptoms of something else, it is important to find the precipitating factor and, if possible, correct it. When this is not feasible, then pharmacologic interventions to remedy the nausea or vomiting can be undertaken.

Most drugs used to control nausea and vomiting have anticholinergic and antidopaminergic effects and are included in the antihistimine, benzodiazepine, and anxiolytic classifications. They usually have antinausea and antiemetic effects as secondary pharmacological properties.

N U R S I N G   A L E R T

Patient Assessment before Administering Magnesium Sulfate

Prior to administration of magnesium sulfate the patient must be carefully assessed. If any of the following are present, magnesium sulfate should not be given:

1. Absent patellar reflexes or knee jerk reflex (as respiratory failure may occur if given after these reflexes disappear)
2. Respirations below 16/min (as respiratory paralysis may occur)
3. Urinary output less than 100 ml during the past 4-hour period (as magnesium is removed from the body solely by the kidneys)
4. Past history of heart block, myocardial damage, prolonged PR or widened QRS intervals (as asystole and heart block can occur)
5. Signs of hypermagnesemia (diaphoresis, flushing, hypotension, hypothermia)

N U R S I N G   A L E R T

Protocols for Antiemetic and Antinauseant Drugs

The nurse must use caution in giving the IV forms of antiemetic and antinauseant drugs because of the rapidly occurring side effects or adverse reactions that can result, including hypotension, respiratory depression, and vertigo. Strict protocols must be followed regarding dilution, admixing, and administration time-frames with many of these drugs as well. Because common side effects include sedation, confusion, and blurred vision, the issue of patient safety must be addressed and protective measures instituted.

Antimicrobials

The nurse who administers intravenous infusion therapy deals with the antimicrobial agents more frequently than any other group of medications. It is very important that she understand how these drugs work and the requirements of correct delivery. It is also important that she relate the underlying principles of infection control and their relationship to the concepts of microbial contamination and resistance.

The **antimicrobials** are natural or synthetic substances that are used in the prevention and treatment of infectious processes caused by microorganisms. They alter the microorganism so it cannot grow or reproduce or kill the microorganism directly.

Microorganisms encompass a broad life-form population not perceptible to the naked eye that include bacteria, fungi, protozoa, rickettsiae, viruses, and other life forms that can gain entrance into the human body. Many are capable of producing disease. **Anti-infective** is a term that refers to an agent that combats an infection and **antibiotic** means destructive to life-forms, generally molds or bacteria. An antibiotic that is **bactericidal** kills bacteria, while one that is **bacteriostatic** inhibits bacterial growth, allowing the host's immune cells to kill the bacteria.

Antimicrobial Selection Criteria

Numerous antimicrobials are available for the prevention and treatment of infectious diseases. When deciding which one is most appropriate, the physician must take into consideration several important factors. These criteria are based on both the patient and the drug.

Clinical Status

When selecting an antimicrobial, the most important factor to consider is patient safety. The patient's clinical status must be carefully weighed against the efficacy of the drug as well as its effect on his body. The patient's clinical status criteria include the following:

1. Age and weight
2. General state of health, especially liver and kidney functioning
3. Severity and pathogenicity of the infection
4. Any underlying medical conditions

Drug Spectrum of Activity

A drug's spectrum of activity refers to the number and type of organisms it can kill. The aim of treatment is to identify the pathogen causing an infectious process (through culture and sensitivity testing) and choose an antimicrobial with the narrowest spectrum of activity that will kill or inactivate it. By focusing treatment toward a more limited range of pathogens, there is minimal disruption of a patient's normal flora and less chance for the development of resistant strains of organisms.

Patterns of Bacterial Resistance

When selecting antimicrobial treatment, the physician must also consider patterns of microbial resistance. Because of the cellular composition of some organisms, they have what is known as a natural resistance to the effects of some antimicrobials (such as gram-negative organisms to penicillin V). There are also microbial resistance patterns that develop over time within individual communities and health care facilities. Since the introduction of antibiotics in the 1940s, bacteria and other microbes that were initially sensitive to various agents have developed mechanisms that enable them to survive in the presence of these drugs. This has become a major problem in treating some infectious diseases. In addition, there is a problem of cross resistance: microbes that are resistant to one agent become resistant to other agents in the same class.

Microbes develop resistance to antimicrobial drugs through two processes: emergence or induction. Emergence resistance, a relatively slow process, occurs during the course of drug therapy and involves selective survival of organisms. Some organisms survive, while the susceptible ones are destroyed by the antimicrobial drug. Random genetic mutations cause certain cells to develop traits that enable them to resist the effects of the drugs that kill their kin. The mutants pass the trait on to their progeny, thus giving rise to the emergence of a new, resistant strain.

Induction resistance occurs when an antimicrobial drug activates microbial genes responsible for resistance to that drug. The drug actually precipitates the appearance of genetically determined bacterial resistance mechanisms. Pathogens that develop resistance as a result of exposure to a drug are said to be inducible. Induction resistance occurs much faster than emergence resistance.

Microorganisms have developed several specific mechanisms that cause them to resist antimicrobial therapy. The most common method is through the production of enzymes (such as the beta-lactamases, which resist cephalosporins and penicillins). Another method of resistance involves alterations in the bacterial cell membranes, which prevents entrance of antimicrobial drugs. This has brought about widespread resistance to the tetracyclines.

A third mechanism of resistance is alteration of target cell–receptor sites. By changing the structure of the binding sites on their ribosomes, many microbes have developed resistance to drugs that inhibit ribosomal synthesis (such as the aminoglycosides). The fourth method of microbial resistance is due to the development of alternative metabolic pathways, thus inactivating drugs that interfere with microbial metabolism. This is how many pathogens have become resistant to the sulfonamide drugs.

Resistance patterns become encoded on microbial DNA. They can be transferred to other microbes through the process of gene transfer, which occurs through transduction, transformation, or conjugation. In transduction, a virus that infects a bacteria can carry portions of bacterial DNA from one bacterium to another (which in turn, pass the new resistance on to their progeny). In transformation, a dying microbe releases its DNA into the environment, and other microbes incorporate it into their own genetic material. In conjugation, there is direct contact (mating) among bacterial cells, and DNA is transferred through bacterial appendages (pili) to many other cells. This method allows the genetic transfer of information from cells (with genes having resistance to multiple drugs) to be transferred rapidly to other cells. This is thought to be how gram-negative bacilli such as *E. coli* may have developed antimicrobial resistance. Plasmids, small particles of DNA found outside the bacterial nucleoid, often contain multiple resistance traits that are transferred by way of conjugation (particularly in gram-negative organisms).

Patterns of bacterial resistance are of tremendous concern, especially in areas of massive IV antibiotic use, such as hospitals (particularly in critical care and oncology areas). Many organisms, especially the gram-negative bacilli, have developed widespread resistance to many antimicrobial agents and are causing great difficulties with treatment regimens. Infections can become very serious, even life-threatening, in a short period of time, necessitating the use of additional antimicrobials.

When there is any suspicion that a particular pathogen has developed resistance to commonly used drugs, an alternative agent must be used. The development of newer intravenous antibiotics has come about in response to the microbial resistances that have evolved.

Pharmacokinetic and Safety Factors

When selecting an antimicrobial treatment regimen, it is important to consider the pharmacokinetic characteristics of the proposed agent. The properties of absorption, distribution, metabolism, and excretion must be looked at in relation to the desired therapeutic effect. These aspects determine the dosing schedule.

An antimicrobial's record of safety must also be assessed in relation to the patient's clinical status. If the adverse effects outweigh the positive attributes, the drug should not be used. Sometimes the infectious process is so severe that it threatens the patient's life, and certain drugs are administered in spite of their adverse side effects (as is often the case when using amphotericin B). The nurse must assess, monitor, and support the patient in these situations and report and record any untoward changes immediately.

Categories of Antimicrobial Therapy

Antimicrobial therapy falls into three categories: prophylactic, empiric, or definitive.

Prophylactic treatment refers to the use of antimicrobials for the prevention of infection. It is used in circumstances where there is a risk for opportunistic organisms to invade and become endogenous pathogens, such as during bowel surgery (where the normal intestinal flora may be released into the abdominal cavity).

Empiric treatment refers to the use of antimicrobials for an infection that has not been identified by culture and sensitivity testing based on the signs and symptoms of the patient. This is usually broad-spectrum or combination therapy in the attempt to treat as many potential pathogens as possible.

Definitive therapy is antimicrobial treatment based on positive identification of the pathogen(s) causing the infectious process. Many times, with IV antimicrobial therapy, empiric treatment is initiated until the results of culture studies are available. Once positive identification is verified, the patient is switched to a narrow-spectrum, pathogen-specific drug. It is best to use a drug with the narrowest spectrum of activity to avoid unnecessary disruption of the body's normal flora and to prevent the body from becoming resistant to agents that may be necessary to combat future infections.

Antimicrobial Classifications

There are several classifications of antimicrobial drugs that the nurse frequently is called upon to prepare and administer. Table 11-3 categorizes and describes them.

Anti-Inflammatory Agents

Anti-inflammatory agents are drugs that relieve the tenderness, swelling, and pain associated with the body's normal response to injury, infection, or irritation of tissue. These drugs do not, in general, treat the cause of inflammation but provide symptomatic relief of inflammation-induced discomfort. They are usually grouped into two categories: the nonsteroidal anti-inflammatory drugs (NSAIDs) and the steroidal anti-inflammatory agents. Only the steroidals are administered intravenously and are grouped in the hormone classification of corticosteroids.

Antihistamines

The antihistamines are drugs that block the effects of histamine 1 (H_1) receptors, responsible for allergic conditions, or histamine 2 (H_2) receptors, responsible for gastrointestinal disorders. These drugs do not interfere with the production or release of histamine, antibody production, or

Table 11-3 | The Antimicrobials

CATEGORY	DESCRIPTION
Aminoglycosides	Aminoglycosides are a group of bacteriocidal antibiotics derived from species of *Streptomyces* or *Micromonosporum* that act by causing misreading and inhibition of protein synthesis on bacterial ribosomes. The main advantages of these drugs are their spectra of activity against nosocomial organisms and their low cost, while the disadvantages are their bacterial resistance and unfavorable side-effect profile. (Gram-negative bacteria develop resistance either by producing enzymes that deactivate these drugs or by altering their ribosomes to prevent binding. Aminoglycosides are associated with high incidences of nephrotoxicity and ototoxicity.)
Antifungals	Antifungals are fungicidals that attach to the sterols of the fungus cell membrane and destroy it.
Antiparasitics	Antiparasitics that counteract malaria act by several modes, some of which are unknown. They may inhibit the erythrocytic stage of parasitic development, bind to and alter DNA properties, or combine with DNA (interfering with its ability to replicate or serve in transcription of RNA) and interfere with protein synthesis.
Antiprotozoals	Antiprotozoals are protozoacidal or act to inhibit the survival/reproduction of protozoa by altering their environment.
Antivirals	Antivirals are not viricidal but act to inhibit viral reproduction by restraint of DNA synthesis.
Carbapenems (Beta-Lactam Antibiotic)	The carbapenems are extremely broad-spectrum (including the CNS) β-lactam antibiotics that are bactericidal due to the presence of a β-lactam ring in their chemical structures that binds with penicillin-binding proteins (PBPs) of bacteria, thus interfering with bacterial cell-wall synthesis. The β-lactam rings of these drugs are different from those of other β-lactams such as the cephalosporins and penicillins. Their main advantages are that they are very stable in the presence of β-lactamase enzymes and have shown minimal bacterial resistance thus far. Their disadvantages are their high cost and association with superinfection. Note: Due to their pharmacokinetic properties, carbapenems are broken down into toxic metabolites in the kidneys by renal enzymes, so they must be administered with cilastatin (a chemical that inhibits renal enzymes).
Cephalosporins (Beta-Lactam Antibiotic)	The cephalosporins are a group of 25+ broad-spectrum, beta-lactam bactericidal antibiotics that are the most commonly used IV antibiotics in acute care settings for empiric therapy and surgical prophylaxis. They destroy susceptible bacteria by binding to their cell membranes and interfering with cell-wall synthesis. Because they vary widely in their spectra of activity, they are grouped based on these differences into subclasses called generations. In general, each successive generation has a broader coverage of gram-negative organisms (but slightly less activity against gram-positive species). The main advantages of the cephalosporins are their safety and efficacy, broad spectra, and infrequent occurrences of hypersensitivity reactions. The disadvantages are their short half-lives, resistance to gram-negative nosocomial pathogens, cross-sensitivity with penicillins (so must be used with caution in penicillin-allergic populations), and their disruption of normal gastrointestinal flora (due to their broad spectra). The third-generation cephalosporins are active against gram-positive, gram-negative, and anaerobic bacteria.
Fluoroquinolones and Quinolones	Fluoroquinolones are the newer, improved version of the original quinolones (to which modifications have been made and a fluorine atom added). The term quinolones is still used, even in reference to the newer, more correct, classification. Quinolones have extremely broad spectra of antimicrobial activity and exert bactericidal effects by interfering with DNA synthesis (by inhibiting the activity of DNA-gyrase, a bacterial enzyme [in bacterial cells] essential for DNA replication). Impaired DNA synthesis results in bacterial death. (They do not interfere with normal human DNA synthesis or replication as human cells do not use DNA-gyrase for genetic replication.) The main advantages of quinolones are associated with their broad spectrum of activity (with high-level bactericidal action), very low minimum inhibitory concentrations (MICs), excellent tissue penetration, long half-lives (resulting in less frequent dosing), and their effectiveness against many nosocomial pathogens that are resistant to other antibiotics. The disadvantages are that they may increase the side effects of certain drugs and are contraindicated in pregnant women and in children.
Macrolides	The macrolides are a group of antibiotics that are bacteriostatic, but, if given in high enough doses, are bactericidal to some organisms. They act by inhibiting bacterial protein synthesis (thus preventing growth and reproduction) by penetrating the bacterial cell membrane and binding with the 50S ribosomal subunit (not the 30S subunit) of sensitive bacteria. Macrolides cannot bind to human ribosomes because human ribosomes have only 30S (but not 50S) subunits. Note: Clindamycin, which is not a macrolide, is often referred to as a macrolide because it has a similar mechanism of action.
Monobactams	The monobactams are a class of β-lactam nuclei that act by inhibiting bacterial cell-wall synthesis.
Penecillins and Penicillin-Related Antibiotics Beta-lactamase-resistant penicillins	The penicillins are a group of bactericidal antibiotics that are biosynthesized from the molds *Penicillium notatum* and *P. chrysogenum*. Based on their spectra of activity, they are grouped into four classes: (1) the natural penicillins (benzathine, penicillin G, and penicillin V), (2) the penicillinase-resistant* penicillins (methicillin, nafcillin, and oxacillin), (3) the broad-spectrum penicillins (ampicillins), and (4) the extended-spectrum penicillins (azlocillin, mezlocillin, piperacillin, and ticarcillin). Penicillins are β-lactam antibiotics that penetrate bacterial cell walls and bind to penicillin-binding proteins (PBPs). During cell division, this binding interferes with the ability of bacteria to construct new cell walls as they divide and reproduce, so death occurs.

(continues)

Table 11-3 | The Antimicrobials (continued)

CATEGORY	DESCRIPTION
	Once in the bloodstream, all penicillins are widely distributed throughout the body, many of them reaching therapeutic levels in the CNS.
	The major advantages of the penicillins are their safety and efficacy, good tissue perfusion, the fact that they can be used for infections in almost every body system, and their low toxicity. Some disadvantages are their very short half-lives, increasing resistance to many bacterial strains, and their ability to produce hypersensitivity (which are compounded by cross-reactivity).
Sulfonamides	The sulfonamides are a group of bacteriostatic compounds derived from sulfanilamide that exert their action by interfering with bacterial enzyme systems needed for metabolism, growth, and replication. They specifically interfere with folic acid synthesis, which is required for cellular growth.
	Prior to the development of the penicillins, the sulfonamides were the backbone of antibiotic therapy. The advantages of these drugs are their coverage of a broad spectrum of pathogens, their ability to penetrate many body tissues and fluids, and their low cost. The disadvantages, however, of widespread bacterial resistance and possible hypersensitivity reactions have limited their use.
	Because so many bacteria have become highly resistant to the sulfonamides, sulfamethoxazole is usually administered in combination with the folic acid-inhibitor trimethoprim. This highly synergistic combination is bactericidally effective and is especially active against *Pneumocystis carinii*, the pathogen implicated in the type of pneumonia that accompanies AIDS.
Tetracyclines	The tetracyclines are a group of chemically related bacteriostatic antibiotics that inhibit bacterial protein synthesis. Their mechanism of action, like the macrolides, is effected by binding with the 30S ribosomal subunit, thus inhibiting protein synthesis. The main advantages of the tetracyclines are their broad spectra of activity and low cost. Because of widespread resistance to these agents (the major disadvantage), especially many strains of *Staphylococci*, *Streptococci*, and *Pseudomonas*, their use has been limited. A possible consequence of tetracycline therapy (which carries with it a history of indiscriminate use) is superinfection due to overgrowth by tetracycline-resistant organisms, especially the yeasts.
Others chloramphenicol sodium succinate	Chloramphenicol is a synthetically produced bacteriostatic and bactericidal antibiotic that is reserved for serious infections due to its high toxicity levels (due to protein synthesis inhibition in rapidly proliferating cells, such as bone marrow). It should never be used for prophylaxis of bacterial infections or to treat colds, flu, or trivial infection because of the possibility of bone marrow depression.
clindamycin phosphate	Clindamycin phosphate is a semisynthetic bacteriostatic and bactericidal antibiotic that suppresses protein synthesis in microorganisms by binding to the 50S ribosomal subunit. It should not be used prophylactically or for the treatment of trivial bacterial or viral infections.
rifampin	Rifampin is a semisynthetic bacteriostatic and bactericidal antitubercular antibiotic derived from *Streptomyces mediterranei* that exerts its effect by binding to the beta subunit of DNA-dependent RNA polymerase, thus preventing attachment of the enzyme to DNA, which results in the blockade of RNA transcription. It is most active against rapidly reproducing organisms.
vancomycin	Vancomycin hydrochloride, a glycopeptide, is a bacteriostatic (for enterococci) and bactericidal antibiotic derived from *Streptomyces orientalis* that exerts its effect by binding to the bacterial cell wall and arresting its synthesis by lysing the cytoplasmic membrane (in a mechanism that differs from that of the cephalosporins and penicillins). It may change the permeability of the cytoplasmic membranes of bacteria, thus inhibiting RNA synthesis.

antigen-antibody reactions. They exert their effect by preventing or reversing the effects of histamine through competitive inhibition (by competing with histamine for histamine receptors). Antihistamines are used for their antitussive effect and to treat allergies, motion sickness, and vertigo. The histamine 2 blockers (H-2 antagonists) are classified separately since they exert their effect only in the digestive system.

Brompheniramine maleate, chlorpheniramine maleate, and diphenhydramine are the three antihistamines administered intravenously. They are administered for the prophylaxis or the treatment of hypersensitivity reactions. Diphenhydramine is also used for the control of parkinsonism in geriatric patients who are unable to tolerate more

---

NURSING ALERT

Antihistamine Side Effects

The safety needs of the patient must always be addressed when administering IV antihistamines. The major side effects of these drugs are dizziness, hypotension (which can precipitate syncope), and sedation.

---

potent drugs. It is given by direct IV bolus, undiluted, at a rate not greater than 25 mg/min. Brompheniramine and chlorpheniramine are used IV only in the 10 mg/ml preparations and may be injected diluted or undiluted. (The 100 mg/ml strength should not be given IV.)

Antineoplastic Agents

Antineoplastic agents are those drugs that prevent the development, growth, or proliferation of malignant cells. For the most part, they are cytotoxic, meaning they are poisonous to both normal and neoplastic cells because cell cycles and methods of division are the same for normal cells and cancer cells. Antineoplastics are often an adjunct to other forms of cancer treatment, such as surgical intervention and radiation therapy.

The choice of which type of antineoplastic agent to use depends on the type of tumor process, its site of origination and growth, and how it interferes with cellular reproduction. Most drugs work by targeting the DNA in some way. The mechanism may cause interference with the DNA itself, interference with enzymes related to DNA or RNA-synthesis, or by destruction of the proteins necessary for cell life. Antineoplastics are classified as cell-cycle–phase specific, which are active on cells that are undergoing cell-cycle division, or cell-cycle–phase nonspecific, which are active on cells that are either in the dividing stage or are in a resting state.

Alkylating Agents and Nitrosoureas

The alkylating agents are the largest group of antineoplastic drugs. They are cell-cycle–phase nonspecific compounds that kill cells by interfering with the structure of cell DNA. They form a molecular bond with the nucleic acids, thus causing interference with nucleic acid reproduction. The outcome is the prevention of mitosis. There are two forms of alkylating agents, the classic alkylating drugs, composed of nitrogen mustard and its derivatives, and the nitrosoureas.

The nitrosoureas are cell-cycle–phase nonspecific and inhibit the synthesis of both DNA and RNA. Because of their lipid-solubility, they cross the blood-brain barrier, making them effective for brain and CNS neoplasms.

Antibiotics

The antibiotic antitumor agents are a group of heterogeneous compounds that are by-products of the fermentation of several bacteria and fungi. (While they exert some antibiotic effect, their toxic side effects contraindicate their use for the treatment of infections.) For the most part (except bleomycin), they are cell-cycle–phase nonspecific and disrupt DNA transcription. They also inhibit DNA and RNA synthesis.

Antimetabolites

An antimetabolite is a chemical analogue of an essential metabolite. It is so similar that the drug is able to enter the metabolite's essential metabolic pathway.

The antimetabolite antineoplastics are a group of cell-cycle–phase specific drugs that act either by blocking the enzymes needed for DNA biosynthesis or by becoming incorporated into the DNA and RNA so that a false message is transmitted. They are divided into three groups, the folate antagonists, the purine antagonists, and the pyrimidine antagonists.

Hormonal Agents

The body's hormones are a group of chemicals secreted by the endocrine glands and are cell-cycle–phase nonspecific. They change the cellular environment by altering cellular membrane permeability. Because the growth of certain tumors is partially dependent on hormones, the hormonal environment may be manipulated in order to suppress tumor growth. They can subdue the growth of certain body tissues without producing cytotoxicity.

The corticosteroids are frequently used with other forms of chemotherapy because of their lack of bone marrow toxicity. They are powerful immunosuppressants, however. Because they have anti-inflammatory effects, they have the disadvantage of masking the signs and symptoms of infectious processes that might be endangering the patient.

Plant Alkaloids

The plant alkaloids are antineoplastic agents with different therapeutic uses and varying levels of toxicity. They are cell-cycle–phase specific and exert their effect primarily during the metaphase period of mitosis by inhibiting spindle formation. They also inhibit DNA and protein synthesis.

Miscellaneous

There are several other forms of antineoplastic therapy that do not fit into the traditional classifications. These include L-asparaginase, an enzyme involved in protein synthesis; cisplatin, a platinum metal that inhibits DNA synthesis; dacarbazine, which functions as an alkylator and acts on the nucleic acids (particularly DNA) of antineoplastic cells; hydroxyurea, a urea derivative that acts by selectively eradicating granulocytes; mitotane, for the treatment of adrenocortical carcinoma, which is cytotoxic to adrenal cortical cells, thus decreasing the secretion of steroids; mitoxantrone, a synthetic drug, which is an anthracenedione, and is cytotoxic through the inhibition of RNA and DNA synthesis; and procarbazine, a hydrazine derivative, which works like an alkylator to inhibit DNA, RNA, and protein synthesis.

Antineoplastic Administration Guidelines

Most forms of antineoplastic therapy are administered intravenously. These agents should be prepared and administered only by trained personnel, as cytotoxic exposure is always a possibility through inhalation, ingestion, or absorption through the skin and mucous membranes. Table 11-4 lists the precautions that should be taken regarding the preparation and administration of antineoplastic agents.

When giving antineoplastic drugs in the home, the nurse must follow strict safety guidelines regarding their preparation and administration. Family members who administer such products must be taught the precautions to be taken to prevent cytotoxic exposure through inhalation, ingestion, or absorption through the skin and mucous membranes. Federal insurance guidelines regarding antineoplastic chemotherapy in the home include administration via an external infusion pump, administration over a period of 24 hours or more, and mandatory delivery of doxorubicin, bleomycin, cytarabine, fluorouracil, vinbastine, or vincristine (Masoorli, 1996).

Anxiolytic Agents

The anxiolytics or antianxiety agents are drugs that relieve both the physiologic and psychological signs and symptoms of anxiety. They are also used to alleviate muscle tension associated with acute and chronic orthopedic conditions.

Table 11-4 | Guidelines for the Preparation and Administration of Antineoplastic Agents

PREPARATION GUIDELINES

1. Preparation of antineoplastic agents should be performed by trained personnel. (Preparation by pregnant women is generally contraindicated.)

2. Preparation should be under a laminar air flow hood.

3. Disposable gloves are to be worn during reconstitution. (Polyvinyl chloride gloves, however, are permeable to some cytotoxic agents.)

4. Goggles, a nonpermeable mask (to cover nose and mouth), and a disposable nonpermeable surgical gown with knit cuffs and closed front should be worn.

5. Use disposable equipment.

6. When reconstituting the drug(s), vent the vial(s) prior to puncture with the needle/syringe used for withdrawal to lower the internal pressure of the vial and reduce the risk of spilling or spraying the drug when the needle is removed from the vial's diaphragm.

7. After withdrawing and preparing the drug, wipe all surfaces of the used syringes and bottles with alcohol sponges. Discard all disposable equipment into the appropriate containers designated for incineration.

8. Prevent contact with skin or mucous membranes. If contact occurs, wash and/or irrigate with water. Eyes should be irrigated with copious amounts of normal saline and immediate consultation with an ophthalmologist should be scheduled. Report and document exposure according to institutional policy and procedure.

9. Wash hands thoroughly before removing gloves and again after removal.

10. Prepare the infusion, using a piggyback setup for the antineoplastic drug connected to a primary infusion. Use an electronic infusion device.

11. If an infusion is not set up because the volume of medication to be administered is relatively small, the triple syringe method (using a winged infusion set) should be used. With this method, normal saline is administered first to verify venous patency and integrity, followed by the medication, after which the vein is flushed with additional normal saline.

ADMINISTRATION GUIDELINES

1. Start the IV in a large vein that has not been previously used, avoiding the veins of the hands, wrist area, or antecubital fossae.

2. Initiate the infusion with an infusate that does not contain the antineoplastic agent.

3. Instruct the patient to report any burning or painful sensations at the infusion site and assess the site frequently for redness, warmth, or edema.

4. In case of extravasation, stop the infusion immediately and follow institutional protocols regarding its management.

POSTADMINISTRATION GUIDELINES

1. Discard all disposable equipment in the appropriate containers designated for incineration.

2. Instruct the family to wear appropriate disposable gloves when handling and discarding the patient's gastrointestinal secretions and excretions.

They include the barbiturates and the benzodiazepines. These drugs do not, however, treat the underlying causes of anxiety, which must be addressed from both a medical and nursing standpoint.

> ### NURSING ALERT
>
> **Determine the Underlying Cause of Anxiety**
>
> Anxiolytic agents do not treat the underlying cause of anxiety, so it is important to determine what is causing the anxiety-producing state and direct primary treatment to this area. It is extremely important to understand that depression, accompanied by suicidal inclinations, is often an adjunct to anxiety.

The barbiturates, although used for many of the symptoms for which the benzodiazepines are administered, have different chemical and pharmacokinetic properties. Because of the hypnotic and sedative effects of these agents, their use for the treatment of anxiety has been largely replaced by the benzodiazepines.

> ### NURSING ALERT
>
> **Barbiturate Cautions**
>
> When barbiturates are used, it is important for the nurse to bear in mind that, unlike the benzodiazepines, these drugs stimulate the same hepatic enzymes that metabolize many other drugs, thus increasing the possibility of numerous drug interactions. The nurse must also assess carefully for the adverse reactions of cardiac, respiratory, and CNS depression, as well as extreme confusion and the paradoxical reactions of nervousness, increased excitability, and hallucinations. Following IV administration, the life-threatening complications of peripheral vascular collapse, seizures, and cardiorespiratory arrest can occur.

The benzodiazepines, as discussed earlier, vary in terms of their selectivity and can exert antianxiety, anticonvulsant, hypnotic, and muscle-relaxant effects. They seem to act on the hypothalamic, limbic, and thalamic regions of the CNS.

Cardiovascular Agents

Agents that affect the heart, its intrinsic conduction system, myocardial contractility, and output, and the blood vessels,

> ### NURSING ALERT
>
> **Benzodiazepine Cautions**
>
> When administering intravenous benzodiazepines, it is important to keep in mind that cardiovascular, CNS, and respiratory depression can occur rapidly and to take the necessary precautions regarding these untoward effects.

as well as the delivery and flow of blood and oxygen throughout the body, fall into the broad category of cardiovascular drugs. These agents, for the most part, also impact the kidneys, since cardiovascular and renal mechanisms work in tandem to regulate blood pressure and preserve the volume and composition of the extracellular fluid.

Antidysrhythmic Agents

Cardiac dysrhythmias are any aberration in the rate and rhythm of the heart. The drugs used to prevent irregularities or return the heart to its normal sinus rhythm fall into the group of drugs called antidysrhythmics (or antiarrhythmics). They normally exert their effect by (one or a combination of actions) decreasing automaticity, altering electrical conductivity, or by changing the myocardial refractory period between contractions (to avert premature stimulation).

There is no single prototype, or universal, dysrhythmic. Instead, these drugs are classified into four groups (Table 11-5), with the first having three subclasses with similar electrophysiologic effects. Adenosine and digoxin, both used as antidysrhythmics, are not currently grouped in this classification system.

> ### NURSING ALERT
>
> **Administration of Antidysrhythmics**
>
> Antidysrhythmics are administered intravenously only to patients who are connected to cardiac monitors and where emergency drugs and equipment are readily available. Unless given by bolus injection, they should be infused using an electronic infusion device.

Antihypertensives

Antihypertensive agents are used to control abnormal elevations in blood pressure. They are often used in con-

Table 11-5 | Antidysrhythmic Classifications

GROUP	DESCRIPTION	NAME	SUBCLASS	DESCRIPTION	NAME
I	Drugs that increase the refractory period through suppression of rapid sodium channel movement	Moricizine (this drug shares some of the actions of groups I-A, I-B, and I-C)	I-A	Drugs that cause reduced automaticity through decreased conduction velocity with augmented action potential	Disopyramide Procainamide Quinidine
			I-B	Drugs that cause increased (or have no effect on) conduction velocity	Lidocaine Mexiletine Phenytoin Tocainide
			I-C	Drugs that depress automaticity by slowing spontaneous depolarization	Encainide Flecainide Indecainide Propafenone
II	Beta-adrenergic blockers that reduce adrenergic cardiac stimulation	Acebutolol Esmolol Propranolol			
III	Drugs that prolong cardiac repolarization without influencing depolarization	Amiodarone Bretylium			
IV	Calcium channel blockers which depress myocardial and smooth muscle contractility, decrease automaticity, and (possibly) slow conduction velocity	Verapamil			

Adenosine and digoxin, both used as cardiac dysrhythmics, are not classified in these groups.

junction with diuretic therapy and other treatment modalities. They may act centrally or peripherally and may be categorized as alpha- or beta-adrenergic blockers (antiadrenergics), angiotensin antagonists, autonomic ganglionic blockers, calcium channel blockers, and vasodilators (Table 11-6).

The antihypertensive agents administered intravenously are generally used to treat hypertensive emergencies. They are indicated when a patient's blood pressure becomes so elevated that severe debilitation or death can occur. These agents include the nondiuretic agents diazoxide, nitroglycerin, sodium nitroprusside, and trimethaphan camsylate. Special precautions must be taken regarding the rate of administration and container and medication incompatibilities that the nurse must be aware before giving these drugs.

Cardiac Glycosides

The cardiac glycosides are natural alkaloids derived from the foxglove plant and include deslanoside, digitoxin, and digoxin. They exert a positive inotropic effect (increased force of contraction) and negative chronotropic (slowed rate) and dromotropic (slowed conduction) effects. They are thought to act by precipitating the release of free calcium in the myocardium, which potentiates the action of the proteins in cardiac muscle (actin and myosin) responsible for myocardial contraction. They alter myocardial electrical conductivity by decreasing conduction velocity and increasing the refractory period of atrial-ventricular conductivity. The outcome is decreased heart rate through increased vagal tone.

Cardiac Stimulants

Cardiac stimulants are adrenergic agents that have a potent pressor effect and increase myocardial contractility. They are administered intravenously to treat patients in emergency situations who are experiencing hypoperfusion and hypotension following cardiac arrest, decompensation, or myocardial infarction. These agents, depending on their degree of adrenergic selectivity, may act to produce peripheral vasoconstriction, skeletal muscle dilation, increased cardiac rate and contractility, increased glycogenolysis or CNS stimulation. They include dobutamine, dopamine, ephedrine sulfate, epinephrine, isoproterenol, levarterenol, mephentermine sulfate, metaraminol bitartrate, methoxamine HCl, norepinephrine, and phenylephrine.

Table 11-6 | Antihypertensive Categories

CATEGORY	MODE OF ACTION
Alpha-adrenergic blocking agents (alpha blockers)	These agents interrupt the action of sympathomimetic agents at alpha-adrenergic receptor sites, resulting in smooth muscle relaxation, increased peripheral vasodilation, and decreased blood pressure.
Beta-adrenergic blocking agents (beta blockers)	These agents inhibit the actions of catecholamines and other sympathomimetic agents at beta-adrenergic receptor sites.
Angiotensin-converting enzyme antagonists (ACE inhibitors)	These agents work by inhibiting the enzyme that that converts angiotensin I to angiotensin II, a potent vasoconstrictor, and decreasing aldosterone release to prevent sodium and water retention.
Angiotensin II Receptor Blockers or antagonists (ARBs)	These agents selectively block the binding of angiotensin II to the AT_1 (Angiotensin II receptor) receptors found in many tissues, thus resulting in blockade of the vasoconstricting and aldosterone-secreting effects of angiotensin II. This results in an antihypertensive effect.
Autonomic ganglion blocking agents	These agents inhibit the action of acetylcholine and block or decrease autonomic nervous system impulse transmission.
Calcium channel blockers	These agents obstruct the flow of calcium ions into the muscle cells and pacemaker cells of the heart.
Vasodilators	These act directly or indirectly to dilate arterial and venous vessels and relax smooth muscle.
Others	These include mixed alpha blockers and beta blockers and norepinephrine-depleting agents.

NURSING ALERT

Toxic Manifestations with Cardiac Glycosides

Cardiac glycosides have a very narrow margin between therapeutic and toxic effects, so patients receiving them require very close monitoring by nurses skilled in identifying toxic manifestations (which include sudden changes in cardiac rate and regularity, anorexia, disorientation, headache, nausea, vomiting, and visual disturbances). Since cardiac monitoring during intravenous administration of cardiac glycosides is not required, it is very important that the nurse take an apical pulse for a full minute prior to injection and at frequent intervals thereafter. If the pulse is below 60 or above 100 or there is evidence of bigeminy, the drug is to be held, and the physician is to be notified. Patients who have hypothyroidism are very sensitive to the cardiac glycosides.

Cholinergic Agents

Cholinergics are parasympathomimetic agents that bring about effects analogous to those produced by acetylcholine

NURSING ALERT

Monitoring Patients During Cardiac Stimulant Therapy

During therapy with cardiac stimulants, the patient's heart, blood pressure, CNS status, and kidney functioning must be meticulously monitored. Strict attention must be paid to fluid-electrolyte balance and acid-base balance. There are numerous preparation and administration guidelines regarding intravenous delivery that the nurse must be aware of and follow. She is usually expected to regulate these drugs to maintain the blood pressure within a specified range. Some of these drugs have vesicant properties, so the infusion site must be carefully monitored. Should extravasation occur, institutional guidelines are to be followed regarding administration of the appropriate counteragent.

in its role as the final neurotransmitter in the parasympathetic nervous system. Acetylcholine acts on the nervous system to produce stimulation (nicotinic effect) of the ganglia, adrenal medulla, and skeletal muscle, and stimulation (muscarinic) of postganglionic nerve endings in glands, cardiac muscle, and smooth muscle.

NURSING TIP

Indications of Cholinergic Drugs

Cholinergic drugs may be direct-acting or indirect-acting. They are indicated for the following:
1. Lower intraocular pressure (in glaucoma)
2. Terminate the curare effects of the neuromuscular blockade associated with surgical anesthesia
3. Stimulate postoperative bladder and intestinal peristalsis
4. Promote diaphoresis and salivation

Direct-Acting Cholinergic Agents

Direct-acting cholinergics, or choline esters, are chemically similar to acetylcholine, but are longer acting. They combine directly with the cholinergic receptors in postsynaptic membranes. They produce the same side effects as parasympathetic stimulation.

Indirect-Acting Cholinergic Agents

The indirect-acting cholinergic agents, or anticholinesterases (cholinesterase inhibitors), do not affect the receptors, but inhibit the action of the enzyme cholinesterase (that normally degrades acetylcholine), thus prolonging the effects of acetylcholine. There is a buildup of acetylcholine at all the sites where it is released.

Diagnostic Agents

Many diagnostic agents, although not classified as such, are considered drugs because they are administered in the same manner and interact with body systems and tissues. They are given to assess the structure and function of various organ systems and vessels, to diagnose, and to monitor the remission, regression, or advancement of disease processes. Biologic in vivo agents are live cultures administered intradermally to determine serologic immunity or to aid in the diagnosis of diseases, such as tuberculosis. Nonbiological in vivo agents are nonliving agents (enzymes, starches, hormones, chemicals, etc.) introduced into the body to test for sensitivity to certain agents, to assess the functional status of various organs and glands, or for diagnostic screening. Radiographic contrast media is administered orally, topically, or parenterally for assessment and diagnostic purposes. Nonbiological in vitro agents are mixed with specimens that have been removed from the body, such as tissues, organs, cells, and secretions, and used to test for a wide variety diseases or conditions or to assess the body's biochemical status.

The diagnostic tests that require the administration of intravenous agents are those involving radiographic contrast media. These include cholecystography, computerized tomographic enhancement, angiography, myelography, urography, and hysterosalpingography. The agents used for these tests are the diatrizoate salts, iodamide meglumines, iothalamate salts, and metrizamide.

NURSING TIP

Pre- and Postexamination Care of the Patient

The nurse seldom administers intravenous diagnostic agents, yet she is responsible for the pre- and postexamination care of the patient. She must, therefore, understand what the patient is being given, why it is indicated, its mechanism of action, the side effects to assess for, and the steps to be taken should any untoward reactions occur.

Diuretics

Diuretic agents increase urine production and water excretion by the kidneys. They are one of the most frequently administered medications. There are five main classifications of these drugs. Each class is established based on the site within the nephron where it exerts its action and effect (Table 11-7).

Table 11-7 | Diuretic Classifications

CLASSIFICATION	DESCRIPTION AND MODE OF ACTION	NAME
Proximal Tubule Diuretics (carbonic anhydrase inhibitors)	These agents act by promoting the reabsorption of sodium and bicarbonate from the proximal tubules. The prototype of this group is acetazolamide, a sulfonamide, that inhibits the action of the enzyme carbonic anhydrase (present in the eyes, kidneys, and other organs), thus reducing the volume of sequestered fluids (especially in the aqueous humor [by >50%], therefore decreasing intraocular pressure).	Acetazolamide Dichlorphenamide Methazolamide
Diluting Segment Diuretics (thiazide and thiazide types)	The primary diuretic agents active within the diluting segments of the kidney are the thiazides, a group of synthetic drugs that compare chemically to the sulfonamides. Thiazides act by inhibiting sodium and chloride reabsorption in the early portion of the distal tubule and may block chloride reabsorption in the ascending loop of Henle.	Bendroflumethiazide Chlorothiazide Hydrochlorothiazide Metolazone Polythiazide
Loop Diuretics	These are potent diuretic agents similar to the thiazides that inhibit the reabsorption of sodium and chloride in the ascending loop of Henle tubules.	Bumetanide Ethacrinic acid Furosemide
Distal Tubule Diuretics and Potassium-Sparing Diuretics	These agents exert their action in the distal tubule by inhibiting potassium excretion. They cause increased sodium and water excretion while retaining potassium.	Amiloride Spironolactone Triamterene
Osmotic Diuretics	These agents can be filtered by the glomeruli but are not reabsorbed into the circulation. They exert their effect by increasing the osmolality of the glomerular filtrate, the tubular fluid, and the plasma, thus promoting the excretion of water, chloride, sodium, and potassium.	Glycerin Isosorbide Mannitol Urea

---

N U R S I N G   A L E R T

Diuretic Cautions

With intravenous administration of diuretics, the nurse must be alert for untoward side effects and adverse reactions. A commonality with these agents are the side effects of weakness, vertigo, and postural hypotension, so the safety needs of the patient must be considered. Fluid and electrolyte imbalances can occur rapidly, so close monitoring of intake and output, weight, and serum electrolyte levels is crucial.

The rapid intravenous administration of furosemide can precipitate ototoxicity, which may or may not be reversible. The rate of administration should never exceed one to two minutes for a 40- to 80-mg bolus.

The loop diuretics are very irritating, causing local pain and irritation. They should only be injected into large veins or diluted adequately and administered slowly. When more than one IV dose is required, different veins should be used to prevent thrombo-phlebitis. With the potent loop diuretics, overdosage can occur rapidly, causing profound water loss, electrolyte depletion, reduced blood volume, and circulatory collapse.

Electrolytes

Electrolytes are frequently administered by intravenous infusion. The indications for each of them were covered extensively in Chapter 2.

N U R S I N G   T I P

Assessing for Fluid and Electrolyte Imbalances

It is the responsibility of the nurse to assess patients for fluid and electrolyte imbalances and be able to recognize deficits or excesses and correlate them with laboratory data and renal functioning so they can be adjusted promptly. Even small fluctuations in levels of calcium, magnesium, and potassium can put patients at great risk.

When administering any electrolyte it is critical that the nurse follow the prescribed guidelines regarding preparation and administration. If there is ever any doubt regarding the proper administration protocols for electrolytes, the nurse must check with an appropriate, current drug reference source or a pharmacist.

N U R S I N G   A L E R T

Administration of Potassium Solutions

It cannot be stressed often enough that potassium solutions must always be well diluted and administered slowly at a rate not to exceed 20 mEq/hr. Potassium is *never* administered by bolus injection, as this can precipitate irreversible, fatal cardiac arrest.

Hematologic Agents

The hematologic agents are those drugs that affect the clotting mechanisms of the blood. They work to inhibit clot formation, overcome coagulation problems, or dissolve clots. Table 11-8 describes each category of these drugs.

N U R S I N G   A L E R T

Side Effects of Anticoagulants

It is important to remember that all anticoagulants are associated with two major side effects: an increased risk of excessive bleeding and hemorrhage. Assessment should be made every 8 to 12 hours (or more often, if indicated) for bruising or bleeding from the nose, mouth, or gums. Stools and urine should be checked for blood and any gastric burning should be evaluated and reported.

With heparin administration, the antagonist, protamine sulfate, should be readily available in case excessive anticoagulant effects occur. When heparin is given by continuous infusion, coagulation studies are usually done every four to six hours during early therapy, then daily, once the PTT is stabilized. The nurse must check these values on a regular basis. When therapy is intermittent, it is the responsibility of the nurse to be sure that coagulation blood levels are drawn at least 30 minutes before a dose of heparin is given, and always taken from the extremity opposite from where the drug is being administered.

Histamine H-2 Antagonists

The H-2 receptor antagonists are competitive blockers of histamine in the gastric parietal cells. They inhibit all facets of gastric acid secretion in both volume and concentration.

Table 11-8 | Hematologic Agents

AGENT	MECHANISMS OF ACTION AND INDICATIONS	NAME
Anticoagulants	The anticoagulant agents are drugs that inhibit one or more of the pathways, or factors, involved in coagulation, thus preventing clot formation. They do not dissolve clots that are already present. Heparin is the prototype and only intravenous preparation is available. It exerts its effect by interfering with the conversion of prothrombin to thrombin. The deficiency of thrombin obstructs the conversion of fibrinogen to fibrin, thus preventing clot formation.	Heparin (IV, SC) Enoxaparin (SC) Anisindione (PO) Dicumarol (PO) Warfarin sodium (PO)
Antihemophilics	The etiology of hemophilia, the disorder (hereditary) in which excessive, uncontrolled bleeding can occur, is a deficiency of one or more plasma protein clotting factors. With type A, Factor VIII (antihemophilic factor, or AHF) activity is impaired, and with type B, the defect is in Factor IX. Specific factor replacement, based on the patient's weight, degree of deficiency, and blood loss, is the treatment. Administration of enough factor to attain 40% of the normal quantity results in hemostasis.	Factor VIII Factor IX
	Some patients develop inhibitors to Factor VIII and do not respond to replacement therapy. They must be given an anti-inhibitor coagulant complex to rectify this problem.	Anti-inhibitor coagulant complex
Antiplatelets	These agents inhibit platelet aggregation (to adhere to themselves or to other biologic or artificial structures) and are used to prevent thromboembolism. They exert their action by inhibiting thromboxane A_2 (the stimulus for platelet aggregation).	Aspirin Clopidrogel bisulfate Dipyridamole Sulfinpyrazone Ticlopidine
Hemorheologics	These agents decrease the viscosity of blood, which increases blood flow to the microcirculation and results in increased tissue oxygenation. It is thought that they exert their effect through decreased thromboxane A_2 synthesis (which decreases platelet aggregation), increased fibrinolysis (to decrease fibrinogen), and decreased aggregation of RBCs and decreased local hypervisosity by increasing cellular ATP.	Pentoxifylline
Hemostatics	These agents are used to arrest excessive bleeding. They may be applied topically to check local hemorrhage concomitant with intravenous administration for systemic control. The systemic hemostatics act by inhibiting the action of fibrinolysin and plasminogen activators. They are competitive antagonists of plasminogen and thereby prevent the formation of plasmin, thus inhibiting the dissolution of clots. The posterior pituitary hormone, desmopressin, increases Factor VIII levels.	Aminocaproic acid (IV, PO) Desmopressin acetate (IV) Topicals: cellulose, collagen, and gelatin products, and thrombin
Thrombolytics	The thrombolytic agents are enzymes that dissolve clots by converting plasminogen to the enzyme fibrinolysin (which dissolves the fibrin clots and plasma proteins contained in emboli and thrombi).	Anistreplase Streptokinase Urokinase
Tissue Plasminogen Activators (t-PA)	Tissue plasminogen activator (t-PA) is an enzyme derived from recombinant DNA that binds to the fibrin in a thrombus and converts the plasminogen in it to plasmin, which causes local fibrinolysis and clot disintegration. It is used to treat acute myocardial infarctions, and its effectiveness depends on how quickly it is injected following the attack.	Alteplase

---

NURSING ALERT

Side Effects of Thrombolytic Agents

Thrombolytic agents can produce serious side effects, including severe internal bleeding, bronchospasm, and angioneurotic edema. Aminocaproic acid should be readily available in the event of excessive bleeding.

It is very important to dilute thrombolytics according to manufacturer directions and administer them at the prescribed rate, using an electronic infusion device. If there is pain or redness at the infusion site, the cannula should be changed, using the opposite extremity, and the drugs should be further diluted to prevent thrombophlebitis. When nurses administer these drugs, they must follow institutional protocols.

They are effective in the prevention and treatment of gastroesophageal reflux, gastric and duodenal ulcers, and hypersecretory conditions.

The drugs in this group that are administered IV include cimetidine, famotidine, and ranitidine, among others. All may be administered by direct IV bolus, intermittent infusion, or continuous infusion. It is important to follow the manufacturer's guidelines regarding bolus injection of each drug, as there are very specific instructions regarding dilution and rate of administration.

Hormones

The endocrine system is composed of all the ductless glands that secrete hormones directly into the blood and lymph.

It works together with the nervous system to regulate and integrate bodily operations.

Hormones, which are either proteins or steroid compounds, control and regulate the functioning of specific organs, tissues and, in some cases, the body as a whole, providing a major contribution to homeostatic processes (Table 11-9). They influence growth and development, adaptation, personality, metabolism, resistance to disease, reproduction, nervous functioning, and stress responses. They exert their effect exercising one of two mechanisms: using either the steroid hormones or the other hormones. The steroids, which originate in the adrenals and reproductive glands, penetrate the cytoplasm of target cells and bind with protein receptors to form a complex. This compound enters the cell nucleus where it mobilizes genes to develop proteins that will do the work of the hormone. All of the other hormones, called first messengers because they attach directly to receptor sites on the cell membranes of their target cells, deliver specific messages themselves. When they bind to these cells, there is an increase in the activity of adenyl cyclase (the enzyme that causes ATP to be converted to cellular cyclic AMP). The cyclic AMP becomes the second messenger and carries out specific functions indicated by the first messenger hormone.

Alterations in endocrine function can result in an immense variety of pathological conditions, each with varying degrees of severity. These are usually the result of either diminished or excessive endocrine secretions or erroneous hormone receptor responses. In medicine and pharmacotherapeutics, exogenous hormones are administered to replace, enhance, or supplement endogenous hormonal supplies that have been altered by disease processes. They are also given for diagnostic purposes.

Since the endocrine system affects so many body systems and functions, numerous drugs might be indicated to adjust irregularities arising from this system. It would not be possible to cover them all here. Nonetheless, it is the responsibility of the nurse who administers such agents to understand what they are, why they are indicated, how they impact the endocrine system and the body as a whole, and how they interact with other agents and metabolic processes.

Hypnotics and Sedatives

Hypnotic agents induce sleep, and sedatives exert a calming effect on the body. They both include the classifications of barbiturates and benzodiazepines, covered earlier under the anticonvulsant and anxiolytic sections.

Table 11-9 | Hormonal Agents

ENDOCRINE GLAND	HORMONAL SECRETION	FUNCTION
Pituitary		
The pituitary gland (or hypophysis) is located in the sella turcica and attaches to the hypothalamus.* It is very small, but is responsible for regulating and coordinating the actions of other endocrine glands and influencing growth and development, thus giving it the designation, "master gland." It contains an anterior and a posterior lobe; both secrete hormones. Both lobes are under hypothalamic control, the anterior (adenohypophysis) being controlled by blood neurohumors that circulate in the blood between it and the hypothalamus, and the posterior (neurohypophysis) via nerve connections between it and the hypothalamus.	Anterior pituitary hormones are secreted in response to hypothalamic substances known as releasing factors (RF), which are specific for the particular hormone to be released (except for the luteinizing hormone). There are two types of cells in the tissue structure of the anterior pituitary that secrete hormones, the acidophils and the basophils.	
	Growth hormone (GH) is secreted by the acidophils.	GH, also called somatotropic hormone, has a growth factor that stimulates the growth of bones, muscles, and organs, and regulates protein anabolism, increases fat catabolism, decreases glucose catabolism and reduces peripheral glucose uptake by muscles and adipose tissue to raise blood sugar (diabetogenic effect).
Posterior pituitary hormones are called *tropic* or stimulating because they cause other glands to secrete their hormones. They work, generally, by a system of negative feedback.	Follicle-stimulating hormone (FSH) is secreted by the basophils.	FSH stimulates follicular growth in the ovaries.

(continues)

Table 11-9 | Hormonal Agents (continued)

ENDOCRINE GLAND	HORMONAL SECRETION	FUNCTION
Pituitary		
	Luteinizing hormone (LH) is secreted by the basophils.	LH, combined with circulating estrogen and FSH, stimulates the mature follicle to break and ovulation to occur, with formation of the corpus luteum.
	Thyrotropic hormone or thyroid-stimulating hormone (TSH) is secreted by the basophils.	TSH stimulates both the growth and secretion of the thyroid gland.
	Lactogenic factor (Prolactin) is secreted by the acidophils.	Prolactin, in association with estrogen and progesterone, stimulates breast formation and milk formation by the mammary glands during pregnancy. The act of sucking continues to stimulate its production.
	Adrenocorticotropic hormone (ACTH)	ACTH stimulates the activity of the adrenal cortex of the adrenal gland, which releases three corticoid hormones. These are the glucocorticoids, mineralocorticoids, and androgens.
	Melanocyte-stimulating hormone (MSH) has a chemical structure similar to ACTH.	MSH may be responsible for normal pigmentation and, under some stressful circumstances, increases pigmentation.
	Posterior pituitary hormones are made by the hypothalamus and stored in the neurohypophysis until the hypothalamus causes their release into the bloodstream.	
	Antidiuretic hormone (ADH) or vasopressin (an ambiguous term because normal physiologic levels of ADH do not cause vasoconstriction).	ADH exerts a stimulating effect on the collecting tubules of the kidneys to increase their permeability and reabsorb water back into the bloodstream.
	The normal stimulus for the release of ADH is any situation that causes dehydration.	Studies suggest this hormone may play a role in learning and memory.
	Oxytocin	Oxytocin stimulates the smooth musculature of the uterus to contract during labor and promotes delivery of the infant and placenta. It also acts on the mammary glands to stimulate the release of milk.
Thyroid		
The thyroid gland is a butterfly-shaped mass of tissue that lies in the anterior neck region. The thyroid produces and secretes thyroxine, triiodothyronine, and calcitonin, the first two being iodine-bearing derivatives of the amino acid tyrosine. The first two are produced in the follicle cells of the thyroid gland and are stimulated by the anterior pituitary hormone, TSH. They require iodine for their synthesis, which they pick up from the circulating blood as it circulates through the thyroid. The iodides combine with the amino acid tyrosine in the thyroid gland to form thyroglobulin. Thyroglobulin is chemically converted to triiodothyronine, and finally to thyroxine before the thyroid releases it into the bloodstream.	Thyroxine or tetraiodothyronine (T_4) works at the cellular level but is released at a much slower rate than T_3.	
	Triiodothyronine (T_3) is the major active form of thyroid hormone at the cellular level.	T_3 controls metabolic rate, cellular oxidation, and heat production (except for the brain and spleen). It plays a major role in the regulation of physical growth, mental development, sexual maturity, and the exchange of water and salts (acting as a diuretic). At the hepatic level, it affects the conversion of glycogen from nonsugar sources, and at the cellular level, it stimulates glucose breakdown.
	Calcitonin, along with parathormone (from the parathyroids), maintains the constant level of calcium in the blood.	Calcitonin controls the calcium ion concentration necessary for blood clotting, cellular integrity, and neuromuscular activity, by sustaining a balanced level (5%) in the blood. (99% of the calcium is stored in the bones.)

(continues)

Table 11-9 | Hormonal Agents (continued)

ENDOCRINE GLAND	HORMONAL SECRETION	FUNCTION
Parathyroids		
The parathyroids are four small, rice-shaped glands attached to the surface of the posterior thyroid.	Parathyroid hormone (Parathormone)	Parathormone, like calcitonin, controls blood calcium levels by stimulating the increased production of osteoclasts which invade bones, digest calcium, and return it to the blood.
Adrenal Glands		
There are two adrenal glands, one located on top of each kidney. Each gland has two parts, the cortex and the medulla. The cortex secretes the hormones known as the corticoids, which include the glucocorticoids, mineralocorticoids, and the androgens. The medulla secretes epinephrine and norepinephrine.	Glucocorticoids	The glucocorticoids (G-Cs) protect against stress (via mechanisms of cortisone and hydrocortisone) and affect carbohydrate and protein metabolism.
	Mineralocorticoids	The mineralocorticoids (M-Cs) are involved in the regulation of fluid and electrolytes through effects on ionic transport and on the renal tubules.
	Androgens	The androgens (male sex hormones), together with those from the gonads, foster the development of masculine characteristics and promote protein metabolism and growth in the male body. (Testosterone is produced in the testes.)
	Epinephrine (adrenaline) is a powerful stimulant.	Epinephrine works by stimulating the release of stored glycogen for muscle action, increasing cardiac rate and contractility force, raising systolic BP, exciting the nervous system, and increasing muscular blood flow.
	Norepinephrine is chemically related to epinephrine but is not as powerful.	Norepinephrine stimulates vasoconstriction and has little effect on cardiac output (even though it is chemically similar to epinephrine.
Pancreas		
The pancreas, located behind the stomach, is an exocrine and an endocrine gland composed of glandular cells (that regulate the release of digestive juices) and the islet cells (which secrete hormones). The islets of Langerhans produce A cells (glucagon), B cells (insulin), D cells (somatostatin), and F cells (pancreatic polypeptide).	Insulin release is stimulated by high levels of blood sugar and growth hormone.	Insulin promotes the utilization of cellular glucose, facilitates protein synthesis, and promotes the transport of amino acids, fatty acids, and fat deposition into the cells.
	Glucagon	Glucagon, an insulin antagonist, increases the blood glucose levels.
	Pancreatic polypeptide	PP inhibits the release of digestive secretions of the pancreas.
	Somatostatin is a GH-inhibiting hormone, the same as is produced by the hypothalamus.	Somatostatin suppresses the release of other hormones from the pancreas and the hormones of the digestive tract. It reduces the rate at which triglycerides are absorbed from the intestine following a high-fat meal.
Ovaries		
The ovaries are the primary female sex organs, located lateral to the uterus on each side of the pelvis. They produce the ova (making them cytogenic), the female germ cells, and the hormones (making them endocrinic) estrogen and progesterone.	Estrogen	Estrogen develops and maintains the female secondary sex characteristics and repairs and thickens the uterine lining by stimulating the production of new epithelial cells.

(continues)

Table 11-9 | Hormonal Agents (continued)

ENDOCRINE GLAND	HORMONAL SECRETION	FUNCTION
Ovaries		
	Progesterone	Progesterone maintains the continued growth of the endometrium for pregnancy maintenance should an embryo implant. It averts the formation of new ovarian follicles by inhibiting the release of FSH and decreases uterine contractions during pregnancy.
Testes		
The testes are the primary male reproductive organs, contained in the scrotum. They produce the male gametes, spermatozoa, and the hormone, testosterone.	Testosterone	Testosterone is the principal male hormone that promotes the growth of male secondary sex characteristics and is essential for the normal growth and development of the male accessory sexual organs and sexual behavior.
Thymus		
The thymus gland is both an endocrine gland and a lymphatic organ, located under the sternum, but anterior and superior to the pericardium.	Homeostatic thymic hormone (HTH)	HTH assists bone marrow cells with immunological abilities.
	Lymphocytosis-stimulating hormones (LSHr and LSH$_R$)	These enhance antigen-antibody responses and stimulate lymphocyte production.
	Thymic factor (TF)	TF stimulates the thymus gland to differentiate and develop T-cells.
	Thymic humoral factor (THF) secretion subsides with age and is ravaged by disease, radiation, and toxins.	THF, a protein, stimulates mitosis.
	Thymic replacing factor (TRF)	TRF restores the immune activity of T-cell–deprived structures.
	Thymopoietin (Thymin)	Thymopoietin obstructs neuromuscular nerve transmission.
	Thymosin	Thymosin enhances T-cell development, assists with the growth and differentiation of thymus lymphoid cells, and activates the secretion of luteinizing hormone releasing factor (LHRF).
	Thymosterin	Thymosterin inhibits lymph cell formation and tumor growth.
Pineal Gland		
The pineal gland, while not classified as an endocrine gland, is located posterior to the third ventricle of the brain. There is a great deal of research being done regarding the hormone melatonin, secreted by this gland, especially in the areas of sleep disorders and the body's problems associated with response to time zone changes ("jet lag").	Melatonin is a precursor of serotonin that is rapidly taken up by the cells and metabolized.	Melatonin is regulatory for the cyclic phenomena of the body and is involved in circadian rhythms. It depresses gonadal function by inhibiting the secretion of LH.

The hypothalamus also secretes somatostatin, a hormone distributed throughout the CNS, that has some bearing on nerve impulse transmission. Somatostatin works to inhibit the secretions of growth hormone, secretions of the intestinal mucosa, and the pancreatic hormones.

Immunobiologic Regulators

The immunobiologic regulators that most people are familiar with are those agents that are used to provide active or passive immunity against diseases when the body's own natural resistance and adaptive responses are inadequate. These, of course, are the common immunizations that are administered throughout the life cycle. When certain disease processes arise in the body, or when people receive organ transplants, other biologic modifiers become necessary, such as the biologic response modifiers, the immunostimulants, and the immunosuppressants.

Biologic Response Modifiers

Biologic response modifiers (BRMs) are used as adjuncts to surgery, chemotherapy, and radiation therapy in the treatment of antineoplastic diseases and are becoming promising modalities in this area. They are divided into three major categories, depending on their mechanism of action:

1. BRMs that augment, modulate, or restore the body's normal immunologic mechanisms
2. BRMs that have antitumor effects
3. BRMs that exert other biologic effects, such as disruption of the metastatic abilities of tumors (either to metastasize, or survive after metastasis), promotion of cell differentiation, or interference with the ability of cells to undergo neoplastic transformation

There are presently five promising areas of cancer research and treatment involving BRMs. These include the colony-stimulating factors, the monoclonal antibodies, the interferons, the interleukins, and tumor necrosis factors.

Immunostimulants

The immunostimulants are agents used to enhance the functioning of the immune system by prompting the formation of antibodies. When given to healthy individuals, they bolster immunity against specific diseases. When given to patients who are ill, they provide passive immunity.

Originally, immunostimulation consisted of the administration of serum (gamma globulin) that contained antibodies produced by another person. Currently, immunostimulation includes nonspecific systemic stimulation, adjuvants, active specific immunotherapy, and adoptive immunotherapy, some modalities of which overlap into areas of biological response modification.

Immune globulin IV, an immune globulin G antibody product, is administered intravenously for immunodeficiency diseases and syndromes. It must be given by a separate IV line, with an EID, and never mixed with other infusates or medications. Epinephrine should be readily available in the event of hypersensitivity or allergic reactions. The same precautions apply for the other immune serums and the antitoxins and antivenins.

Immunosuppressants

Immunosuppressants are agents administered to suppress the body's natural immune response to antigens. These are used to control autoimmune diseases and to enhance the survival of foreign tissue grafts and transplants. They supposedly act by suppressing the T-lymphocytes and are often administered in conjunction with corticosteroid preparations, which enhance their effectiveness.

Muscle Relaxants

Muscle relaxants are agents that relax or inactivate one or more muscles. They act by either competitively blocking acetylcholine at the neuromuscular junction or by depressing areas of the CNS (basal ganglia, brain stem, and internuncial neurons of the spinal cord).

NURSING ALERT

Monitoring Patients Who Receive Neuromuscular Blocking Agents

Patients who receive neuromuscular blocking agents require meticulous monitoring, since these agents can produce cardiac collapse, respiratory paralysis, or both. There is a narrow margin of safety between the dose that induces muscle relaxation and the amount that results in a toxic dose. The antidotes edrophonium, neostigmine, or pyridostigmine, along with atropine and cardiac and respiratory life-support equipment, must be readily available to reverse any untoward effects that may develop. Vital signs must be frequently monitored. The nurse must also be aware that many other agents interfere with, or potentiate, the effect of these drugs. Low serum potassium levels antagonize them, and their effects are potentiated by acidosis.

The neuromuscular blocking agents are used to inactivate or relax one or more muscles to facilitate surgery, prevent laryngospasm affiliated with endotracheal intubation, or to control severe muscle spasms associated with certain disease processes. They are also used during electroconvulsive therapy to reduce excessive muscular contractions. These agents are ineffective for the muscle rigidity and spasticity that is associated with neurological disease or trauma. These drugs are generally given intravenously, with the initial dose being administered by a physician.

The centrally acting muscle relaxants do not alter muscle excitability, nerve conductivity, or neuromuscular impulse transmission. These agents are used to treat the muscle spasms related to severe sprains, strains, and other traumatic situations. They also are used to treat conditions that are characterized by the involuntary spasms accompanying some neurological diseases as well as the chronic pain of the arthritic and rheumatoid diseases.

Parenteral administration of these drugs is five to ten times more effective than by the oral route. The major side effect to assess for, however, is the degree of sedation, which may compromise patient safety.

Nutritional Agents

The nutritional agents include the carbohydrates, proteins, fats, vitamins, minerals, some organic salts, and the trace elements. When they are administered intravenously, they are usually a component of total parenteral nutrition therapy (see Chapter 13).

Respiratory Agents

The respiratory agents are those preparations used in the prevention and treatment of disorders involving the internal and external exchange of oxygen and carbon dioxide between the body and the external environment. Some exert their effect on specific respiratory structures, while others are centrally acting. These agents include the antitussives, bronchodilators, decongestants, expectorants, and mucolytics. Some antitussives and bronchodilators are administered intravenously, while the decongestants, expectorants, and mucolytics are generally administered by other routes.

Antitussives

The antitussives prevent or relieve cough. Although they have no effect on the underlying cause of coughing, they relieve the discomfort and irritation associated with it and allow the patient to rest.

The nonnarcotic antitussives exert their effect by acting on receptors in the pulmonary tree and the pleura to anesthetize and stretch them, thus inhibiting their activity and reduce the cough reflex. The narcotic agents depress the cough center in the medulla, which results in an increased threshold for incoming cough impulses.

Bronchodilators

The bronchodilators improve air flow in the bronchi and bronchioles in order to facilitate breathing. They are indicated for the treatment of asthma and obstructive pulmonary conditions. In general, they are adrenergic (sympathomimetic) agents, but some are also xanthines. The sympathomimetics act on the alpha-adrenergic receptors to induce vasoconstriction (which reduces bronchial mucosal edema) and on the $beta_2$-adrenergic receptors (to induce smooth muscle relaxation in the bronchi). The xanthines break down the cyclic AMP cycle which, in turn, results in bronchial smooth muscle relaxation and bronchodilation. They include the theophylline derivatives, which are administered in accord with serum blood levels, which the nurse must monitor.

> ### NURSING ALERT
>
> #### Effects of Bronchodilating Agents
>
> Remember that bronchodilating agents also exert $beta_1$ stimulation (which increases cardiac rate and contractility). They may produce cardiac, cerebral, and skeletal muscle stimulation as well as coronary vasodilation and diuresis. The nurse must assess for anorexia, anxiety, cardiac dysrhythmias, confusion, headache, nausea, and tremors, all adverse reactions to bronchodilating agents.

Decongestants, Expectorants, and Mucolytics

Decongestants act to dilate the arterioles of the nasal mucosa by stimulating the alpha-adrenergic receptors of vascular smooth muscle. Expectorants stimulate the removal of lower respiratory tract secretions by decreasing secretion viscosity and facilitating their removal by enhancing cough productivity. The mucolytics reduce the viscosity of respiratory secretions by dividing the disulfide chemical bonds of mucous. These agents, although not administered intravenously, are mentioned here because they are often administered as adjuncts to the antitussives and bronchodilators. It is important for the nurse to understand that these preparations have many of the same side effects as the parenteral products and may potentiate or interact with them.

Volume Expanders

The volume expanders are nonblood products indicated to replace plasma volume. They are indicated for hypovolemic conditions resulting from burns, hemorrhage, sepsis, and surgery. The two commonly prescribed products are dextran and hetastarch (see Chapter 14).

DRUG COMPATIBILITY AND INTERACTIONS

For medications and infusates to be administered intravenously they must be chemically, physically, and therapeutically compatible with each other in order to avoid serious complications that can result from interactions. **Incompatibility** refers to any undesirable chemical or physical interaction or reaction between two or more medications or medications and infusates when they are admixed. Incompatibilities can occur for any combination of reasons, but usually are the result of:

1. Acidity or alkalinity of the admixture
2. Exposure to light prior to or during administration
3. Extremes of temperature
4. Length of time in solution prior to administration or the duration of infusion
5. Order in which drugs are mixed

Pharmacokinetic incompatibilities can result from a variety of physical or chemical interactions that alter the way any of the components in an admixture exert, or fail to exert, their effect. These may be chemical, which include complications resulting from hydrolysis, oxidation-reduction reactions, precipitation, and others, or physical, in which an actual visual change is evident. Many incompatibilities are the result of acid-base irregularities.

Therapeutic incompatibilities are those that occur once the medications come in contact with the body. These include any alterations in the intended effects of the products administered. Examples of these are allergy, antagonism (unintended), idiosyncrasy, potentiation, paradoxical effects, and any other unpredictable drug responses.

It is the responsibility of the nurse who prepares and administers medications and infusates to ascertain compatibility. There are many compatibility charts prepared by various pharmaceutical and product manufacturers, as well as those created within various agencies. This book, along with literature accompanying medications and infusates, appropriate drug references, and consultation with pharmacists, are all methods the nurse should be familiar with and use to ensure patient safety when administering medications.

Key Concepts

❋ Before preparing or giving any medication or intravenous infusion, the nurse must have a practical, working knowledge of the pharmacokinetics and principles of drug action associated with the products she is administering.

❋ It is important for the nurse to have a working knowledge of the intravenous drug classifications, along with the precautions and nursing actions and interventions associated with their administration.

❋ Because of indiscriminate use of antibiotics and carelessness among health care workers, many microbes have become resistant to standard treatment and eradication regimens.

❋ Prior to administering any medication or infusate, the nurse must verify compatibility with other agents the patient is receiving. This means that she must be able to understand and properly use approved compatibility charts.

Review Questions and Activities

1. Using a current nurses' drug handbook or the *Physicians' Desk Reference,*® look up three drugs that are administered intravenously (e.g., ampicillin sodium, phenytoin, and digoxin). Formulate a chart that diagrams the pharmacokinetics of these drugs, illustrating the following:

   (a) Uptake and absorption

   (b) Biotransformation

   (c) Local and systemic distribution

   (d) Duration of action

   (e) Mode and routes of excretion

2. Explain the concepts of drug action in terms of the following:

    (a) Target cell–receptor site interaction

    (b) Enzymatic interaction

    (c) Physiochemical composition changes

    (d) Metabolic pathway alterations

    (e) Biotransformation

    (f) Time-response reactions

3. Explain how the following factors are considered when antimicrobial therapy is prescribed:

    (a) Clinical status of the patient

    (b) Activity spectrum of the drug

    (c) Patterns of bacterial resistance

    (d) Pharmacokinetics and safety

    (e) Categories for use: prophylaxis, empirical treatment, or definitive therapy

4. Explain the nurse's role in the preparation and administration of antineoplastic agents.

5. What precautions must be taken with the intravenous administration of potassium? Why?

6. What side effects common to most diuretic agents must the nurse assess for, especially when they are administered intravenously?

7. Describe the concepts of incompatibility as they relate to intravenous medication administration.

8. Formulate an intravenous compatibility chart for the following medications:

    - Albumin
    - Aminophylline
    - Atropine
    - Calcium chloride
    - Dextran
    - D_5W
    - Diazepam
    - Digoxin
    - Dopamine
    - Epinephrine
    - Furosemide

    - Gentamycin
    - Heparin sodium
    - Insulin (regular)
    - Lidocaine
    - Morphine
    - Nitroglycerin
    - Normal saline
    - Phenobarbital
    - Potassium chloride
    - Phenytoin
    - Ringer's lactate

Chapter 12

Central and Peripherally Placed Vascular Access Devices and Advanced Medication Delivery Systems

COMPETENCIES

Upon completion of this chapter, the reader should be able to:

✳ List the major indications for placement of a central venous catheter (CVC).

✳ List the major contraindications for placement of a central venous catheter.

✳ Locate the insertion pathways and dwelling positions for centrally placed venous catheters, peripherally inserted central catheters, midline catheters, and centrally and peripherally implanted subcutaneous ports.

✳ Identify the signs and symptoms of the immediate and delayed risks and complications associated with central line placement.

✳ Analyze the nursing interventions related to the complications that may occur subsequent to central venous catheter placement and use.

✳ Review the preventive measures, signs, symptoms, and emergency nursing interventions associated with a CVC-related air embolism.

✳ Examine the protocols regarding the care of single and multilumen nontunneled and tunneled central catheters.

✳ Explain the differences in pressure gradients associated with the use of small-barrel and large-barrel syringes in irrigating central lines.

✳ List the major indications and advantages for placement of peripherally inserted central catheters (PICCs) and midline catheters (MLCs).

✳ List the major contraindications and disadvantages for placement of PICCs and MLCs.

✳ Differentiate between peripherally inserted central catheters and midline catheters in terms of placement and the infusates that can be administered through them.

✳ Review the protocols for the insertion, use, and maintenance of subcutaneously implanted vascular access ports.

✳ Explain the placement and use of central venous catheters in hemodynamic monitoring.

✳ Outline the advanced access routes used for the delivery of infusates and medications other than those used for peripheral and central venous access.

KEY TERMS

air embolism	chylothorax	intraosseus
arterial laceration	epidural	intrathecal
brachial plexus injury	extracorporeal	mediastinal injury
cardiac tamponade	hemothorax	pneumothorax
catheter embolism	hydromediastinum	sepsis
catheter malposition	hydrothorax	thrombosis

Note to the Reader

Within this chapter there are many illustrations and step-by-step guidelines for using various vascular access devices and delivery systems. They are included to visually acquaint the reader with such products and to illustrate the principles and procedures that the nurse may use in working with them. This is especially important for the student using the material in this chapter to prepare for a clinical practicum. It provides a means to correlate theoretical principles with actual nursing practice and acquaints the learner with a general knowledge of the types of vascular devices that may be encountered during clinical rotations. In actual professional practice, however, the nurse is expected to be familiar with the products, as well as the procedures and protocols for their use, based on manufacturer's instructions and agency or institutional policy.

Permission has been granted to illustrate each of the products cited. While credit is given to each manufacturer's device, the author and publisher are not endorsing any of these particular products over other, similar ones that are on the market.

When patients are in need of long-term infusion therapy or, because of their condition or disease processes, require special types of medication and treatment, the commonly used peripheral vascular access routes indicated for relatively short-term use are not practical. In such situations, central venous access may be required, using specialized catheters or ports. Today, in fact, a central line may be the first choice for vascular access in many patients.

With nurses providing care in such varied settings today, they are coming in contact with central venous access devices (CVADs) that, until recently, were seen only in acute care settings. Nurses assist with the insertion of many of these products and are being trained to insert some of them. Regardless of the situation pertaining to when or where they are inserted, or by whom, nurses are expected to know how to care for patients who have central venous access devices in place. It is becoming more and more common for nurses to administer medications, fluids, and blood through these access routes, to troubleshoot and correct complications, and to teach family members in the home how to use these devices and care for patients who have them. With the increasing health care shift (from the hospital) to a community-based setting, more and more in recent years, patients and their caregivers are now required to take a proactive stance in their infusion-related care.

CENTRAL VENOUS THERAPY

Central venous routes are accessed in order to deliver fluids, medications, blood or blood products, chemotherapy, nutritional agents, and for the withdrawal of blood samples when frequent laboratory tests are required. They are also used to assess cardiac and pulmonary function parameters. Such routes provide a reliable means of vascular access that can be used repeatedly and for long periods of time.

Central venous access is achieved using one of four devices: centrally inserted catheters, peripherally inserted catheters, centrally implanted ports, or peripherally inserted ports. Some devices have been on the market for years and are reliable, safe, and efficacious. Newer products have various characteristics of the original devices, with more advanced features. An estimated 5 million CVADs are placed each year in the U.S., with the number increasing as the population ages (Genentech, 2002).

Indications

The major indications for placement of a central venous catheter include the following:

1. Inadequate peripheral vascular access.
2. Complex treatment regimens requiring frequent vascular access for analgesics, antibiotics, chemotherapy, hematologic agents, or long-term rehydration. By putting a central line in place, the peripheral veins are spared, and the patient is saved the discomfort and stress associated with multiple needlesticks.
3. Hyperosmolar infusions. The greater hemodilution of a central vessel precludes the vein irritation that occurs when hypertonic infusates are administered through peripheral veins.
4. Infusion of irritating or vesicant drugs. Any drug with a pH below 5, above 9, or with an osmlarity greater than 500 mOsm can cause severe venous irritation and subsequent chemical phlebitis. Some drugs with a safe pH range (such as erythromycin, lidocaine, and others) may cause chemical irritation. Others, such as morphine, potassium, and others are irritating if they are not adequately diluted. Vesicants bind with cellular DNA and cause tissue necrosis. The high degree of hemodilution in large central vessels reduces these complications.
5. Rapid absorption and rapid blood and tissue perfusion.
6. Long-term IV therapy in the hospital, home, or outpatient clinic setting.
7. Patient preference. Based on lifestyles, especially those related to occupation and recreational or sports activities, patients choose the convenience of certain central devices over others.

Contraindications

The major reasons for not inserting a central venous catheter are related to the patient's condition, underlying disease processes, or anatomic structural deviations or pathologies. The contraindications include:

1. Altered skin integrity
2. Anomalies of the central vasculature
3. Cancer at the base of the neck or apex of the lung
4. Chronic immunosuppression
5. Coagulopathies
6. Fractured clavicle
7. Hyperinflated lungs secondary to mechanical hyperventilation or pathophysiology
8. Radiation to the insertion site area
9. Septicemia
10. Superior vena cava syndrome
11. VAD complication history

Insertion Pathways and Placement

The usual sites of insertion for central catheters are the subclavian vein or the internal and external jugulars. Although these exist bilaterally, access from the right side is preferable because the path to the superior vena cava is less tortuous and associated with less chance of tension pneumothorax than from left-sided entry. The subclavian is the preferred vein because it is easier to access (supra- or infraclavicular approaches), is a high-flow vessel, is easier to secure without major discomfort to the patient, is associated with a lower risk of infection, and presents less likelihood of catheter tip movement. Its disadvantages are its close proximity to the lung apex (pneumothorax risk) and subclavian artery (laceration risk), and the fact that it is a noncompressible vessel, making bleeding control difficult. The internal jugular is a large vessel, easy to access with a short, straight pathway to the superior vena cava (although it is in close proximity to the carotid artery). It is acceptable but, because of its location, it is difficult to immobilize and secure the catheter, and there is a greater risk of infection because of its proximity to oropharyngeal secretions (having the highest infection rate of all the insertion sites). It is also more uncomfortable for the patient, especially if he is mobile and in need of it for long-term therapy. Mechanical complications associated with insertion are less of a problem with the internal jugular than the subclavian. The external jugular is not often used, although its superficial location makes it easy to see and locate. It is difficult to cannulate because of its tortuous path and valves, and because it tends to roll.

If the veins of the upper body are unsuitable or difficult to access, the catheter is inserted into the femoral vein and threaded into the inferior vena cava. This site is only recommended for short-term, emergency use, as it carries an increased rate of thrombosis, phlebitis, and infection, and is difficult to dress. The femoral vein cannot be used for central venous pressure (CVP) line insertion because the catheter tip rests in the inferior vena cava.

For peripherally inserted central lines, the three commonly used veins of the arm are the basilic (preferred because it is larger and maintains a straighter path), the cephalic, and the median cubital. For implantable ports, surgical cutdown on the cephalic or jugular veins provides a passageway into the superior vena cava. Peripherally placed ports are accessed via the basilic or cephalic veins. Figure 12-1 shows the location of some major veins of the upper body and trunk and Figure 12-2 illustrates the length and diameter of the upper extremity veins in relation to the diameter of a 4.0 French catheter.

A central venous catheter needs to be positioned so the tip terminates in the superior vena cava, within 3 to 4 cm of the right atrial-superior vena cava junction. The tip of a femoral line resides in the inferior vena cava. It must be free-floating and lie parallel to the vessel wall without any looping or kinking. The catheter tip must never rest within the right atrium, where it could traverse the sinoatrial node and trigger a dysrhythmia or become entrapped in the tricuspid

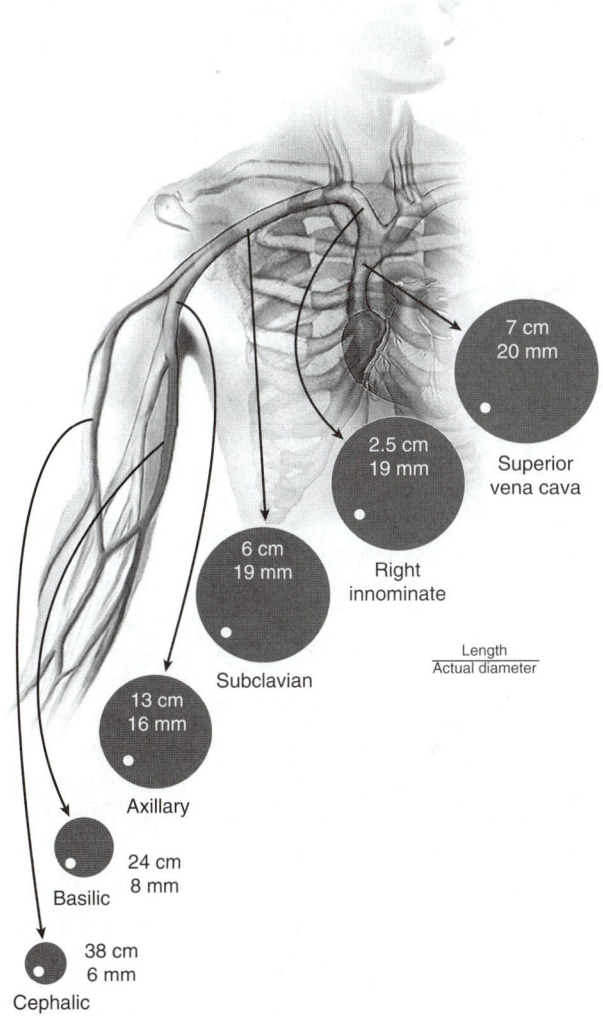

Figure 12-2 | Upper extremity vein sizes. The white dot represents the size of a 4.0 French catheter in relation to the diameter of these vessels. Courtesy of GESCO® International

valve and cause damage that could result in the need for valvular replacement surgery. Placement must always be confirmed by x-ray before any infusate is administered, even if verification with calibrated pressure transducers or right atrial cardioelectrographics is done. (The policy in some agencies allows infusion at a KVO rate of 10 to 50 ml/hr until radiological verification of placement can be obtained. This is not necessary, as the central line lumen(s) should have been primed with 0.9% sodium chloride prior to insertion to maintain patency.)

Proper positioning of a CVC in the superior vena cava provides the following:

1. Optimum dilution of infusates
2. Large volume infusate administration
3. Rapid administration when needed

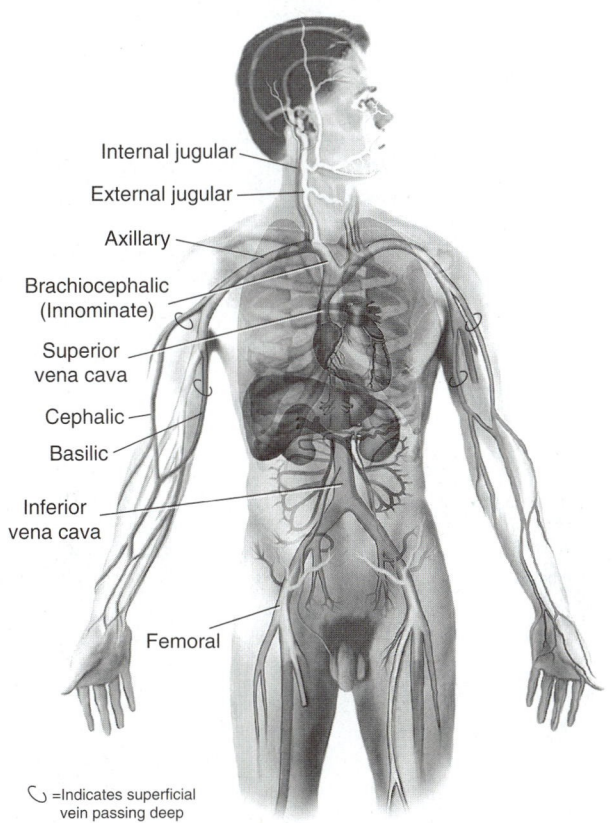

Figure 12-1 | Veins of the upper body and trunk

4. Accurate CVP monitoring (within 1 mm Hg of actual right atrial pressure in the supine patient)
5. The least risk of vascular or cardiac trauma or perforation

Risks and Complications

Although the advantages of CVC use far outweigh the disadvantages, the potential for complications and adverse reactions associated with central venous therapy must always be an uppermost consideration. The general complications related to infusion therapy were covered in Chapter 5, but Table 12-1 reviews those that are specifically associated with central venous catheters. The immediate complications are

Table 12-1 | Risks and Complications Associated with Central Venous Catheters

IMMEDIATE COMPLICATIONS		
Problem and Etiology	**Signs and Symptoms**	**Interventions**
Air Embolism: The entry of air into the circulatory system during CVC insertion, tubing change, or removal, or due to catheter damage or breakage. Death ensues from the rapid injection of 100 cc to 200 cc of air, with the average lethal dose being 70 cc to 150 cc or 5 cc/kg. to 15 cc/kg. As little as 10 cc can be lethal to a gravely ill person.	• Chest pain • Confusion • Dyspnea • Elevated CVP • Hypotension • Light-headedness • Pallor • Precordial churning murmur • Tachycardia • Tachypnea • Thready pulse • Unresponsiveness	• Place patient in left lateral Trendelenburg position • Clamp catheter • Administer oxygen (100%, if possible) • Notify physician • Monitor vital signs • Document incident ***Note:*** In only 1 sec, 100 cc of air can be inspired by a patient sitting upright with an open 14-gauge CVC.
Arterial Laceration: The inadvertent cut or puncture of an artery by the insertion needle or guide wire during CVP insertion.	• Hematoma formation • Hemothorax, if subclavian artery is perforated • Hypotension • Loss of consciousness • Respiratory distress • Tachycardia • Tracheal compression	• Apply pressure (depending on which vessel is lacerated) • Monitor vital signs • Assist with preparation for surgical intervention if carotid is lacerated
Cardiac Tamponade: Perforation of the pericardium by a CVC, resulting in compression of the heart because of leakage of blood or infusates into the pericardial sac.	• Cardiovascular collapse • Hypotension • Elevated CVP (neck vein distension) • Pulsus paradoxus • Quiet heart (muffled heart sounds due to fluid)	• Assist with aspiration of the pericardial sac • Assist with emergency resuscitation measures • Monitor vital signs • Support the patient
Catheter Embolism: Breakage of a portion of the CVC, due to improper insertion technique, improper administration of infusates (using excessive pressure), or pinch-off	Signs and symptoms are dependent on where the severed portion of the CVC lodges and blocks circulation and may include the following: • Cardiac arrest • Chest pain • Cyanosis • Dyspnea • Hypotension • Loss of consciousness • Respiratory arrest	• Institute emergency measures in accord with symptoms • Maintain bed rest • Monitor vital signs • Prepare the patient for x-ray • Prepare for surgery

continues

Table 12-1 | Risks and Complications Associated with Central Venous Catheters (continued)

IMMEDIATE COMPLICATIONS		
Problem and Etiology	**Signs and Symptoms**	**Interventions**
Catheter Malposition: Intravascular malposition outside of the superior vena cava is usually due to improper positioning of the patient during insertion. Extravascular malposition occurs when the CVC exits the vein due to perforation of the vessel during insertion.	• Arm, neck, or shoulder discomfort • Difficulty or inability to aspirate or deliver infusions • Neck or shoulder edema • Neurologic deficits • Arm or neck swelling • Chylothorax • Hemothorax • Hydrothorax • Pneumothorax	• Assist the physician during guide wire exchange • Flush to reposition (20 ml of 0.9% NaCl over a 5-second period) silicon CVCs if there is no resistance to flow • Administer oxygen • Assist with catheter removal • Assist with chest tube insertion • Assist with coughing and deep breathing • Monitor vital signs • Position to promote ease of breathing
Chylothorax: Lymph (chyle) accumulation in the thoracic cavity due to laceration or perforation of the thoracic duct (where it enters the subclavian vein) during CVC insertion	• *See note • Chest pain • Dyspnea • Withdrawal of milky chyle during CVC insertion as thoracic duct is pierced • Leakage of chyle around CVC insertion site	• Administer oxygen • Assist with catheter removal • Assist with chest tube insertion • Monitor vital signs • Collect specimen of cloudy leakage for analysis
Hemothorax: Blood accumulation in the pleural cavity due to vessel laceration or perforation during CVC insertion	• *See note • Chest pain • Cyanosis with dusky pallor • Decreased or absent breath sounds • Dullness with percussion over affected area • Dyspnea • Hemoptysis • Reduced hemoglobin from blood pooling	• Administer oxygen • Assist with catheter removal • Assist with chest tube insertion • Monitor vital signs • Position for breathing ease • Provide frequent mouth care
Hydrothorax: Fluid accumulation in the thoracic cavity due to vessel laceration or perforation during CVC insertion	• *See note • Chest pain • Cyanosis • Dyspnea • Flat, dull sound over fluid • Murmur over fluid • Vesicular breath sound absence	• Administer oxygen • Assist with catheter removal • Assist with aspiration of pleural space fluid • Assist with chest tube insertion • Monitor vital signs • Position for breathing comfort
Pneumothorax: Air accumulation in the pleural cavity due to perforation of the visceral pleura during CVC insertion, usually due to improper patient positioning	• Absent breath sounds • Chest pain (sudden) • Cyanosis • Distended unilateral chest • Dyspnea with gasping respirations • Hypotension • Mediastinal shift • Pallor • Tachycardia • Tachypnea • Tympanic resonance	• Administer oxygen • Assess breath sounds, chest expansion, and vital signs • Assist with chest tube insertion • Instruct and assist with deep breathing and coughing • Maintain hydration and nutrition • Maintain range of motion • Position patient in semi-Fowler's position for ease of breathing • Provide rest
Brachial Plexus Injury: Results from damage incurred during CVC insertion and involves the cervical and upper dorsal spinal nerves that extend into the arms and hands.	• Hand and finger numbness and tingling • Arm, wrist, and hand pain • Paralysis of the arm	**Note:** Injury may be permanent and treatment is palliative. • Administer medication for pain control • Encourage compliance with physical therapy regimens • Reposition for comfort • Teaching regarding safety measures related to loss of function

continues

Table 12-1 | Risks and Complications Associated with Central Venous Catheters (continued)

IMMEDIATE COMPLICATIONS

Problem and Etiology	Signs and Symptoms	Interventions
Mediastinal Injury and Hydromediastinum: Results from inadvertent puncture of the interpleural cavity (that contains the heart and its large vessels, esophagus, trachea, thymus, lymph nodes, and connective tissue) with the introducer needle or guide wire and the passage of infusate into the mediastinum.	Symptoms may be similar to those of cardiac tamponade, with the following: • Dyspnea • Chest pain with pressure • Hypotension • Neck vein distension • Pallor • Tachycardia • Tachypnea	• Administer oxygen • Assess vital signs • Assist with emergency resuscitation measures • Assist with removal of CVC • Position to promote breathing ease

Thoracic Duct Laceration: See chylothorax

DELAYED OR LONG-TERM COMPLICATIONS

Problem and Etiology	Signs and Symptoms	Interventions
Air Embolism: See Immediate Complications. This can occur at any time during the course of central therapy and CVC removal.		**Note:** Air embolism can occur 24–48 hours after removal if site is not dressed with an occlusive dressing.
Catheter Migration or Dislodgement: Occurs when the CVC moves from its insertion placement site to another location (usually to the axillary and internal jugular vein or the right atrium) or comes out. It may result from improper suturing, insertion site trauma, disease processes, changes in intrathoracic pressure (such as occurs with forceful coughing, sneezing, or vomiting), forceful catheter flushing, tumor progression, or venous thrombosis. Migration can also occur spontaneously for no apparent reason or when patient is physically active.	• Aspiration or infusion difficulties • Burning sensation, discomfort, or pain during infusion • Cardiac dysrhythmias (indicative of migration to the right atrium) • Coiling of the catheter in the exit site tunnel (seen or palpated) • Edema of the chest or neck during infusion • Increased external catheter length or exposure of the anchoring cuff • Leaking around the insertion site • Palpation of the catheter in the internal jugular vein • Patient complaints of a gurgling sound in the ear (indicative of internal jugular migration)	• Prepare patient for x-ray to verify position • Assist with CVC removal • Assist with new CVC placement For catheter dislodgment from the body, a sterile, occlusive dressing must be immediately applied to the site, with pressure maintained until bleeding stops. The patient should be placed in a supine position and assessed for signs and symptoms of air embolism.
Local Infection: Occurs at the CVC insertion site as a result of deficient asepsis during catheter insertion and placement of the initial dressing, improper routine hand hygiene, or inadequate site care. It can also occur because of a compromised immune state. A local infection may precede or occur concomitantly with sepsis. Local infection includes exit site, pocket, or tunnel infections.	• Cording of the vein • Site drainage • Site edema • Site redness • Site tenderness • Site warmth	• Immediate notification of physician at first sign of local infection • Draw blood cultures from CVC • Obtain peripheral blood cultures • Administer antibiotics as ordered • Administer anticoagulants as ordered
Sepsis: Occurs for the same reasons as local infections, as well as catheter or infusate contamination, the formation of a fibrin sheath that increases the potential for microbial growth, or another infectious process not related to the CVC. It occurs more frequently in patients who are immunocompromised, malnourished, or are undergoing steroid and total parenteral nutrition therapy.	• Chills • Cyanosis • Fever • Facial flushing • Glucosuria • Headache • Leukocytosis • Malaise • Nausea and vomiting • Positive blood cultures • Tachycardia • Tachypnea	• Assess for all sources of infection • Assess vital signs • Draw central and peripheral blood cultures (to verify that CVC is the primary source of sepsis) • Assist with removal and replacement of CVC and culture removed catheter • Administer antibiotics • Administer anticoagulants • Administer antipyretics and institute other fever-reducing measures

continues

Table 12-1 | Risks and Complications Associated with Central Venous Catheters (continued)

DELAYED OR LONG-TERM COMPLICATIONS		
Problem and Etiology	**Signs and Symptoms**	**Interventions**
Sepsis: *(continued)*	The signs of septic shock include the signs of septicemia combined with the following: • Altered mental function • Hypotension • Inadequate organ perfusion • Petechiae • Purpuric pustules	• Cardiovascular/BP support • Respiratory support • Prevention of acidosis • Platelet and clotting factor replacement • Emergency resuscitation measures
Thrombosis: The formation of blood clots within the vessel as a result of the following: • Catheter placement outside of the superior vena cava • Fibrin sheath formation • Platelet aggregation on the catheter surface • Precipitate formation on the catheter surface • Preexisting cardiovascular disease • Preexisting hematopoietic pathology • Preexisting limb edema • Prolonged use of the same vessel • Stasis and sluggish flow rate resulting from disease processes • Use of thrombogenic catheter materials (such as PVC) • Vessel wall injury at the catheter insertion site • Vessel wall injury from mechanical irritation of the catheter tip or the infusion of irritating products	• Chills • Earache or jaw pain • Fever • Insertion site edema • Insertion site redness • Malaise • Tachycardia • Tachypnea • Unilateral arm or neck pain • Edema Signs and symptoms of pulmonary obstruction following thrombosis include the following: • Chest pain (sudden and severe) • Hemoptysis • Pleural friction rub • Signs of consolidation Signs of kidney obstruction following thrombosis include the following: • Hematuria • Petechiae Signs of thrombotic obstruction evidenced in the extremities include the following: • Absence of pulse distal to the obstruction • Coldness • Cyanosis • Dusky pallor • Necrosis of the digits or the limb If there is splenic obstruction, the patient will have left upper quadrant abdominal pain and tenderness.	• Administer analgesics • Administer anticoagulants • Administer oxygen • Apply moist, warm compresses locally, if indicated • Apply surgical stockings • Assess vital signs • Assist with catheter removal • Avoid use of limb on affected side for blood pressure and venipuncture • Position patient in a semi- to high-Fowler's position for breathing ease • Prepare to institute emergency resuscitative measures • Prepare patient for operative thrombectomy, insertion of vena cava filter or vena caval interruption, if indicated • Prevent formation of pressure sores to edematous limbs • Provide emotional support • Provide frequent mouth care

Note: The patient may be asymptomatic or the signs and symptoms will depend on the severity of the effusion.

usually related to problems involving insertion of the line, while long-term complications are often the result of inadequate catheter care or the patient's clinical situation. The nurse must be thoroughly familiar with principles and products involved in central vascular access in order to assess and evaluate appropriately and avert problems before they occur or become serious. He must also know what interventions to take once complications set in. The home care nurse must be especially adept at anticipating problems, troubleshooting, and taking charge in emergency situations.

It is very important to remember that air embolism is a major preventable complication that can occur at any time during therapy, including the 24-hour period following CVC removal. The rate of air entry into a central line is very critical, more so than the volume. Air absorption depends on the ability of the red blood cells (hemoglobin) to effect a gas

NURSING ALERT

Air Bolus Effects

A 100 cc/sec influx of air can occur through a breach in a 14-ga. central venous catheter in a patient sitting in an upright position. This bolus of air proceeds to the heart where it usually lodges against the pulmonic valve and blocks pulmonary blood flow. With the pumping force of the right ventricle, the air bolus may break up into smaller bubbles that enter the pulmonary circulation, causing further blood obstruction, which leads to localized tissue hypoxia, decreased cardiac output, and a generalized decrease in tissue perfusion. Without intervention, the condition rapidly progresses to shock and death.

exchange. In the normal adult the average lethal dose of air is 70 to 150 cc of air or 5 to 15 cc/kg of body weight. Death ensues from the rapid bolus injection of 100 to 200 cc of air. While the normal adult may be able to tolerate the inadvertent intake of 200 cc of air into the circulation, the gravely ill person may not be able to tolerate even 10 cc. The mortality rate from air embolism ranges from 29% to 50% (Thielen, 1996).

CENTRALLY INSERTED SINGLE AND MULTILUMEN NONTUNNELED CENTRAL VENOUS ACCESS CATHETERS

Central venous catheters are flexible single or multilumen cannulas with open- or closed-end tips that are radiopaque; some have radiopaque stripes that extend the full length of the catheter. They are usually called central lines or CVCs, but are often referred to as permanent indwelling catheters or percutaneous central venous catheters. They are generally made of medical grade silicone elastomers (SE), thermoplastic polyurethane (TPU), or PVC, and range in size from 24 ga., 3½ in. (8.75 cm) lengths to 14 ga., 12 in. (30 cm) catheters. The polyurethane catheter is commonly used because of the material's versatility, malleability (tensile strength and elongation characteristics), and biocompatibility.

Although the incidence of local or bloodstream infections (BSIs) associated with peripheral venous catheters is usually low, serious infectious complications produce considerable annual morbidity because of the frequency with which such catheters are used. However, the majority of serious catheter-related infections are associated with central venous catheters (CVCs), especially those that are placed in patients in ICUs (CDC, 2002a).

A total of 250,000 cases of CVC-associated BSIs have been estimated to occur annually in the USA, with the cost per infection amounting to an estimated $34,508–$56,000. The annual cost of caring for patients with CVC-associated BSIs ranges from $296 million to $2.3 billion. The attributable mortality is an estimated 12%–25% for each infection, and the marginal cost to the health care system is $25,000 per episode (CDC, 2002a).

The incidence of CRBSI varies considerably by type of catheter, frequency of catheter manipulation, and patient-related issues, such as underlying disease processes and other illness-related factors. Significant pathogenic determinants of catheter-related infection are (1) the material with which the device is made and (2) the natural virulence factors of the infecting organism. Some catheter materials have surface irregularities that enhance the microbial adherence of certain species (e.g., coagulase-negative staphylococci, *Acinetobacter calcoaceticus*, and *Pseudomonas aeruginosa*) and others are made in such a way to make them more thrombogenic than others—a characteristic that also might predispose to catheter colonization and catheter-related infection (CDC, 2002a).

In vitro studies demonstrate that catheters made of polyvinyl chloride (PVC) or polyethylene are less resistant to the adherence of microorganisms than are catheters made of Teflon®, silicone elastomer, or polyurethane. Therefore, the majority of catheters sold in the United States are no longer made of PVC or polyethylene (CDC, 2002).

Manufacturers have worked to develop state-of-the-art catheters, such as the ARROWgard™, a catheter with colonization-resistant chlorhexidine and silver sulfadiazine antiseptic surface molecularly bonded into the polyurethane catheter along its indwelling length.

Because infections often arise from organisms pervading the catheter tract around the external surface, the VitaCuff® (Figure 12-3) and the VitaSleeve® were developed. The cuff, that is a component of many catheters (and works in conjunction with the Dacron® cuff, an inherent component of some catheters), is positioned beneath the skin surface during catheter placement. It is a collagen band impregnated with silver ions that are released over several weeks, providing protection during the critical postimplant healing period until the collagen is completely absorbed into the tissue. It creates a physical barrier to bacteria by swelling to about twice its original size and facilitating tissue growth into its porous collagen, resulting in a catheter seal at the exit site. Once tissue ingrowth has occurred, there is long-term

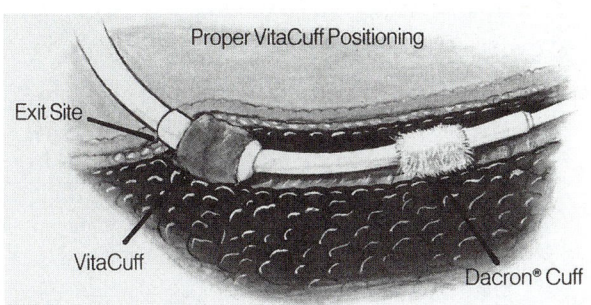

Figure 12-3 | VitaCuff® Antimicrobial Cuff *Courtesy of BARD Access Systems*

catheter securement and a barrier to catheter-related infections. Silver ions have broad-spectrum activity against many of the bacteria and fungi that are related to catheter infections.

Catheters coated with chlorhexidine/silver sulfadiazine only on the external luminal surface have been studied as a means to reduce CRBSI. Two meta-analyses demonstrated that such catheters reduced the risk for CRBSI compared with standard noncoated catheters (CDC, 2002). A second-generation catheter is now available with chlorhexidine coating on both the internal and external luminal surfaces. The external surface has three times the amount of chlorhexidine and extended release of the surface-bound antiseptics than that in the first generation catheters. The external surface coating of chlorhexidine is combined with silver-sulfadiazine, and the internal surface is coated with chlorhexidine alone. Preliminary studies indicate that prolonged anti-infective activity provides improved efficacy in preventing infections (CDC, 2002).

Single-lumen central lines are usually inserted for emergency or short-term central venous access or for single-purpose therapy or CVP monitoring. Although they continue to be used (often because of the preference and established routines of some surgeons) it is now becoming more common to insert multilumen lines in anticipation of more complex infusion needs, should they arise. The CDC recommends using a CVC with the minimum number of ports or lumens essential for the management of the patient (CDC, 2002).

The multilumen central line consists of a main catheter stem, marked in length increments, containing separate lumens (double, triple, or quad-lumen) that extend into various portions of the catheter length. The lumens are situated to exit the catheter stem around its circumference and usually are separated by a 2- to 3-cm distance for optimal mixing of infusates. Each lumen is attached to a clear, see-through extension, called a pigtail, that exits the body. Each pigtail is a different length and has a different color-coded hub for easy identification. At the site where the

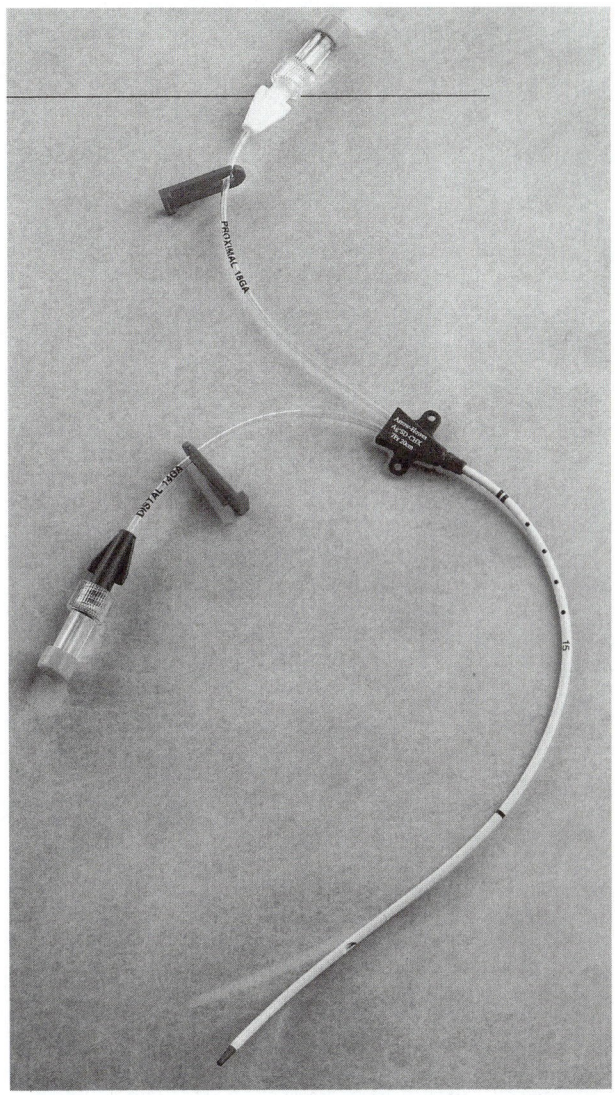

A.

Figure 12-4 | Multilumen central venous catheters: (A) double-lumen CVC; (B) triple-lumen CVC; (C) quad-lumen CVC *Courtesy of ARROW® International, Inc.* (continues)

catheter exits the body and joins with the pigtails, there is a color-coded triangular junction that states the name and size of the line and has integral suture rings and side wings where the device can be sutured to the skin (Figure 12-4). In addition, if the full length of the catheter is not inserted into the body up to the triangular junction, a winged rubber catheter clamp with suture rings is placed over the catheter where it exits the body, and it is covered by a rigid fastener (Figure 12-5A). Both the clamp and fastener are sutured in place to prevent catheter migration (Figure 12-5B). Another option is the use of a device such as the STATLOCK CV® (VENETEK International), which eliminates the need to

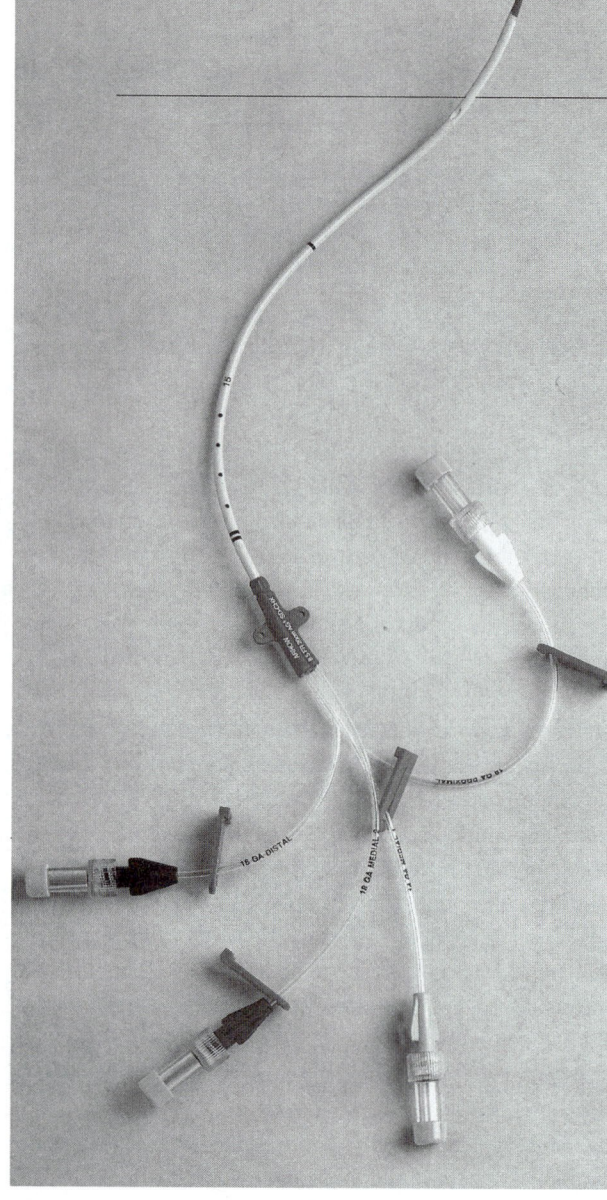

B.

C.

Figure 12-4 | continued

suture-secure and tape the CVC. It can be used in conjunction with the STATLOCK CV PLUS®, which retains the pigtail lumens in place (Figure 12-6). These devices are made of various molded-plastic, adhesive-backed anchors. Sutures not only present a risk to the practitioner for accidental needlesticks, they also contribute to bloodstream infections, at the cost of $28,000 to $40,000 per episode (Kite, 1999), so sutureless devices are now being used in some settings as a means to stabilize CVCs. The CDC has no recommendations regarding the use of sutureless devices (CDC, 2002).

Multilumen catheters come in a wide variety of sizes, with an ample variety of lumen diameters, the selection of which depends on the clinical needs of the patient (Figure 12-7). Each lumen opens at a different point on the catheter for adequate dilution within the vessel during simultaneous administration of different infusates (Figure 12-8). The rationale behind using these catheters is that, in addition to conserving puncture sites, they allow greater treatment variety. Each lumen opens to the bloodstream at a different point on the catheter, so the following procedures may be performed through one device, some simultaneously:

1. Blood sampling
2. Central venous pressure (CVP) monitoring

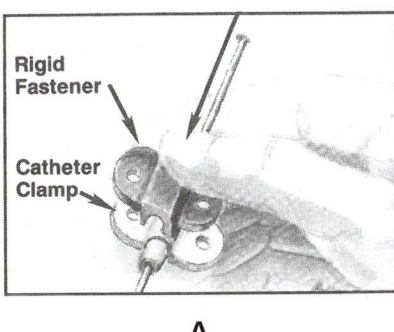

A.

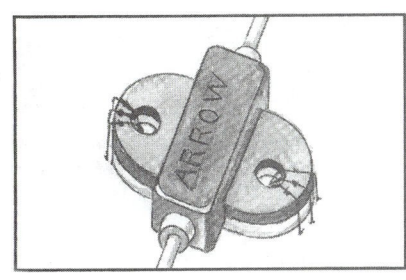

B.

Figure 12-5 | Central venous catheter clamp and fastener *Courtesy of ARROW® International, Inc.*

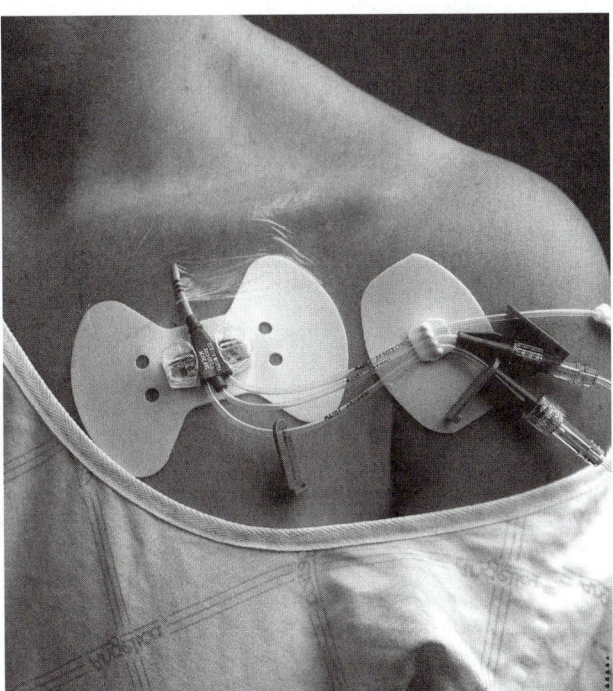

Figure 12-6 | STATLOCK CV PLUS® *Courtesy of Venetek International*

3. Continuous or intermittent drug infusions
4. Diagnostic testing
5. Simultaneous infusion of several medications, even those that are incompatible with each other
6. Administration of viscous or high-volume fluids
7. Blood or blood product administration
8. Short-term or long-term parenteral nutrition
9. High-flow fluid administration in trauma or emergency situations

Port Designation for Multilumen CVCs

The ports of multilumen CVCs should be labeled for designated use and the information must be entered into the chart. The reason for port designation is to ensure uniform use of the catheter by all nurses.

Port designation protocols currently used are based on the following:

1. Distal port: CVP monitoring (and high volume or viscous fluids, colloids, or medications)
   Rationale: Largest lumen; closest to the heart
2. Proximal port: Blood sampling (medications and blood component administration)
   Rationale: Rapid flow of blood within the large central vein quickly carries infusates from the more distal lumens that might affect laboratory tests away from the proximal sampling port.
3. Medial port: Reserved exclusively for TPN
   Rationale: Prevention of catheter-related infections (If TPN is not used, administer medications through this port.)
4. Fourth lumen: Infusion of fluids or medications (Arrow, 1996)

When using multilumen central catheters, the choice of lumen depends on the patient's treatment regimen. The largest diameter lumen is generally used for high-flow or viscous infusions, whereas the others are used for all additional modalities. Each lumen should be labeled as to its intended use.

Insertion Protocols for Central Venous Catheters

Sterile technique is maintained during central venous catheter insertion. Any person who is directly involved in the procedure must follow recommended CDC barrier precautions. Such safeguards include maximal sterile barrier precautions during catheter insertion, including the use of a cap, mask, sterile gown, sterile gloves, and a large sterile sheet, for the insertion of CVCs (including PICCS) or guidewire exchange (CDC, 2002). Anyone else in the area must wear a mask. If a patient is intubated, has a tracheostomy, or is otherwise compromised, potential sources of contamination must be screened with a

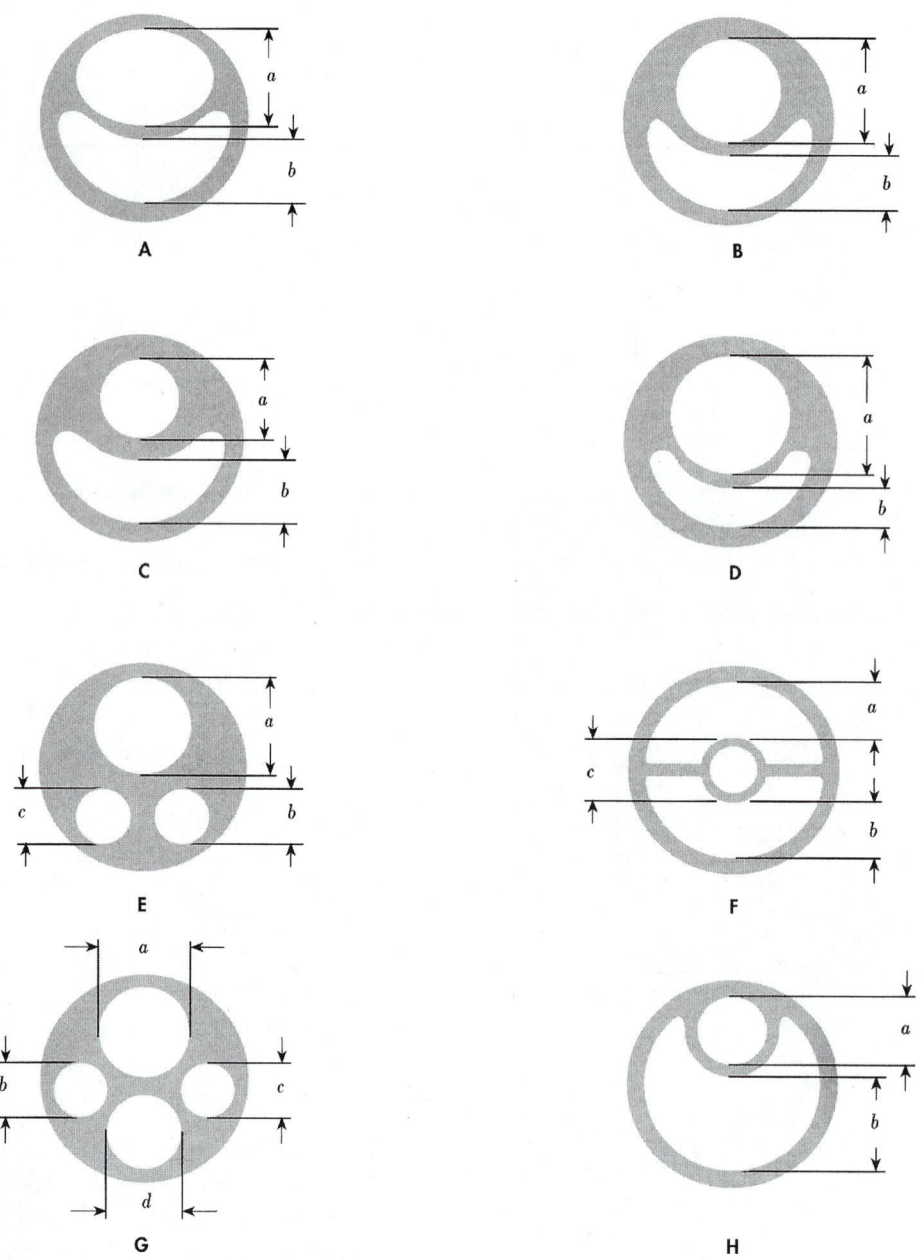

Figure 12-7 | Cross-sectional views of multilumen CVCs *Courtesy of ARROW® International, Inc.*

sterile towel or drape. Table 12-2 lists the general protocols for CVC insertion in terms of the responsibilities of the physician and the nurse. For skin antisepsis, in the United States, povidone-iodine has been the most widely used antiseptic for cleansing arterial catheter and CVC insertion sites. However, in one study, preparation of central venous and arterial sites with a 2% aqueous chlorhexidine gluconate lowered BSI rates compared with site preparation with 10% povidone-iodine or 70% alcohol (CDC, 2002). Commercially available products containing chlorhexidine have not been available until recently;

in July 2000, the U.S. Food and Drug Administration (FDA) approved a 2% tincture of chlorhexidine preparation for skin antisepsis. Other preparations of chlorhexidine might not be as effective. Tincture of chlorhexidine gluconate 0.5% is no more effective in preventing CRBSI or CVC colonization than 10% povidone-iodine, as demonstrated by a prospective randomized study of adults. A 1% tincture of chlorhexidine preparation is available in Canada and Australia, but not yet in the United States. No published trials have compared a 1% chlorhexidine preparation to povidone-iodine.

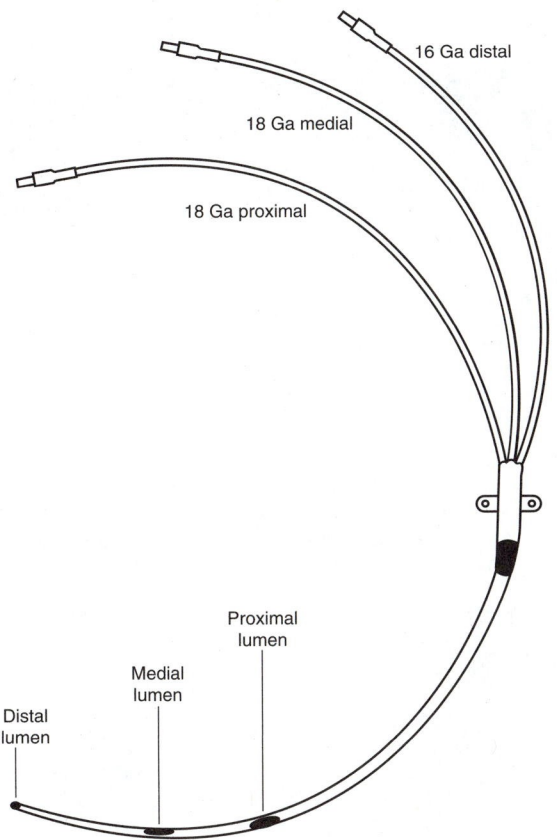

Figure 12-8 | Exit Sites of the Different Lumens on the Multilumen CVC Stem

The Valsalva Maneuver

Prior to the insertion of a central line, the patient (if able) should be instructed regarding performance of the Valsalva maneuver to reduce the risk of air embolism. This is a forced expiratory effort against a closed airway that is used to increase intrathoracic pressure (from a normal of −3 to −4 mm Hg to 60 mm Hg or higher), raise venous pressure, impede venous return to the right atrium, and slow the pulse rate. Its use prevents air from entering the circulation and embolizing when a large vessel is cannulated. The Valsalva maneuver is to be executed during insertion of the CVC and for any treatment or maintenance procedures thereafter if there is the potential for air to enter the circulation, including the period during and after catheter removal.

It is the responsibility of the nurse to teach the patient how to perform the Valsalva maneuver and ensure that he understands it and does it correctly. Using terminology the patient can understand, he is to be instructed to take a deep breath, hold it (with mouth closed), and bear down for 10 seconds, after which he can exhale and breathe normally. If he is unable to perform the maneuver, the nurse may instruct him to take a deep breath and hold it, allowing her to carry out necessary procedures while he slowly exhales. For the unresponsive patient it may be necessary to deliver positive pressure with a resuscitation bag. Use of the Valsalva maneuver is contraindicated in patients with increased intracranial pressure or who have had recent eye surgery, a

Table 12-2 | Medical and Nursing Insertion Protocols for Central Venous Catheters

MEDICAL RESPONSIBILITIES	NURSING RESPONSIBILITIES
	Explain the procedure to the patient and obtain signed consent. (If an antiseptic surface catheter is to be used, verify patient's allergy status. It is contraindicated in anyone with known sensitivity to chlorhexidine, silver sulfadiazine, and/or sulfa drugs. The VitaCuff® should not be used on those with sensitivities to silver ions or collagen.)
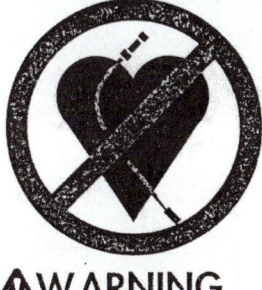 **⚠WARNING** DO NOT PLACE THE CATHETER INTO OR ALLOW IT TO REMAIN IN THE RIGHT ATRIUM OR RIGHT VENTRICLE. FAILURE TO FOLLOW THESE INSTRUCTIONS CAN RESULT IN SEVERE PATIENT INJURY OR DEATH.	Secure all the necessary supplies needed for insertion of the CVC, including masks, caps, goggles, and sterile gowns and gloves.
	Set up the prescribed infusion and prime the administration set tubing.
	Physically prepare the area where the procedure will be performed. Provide privacy.
	Wash insertion area with soap and rinse well with water and dry. Review the procedure for performing the Valsalva maneuver with the patient.
	Assess vital signs and LOC (level of consciousness).
Assess for measurement from the proposed insertion site to the junction of the superior vena cava and the right atrium (as the catheter tip will lie parallel to the superior vena cava vessel wall above the junction of the right atrium).	Place patient in a 20° Trendelenburg position, if he can tolerate it, with a rolled towel between the shoulder blades.

continues

Table 12-2 | Medical and Nursing Insertion Protocols for Central Venous Catheters (continued)

MEDICAL RESPONSIBILITIES	NURSING RESPONSIBILITIES
Apply mask, cap, sterile gown, goggles, and sterile gloves.	Apply mask, cap, goggles, gown, and gloves.
Prep and drape puncture site as required.	Assist the physician and reassure the patient throughout the procedure.
Perform skin wheal.	
Locate a central vein with a 22-ga. locator needle and syringe.	Instruct patient to perform Valsalva maneuver.
Insert introducer catheter/needle assembly with attached syringe into vein along side of locator needle and aspirate.	
Remove locator needle.	
Remove introducer needle.	
If no free flow of venous blood is observed, attach syringe to catheter and aspirate until venous blood flow is established. (The needle is not to be reinserted into the catheter.)	
Insert desired tip of spring wire guide through the guide wire introducer needle into the vein. (If the 'J' tip is used, prepare for insertion by sliding the plastic tube over it to straighten it.)	
Advance the spring wire guide to the required depth. (Advancement of the 'J' tip may require a gentle rotating motion.)	
Hold the spring wire guide in place and remove the introducer needle or catheter, maintaining a firm grip of the spring wire guide at all times.	
Enlarge the cutaneous puncture site with a scalpel. Do not cut the wire guide. Use the vessel dilator to enlarge the site as required. (Do not leave the vessel dilator in place as an indwelling catheter, to avoid possible vessel wall perforation.)	
Prepare the CVC for insertion by flushing all of the lumens and connecting respective port(s) to the desired line(s). Unused ports may be heparin locked through the injection cap(s), using standard hospital protocols.	Assist with drawing up of the heparin solution (according to agency protocols).
Thread the tip of the CVC over the spring wire guide. Grasping near the skin, advance the catheter into the vein with a slight twisting motion. (Sufficient wire guide length must remain exposed at the hub end of the catheter to maintain a firm grip on the wire guide.)	
Using the centimeter marks on the catheter as positioning reference points, advance the catheter to its final dwelling position.	
Hold the catheter at the desired depth and remove the spring wire guide. (Use extreme care when removing the spring wire guide. If resistance is encountered, remove the spring wire guide and catheter simultaneously. Use of excessive force may damage the spring wire guide.)	
Attach a syringe and aspirate until a free flow of venous blood is observed.	
Connect the distal hub to the appropriate line as required. Close the slide clamps on the pigtails to occlude the flow through each lumen.	
Secure the catheter to the patient using the triangular juncture hub with integral suture ring and side wings as the primary suture site. The additional suture clamp (where provided) should be utilized as a secondary suture site as necessary. Secure the catheter in the white suture clamp by suturing around the rings. A purse-string suture may also be placed at the insertion site as necessary	Dress the site, per agency policy.

continues

Table 12-2 | Medical and Nursing Insertion Protocols for Central Venous Catheters (continued)

MEDICAL RESPONSIBILITIES	NURSING RESPONSIBILITIES
Catheter placement must be documented by chest x-ray	Label all pigtails according to intended use.
Document insertion length of catheter.	Document patient's response to the procedure in the nurse's notes.

Note: The preceding protocols are provided by ARROW® International for use on their multiple lumen central venous catheterization products. They are essentially the same as those for any central line insertion. Always follow manufacturer's guidelines.

myocardial infarction, or are experiencing bradycardia or respiratory distress.

Catheter Site Management

The CDC recommendations regarding catheter site care regimens are that the routine application of topical antimicrobial ointments or creams to CVC insertion sites is not considered safe (except for dialysis catheters) because of their potential to promote fungal infections and antimicrobial resistance (CDC, 2002). A meta-analysis has assessed studies that compared the risk for catheter-related BSIs for groups using transparent dressings versus groups using gauze dressings. The risk for CRBSIs did not differ between the groups. The choice of dressing can be a matter of preference. The CDC concludes that "transparent dressings reliably secure the device, permit continuous visual inspection of the catheter site, permit patients to bathe and shower without saturating the dressing, and require less frequent changes than do standard gauze and tape dressings; the use of these dressings saves personnel time. If blood is oozing from the catheter insertion site, gauze dressing might be preferred" (CDC, 2002). Dressings are to be replaced if they become damp, loosened, or visibly soiled, or if inspection of the site requires removal. Dressings are to be changed at least weekly for adult and adolescent patients, depending on the circumstances of the individual patient (CDC, 2002). CVCs are not to be submerged under water. Showering should be permitted if precautions can be taken to reduce the likelihood of introducing organisms into the catheter (e.g., if the catheter and connecting device are protected with an impermeable cover during the shower).

Organic solvents such as acetone or ether, to remove skin lipids, should not be applied to the skin before insertion of parenteral nutrition catheters as they neither confer added protection against microbial colonization nor decrease the incidence of catheter-related infections (CDC, 2002). In addition, catheters that come in contact with 100% acetone solution are prone to weakening and possible leakage.

When a CVC dressing needs to be changed, it should be done by specially trained personnel who are well versed in the principles and practice of infusion therapy as it relates to insertion,

maintenance, monitoring, and discontinuation. Research findings from studies and reports spanning the past two decades have consistently substantiated that the risk for infection declines following standardization of aseptic care and that insertion and maintenance of intravascular catheters by inexperienced staff might increase the risk for catheter colonization and catheter-related BSIs (CDC, 2002). "Specialized 'IV teams' have shown unequivocal effectiveness in reducing the incidence of catheter-related infections and associated complication and costs . . . infection risk increases with nursing staff reductions below a critical level" (CDC, 2002). It is the responsibility of the nurse to follow current CDC guidelines, the INS Standards of Care, and to comply with employer policies regarding infusion therapy procedures. The general protocols for dressing changes and catheter site care follow.

Procedure for Central Venous Catheter Dressing Change and Site Care

This procedure should be performed only by nurses who are specially trained and authorized by the agency. The CDC recommends the use of either sterile gauze or a sterile, transparent, semipermeable dressing to cover the catheter site. Tunneled CVC sites that are well healed might not require dressings. If the patient is diaphoretic, or if the site is bleeding or oozing, a gauze dressing is preferable to a transparent, semipermeable dressing. The catheter-site dressing is to be changed at least weekly for adult and adolescent patients, depending on the circumstances of the individual patient. It is to be replaced if the dressing becomes damp, loosened, or visibly soiled or if inspection of the site requires removal of the dressing (CDC, 2002). Clean skin is to be disinfected with an appropriate antiseptic before catheter insertion and during dressing changes. Although a 2% chlorhexidine-based preparation is preferred, tincture of iodine, an iodophor, or 70% alcohol can be used. The antiseptic is to remain on the insertion site and allowed to air dry (CDC, 2002). The nurse is required to follow the policies and protocols of the agency regarding catheter site care and maintenance procedures. See Skill 12-1 for the procedure for changing dressings on CVCs.

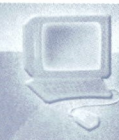

SKILL 12-1

CVC Dressing Change and Site Care

Equipment Needed:

Masks (for nurse and patient)

Disposable gloves

Sterile gown

CVC dressing kit (which includes antiseptic agents [three povidone-iodine/ betadine swab sticks and three 70% isopropyl alcohol swab sticks] for cleaning, tape, gauze, scissor, labels, and all items needed for dressing change).

Agency-approved CVC dressing (if not in kit)

Written instructions (as appropriate) for client

Implementation/Action	Rationale
1. Check the physician's order.	A physician's order is a legal requirement for infusion therapy.
2. Introduce yourself to the patient.	By introducing yourself, you convey courtesy, establish/promote the nurse-patient relationship, instill patient trust, and thus alleviate anxiety.
3. Identify the patient by checking the wrist band against the doctor's order and asking the patient, if conscious, to state his/her name.	Proper identification ensures that the procedure is being performed on the correct patient.
4. Verify the allergy status of the patient.	This is a patient safety measure.
5. Explain the proposed procedure in terms the patient can understand.	The patient has the right to know what is being done and the right to refuse care.
6. Carry out proper hand hygiene.	Good hand hygiene is the single most important means of preventing the spread of infection.
7. Provide privacy.	To maintain patient dignity.
8. Elevate the bed level.	Conducive to successful access and alleviates back strain for the nurse.
9. Secure all necessary supplies (Figure 12-9).	To economize time and promote efficiency.

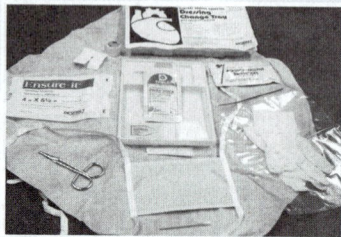

Figure 12-9 | Supplies for changing the dressing on the CVC

Implementation/Action	Rationale
10. Carry out proper hand hygiene.	To promote asepsis and reduce the spread of microorganisms.
11. Nurse and patient don masks.	To prevent the spread of respiratory contaminants to the CVC site.
12. Don clean, disposable gloves.	To prevent contact with body fluids.
13. Gently remove the soiled dressing, maneuvering the skin from the dressing, in the direction of (toward) the catheter insertion site, rather than from the insertion site outward. Use the stretch method if the dressing is	To reduce the risk of trauma to the site and dislodgement of the CVC.

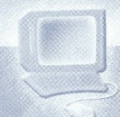

S K I L L   12-1

CVC Dressing Change and Site Care

Implementation/Action	Rationale
a transparent semipermeable membrane dressing. Do not touch the catheter insertion site (Figure 12-10).	

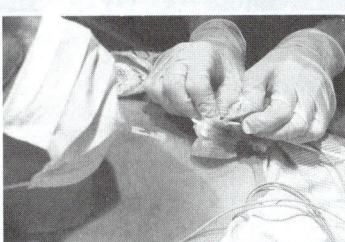

Figure 12-10 | Removing the soiled dressing from the CVC

14. Examine the dressing for purulent drainage or foul odor.	These are signs of infection and may warrant a culture of the drainage.
15. Remove disposable gloves and carry out proper hand hygiene.	To maintain asepsis.
16. Examine the catheter site for abnormalities (Figure 12-11), such as the following:	Any of these signs warrant notification of the physician and appropriate personnel, as they are all considered to be complications associated with a CVC.

   a. catheter malposition or slippage

   b. erythema

   c. dilated vessels

   d. drainage (Notify physician and obtain specimen for culture and sensitivity [C & S], per agency policy.)

   e. induration

   f. loose or absent sutures (Notify physician or appropriate personnel regarding resuturing, or obtain Steri-Strips, per agency policy.)

   g. tenderness

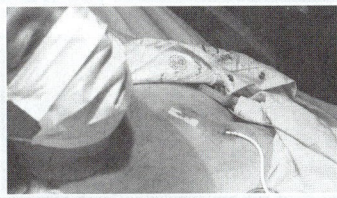

Figure 12-11 | Inspect the site for redness, swelling, and tenderness

(continues)

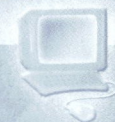

SKILL 12-1

CVC Dressing Change and Site Care *(continued)*

Implementation/Action	Rationale
17. Remove outer plastic wrap from the kit and tape it to the bedside.	For disposal of equipment.
18. Aseptically open the supplies.	To ensure no contamination of equipment and maintain the health and safety of the patient.
19. Don sterile gloves.	Provides asepsis.
20. Clean the CVC site slowly, using friction and moving from the insertion site outward (including the catheter and catheter junction hub), in a concentric circle, to include the full area that will be covered by the final dressing. The sequence for cleaning is as follows:	
a. Clean, first with the alcohol swabsticks, removing all debris. Use each side of each swab. Use all three swabsticks. Do not use organic solvents, such as acetone or ether.	These solvents can damage the CVC.
b. Allow the alcohol to dry completely.	
c. Clean with 2% aqueous chlorhexidine gluconate or the iodophor, using all that are in the dressing kit (Figure 12-12). Use each side of the swabstick.	To ensure proper and thorough cleaning and removal of debris.

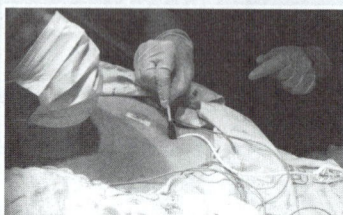

Figure 12-12 | Cleansing the exit site of the CVC

Implementation/Action	Rationale
d. Allow the area to dry completely before applying the dressing.	
21. Apply an agency-approved dressing. If a transparent semipermeable membrane (TSM) dressing is used, be sure it molds around the catheter and junction of the hub (and do not stretch it during application).	To secure an even, smooth fit and inhibit entry of microorganisms under the dressing.
22. Remove the gloves and discard. Dispose of all used materials.	Reduces microbial contamination.
23. Secure the CVC pigtails to the skin above the dressing site.	So as not to place pressure over the CVC entry site and to prevent undue pressure on the skin.

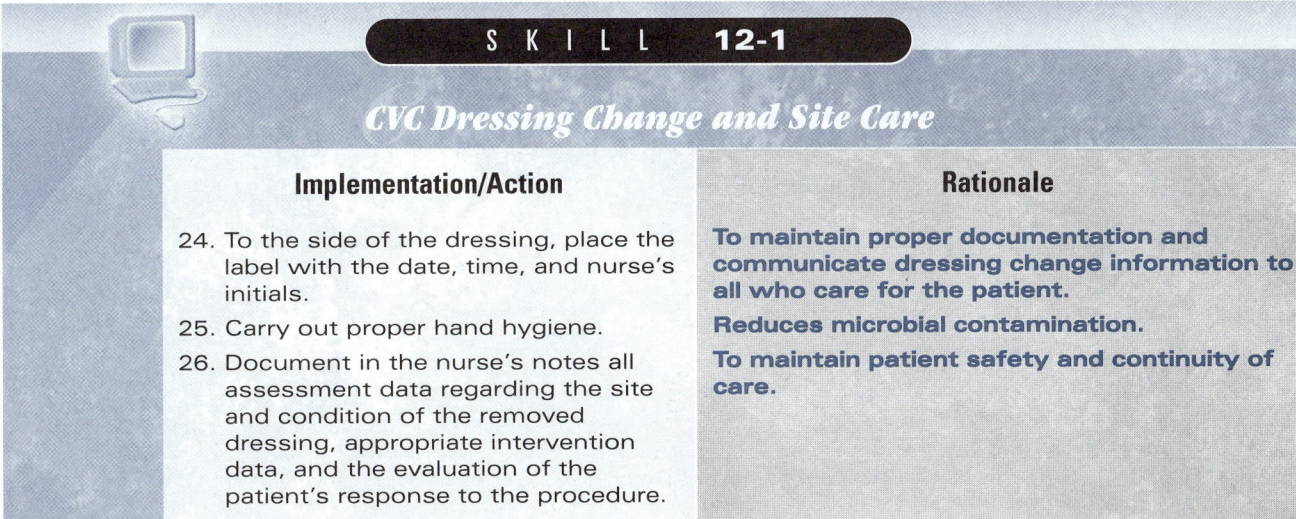

SKILL 12-1

CVC Dressing Change and Site Care

Implementation/Action	Rationale
24. To the side of the dressing, place the label with the date, time, and nurse's initials.	**To maintain proper documentation and communicate dressing change information to all who care for the patient.**
25. Carry out proper hand hygiene.	**Reduces microbial contamination.**
26. Document in the nurse's notes all assessment data regarding the site and condition of the removed dressing, appropriate intervention data, and the evaluation of the patient's response to the procedure.	**To maintain patient safety and continuity of care.**

Infusion Delivery

Infusions via central lines must be monitored carefully. If left unattended, and the control clamp is inadvertently opened fully, anywhere from 1,700 to 4,000 ml of fluid can infuse in an hour's time (depending on the size of the CVC lumen). It is preferable that all IVs ordered for patients with CVCs be administered using an electronic infusion pump to maintain a consistent rate of delivery.

To avert the possibility of disconnection and the risk of air embolism or hemorrhage, the administration of infusates into any lumen of a central line must be via a threaded device such as a Luer-Lok® administration tubing (or extension tubing) attached to a catheter pigtail or through a Luer-Lok® intermittent injection cap connected to the pigtail. Even with these locking connectors, many institutions still require that all connections be taped. Whenever a central line is disconnected for any reason, the pigtail must be closed off with the attached slide clamp, and the patient should perform the Valsalva maneuver. A hemostat must never be used to clamp the line as it may cut it.

Flushing/Irrigating

Flushing, or irrigating, is one of the most important mechanisms used to maintain the patency of a central line and prevent occlusion. Whenever it is necessary to flush, or irrigate, a central venous catheter, the nurse must remember that excessive pressure can damage the line. If resistance is met, the irrigant must never be forced into the vessel because this can result in an embolism if a thrombus is present.

Syringes with barrel capacities of less than 10 ml must never be used to irrigate central lines. Smaller syringes generate more pressure than larger ones. Force equivalent to a 3-lb weight on the barrel of a 3-ml syringe generates pressure in excess of 25 psi, while the same force on the barrel of a 10-ml syringe pro-

duces less than 10 psi of force. It is very important to explain this to patients and family members who care for their central lines in the home care setting. Flushing of any device must be performed in a method that is within manufacturer-recommended pressure limits. Excessive internal pressures in the line can weaken and damage the cannula.

A central line should be flushed with at least 10 ml of normal saline whenever it is irrigated. Some agencies advocate using at least 20 ml. When pressure is exerted on the plunger of the syringe, the pulsatile push-pause method should be used rather than a continual, even push of saline into the catheter. The latter method creates laminar flow, the regular, continuous, nonturbulent movement of fluid in a single direction, and may not remove particles that adhere to the lumen of the catheter. The push-pause technique creates turbulence, with a swirling effect within the catheter lumen, thus removing fibrin and residues of medications or other infusates. A true flushing is accomplished using the pulsatile method. The push-pauses are done in rapid succession, instilling 1 to 2 ml each time force is exerted with a push on the syringe plunger. Positive end-pressure is to be maintained within the catheter lumen after flushing to prevent blood reflux into the cannula lumen. Skill 12-2 outlines the steps used when flushing the CVC.

> **NURSING ALERT**
>
> ### *Syringe Capacity Minimum for Irrigation*
>
> Never irrigate a central venous catheter with a syringe that has a barrel capacity of less than 10 ml. The smaller syringe barrel discharges excessive pressure when force is exerted on the plunger that can damage (rupture, shear, or tear) the catheter or propel small thrombi into the bloodstream, causing embolization.

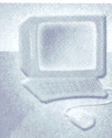

S K I L L 12-2

Flushing the CVC

Equipment Needed:

Gloves

Alcohol swabs

Povidone-iodine swabs

20 ml syringe (with appropriate access needle or needleless adapter), filled with 10 ml of normal saline [or amount recommended by agency or manufacturer for injection]

Heparin (100 units/ml—agency-accepted volume) in a 10-ml syringe (with appropriate needle or needleless adapter), filled with the amount needed to fill the CVC line

Implementation/Action	Rationale
1. Check the physician's order.	A physician's order is a legal requirement for infusion therapy.
2. Introduce yourself to the patient.	By introducing yourself, you convey courtesy, establish/promote the nurse-patient relationship, instill patient trust, and thus alleviate anxiety.
3. Identify the patient by checking the wrist band against the doctor's order and asking the patient, if conscious, to state his/her name.	Proper identification ensures that the procedure is being performed on the correct patient.
4. Verify the allergy status of the patient.	This is a patient safety measure.
5. Explain the proposed procedure in terms the patient can understand.	The patient has the right to know what is being done and the right to refuse care. Thorough explanations reduce anxiety and promote patient compliance.
6. Carry out proper hand hygiene.	Good hand hygiene is the single most important means of preventing the spread of infection.
7. Gather equipment. Have all necessary saline and heparin drawn up before beginning the procedure (Figure 12-13).	Saves time, prevents interruptions during the procedure.

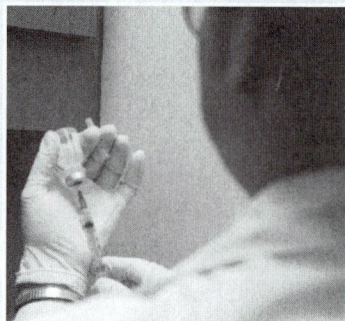

Figure 12-13 | Preparing syringes with saline and heparin

8. Provide for privacy.	Maintains patient dignity.
9. Set up equipment.	Allows for the procedure to be completed quickly and efficiently.
10. Put on gloves.	Prevents the spread of infection.
11. Cleanse the central venous catheter cap with 70% isopropyl alcohol followed by povidone-iodine (or per agency policy). Allow each solution to air dry.	Prevents the introduction of microorganisms into the system.
12. Attach a syringe containing normal saline to the CVC.	To administer irrigation.
13. Instruct the patient to perform the Valsalva maneuver and open the CVC clamp.	To prevent air embolism.

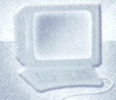

SKILL 12-2

Flushing the CVC

Implementation/Action	Rationale
14. Flush the line with normal saline. Use the pulsatile, push-pause method. Clamp the line (Figure 12-14).	Prevents a nidus for microbial growth, cleans the lumen of the CVC, and prevents occlusion of the line.

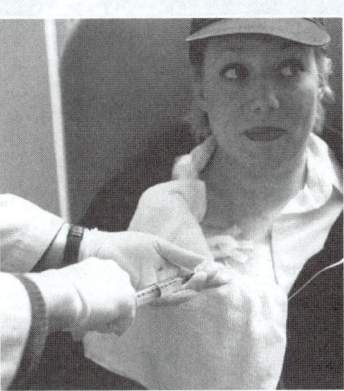

Figure 12-14 | Flush the line with normal saline

NOTE: Should the catheter not flush, it may be occluded. The physician should be notified and the physician/agency-approved protocols are to be followed.

Implementation/Action	Rationale
15. Attach the syringe with the heparin.	
16. Instruct the patient to perform the Valsalva maneuver and open the CVC clamp. Flush the line with the heparin. Clamp the line while infusing the last 0.5 ml of solution.	Prevents the IV from occluding. To heparinize the line and prevent occlusion.
17. Document the procedure.	To maintain patient safety and continuity of care.

NURSING TIP

Pulsatile (Push-Pause) Flushing

When irrigating or flushing a central line, a rapid succession of pulsatile push-pause-push-pause movements should be exerted on the plunger of the syringe barrel. This creates a turbulence within the catheter lumen that causes a swirling effect (a true flush) to move any debris (residues of fibrin, medication, lipids, or other adherents) attached to the catheter lumen.

NURSING TIP

CVC Infusion Guidelines

- Medications containing high concentrations of alcohol should not be infused through polyurethane catheters.
- Medications and infusates such as Taxol® or lipid infusions should not be infused through catheters made of polymers that contain plasticizers, e.g., PVC. (Polyurethane does not contain plasticizers.)
- Consideration must be given to dosages of medications such as nitroglycerin or insulin that are absorbed by certain polymers (e.g., PVC).

Injection Caps

There are no CDC recommendations regarding the frequency of injection cap changes. Most facilities advocate changing them every 72 hours (although some go as long as 7 days) or when they are damaged from excessive punctures. The pro-

cedure for changing intermittent injection caps is outlined in Skill 12-3.

Prior to accessing an injection cap, the top should be cleansed with 70% alcohol, followed by 10% povidone-iodine or iodine. With the use of needleless systems, the blunt-end devices with reflux valves or Luer-activated valves are used

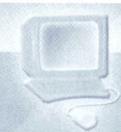

SKILL 12-3

Changing Injection Caps on the CVC

Equipment Needed (for one injection cap replacement):	Implementation/Action	Rationale
Luer-Lok® intermittent injection cap, primed with sterile normal (0.9%) saline per manufacturer's guidelines	1. Check the physician's order.	A physician's order is a legal requirement for infusion therapy.
	2. Verify the schedule.	
	3. Introduce yourself to the patient.	By introducing yourself, you convey courtesy, establish/promote the nurse-patient relationship, instill patient trust, and thus alleviate anxiety.
	4. Identify the patient by checking the wrist band against the doctor's order and asking the patient, if conscious, to state his/her name.	Proper identification ensures that the procedure is being performed on the correct patient.
2 × 2-inch gauze dressing (optional)	5. Verify the allergy status of the patient.	This is a patient safety measure.
	6. Explain the proposed procedure in terms the patient can understand.	The patient has the right to know what is being done and the right to refuse care. Thorough explanations reduce anxiety and promote patient compliance.
Needleless male Luer-Lok® adapter	7. Gather all necessary equipment.	This serves to economize time and reduce patient anxiety.
2% aqueous chlorhexidine gluconate,	8. Carry out proper hand hygiene.	Good hand hygiene is the single most important means of preventing the spread of infection.
10% povidone-iodine, or 2% tincture of iodine swabs (or agency-approved iodophor)	9. Verify the schedule for injection cap replacement.	Routine changing helps prevent complications.
	10. Provide for privacy.	Privacy allows the patient to maintain dignity.
	11. Instruct the patient to position the head to the side opposite the CVC insertion site.	This will prevent bacteria from the respiratory tract from contaminating the CVC site.
	12. Aseptically open the injection cap package.	Aseptic technique maintains the sterility of the device.
	13. Prime the injection cap with normal saline per manufacturer's guidelines.	This removes any air in the device and prevents air from entering the patient's bloodstream causing an embolus.
70% isopropyl alcohol swabs	14. Don gloves.	This prevents exposure to body fluids.
	15. Close the slide clamp on the catheter pigtail.	This prevents air from entering circulation.
(continues)	16. Grasp the hub of the pigtail with the nondominant hand and the injection cap with the other. (For enhanced traction, use 2 × 2-inch gauze [optional] to hold the hub and injection cap.)	This aids in removing the cap without exerting undue traction on the CVC line.

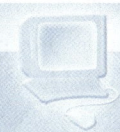

S K I L L 12-3

Changing Injection Caps on the CVC

Equipment Needed (for one injection cap replacement):

10-cc syringe containing 5-cc of sterile normal saline, with air purged from the system

10-cc syringe with 20 ga., 1-inch needle or needleless adapter containing 3 ml of heparin (100 units/ml strength) with air purged from the system

Disposable gloves

Sterile Luer-Lok® injection cap cover (if applicable) for the needleless adapter (depending on the type used by the agency)

Sharps container

Implementation/Action	Rationale
17. Instruct the patient to perform the Valsalva maneuver and, as the breath is held, quickly twist off (counter-clockwise direction) and remove the used cap and connect the new cap. Be sure the Luer-Lok® is secure (clockwise twisting direction).	**To prevent air entry into circulation and air embolism.**
18. Instruct the patient to resume her usual breathing pattern.	**Promotes patient comfort.**
19. Open the slide clamp.	**Allows for proper operation of the CVC.**
20. Prep the top of the injection cap (or remove the sterile cap from the needleless system, if applicable), first with the 70% isopropyl alcohol, then with the CHG or povidone-iodine (or agency-approved iodophor).	**Prevents infection.**
21. Attach the 10-ml syringe containing the normal saline to the Luer-Lok® connection. Aspirate to confirm placement of the CVC. (There may not always be a blood return.) When aspirating, allow the blood to flow only a short distance into the pigtail. Do not aspirate blood back into the syringe.	**Ensures that the position of the CVC has been maintained.** **Prevents a nidus for microbial growth.**
22. Inject 4.5 ml of NS with a continuous forward motion on the plunger, exerting the pulsatile flush movement on the plunger. If resistance is encountered while injecting, *do not exert pressure on the CVC by exerting force on the syringe plunger. No further attempts to flush should be made. NOTIFY THE PHYSICIAN.*	**Maintains positive pressure within the line and provides a true flush of the line.** **The catheter could rupture.**
23. Attach the 10-ml syringe containing the heparin solution to the Luer-Lok® connection. Inject the 2.5 ml of heparin solution (except for Groshong® CVCs), injecting only part of the last 0.5 ml, following the guidelines for needle and needleless systems.	**Maintains positive pressure within the line.**
24. Change all other caps, if present, following the same guidelines.	**All injection caps on a CVC should be changed at the same time; this ensures uniformity, safety, and continuity of care.**
25. Discard the used injection cap and any syringes/needles used in the sharps container.	**Proper disposal prevents the threat of infection.**
26. Remove gloves.	**Prevents cross-contamination.**
27. Carry out proper hand hygiene.	**Prevents the spread of infection.**
28. Document the procedure.	**Validates that the procedure was carried out, provides continuity of care, and communicates to other members of the health care team.**

instead of injection caps. The changing schedules for both types of caps are usually the same, as are the general protocols for antisepsis, and accessing and flushing them.

Heparin Lock Management

The pigtails of each central catheter lumen must be heparinized to maintain patency. For cannulas not in use, heparin flushing should be done every 8 to 12 hours. The strength of the heparin solution used for central lines is usually 100 units/ml, but may range from 10 units/ml to 1000 units/ml, depending on the condition of the patient and policy of the agency. The patient's clotting factors should be monitored so that they are not altered by the heparin dosage used. "The concentration of heparin should be the lowest possible that will maintain patency" (INS, 2000, Standard 56, S54). The procedure for heparin-locking a central line lumen is outlined in Skill 12-4.

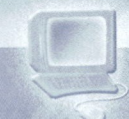

S K I L L   12-4

Heparin-Locking the CVC

Equipment Needed:	Implementation/Action	Rationale
For each lumen of the CVC that needs to be locked, obtain the following: Two (three for SASH) 2% aqueous chlorhexidine gluconate or iodophor swabsticks Two (three for SASH) 70% isopropyl alcohol swabsticks Disposable gloves Sterile injection cap covers (if applicable) for needleless adapters (depending on the type) *(continues)*	1. Check the physician's order.	A physician's order is a legal requirement for infusion therapy.
	2. Introduce yourself to the patient.	By introducing yourself, you convey courtesy, establish/promote the nurse-patient relationship, instill patient trust, and thus alleviate anxiety.
	3. Identify the patient by checking the wrist band against the doctor's order and asking the patient, if conscious, to state his/her name.	Proper identification ensures that the procedure is being performed on the correct patient.
	4. Verify the allergy status of the patient.	This is a patient safety measure.
	5. Explain the proposed procedure in terms the patient can understand.	The patient has the right to know what is being done and the right to refuse care.
	6. Gather all necessary equipment.	This serves to economize time and reduce patient anxiety.
	7. Carry out proper hand hygiene.	Good hand hygiene is the single most important means of preventing the spread of infection.
	8. Provide privacy.	To maintain patient dignity.
	9. Review the Valsalva maneuver with patient.	To ensure compliance while the procedure is performed.
	10. Elevate the bed level.	Conducive to a successful procedure and alleviates back strain for the nurse.
	11. Carry out proper hand hygiene.	To reduce cross-contamination and the spread of microorganisms.
	12. Set up all the necessary supplies on the bedside stand or overbed table in the order in which they will be used.	Maintains order, lessens the chance of contamination, and conserves time.
	13. Assess the site.	To be sure the area is clean, dry, and free of infection.
	14. Don gloves.	Protects the nurse from contamination should hands come in contact with blood.
	15. Swab the injection port with alcohol and let it air dry.	To promote antisepsis.
	16. Swab the injection port with the 2% CHG or iodophor; allow it to air dry.	To inhibit microbial growth and maintain prolonged antisepsis.

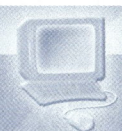

S K I L L 12-4

Heparin-Locking the CVC

Note: If needles are used (in lieu of needleless systems), a 20-ga., 1-inch needle (or smaller) is to be attached to each syringe.

One (two for SASH)10-ml syringe filled with sterile normal (0.9%) saline

10-ml syringe with medication to be given (if applicable)

10-ml syringe filled with appropriate volume/strength of heparin

Note: The volume of the flush should be equal to the volume capacity of the cannula plus any add-on devices. Some agencies recommend using double the capacity of the cannula and add-on devices.

Implementation/Action	Rationale
17. Open the slide clamp and insert the syringe containing the normal saline, have the patient perform the Valsalva maneuver, unclamp the line, and aspirate.	To verify patency of the line.
18. Instill the sterile normal saline, using the pulsatile, push-pause method of plunger movement, and close the slide clamp.	To verify placement and venous function and exert a true flush of the line.
19. Remove the syringe, maintaining positive pressure in the line, and clamp.	Backflow of blood into the cannula hub or injection cap provides a nidus for microbial growth.
20. Ask the patient to perform the Valsalva maneuver and unclamp the line.	To prevent air embolism.
21. Instill the prescribed dose of medication, maintain positive pressure in the line, clamp the line, and remove the syringe.	To maintain the patient's medication regimen.
22. Prep the port as described in steps 12 and 13.	
23. Ask the patient to perform the Valsalva maneuver. Attach the syringe of normal saline, unclamp the line, and instill 3 ml of normal saline, maintaining positive pressure in the line. Clamp the line and remove the syringe.	To prevent air embolism, maintain patency of the vein, and prevent backflow of blood into the lock.
24. Prep the port, attach the syringe of heparin, and unclamp the line. Administer the heparin. Clamp, maintaining positive pressure in the line, and remove the syringe.	Maintains patency in the line.
25. Dispose of all used equipment and place used syringes in sharps container.	Promotes safety and asepsis.
26. Remove gloves and carry out proper hand hygiene.	To prevent microbial contamination.
27. Lower the bed and raise the side rails.	Promotes patient safety.
28. Document the procedure in the MAR. Report any problems encountered in the nurse's notes.	Validates that the procedure was carried out.

Phlebotomy

When blood sampling is required for a patient with a central venous catheter, the phlebotomy is usually performed using the CVC, rather than a peripheral vein. If a multilumen line is in place, the proximal lumen is usually designated for phlebotomy purposes.

It is very important that certain protocols be instituted to prevent erroneous laboratory values, unnecessary blood loss, and repetitive heparin locking. In most agencies, only registered nurses who are trained to work with central lines and care for patients who have them are authorized to draw blood specimens. In this case an alert sign stating that RNs only are to draw blood is placed over the head of the patient's bed and on the chart so that needless attempts at peripheral blood sampling are prevented. It is extremely important that infusates containing glucose or electrolytes be turned off at least one full minute prior to drawing blood for these levels. Whenever blood values are unusually high, especially in a previously stable patient, it is important to question whether or not samples were drawn while the infusions containing the components being evaluated were still running. When results are suspect, lab values should always be repeated, following strict CVC phlebotomy protocols, before instituting treatment to correct the abnormalities.

Whenever blood is drawn from a CVC, it is important that blood is not left in the pigtail or the cap, as this may enhance microbial growth and increase the risk of clotting and infection. The catheter must always be appropriately flushed with at least 20 cc of normal saline and heparinized following phlebotomy. End positive pressure must always be maintained in the cannula lumen to prevent blood reflux. Skill 12-5 illustrates the steps for drawing blood from a CVC.

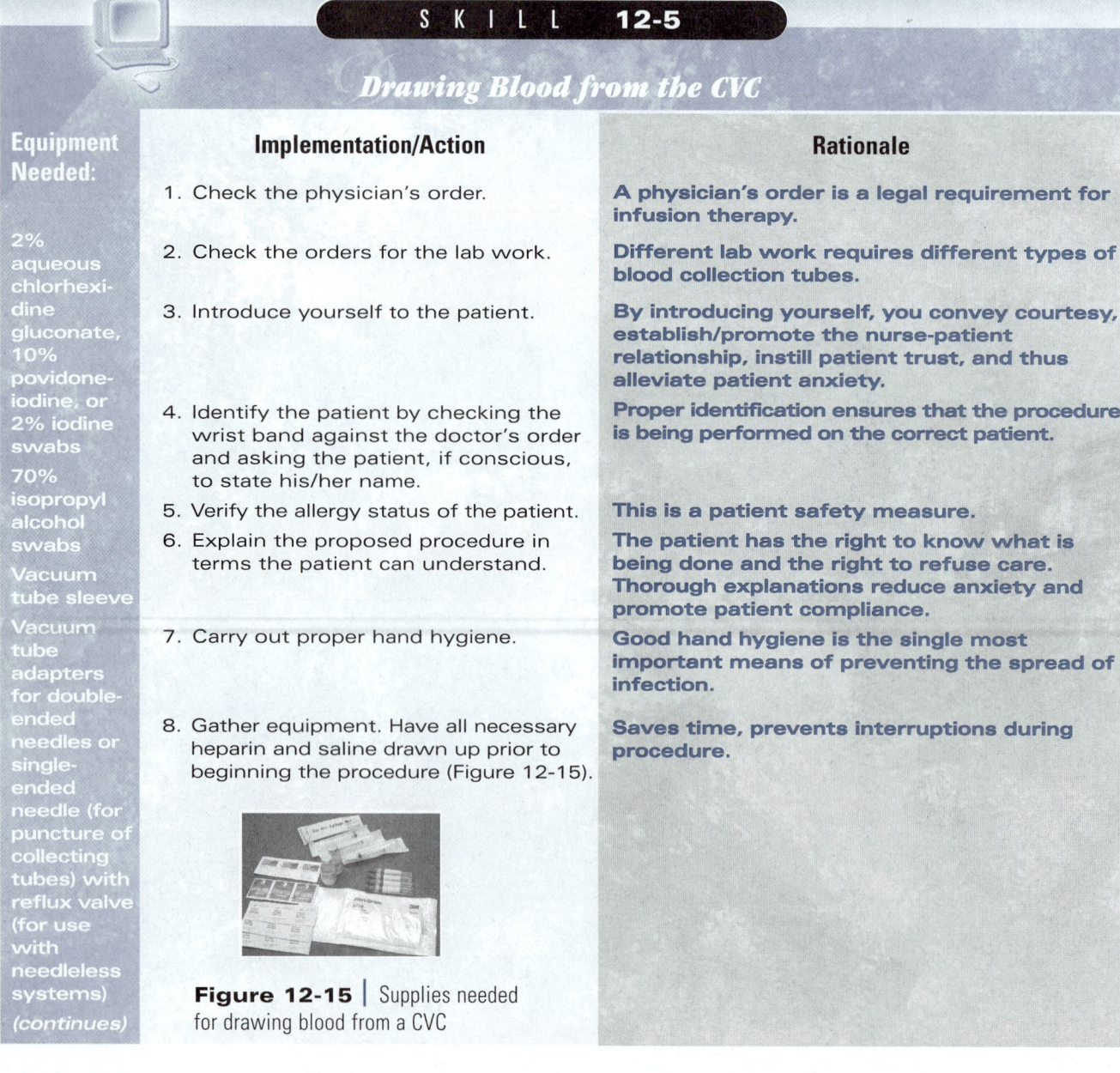

SKILL 12-5

Drawing Blood from the CVC

Equipment Needed:	Implementation/Action	Rationale
2% aqueous chlorhexidine gluconate, 10% povidone-iodine, or 2% iodine swabs	1. Check the physician's order.	A physician's order is a legal requirement for infusion therapy.
	2. Check the orders for the lab work.	Different lab work requires different types of blood collection tubes.
	3. Introduce yourself to the patient.	By introducing yourself, you convey courtesy, establish/promote the nurse-patient relationship, instill patient trust, and thus alleviate patient anxiety.
	4. Identify the patient by checking the wrist band against the doctor's order and asking the patient, if conscious, to state his/her name.	Proper identification ensures that the procedure is being performed on the correct patient.
70% isopropyl alcohol swabs	5. Verify the allergy status of the patient.	This is a patient safety measure.
Vacuum tube sleeve	6. Explain the proposed procedure in terms the patient can understand.	The patient has the right to know what is being done and the right to refuse care. Thorough explanations reduce anxiety and promote patient compliance.
Vacuum tube adapters for double-ended needles or single-ended needle (for puncture of collecting tubes) with reflux valve (for use with needleless systems)	7. Carry out proper hand hygiene.	Good hand hygiene is the single most important means of preventing the spread of infection.
	8. Gather equipment. Have all necessary heparin and saline drawn up prior to beginning the procedure (Figure 12-15).	Saves time, prevents interruptions during procedure.

Figure 12-15 | Supplies needed for drawing blood from a CVC

(continues)

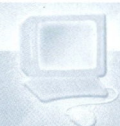

SKILL 12-5

Drawing Blood from the CVC

Equipment Needed:

Assorted blood collecting tubes or appropriate number of empty 10- to 20-ml syringes (if vacuum system is not used)

Two or three 10-ml syringes filled with sterile normal saline

30-ml syringe filled with 20 ml of sterile normal saline

10-ml syringe filled with 3 ml of heparin (100 units/ml)

Disposable gloves

Sterile injection cap (if applicable)

Implementation/Action	Rationale
9. Provide for privacy.	Maintains patient dignity.
10. Set up equipment.	Allows for the procedure to be completed in an efficient and timely manner.
11. Put on gloves.	Protects the nurse from contamination.
12. If an infusion is running, and the patient has a single lumen CVC, do the following:	To prevent air entry and embolism and maintain sterility of connection points.
a. Close the slide clamp on the pigtail.	
b. Instruct the patient to perform the Valsalva maneuver, then quickly disconnect the administration set tubing from the pigtail, cap the pigtail with the injection cap, and cap the distal end of the administration set with the sterile cap.	To prevent air entry into circulation and air embolism.
13. For multilumen CVCs, use the proximal lumen to draw blood and turn off all electrolyte and glucose-containing infusates that are infusing into other lumens for one full minute.	So the blood will be unadulterated.
14. Prep the injection cap of the pigtail with the alcohol followed by the 2% CHG or iodophor.	To prevent contamination.
15. Attach a 10-ml saline-filled syringe. Open the slide clamp and ascertain placement and patency of the CVC, then vigorously flush with 10 ml of NS using the pulsatile, push-pause method. Clamp.	To ascertain patency of the line and exert a true flush.
16. Attach the vacuum container to the injection cap (Figure 12-16). Unclamp.	To obtain the blood samples needed.

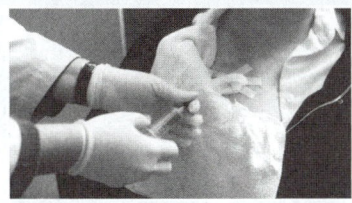

Figure 12-16 | Attach the vacutainer tube.

17. Draw 5 to 10 ml of blood into the discard tube. (The first flow of fluid into the tube will be clear, as it is that which is in the pigtail.)	So the blood will be unadulterated.
18. Quickly insert and fill the required blood collection tube, then close the slide clamp on the pigtail and remove the vacuum container collecting device (Figure 12-17). Clamp.	To obtain the required specimen.

(continues)

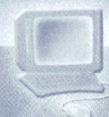

SKILL 12-5

Drawing Blood from the CVC (continued)

Implementation/Action	Rationale

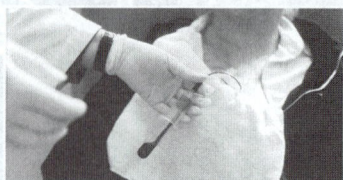

Figure 12-17 | Allow the blood to flow into the vacutainer tube.

19. Prep the injection cap, open the slide clamp, and vigorously flush the line with at least 20 ml of NS to remove any residual blood (Figure 12-18). Clamp.

To clear the line and eliminate a site for microbial growth.

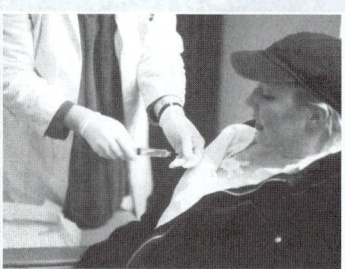

Figure 12-18 | Flush with normal saline.

20. Reconnect the infusion line and unclamp so the infusion may run (or unclamp, heparin-lock the pigtail, and then clamp).

To resume the ordered infusate or to prevent occlusion of the CVC line.

21. Label the blood tubes and deliver the sample to the laboratory as soon as the blood draw is complete and the integrity of the CVC is ensured (Figure 12-19).

The blood for the correct patient will be delivered in a timely manner so that results can be obtained as soon as possible.

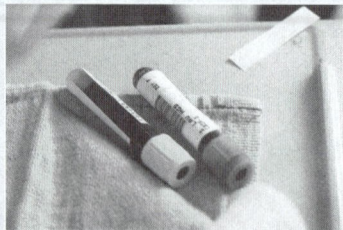

Figure 12-19 | Label the blood specimen tubes.

22. Dispose of used equipment and carry out proper hand hygiene.

To avoid needlestick injury and prevent the transmission of microorganisms.

23. Document the procedure.

To maintain patient safety and continuity of care.

Occluded Central Lines

CVCs can become occluded for various reasons. Withdrawal (or aspiration) occlusion (which is not a true occlusion because there is no obstruction to infusion passage) is usually the result of fibrin sheath or fibrin tail formation or because the catheter tip or lumen opening is pressed against the wall of the vessel. The latter situation can usually be alleviated by repositioning the patient or having him perform the Valsalva maneuver.

Possible causes of true catheter occlusion include the following:

- Clot formation at the lumen exit
- Obstruction by drug precipitates
- Obstruction by lipid deposition
- Catheter displacement
- Restriction of catheter flow by sutures that have tightened around the circumference of the catheter
- Coiling, kinking, or pinching of the catheter between the clavicle and the first rib
- Catheter damage or transection from the repeated pressure of the clavicle and the first rib on the catheter during normal movement, if it is placed through the "pinch-off" area.

Catheter Pinch-off

Catheter pinch-off is the anatomic compression of a vascular access device between the clavicle and the first rib. It can occur when the CVC enters the costoclavicular space medial to the subclavian vein and is positioned outside the lumen of the subclavian vein in the narrow area bounded by the clavicle, first rib, and costoclavicular ligament. Anatomic compression of the catheter occurs when movement of the arm and shoulder further narrows the costoclavicular space, resulting in intermittent occlusion. It is diagnosed by chest x-ray and the clinical signs of inability to aspirate blood or administer infusates unless the patient's position is altered. Catheter fracture can result from pinch-off, which may result in extravasation of vesicants, dysrhythmias, thromboembolic formation, or catheter fragment embolization (Figure 12-20).

Catheter Occlusion

The treatment of any occlusion involves eliminating the cause. The nurse may aspirate a blood clot or dissolve it. The procedures for clearing catheters occluded by clots, lipids, and some precipitates follow. Constricting sutures must be removed and the catheter re-anchored. The catheter may even have to be repositioned or removed.

Before using a declotting solution, it is useful to attempt to remove the occlusion in the catheter lumen using the POP

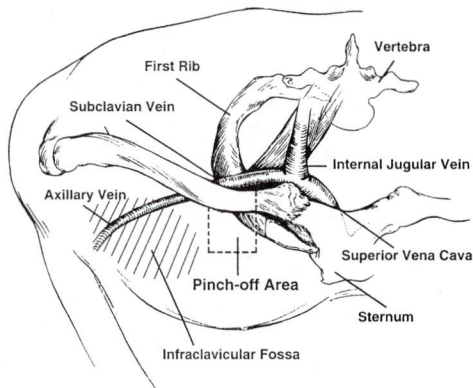

Figure 12-20 | Catheter "pinch-off" area

NURSING TIP

Clearing Occluded Catheters

Thrombolytic or fibrinolytic agents are the products of choice to clear occluded catheters. Urokinase, once widely-used as a fibrinolytic and derived from pooled human donors, was withdrawn from the market in January 1999 due to the possibility of viral contamination. Tissue plasminogen activator (tPA) is the main agent that has replaced urokinase as the fibrinolytic agent of choice for the clearing of thrombosed central lines. It is an enzyme produced by recombinant DNA that binds to the fibrin in a clot and enhances the conversion of plasminogen to plasmin in the presence of fibrin. Plasmin digests fibrin, thereby dissolving the thrombus (fibrinolysis). The product Cathflo Activase is also commonly used to clear occluded catheters.

method developed by infusion specialist Sharon Mazur, RN, CRNI. This is often successful and saves the cost and potential ill-effects of using the declotting solution.

For a CVC (other than one made of polyurethane) that is a 4 French or larger:

- Draw up 5 ml of 0.9% sodium chloride (NS) into a 20-ml syringe.
- Using aseptic technique, attach the hub of the syringe to the occluded CVC lumen.
- Pull back on the syringe plunger to the 15-ml mark and let go of the plunger. A popping sound results. Repeat the maneuver several times in rapid succession.

The negative pressure may pull the clot(s) or infusate residue back into the syringe. The CVC occlusion will be removed as evidenced by a blood return or diminished resistance with flushing.

If the POP method is unsuccessful, then use an approved declotting solution. Follow agency and medically approved guidelines when clearing any IV line.

Another method of declotting, the stopcock-negative pressure method, was developed by infusion specialists Ronald Bonstell and Joseph Brown. This technique eliminates the problem of inadvertent positive pressure catheter rupture. When negative pressure is applied (by opening the stopcock port to the syringe containing a declotting agent), a vacuum is created within the CVC lumen, thus drawing the medication into the catheter to the clot or obstruction. The CVC is not expanded beyond its normal size and only the volume of medication that is needed is administered because only the dead space created by aspiration is filled.

Clearing Occluded Catheters

For dosage accuracy, use a tuberculin syringe to draw up the medication. The volume of the agent instilled should approximate the volume of the catheter so that the agent remains in the catheter and is not advanced into the bloodstream. Transfer the drug to a 10-ml syringe for administration into the catheter lumen to prevent rupture from positive pressure. *Never aspirate or inject into any central line using a syringe* *with a barrel capacity less than 10 ml.* The patient is to use the Valsalva maneuver, as appropriate.

Clots	Normal saline—0.9%NaCl (5 ml) for POP method tPA 2mg/ml (1 ml)
Lipid deposits:	Ethanol 70% (1 ml) following procedure for instillation of thrombolytic
Decreased pH (acid residues; minerals such calcium phosphate; cipitates; most antibiotics)	Hydrochloric acid 0.1 N/ml (1 ml) following procedure as for instillation of thrombolytic
Increased pH (alkaline residues)	Sodium bicarbonate 1 mEq/ml (1 ml) following procedure for instillation of thrombolytic

Note: The physiologic mechanism by which precipitates are resolved is that of returning the precipitate back into a solution by modifying its pH.

Use the POP method before trying a declotting solution when there is resistance or inability to flush due to a suspected clot or fibrin buildup. Do not use this method with polyurethane catheters. Skills 12-6 through 12-8 outline procedures for clearing an occluded catheter.

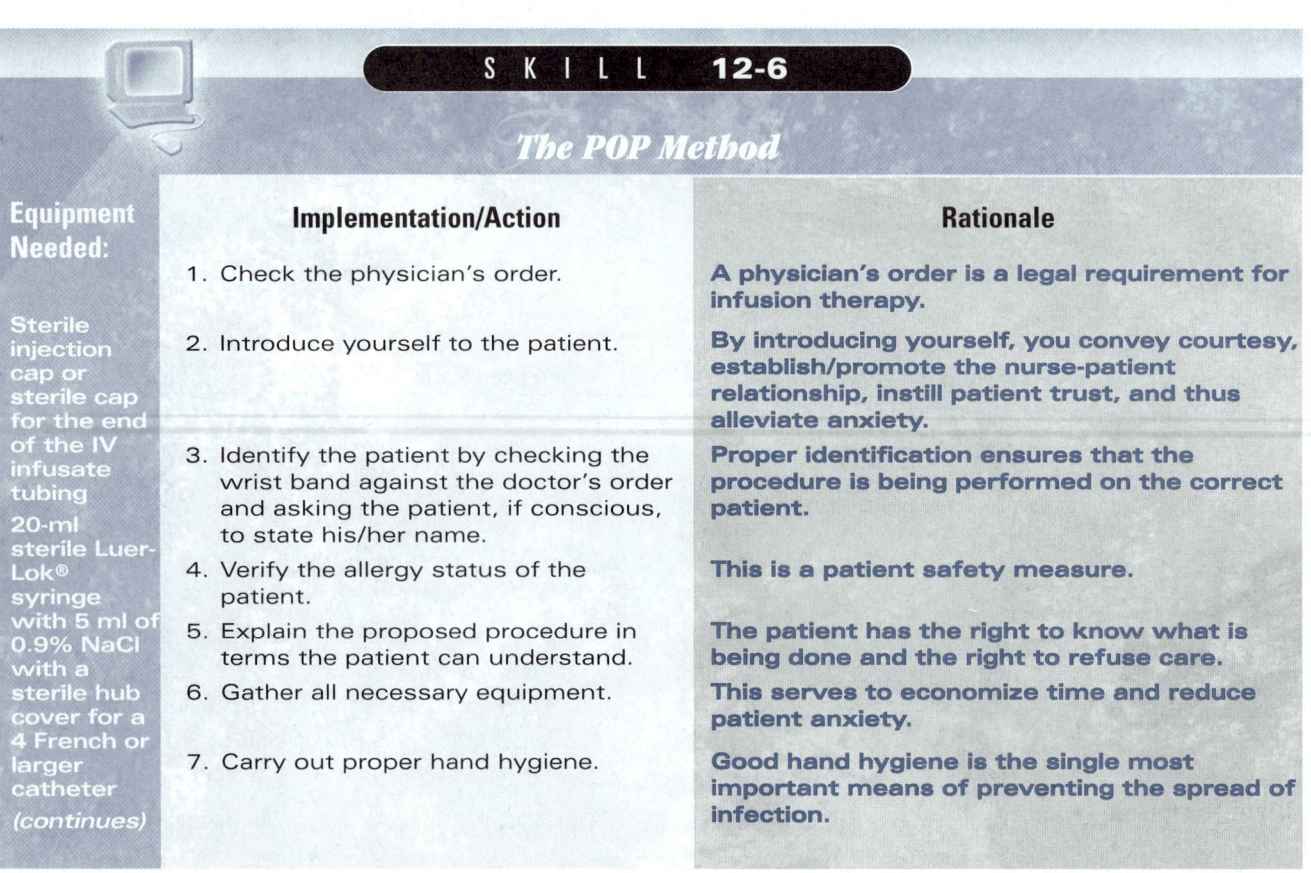

SKILL 12-6

The POP Method

Equipment Needed:	Implementation/Action	Rationale
Sterile injection cap or sterile cap for the end of the IV infusate tubing	1. Check the physician's order.	A physician's order is a legal requirement for infusion therapy.
	2. Introduce yourself to the patient.	By introducing yourself, you convey courtesy, establish/promote the nurse-patient relationship, instill patient trust, and thus alleviate anxiety.
20-ml sterile Luer-Lok® syringe with 5 ml of 0.9% NaCl with a sterile hub cover for a 4 French or larger catheter	3. Identify the patient by checking the wrist band against the doctor's order and asking the patient, if conscious, to state his/her name.	Proper identification ensures that the procedure is being performed on the correct patient.
	4. Verify the allergy status of the patient.	This is a patient safety measure.
	5. Explain the proposed procedure in terms the patient can understand.	The patient has the right to know what is being done and the right to refuse care.
	6. Gather all necessary equipment.	This serves to economize time and reduce patient anxiety.
(continues)	7. Carry out proper hand hygiene.	Good hand hygiene is the single most important means of preventing the spread of infection.

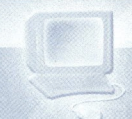

S K I L L 12-6

The POP Method

Equipment Needed:	Implementation/Action	Rationale
(and a 10-ml syringe with 3 ml of NS for a 3 French or smaller catheter)	8. Follow the medical order or agency policy regarding clearing occluded CVCs.	
	9. Gather equipment.	**Saves time, prevents interruptions during procedure.**
20-ml sterile Luer-Lok® syringe filled with NS for a 4 French or larger CVC (and 10-ml syringe filled with NS for 3 French or smaller) with sterile hub cover	10. Provide for privacy.	**Maintains patient dignity.**
	11. Set up equipment.	**Allows for the procedure to be completed quickly and efficiently.**
	12. Put on gloves.	**To protect nurse from contamination.**
	13. Cleanse the central venous catheter cap with 70% isopropyl alcohol followed by 2% CHG or povidone-iodine. Allow each solution to air dry.	**Prevents the introduction of microorganisms into the system.**
70% isopropyl alcohol swabs	14. Instruct the patient to perform the Valsalva maneuver, then open the CVC clamp.	**To prevent air embolism.**
2% aqueous chlorhexi-dine gluconate or povidone-iodine swabs	15. Disconnect the catheter cap or IV infusion line (covering the tubing end with a sterile cap) and attach the 20-ml syringe containing the 5 ml of NS to the catheter hub. Tell the patient to breathe normally.	
Gloves	16. Open the slide clamp.	**So there is access to the system.**
Heparin flush	17. Pull back on the syringe plunger to the 15-ml mark and let go of the plunger. A popping sound results. Repeat the maneuver several times in rapid succession. (Follow the same procedure for the 3 French catheter, but pull back to the 10-ml mark on the syringe.)	**To pull clot/residue(s) back into the syringe.**
	18. Ask the patient to perform the Valsalva maneuver.	**To prevent air embolism.**
	19. Remove the syringe and attach the syringe filled with the 20 ml of NS to the hub (or smaller syringe for smaller CVC). Tell the patient to breathe normally.	**If successful, there should be a blood return (or diminished pressure) with flushing.**
	20. Open the slide clamp.	**So there is access to the system.**
	21. Attempt to flush. If no resistance is felt, flush vigorously, using the pulsatile, push-pause method.	**To irrigate/flush the line.**
	22. Close the slide clamp.	**To maintain patency of the line.**
	23. Ask the patient to perform the Valsalva maneuver.	**To prevent air embolism.**
	24. Attach the sterile injection cap to the catheter hub and heparin-lock the catheter or attach the IV line to the catheter hub and regulate the infusion.	**To keep the declotted line patent.**
	25. Tell the patient to breathe normally.	**For patient comfort.**
	26. Document in the nurse's notes.	**For patient safety and to maintain continuity of care.**

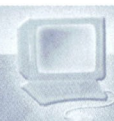

S K I L L   12-7

The Positive Pressure Method

Equipment Needed:	Implementation/Action	Rationale
Sterile injection cap or sterile cap for the end of the IV infusate tubing	1. Check the physician's order.	A physician's order is a legal requirement for infusion therapy.
	2. Introduce yourself to the patient.	By introducing yourself, you convey courtesy, establish/promote the nurse-patient relationship, instill patient trust, and thus alleviate anxiety.
10-ml syringe with prescribed volume of Activase (or other declotting agent) with sterile hub cover	3. Identify the patient by checking the wrist band against the doctor's order and asking the patient, if conscious, to state his/her name.	Proper identification ensures that the procedure is being performed on the correct patient.
	4. Verify the allergy status of the patient.	This is a patient safety measure.
	5. Explain the proposed procedure in terms the patient can understand.	The patient has the right to know what is being done and the right to refuse care.
	6. Gather all necessary equipment.	This serves to economize time and reduce patient anxiety.
10-ml (or 20-ml) syringe filled with 0.9% NaCl with sterile hub cover	7. Carry out proper hand hygiene.	Good hand hygiene is the single most important means of preventing the spread of infection.
	8. Follow the medical order or agency policy regarding clearing occluded CVCs.	
	9. Provide for privacy.	Maintains patient dignity.
10-ml syringe with sterile hub cover (empty)	10. Set up equipment.	Allows for the procedure to be completed quickly and efficiently.
	11. Put on gloves.	Prevents the spread of infection.
Heparin flush	12. Cleanse the central venous catheter cap with 70% isopropyl alcohol followed by 2% CHG or povidone-iodine. Allow each solution to air dry.	Prevents the introduction of microorganisms into the system.
70% isopropyl alcohol swabs	13. If the CVC is connected to an infusion line, close the slide clamp, have the patient perform the Valsalva maneuver, disconnect the catheter cap or IV infusion line (covering the tubing end with a sterile cap), and attach the empty syringe to the CVC hub. Tell the patient to breathe normally.	To prevent air entry into the circulation and air embolism.
2% aqueous chlorhexi-dine gluconate or povidone-iodine swabs	14. Open the slide clamp and attempt to aspirate. If successful, withdraw the clots/residue(s), close the slide clamp, detach the syringe, and proceed to the next step.	If the CVC is patent, declotting is unnecessary.
Disposable gloves	If aspiration is unsuccessful, close the slide clamp. Have the patient perform the Valsalva maneuver, then detach the syringe and proceed to step # 13.	Declotting is necessary.

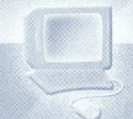

S K I L L   12-7

The Positive Pressure Method

Implementation/Action	Rationale
15. Attach the syringe containing the 10 ml (or 20 ml) of NS and flush vigorously, using the pulsatile, push-pause method. Then, do one of the following:	
• Close the slide clamp, have the patient perform the Valsalva maneuver, attach the syringe with the heparin flush, have the patient breathe normally, open the slide clamp, heparin-lock the line, and close the slide clamp.	
• Close the slide clamp, have the patient perform the Valsalva maneuver, connect the IV tubing to the CVC hub, have the patient breathe normally, unclamp, and regulate the infusion.	
16. Attach the syringe containing the thrombolytic agent (or other declotting agent) and have the patient breathe normally. Open the slide clamp.	**To prepare for declotting.**
17. Open the slide clamp.	**To provide access to the CVC lumen.**
18. Slowly and gently inject the declotting agent into the catheter, using a push-pull motion. Do not force the entire amount into the catheter if strong resistance is encountered.	**To achieve maximum mixing. This could cause the CVC to rupture, causing the obstruction and/or a segment of the catheter to embolize.**
19. Leave the syringe attached to the catheter for 30 to 90 minutes (or per physician's order or agency policy) and do not attempt to aspirate during this period.	**The declotting agent must be in contact with the obstruction long enough to dissolve it.**
20. Attempt to aspirate after the prescribed amount of time. If unsuccessful, repeat the procedure or notify the physician, depending on agency policy.	
If patency is restored, aspirate 5 ml to 10 ml of blood.	**To ensure removal of all of the declotting agent and the clots/residues.**
21. Close the clamp.	**To prevent air from entering the line.**
22. Have the patient perform the Valsalva maneuver, attach the 20-ml NS-filled syringe, have the patient breathe normally, and open the clamp.	
23. Flush the line vigorously, using the pulsatile, push-pause method, then close the slide clamp.	**To reinstate the patency and function of the CVC.**
24. Attach the injection cap and heparin-lock the catheter or attach the IV line and regulate the infusion.	
25. Document the procedure.	

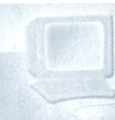

SKILL 12-8

The Stopcock–Negative Pressure Method

Equipment Needed:	Implementation/Action	Rationale
Three-way stopcock with Luer-Lok® connection	1. Check the physician's order.	A physician's order is a legal requirement for infusion therapy.
Sterile injection cap or sterile cap for end of IV infusate tubing	2. Introduce yourself to the patient.	By introducing yourself, you convey courtesy, establish/promote the nurse-patient relationship, instill patient trust, and thus alleviate patient anxiety.
	3. Identify the patient by checking the wrist band against the doctor's order and asking the patient, if conscious, to state his/her name.	Proper identification ensures that the procedure is being performed on the correct patient.
20-ml sterile syringe (empty) with sterile hub cover	4. Verify the allergy status of the patient.	This is a patient safety measure.
	5. Explain the proposed procedure in terms the patient can understand.	The patient has the right to know what is being done and the right to refuse care. Thorough explanations reduce anxiety and promote patient compliance.
20-ml sterile syringe with appropriate volume of declotting agent with sterile hub cover	6. Gather all necessary equipment.	This serves to economize time and reduce patient anxiety.
	7. Carry out proper hand hygiene.	Good hand hygiene is the single most important means of preventing the spread of infection.
20-ml syringe filled with NS with sterile hub cover	8. Follow the medical order or agency policy regarding clearing occluded CVCs.	
	9. Provide for privacy.	Maintains patient dignity.
Heparin flush	10. Set up equipment.	Allows for the procedure to be completed quickly and efficiently.
70% isopropyl alcohol swabs	11. Put on gloves.	Protects the nurse from contamination.
	12. Cleanse the central venous catheter cap with 70% isopropyl alcohol followed by 2% CHG or povidone-iodine. Allow each solution to air dry.	Prevents the introduction of microorganisms into the system.
2% aqueous chlorhexidine gluconate or povidone-iodine swabs	13. If the CVC is connected to an infusion line, close the slide clamp, have the patient perform the Valsalva maneuver, disconnect the catheter cap or IV infusion line (covering the tubing end with a sterile cap), and attach the empty syringe to the CVC hub. Tell the patient to breathe normally. Turn the three-way stopcock to the *off* position before it is attached to the CVC hub.	To maintain a closed central line until ready for declotting.
Disposable gloves	14. Close the slide clamp, instruct the patient to perform the Valsalva maneuver, attach the closed stopcock to the CVC hub, and open the CVC clamp. Tell the patient to breathe normally.	To prevent air embolism.
	15. Cleanse one port of the stopcock with alcohol and 2% CHG or povidone-iodine (if sterility has been breached) and attach it to the empty 20-ml syringe.	

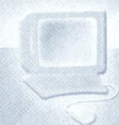

SKILL 12-8

The Stopcock–Negative Pressure Method

Implementation/Action	Rationale
16. Cleanse the other port of the stopcock, as before (if sterility has been breached), and attach it to the 20-ml syringe containing the declotting agent.	
17. Turn off the stopcock to the syringe containing the declotting agent and open it to the empty 20-ml syringe.	
18. Open the slide clamp on the CVC.	
19. Gently aspirate the CVC until the plunger is pulled back to the 15-ml marking.	**This evacuates anything lying between the hub and the clot/obstruction and provides a clear path for the declotting agent.**
20. With the plunger retracted to the 15-ml mark, turn off the stopcock to the plunger-aspirated syringe.	**This allows the negative pressure to be maintained until released by the syringe containing the declotting agent.**
21. Open the stopcock (*on* position) to the syringe containing the declotting agent.	
22. Turn the stopcock to the *off* position, leaving the declotting agent in the CVC lumen for the prescribed time (per manufacturer/agency/physician recommendations).	**This allows it to effect its thrombolytic action.**
23. Open the stopcock and aspirate for a blood return. If blood is returned, aspirate a waste volume of 5 to 10 ml.	**To remove the declotting agent and clot particles or residues.**
Close the catheter clamp and proceed to the next step.	**If there is no blood return, repeat the procedure for negative pressure declotting.**
24. Have the patient perform the Valsalva maneuver, remove the stopcock, and attach the 20-ml syringe containing the NS to the catheter hub. Tell the patient to breathe normally.	
25. Open the catheter slide clamp and vigorously flush the catheter, using the pulsatile, push-pause method. Close the slide clamp.	
26. Have the patient perform the Valsalva maneuver, then do one of the following:	
Open the slide clamp, and attach the heparin flush syringe. Have the patient breathe normally. Instill the heparin solution and close the clamp.	
After removing the syringe, connect the IV infusion line, open the slide clamp, and regulate the infusion.	
27. Document the procedure.	

Emergency Measures

All central catheters and their pigtails should be handled with care and not be allowed to kink. It is especially important to prevent bending at the catheter exit site or at the connection between the catheter and its junction with the pigtails. Excessive external force (as with superfluous twisting during injection cap changes) or use of too much internal pressure during flushing can result in a torn or broken pigtail, cracked catheter hub, or broken suture. The patient and family should have a full understanding as to how these devices function and the safety measures associated with their use. The home infusion patient should have step-by-step written information regarding care/maintenance of the device and documented teaching methods related to patient education outcomes.

Cannula Clamps

An atraumatic, nontoothed cannula clamp should be kept in close proximity to any patient with a central catheter. This is a special clamp designed for use with CVCs. A clamp with

teeth must never be used on the catheter or pigtails as it may sever them. In the event of pigtail injury (break, leak, or tear) the clamp must be applied to the area between the patient and the damaged area. If a breach occurs in the catheter stem or at the stem-pigtail junction, the clamp must be affixed between the catheter exit site and the damaged area and must remain clamped until after it is repaired. The physician must be notified if the catheter stem is not usable. With multilumen CVCs, a nonfunctional pigtail may be clamped and labeled accordingly.

Catheter Repair

Catheter repairs consist of pigtail hub replacement, pigtail repair, and catheter stem repair. Catheter repair kits specific to individual CVCs are available and should be used in accordance with the manufacturer's directions. On some catheters, such as Strato's Infuse-a-Cath,™ the number of the required repair kit is printed on the clamp of the extension assembly. There are also universal repair kits that can be adapted for use with many different CVCs. Figure 12-21

Purpose

To repair a damaged or loose connector.

NOTE: Catheter should have been clamped with an atraumatic non-toothed clamp between the catheter exit site and the damaged area when damage or connector separation occurred and **must remain clamped** during repair.

Supplies

- 1-Replacement connector
- 3-Isopropyl alcohol wipes
- 1-Povidone-iodine wipe
- 1-Sterile scissors
- Pr. sterile gloves
- 10 cc syringe with attached 1in. needle filled with 5 cc sterile 0.9% sodium chloride (normal saline)

Procedure

1. Obtain a new sterile replacement connector of the correct size (color-coded).
2. Determine where the damaged catheter is to be cut off. Do not cut at this time. Be sure to retain as much of the original external segment as possible. If the external segment needs to be lengthened, see the Single Lumen or Dual Lumen Body Repair Procedure.
3. Thoroughly clean the catheter with alcohol and povidone-iodine wipes at the point where it is to be cut.
4. Wearing sterile gloves and using sterile scissors, cut the catheter off at a 90°angle, 1/2 in. distal to the location of the previous connector or damaged site to remove any damaged catheter material.

5. Transfer the clear sleeve (A) onto catheter from connector.

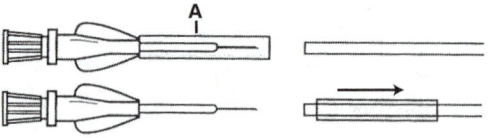

6. Firmly push catheter onto adapter to Position B.

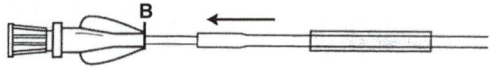

7. Slide the clear oversleeve over the catheter and hub to Position B. If catheter starts to bunch up, swab the catheter with an alcohol wipe before sliding sleeve over it.

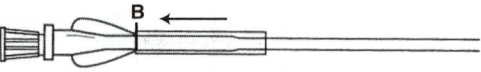

8. Remove and discard stylet.

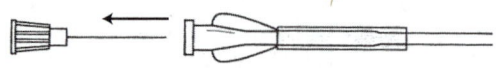

9. Attach injection cap and flush catheter with normal saline, or flush catheter with normal saline and attach IV tubing.

Figure 12-21 | The connector repair procdure for the Groshong® CVC. *Courtesy of BARD Access Systems*

shows the connector repair procedure for the Groshong® tip CV. When kits are not used, short-term repairs are sometimes executed by cutting off the damaged portion of catheter and inserting a blunt-end needle (with Luer-Lok® injection cap attached to the hub) into the viable catheter portion, then tying suture material around it. Depending on policy, most agencies authorize specially trained nurses to repair damaged CVCs. Some general precautionary guidelines (from BARD Access Systems) that apply to most repairs include the following:

- Repair kits should be used to repair only those catheters or catheter segments for which they are intended.
- Repair kits are indicated only for repair of the external portion of the catheter.
- Catheter repair is a sterile procedure.
- Antisepsis with 70% isopropyl alcohol and 2% CHG or povidone-iodine is recommended.

- When cutting the damaged external catheter segment, a sufficient length of the external catheter segment (at least 2 inches or 4.4 cm) must remain to permit repair and prevent catheter retraction under the skin line.

Removal and Discontinuation

It is the policy in most agencies that the registered nurse may take out a nontunneled central line, once a physician has written the order to discontinue it. Central catheters may be removed by the RN in accordance with established organizational policy and procedure and State Nurse Practice Acts. The removal of tunneled/implanted catheters is a medical act" (INS, 2000, Standard 55.V, S52). The basic procedure for the withdrawal of a nontunneled CVC and the nursing assessments and interventions that must be instituted during and after removal can be found in Skill 12-9.

S K I L L 12-9

Removal of the CVC

Equipment Needed:	Implementation/Action	Rationale
Disposable gloves	1. Check the physician's order.	A physician's order is a legal requirement for infusion therapy.
Sterile gloves	2. Introduce yourself to the patient.	By introducing yourself, you convey courtesy, establish/promote the nurse-patient relationship, instill patient trust, and thus alleviate patient anxiety.
Suture removal kit	3. Identify the patient by checking the wrist band against the doctor's order and asking the patient, if conscious, to state his/her name.	Proper identification ensures that the procedure is being performed on the correct patient.
70% isopropyl alcohol swabs or adhesive solvent	4. Verify the allergy status of the patient.	This is a patient safety measure.
2% aqueous chlorhexidine gluconate or povidone-iodine swabs	5. Explain the proposed procedure in terms the patient can understand.	The patient has the right to know what is being done and the right to refuse care. Thorough explanations reduce anxiety and promote patient compliance.
	6. Gather all necessary supplies.	This serves to economize time and reduce patient anxiety.
Plastic disposal container or sheet of plastic	7. Carry out proper hand hygiene.	Good hand hygiene is the single most important means of preventing the spread of infection.
	8. Gather supplies.	To complete the skill in a timely manner.
4 × 4-inch sterile gauze	9. Provide privacy.	To maintain patient dignity.
	10. Review the procedure for performing the Valsalva maneuver.	To prevent air embolism.
(continues)	11. Elevate the bed level.	Conducive to successful procedure and alleviates back strain for the nurse.

(continues)

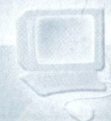

SKILL 12-9

Removal of the CVC (continued)

Equipment Needed:

Sterile air-occlusive dressing (such as petrolatum-impregnated or antiseptic ointment-impregnated)

Tape

Scissors

Sharps container

Culture container for catheter tip, if indicated

Culture container for cannulation site culture, if indicated

Implementation/Action	Rationale
12. Position bed in Trendelenburg or flat position.	To raise intrathoracic pressure, which reduces chance for air entry into system and embolism.
13. Attach the plastic disposal bag to the side of the bed or overbed table or place the plastic sheeting in close proximity to the patient.	For disposal of contaminated items.
14. Carry out proper hand hygiene.	To reduce cross-contamination and the spread of microorganisms.
15. Clamp infusion tubing and turn off the electronic infusion device (if appropriate).	The infusion must cease to infuse prior to removal of the CVC.
16. Close the slide clamp on the CVC.	The CVC is no longer needed.
17. Apply disposable gloves.	To protect the nurse from body fluid contamination.
18. Remove the dressing, following the guidelines for dressing removal as described in *CVC Dressing Change and Site Care.*	Removal is to be done in a manner that will not compromise the skin and cannula exit site.
19. Inspect the dressing for purulent drainage or foul odor.	If there is abnormal drainage or odor, the cannulation site is to be cultured per agency policy.
20. Discard the dressing in the plastic bag or on the plastic sheeting.	To prevent contamination of patient's clothing and linens.
21. Remove gloves and carry out proper hand hygiene.	Prevent cross-contamination.
22. Place 4 × 4-inch gauze, skin antiseptics, suture removal kit, and dressing materials in close proximity to the patient and open them, using aseptic technique (Figure 12-22).	For efficiency of CVC removal, to economize time, and to prevent contamination of site.

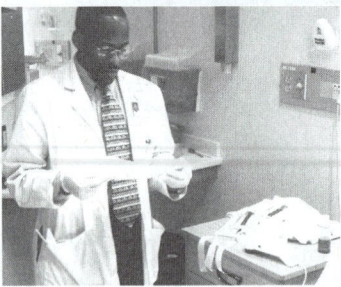

Figure 12-22 | Set up supplies using a sterile technique.

23. Don sterile gloves, leaving the inside (sterile portion) of the wrapper at the bedside.	To place the CVC on once it is removed, so it can be inspected and placed in a culture specimen tube, if necessary.
24. Inspect the site around the cannula insertion area.	In order to culture any purulent drainage at the skin-cannula junction site before cleansing the site.

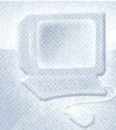

SKILL 12-9

Removal of the CVC

Implementation/Action	Rationale
25. Cleanse the CVC insertion site and surrounding area, including the catheter and sutures, in a concentric circle, starting at the catheter exit site. Clean first with the alcohol, repeating as needed, to remove all debris. Use adhesive remover, if necessary, to eliminate any tape deposits. Follow with thorough cleansing with the 2% CHG or povidone-iodine and allow the area to air dry.	This is necessary to remove any contaminants on or around the exit site that could migrate into the CVC removal site and cause contamination after catheter discontinuation.
26. Carefully clip and remove sutures, while securing the CVC (Figure 12-23).	To prevent undue trauma to the skin.

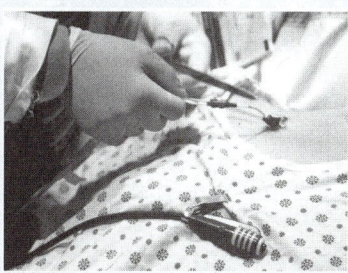

Figure 12-23 | Remove the sutures.

27. Place the 4 × 4-inch sterile gauze over the CVC exit site, holding in place with the nondominant hand. Instruct the patient to perform the Valsalva maneuver.	To prevent air embolism.
28. As the patient performs the Valsalva maneuver, withdraw the CVC from the vein in one smooth, steady motion, continuing to hold the 4 × 4-inch gauze in place (Figure 12-24). Exert firm pressure over the exit site for one to five minutes after the catheter is out and discard the catheter on the	The cannulation site must be held secure to prevent air entry into the vein. The CVC must be placed on a sterile field until it can be inspected and a valid culture can be obtained if there is any abnormal drainage or odor.

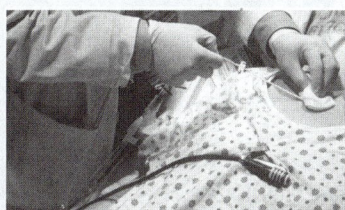

Figure 12-24 | Gently pull the catheter in a fluid motion to remove it.

(continues)

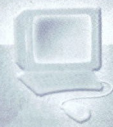

Removal of the CVC (continued)

Implementation/Action	Rationale
sterile inner wrapper from the gloves. Instruct the patient to breathe normally. Continue to apply pressure until any bleeding stops (Figure 12-25).	

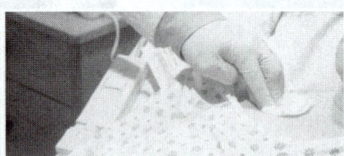

Figure 12-25 │ Apply pressure over the site to stop bleeding.

Implementation/Action	Rationale
29. Apply the sterile air-occlusive dressing over the site and secure the edges so that air cannot enter.	To prevent post-removal air embolism.
30. Leave the dressing in place for 24 to 72 hours.	
31. Examine the removed CVC and assess it for drainage, odor, integrity, and length. If there is any breach in the CVC structure, instruct the patient to maintain complete bed rest, save the catheter, and notify the physician immediately. If there is any drainage or foul smell, cut off the tip (2-3 inches) and place the tip portion of the CVC in a sterile specimen container for culture studies (Figure 12-26).	To assess for infection and catheter embolization.

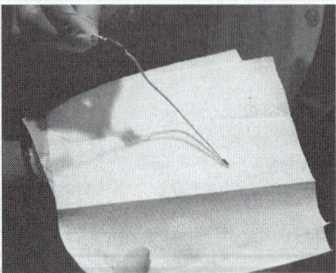

Figure 12-26 │ Examine the catheter to be sure all of it has been removed.

Implementation/Action	Rationale
32. Dispose of used equipment and carry out proper hand hygiene.	To prevent the spread of microorganisms.
33. Assess the dressing every 15 minutes for the first hour after removal, then hourly for the first 24 hours, post removal. The patient should maintain bedrest, as needed, until the exit site has epithelialized.	To assure proper wound healing and maintain patient safety.
34. Document the patient's response to CVC removal, the appearance of the site, dressing regimen, and the condition and length of the catheter as well as any associated interventions.	For patient safety and to maintain continuity of care.

CENTRAL VENOUS TUNNELED CATHETERS

A central venous tunneled catheter (CVTC) is usually made of soft, medical-grade silicon. It has a Dacron® cuff near the subcutaneous exit site of the catheter that anchors it in place, acts as a securing device, and serves as a microbial barrier (due to the formation of granulation tissue around it). There may also be a VitaCuff® surrounding the catheter that sits proximal to the Dacron® cuff. The CVTC is surgically inserted via percutaneous cutdown under local or general anesthesia. The distal catheter tip is advanced into the vessel and is placed in the superior vena cava, while the proximal end is subcutaneously tunneled to an incisional exit site on the anterior or posterior trunk of the body (Figure 12-27). The usual exit sites for CVTCs are in the mid to lower thoracic or upper abdominal regions, making them convenient to care for (by the patient) and allowing them to be concealed under clothing.

Tunneled CVCs may be single or multilumen and the general guidelines for caring for patients with them are essentially the same as for the nontunneled products, except that there are two exit-site incisions to care for. Insertion and removal are surgical procedures performed by a physician. CVTCs are left in place for an indefinite period of time. In some agencies, dressings are not used over the exit site of a CVTC once the cuff has epithelialized. With the exception of the closed-tip Groshong,® the methods of access, flushing, and heparinizing are the same as for the nontunneled CVCs. There are many different brands available, all with minor variations. The Broviac,® Hickman,® Leonard,® and Groshong®

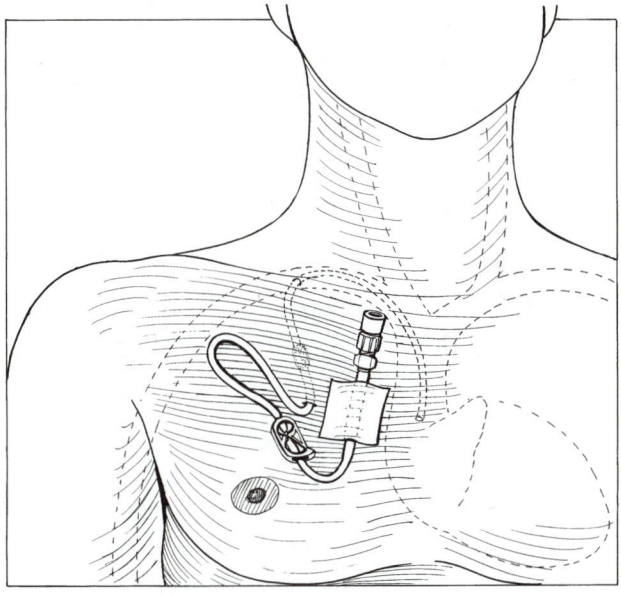

Figure 12-27 | Insertion and exit sites of a central venous tunneled catheter (CVTC)

were prototypes of many of the more recently developed CVTCs and will be covered briefly here.

Broviac,® Hickman,® and Leonard® Catheters

The Broviac,® Hickman,® and Leonard® CVCs are members of the same family, size being the main difference (Figure 12-28). They are made of biocompatible silicone, have a Dacron® cuff, and are indicated for long-term venous access in the hospital or at home. The Broviac,® which is used mainly in pediatric patients or adults with small central vessels, has the smallest diameter (2.7–6.6 French), lengths of either 71 cm or 90 cm, and only one lumen. The Hickman® ranges in size from 9.6 to 14.4 French and may be single or multilumen, with lengths ranging from 65 to 90 cm. The Hickman® is indicated for multipurpose infusion therapy, CVP monitoring, and blood sampling. The Leonard® is a single or dual-lumen catheter that only comes in a 10 French, 90 cm length. There is also a Hickman/Broviac® combination CVTC that incorporates a double-lumen Hickman® catheter with a single-lumen Broviac.®

Groshong® Tip Catheters

The Groshong® tip catheter is a soft, medical-grade silicone long-term catheter with a closed-end, atraumatic rounded tip (Figure 12-29). It is placed into one of the large central veins so that the tip lies in the superior vena cava and is tunneled subcutaneously for several inches to the desired exit site. It has the SureCuff® Tissue Ingrowth Cuff that is positioned in the tunnel to promote tissue ingrowth and secure the catheter in place.

The Groshong® tip differs from other CVCs (which are open-ended) in that it has a patented three-position, pressure-sensitive valve (or valves), which allows fluids to flow in or out, but stays closed when not in use (Figure 12-30), thus reducing the need for clamping. The valve is located near the rounded, closed, radiopaque catheter tip and allows fluid infusion and blood aspiration. When not in use, the valve restricts blood backflow (bleedback) and air embolism by remaining closed. With the Groshong® CVC there is virtual elimination of heparin flushing to maintain catheter patency, as only saline is needed after use to maintain the valve in its normal closed position. The use of heparin, however, is not contraindicated and is used by some practitioners. When the catheter is not in use, it only needs to be flushed with normal saline every seven days. Figure 12-31 provides a troubleshooting guide for the Groshong® CVC.

The Groshong® valve is available in cuffed (tunneled) CVCs designed for long-term use as well as noncuffed (nontunneled) short-term use CVCs and PICCs.

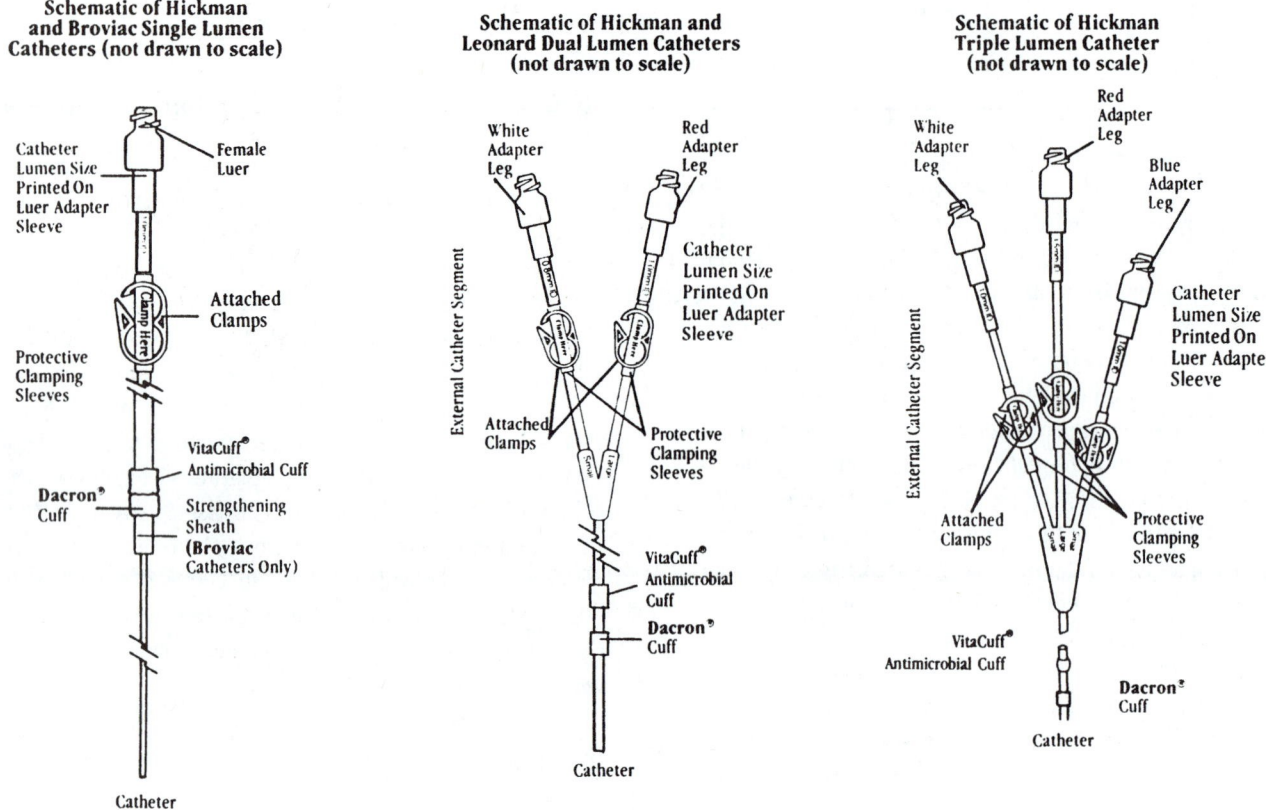

Figure 12-28 | Broviac,® Hickman,® and Leonard® CVCs *Courtesy of BARD Access Systems*

The PASV™ Catheter

The one-valved PASV™ catheter has a valve located within the catheter hub. The valve remains closed when the catheter is not in use and when subjected to normal central venous pressures. When positive fluid pressure is exerted through the Luer-Lok® hub, the valve opens, thus allowing infusion through the catheter. When negative pressure (as with aspiration) is applied, the valve also opens, permitting the withdrawal of blood into a syringe. The catheter has a polyester Tissue Ingrowth Cuff that is surgically tunneled under the skin, inside the body, and exits the chest wall. This supports the ingrowth of tissue, prevents dislodgement, and provides a barrier to the introduction of microorganisms. A dressing is applied until tissue has grown into the cuff, after which a covering is not required (even though some physicians prefer that the site is dressed). The PASV™ is available as a single or double lumen catheter and requires saline flushes. The use of heparin, however, is not contraindicated for flushing.

PERIPHERALLY INSERTED CENTRAL CATHETERS

A peripherally inserted central catheter (PICC) is a percutaneous IV line composed of silicone elastomers or polyurethane. It may be single or multilumen with sizes ranging from 50 to 60 cm in length and diameters of 16 to 23 ga. Insertion may be through the needle, through a peel-away introducer, through an intact cannula, or with a guide wire.

Legal Issues

PICC lines should only be inserted by persons who are specially trained and qualified in the theory, placement, and maintenance of such devices. Since 1994, no nurse practice act in any of the fifty United States has stated that PICC line insertion is not within the scope of practice for the registered nurse (although some states have specifically included it and others have made no declaration either way). (Some states prohibit placement of PICC lines in the home care setting and some have restrictions regarding the use of lidocaine, suturing, and catheter placement in the superior vena cava.)

SCHEMATIC OF GROSHONG CATHETERS
(not drawn to scale)

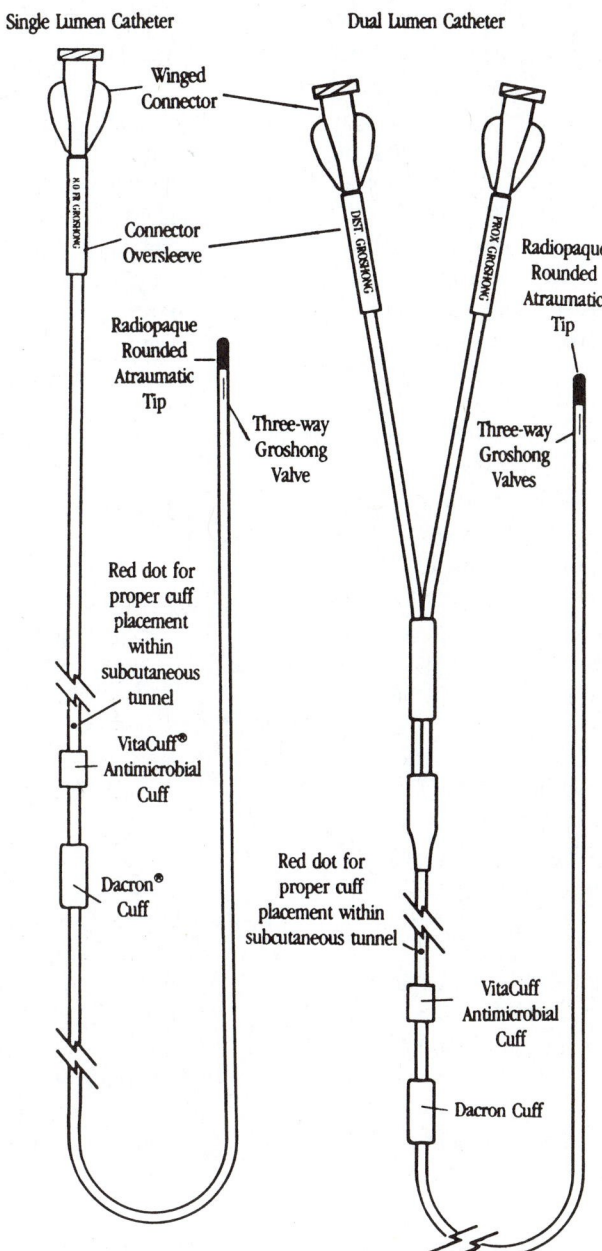

Figure 12-29 | Single- and dual-lumen Groshong® CVCs
Courtesy of BARD Access Systems

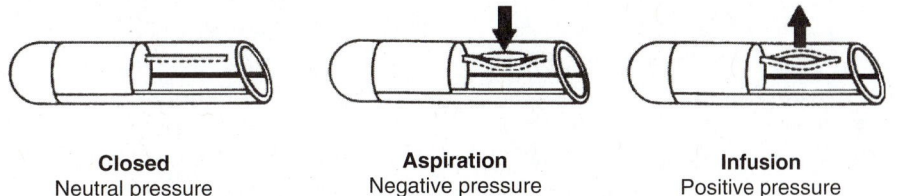

Closed
Neutral pressure

Aspiration
Negative pressure

Infusion
Positive pressure

Figure 12-30 | The three-way Groshong® valve remains closed when not in use, opens inward for aspiration, and opens outward for infusion *Courtesy of BARD Access Systems*

I. Aspiration Difficulties
A. Possible Causes
1. Failure to flush according to catheter Irrigation Procedure, resulting in lumen obstruction.
2. Catheter opening may suck up against vein wall with aspiration.
3. Blood clot, fibrin sheath, or particulate matter obstructing valve when catheter is aspirated.
   - A clot or other obstruction in the catheter lumen can produce a one-way valve effect. During infusion, the catheter wall expands slightly and allows fluid to flow around the obstruction. During aspiration, the catheter wall contracts slightly, tightening down around the obstruction and preventing aspiration.
   - Fibrin sheaths usually begin to form within a few days after the insertion of a central venous catheter. When it has grown enough to extend to the tip of the catheter, it may be pulled into and obstruct the catheter valve when aspiration is attempted, but offer no resistance to infusion.
4. Compression or transection of the catheter between the clavicle and the first rib ("pinch-off area").
5. Kinked catheter outside or inside the body.
   - Suture constriction at the catheter skin exit site, cuff, or vessel insertion site.
   - Catheter may be pulled too tight through skin tunnel, causing kink at vessel insertion site, or where it curves into the subcutaneous tunnel.
   - Catheter may be curled or kinked within the vessel, or under the dressing.
6. Malposition of catheter (i.e., jugular vein, outside of vein).

B. Possible Solutions
1. Visually check catheter for any exterior kinks, or constricting sutures. Check operative report, or with placement physician for placement of sutures. If sutures are present, their removal may release the constriction and allow aspiration. A removable suture wing is supplied with the insertion tray to prevent suture constriction at the exit site.
2. If no resistance to infusion is felt, attempt to flush with 10 cc normal saline. Then pull back gently on syringe plunger 2–3 cc, pause and proceed with aspiration.
3. If resistance to infusion is felt, check for signs of extravasation. If present, notify physician of possibility of catheter leakage or transection and embolization. If not present, see Step 5.
4. Attempt to aspirate with a 20-cc syringe (creates a greater vacuum).
5. Move patient's arm, shoulder, and head to see if a change in position will allow aspiration. If aspiration can only be accomplished with the patient in a certain position, the patient should be examined to see if the catheter has been placed in the "pinch-off" area. See Step 7.
6. Obtain physician's order and instill urokinase 5,000 IU/ml per Clearing Occluded Catheters Procedure.
7. Obtain physician's order for chest x-ray to verify catheter placement.
   - If the insertion into the subclavian vein is between the clavicle and first rib ("pinch-off" area), the catheter may be occluded mechanically enough to allow low-volume infusion, but prevent aspiration due to compression between the clavicle and first rib. The more medial the insertion site, the greater the potential for "pinch-off." Catheters in this area are at risk for catheter transection and embolization and the physician should evaluate the patient for catheter replacement.
   - If the catheter tip is not in the superior vena cava, it should be repositioned.
   - If the catheter tip is out of the vein, it should be replaced.

II. Bleedback in Catheter
A. Possible Causes
1. A blood clot or particulate matter may be holding the valve open.
2. Migration or placement of the catheter tip in the internal jugular vein, or vessel other than the superior vena cava, or coiling of the catheter in a vein may position the catheter tip where the valve is pushed open.
3. Placement of the catheter in the right atrium or ventricle:
   - Contractions of the heart muscle can force the catheter valve open.
   - Impingement of the catheter tip on the tricuspid valve, heart wall, or apex of the heart can force the catheter valve open.
4. Catheter valve tip cut off in error during catheter placement.

B. Possible Solutions
1. Attempt to aspirate clot out of the lumen.
2. If no resistance felt, flush with 10 cc normal saline. If resistance is felt, see Step 3.

Figure 12-31 | Troubleshooting guide for the Groshong® CVC *Courtesy of BARD Access Systems*

3. Obtain physician's order and instill urokinase or other solution per Clearing Occluded Catheters Procedure to clear lumen and valve of blood clots or precipitates.
4. Obtain physician's order for chest x-ray or dye study to determine catheter position.
   - Check for radiopaque tip to verify if it is still in place. If not, treat catheter as an open-ended catheter, using heparin and clamping with an atraumatic clamp when opening it to the air until it is repositioned.
   - If malpositioned, coiled or kinked, catheter should be repositioned with the tip in the superior vena cava. If unable to reposition for some reason, treat catheter as an open-ended catheter, using heparin and clamping with an atraumatic clamp when opening it to the air.

III. **Catheter Occlusion**
   A. **Possible Causes**
   1. Blood clot completely obstructing lumen.
   2. Drug precipitate or lipid deposition completely obstructing lumen.
   3. Catheter may be kinked, coiled, damaged, or pinched between the clavicle and first rib.
   4. Catheter valve may not be within vein.
   5. If sutures were used during the placement of the catheter, they can tighten and restrict flow.
   6. Catheter may be partially or completely transected. Transection can occur from the repeated pressure of the clavicle and the first rib on the catheter during normal movement if it is placed through the "pinch-off" area.
   B. **Possible Solutions**
   1. Attempt to aspirate blood clot.
   2. Move patient's arm, shoulder, and head to see if position change affects ability to infuse. If so, see Step 5 (could be pinch-off).
   3. Inspect patient and operative report for presence of sutures around the catheter. If sutures are present, they should be removed. Removable suture wings are available in the insertion tray for holding long-term catheters in place until the SureCuff Tissue Ingrowth Cuff heals in enough to anchor the catheter.
   4. Obtain physician's order and instill urokinase or other solution per Clearing Occluded Catheters Procedure.
   5. Obtain physician's order for a chest x-ray or dye study to determine the position of the catheter.
      - If the catheter tip is not in the superior vena cava, the catheter should be repositioned.

   - If the catheter tip is not in the vein, the catheter should be replaced.
   - If the catheter has been placed through the "pinch-off" area, between the clavicle and the first rib, and is being compressed enough to interfere with infusion or aspiration, it is at risk for catheter transection and embolization. The physician should evaluate the patient for catheter replacement.

IV. **Catheter Damage**
   A. **Possible Causes**
   1. Repeated clamping.
   2. Contact with a sharp object.
   3. Rupture from attempt to irrigate an occluded catheter with a small syringe (i.e., 1- or 3-cc syringe).
      - Small syringes can generate very high internal pressures with very little force. The back pressure from an occlusion may not be felt when using a small syringe until damage to the catheter has occurred.
   B. **Possible Solutions**
   1. Always fold the catheter between the patient and the damaged area and tape it together, or clamp the catheter between the patient and the damaged area with a smooth-edged, atraumatic clamp.
   2. Determine the site of damage and the size and type of catheter.
   3. Refer to the appropriate Catheter Repair Procedure to repair the damage. At least 2 in. of intact catheter beyond the skin exit site is needed to be able to repair the body of the catheter. use the appropriate size repair kit to assure a good repair.
   4. Always use a 10-cc syringe or larger when infusing into the catheter.

V. **Air in Line**
   A. **Possible Causes**
   1. Hole in catheter.
   2. Injection cap not prefilled with normal saline.
   3. Loose connections (injection cap, IV tubing).
      - If the oversleeve has not been put on the catheter connector at all, or if it or the catheter has not been slid all the way onto the hub, air and fluid leakage can occur.
   4. "Manometer effect"—holding the catheter connector end above the level of the heart while it is open to the air creates a manometer effect, with fluid dropping to a level of 8–10 cm above the Groshong valve at the tip of the catheter. Air will not enter the bloodstream unless the valve has

(continues)

Figure 12-31 | continued

been propped open by a blood clot or drug precipitate, or the catheter tip has been placed where mechanical pressure forces the valve open.

5. Diffusion and evaporation of water through the external catheter segment due to silicone permeability. This may be noticed in the Groshong catheter because it is flushed less frequently than other silicone catheters, and it is clear, allowing the visualization of air, which is not possible with other silicone catheters.

- Silicone has an open matrix that allows water vapor and gases to diffuse through the membrane.
- The amount of diffusion that takes place is dependent on many factors. Therefore, not all patients with silicone catheters will demonstrate this phenomenon.
- The air will stay in catheter's external segment. It does not extend below the level of the skin. The air can be aspirated once a week when routine flushing is done. There is no danger of air embolism from silicone permeability.

B. Possible Solutions

1. Check catheter for leakage by flushing well with normal saline.
2. Prefill injection cap with normal saline before attaching it to the catheter.
3. Check for loose connections (injection cap, IV tubing). Check for the presence of the oversleeve. If present, check for proper attachment of the catheter, the connector, and oversleeve (see Connector Repair Procedure).
4. If the catheter is not damaged, aspirate the air and then irrigate the catheter with 10 cc normal saline to flush out any aspirated blood. Air present in the catheter due to silicone permeability will only be present in the external catheter segment and will not migrate into the patient's bloodstream unless injected.
5. Perform procedures requiring the catheter to be opened to the air with the connector end below the level of the patient's heart.

VI. Fluid Leakage from Catheter Exit Site

A. Possible Causes

1. Catheter punctured by sharp object (i.e., scalpel, suture needle, trocar) just prior to placement.
2. Catheter ruptured from attempt to irrigate an occluded catheter with a small syringe (i.e., 1-cc or 3-cc syringe).
   - Small syringes can generate very high internal pressures with very little manual force. The back pressure from an occlusion may not be felt when using a small syringe until the damage to the catheter has occurred.
3. Catheter may have become encapsulated by a fibrin sheath, which is preventing infused fluid from entering the venous system. The fluid will then take the path of least resistance, flowing back along the outside of the catheter to the skin exit site.
4. Central vein thrombosis or tumor growth occluding the vein can cause infused fluid to flow back along the outside of the catheter to the skin exit site.
5. Catheter may have been transected by the clavicle and the first rib due to placement through the "pinch-off" area, allowing fluid infused to flow back along the outside of the catheter to the skin exit site.

B. Possible Solutions

1. Infuse 10 cc of normal saline and observe for signs of fluid extravasation under the skin.
2. Obtain physician's order for a dye study through the catheter to determine path of fluid flow.
3. Remove the catheter if a leak or transection is discovered inside the body. If a transection has occurred, the embolized fragment may have to be retrieved with a snare. Please report such incidents to BARD Access Systems (800-443-3385).
4. If a leak is discovered in the catheter outside the body, repair it following the Catheter Repair Procedure appropriate for the catheter type and the location of the damage.

Figure 12-31 | continued

Since it is within the scope of nursing practice, it is the responsibility of every nurse to know and follow nursing board guidelines and employer policies and procedures regarding PICC insertion, maintenance, and patient care. Certification to insert PICCs can be granted only by the nurse's employer after minimum educational requirements

are met and evidence of competency in the successful placement and maintenance of PICCs has been demonstrated and supervised by a qualified individual. It is advisable that nurses who insert and maintain PICCs undergo continuing education and routine retraining to maintain competence. With any PICC placement, there must be a physician's order and appropriate medical staff coverage. LVNs and LPNs should be involved only in observational assessments of PICCs, not in hands-on insertion or maintenance of PICCs. The INS PICC task force has developed position papers on these devices and has a recommended educational curriculum. The curriculum highlights the INS position papers and prepares the nurse to assess potential PICC candidates, comprehend the procedure, and initiate appropriate care and maintenance.

Indications and Advantages

PICC lines are indicated for the administration of fluids, blood or blood products, and medications in patients who lack suitable veins for repeated peripheral vascular access. Placed in the superior vena cava, they are also used to draw blood for sampling and administer chemotherapy and parenteral nutrition preparations. They are usually intended for patients who require therapy for periods of 1 to 12 weeks but some PICCs have remained in place for four years or longer. Patients who are candidates for PICCs must have peripheral antecubital veins large enough to accept a 14- to 16-ga. introducer needle. To be most cost effective, therapy should be required for at least 7 days.

The advantages associated with PICC lines include the following:

1. Avoidance of the discomfort and stress affiliated with multiple peripheral sticks
2. Least traumatic due to avoidance of the risks associated with insertions in the neck and chest regions such as pneumothorax and great vessel perforation
3. Insertion on an outpatient basis
4. Reduced risk of infiltration
5. Lowest incidence of complications upon insertion compared to other central lines
6. Decreased risk of phlebitis
7. Preservation of peripheral veins
8. Cost effectiveness
9. No age barrier

Contraindications and Disadvantages

PICC lines are contraindicated in the following patient populations:

1. Those with inadequate antecubital veins
2. Those who have pre-existing skin infections
3. Anyone with anatomical distortions related to injury, surgical dissection, or trauma
4. Individuals with coagulopathies
5. Those with severe peripheral edema
6. Confused or noncompliant patients
7. Those requiring high-volume or high-pressure infusions
8. Those who cannot change the dressings
9. Those whose lifestyles/occupations involve being in water

There are very few disadvantages associated with PICC lines. The few that do exist, however, make them inappropriate for use in some patients. PICC line maintenance in the home care patient requires a degree of responsibility for self-care that some persons cannot undertake, especially if they have physical or mental impairments or do not have anyone to help them. In addition, there is some limitation of activity related to arm movement for recreational and sports activities, such as swimming. Otherwise, they are an ideal alternative to CVCs for many people.

Insertion and Placement Sites for PICCs

The preferred veins for peripheral insertion of a central line are the large antecubital basilic or cephalic veins or the median cubital vein (Figure 12-32). These routes are ideal because they are associated with fewer insertion complications than other veins (Table 12-3).

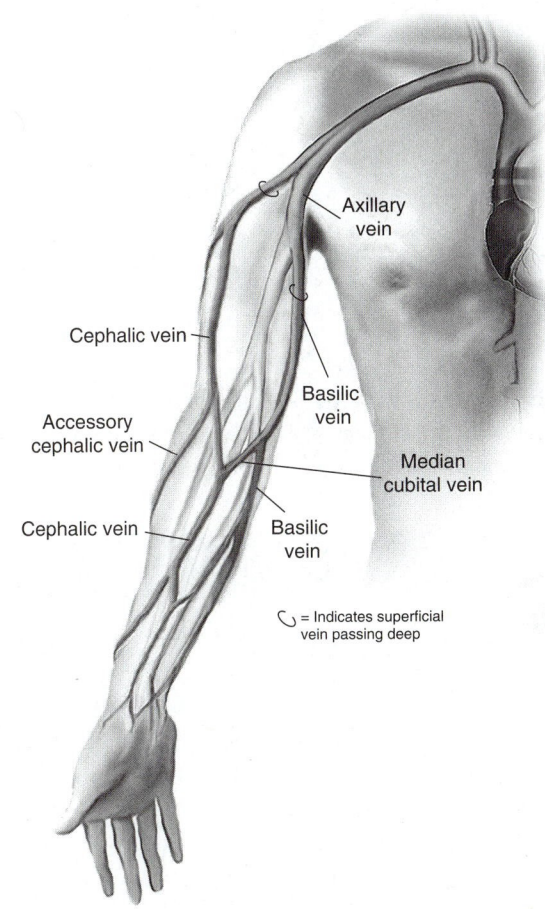

Figure 12-32 | PICC line vein selection

Table 12-3 | PICC Line Venous Insertion Site Selections

BASIC VEIN
(USUALLY THE FIRST CHOICE)

Advantages	Disadvantages
• Large size	• Usually requires palpation to locate because it is not as superficial as the cephalic.
• Follows a straight path	• Lies in close proximity to the brachial artery and some of the branches of the internal cutaneous nerve, so care must be taken not to injure these structures during venipuncture.
• Facilitates passage of the catheter into the axillary vein, subclavian, brachiocephalic (innominate), and superior vena cava	• Should not be used for patients on crutches.

CEPHALIC VEIN

Advantages	Disadvantages
• Superficial	• Difficulty may be encountered with catheter threading due to the sharp angle where it joins the axillary vein and because of narrowing due to valves. With this vein there is the greatest chance for malposition by entering the jugular or thoracic vein, or turning back into the arm.
• Easy to enter at the antecubital fossa	
• The vein of choice for patients on crutches	

Basilic Vein

The basilic vein is the vein of choice for a PICC insertion. It originates on the ulnar side of the forearm, moves anteriorly near the antecubital region, and then continues upward toward the medial aspect of the arm to the antecubital area. Above the antecubital fossa, the basilic vein pierces the deep fascia (making visualization and palpation exacting) and travels up the inner aspect of the upper arm. It junctures with the deep brachial vein to form the beginning of the axillary vein near the shoulder. For this reason, the basilic vein should not be cannulated for a PICC in a patient who ambulates or supports her upright body weight using crutches. The axillary vein continues on to become the subclavian vein.

Cephalic Vein

The cephalic vein, which is smaller than the basilic, arises on the radial (thumb) side of the forearm at the wrist and moves up laterally on the forearm into the antecubital area. The cephalic vein is more superficial above and below the antecubital fossa, making it easier to palpate than the basilic. It continues upward over the biceps to the shoulder, crosses the shoulder, and merges with the axillary vein just distal to the clavicle. At the top of the shoulder, the cephalic vein usually narrows, because of its valves, at the point where it starts to terminate in the axillary vessel. Because of this and the sharp angle of entry into the axillary vein, there is the potential for catheter malposition, with the chance that the catheter will be threaded into the jugular vein or the thoracic vein, or turn back and loop into the arm vessel. In some individuals, there may be variations in the vein's anatomy.

Median Cubital Vein

The median cubital vein serves as the connection between the basilic and the cephalic veins. It is usually located in the antecubital fossa at the bend of the arm where, if cannulated, it may limit movement. It is usually easy to see and palpate.

NURSING TIP

Crutch Walking and Basilic Vein PICCs

For patients who use crutches, the cephalic or median cubital vein should be used for PICC cannulation instead of the basilic vein. The basilic vein follows an inner arm pathway to juncture with the deep brachial vein and form the axillary vein. Because of this anatomic course, blood flow would be compromised in the vessel due to compression from the crutch.

NURSING TIP

The Veins of Choice for PICC Cannulation

REMEMBER:
Basilic: Best (route); Biggest; Baby finger
Cephalic: Curved (route); Chance for malposition; Crutches

PICC Insertion and Maintenance Procedures

Once the order is obtained to use a PICC line, the nurse is expected to follow the policy and procedural guidelines of his employer and adhere to the insertion techniques provided by the manufacturer of the specific catheter being used. There are many varieties of these devices available, all with similar characteristics, but with varying insertion and maintenance guidelines. It cannot be stressed enough that individual manufacturer's directions must be followed exactly in order to safely and correctly insert any line.

The area of proposed PICC access should not be phlebitic or sclerosed. The nurse should always ask the patient if she has ever had a clot or thrombus develop in the arm or chest on the side of intended access. If the patient has had a mastectomy with axillary dissection and any history of edema, it is best to avoid using that side. Assess both arms carefully.

The veins in the arm of the patient's dominant hand are usually more prominent. If the PICC is being placed for preoperative major surgery, use the left arm, as central lines or Swan-Ganz catheters are usually accessed through the right side. For pacemaker candidates, use the right arm, as pacers are usually placed on the left side.

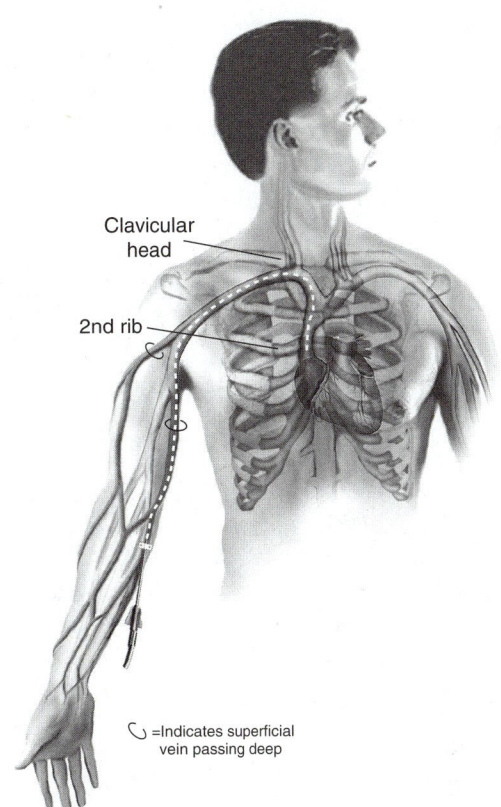

Figure 12-33 | PICC line placement in the superior vena cava

NURSING TIP

Edema and PICC Insertion

For a patient who has edema of the arms, a PICC can still be inserted. Using the heel of his hand, the nurse applies pressure to the patient's arm, over the area of proposed vessel cannulation, and holds it in place for 60 seconds. With release of the pressure, the edema will be displaced so the vein can be palpated or visualized.

Placement

Up until recently, it was considered acceptable to place a PICC line so that its tip was located in the subclavian or midclavicular position, which did not require radiologic verification of tip placement prior to use. The Food and Drug Administration Central Venous Catheter Task Force, the Infusion Nurses Society, and the National Association of Vascular Access Networks now recommend that catheter tip placement, for all PICC lines, be in the superior vena cava. This location provides optimal dilution of infusates and catheters maintain a longer dwell time with minimal complications. Placement in the superior vena cava is the preferred location because of the vessel's large, 20-mm diameter above its junction with the right atrium. An open-ended PICC implemented with a pressure pump can be used for CVP readings when situated in the SVC. Midclavicular placement in the brachiocephalic (innominate) or subclavian vein, is no longer used.

To measure for placement of the catheter tip in the superior vena cava (Figure 12-33), follow agency or manufacturer guidelines.

It is important that the nurse follow manufacturer guidelines and employer policy regarding the protocols for measuring the distance from the insertion site to the prescribed tip location. Placement must be confirmed by chest x-ray prior to the administration of infusates into any PICC line.

PICC Insertion and Gloves

The sterile gloves used to insert a PICC or midline catheter should be powderless. The starch powder on gloves, if not thoroughly rinsed, can enter the cannulation site. The residue serves as a foreign body and can precipitate an inflammatory response or a talc phlebitis. If used in conjunction with latex gloves, the powder, which becomes coated with latex protein, can act as a vector for latex allergens, thus jeopardizing the safety of both the patient and the nurse. Ninety percent of all latex allergies are thought to be caused by powdered latex gloves (Medical Educational Services & Kellett, 1996).

Rinsing off powdered gloves with sterile water or saline may not be effective in removing the powder. Washing or rinsing still leaves a significant residue of starch powder. The US Food and Drug Administration (FDA) advises that glove powder should be washed off before use (Cuming, 2002).

Research reveals, however, that most attempts to wash powder off are ineffective at best and, at times, may be more harmful. The problem is that the washing process causes residual powder to clump together, which could lead to a concentrated amount of cornstarch being deposited into the surgical wound (Edlich, 1997).

If latex gloves are used, it is best to use those that are powder-free with reduced protein content. Such gloves reduce exposures to latex protein and thus reduce the risk of latex allergy. Skill 12-10 outlines the steps involved in PICC insertion.

S K I L L 12-10

Insertion of the Peripherally Inserted Central Catheter

Equipment Needed:	Implementation/Action	Rationale
Non-sterile tape measure	1. Check the physician's order and institutional policy regarding insertion of a PICC.	A physician's order is a legal requirement for infusion therapy.
Two pairs of sterile gloves	2. Introduce yourself to the patient.	By introducing yourself, you convey courtesy, establish/promote the nurse-patient relationship, instill patient trust, and thus alleviate anxiety.
Two sterile drapes	3. Identify the patient by checking the wrist band against the doctor's order and asking the patient, if conscious, to state his/her name.	Proper identification ensures that the procedure is being performed on the correct patient.
Sterile scissors	4. Verify the allergy status of the patient.	This is a patient safety measure.
Tourniquet	5. Explain the proposed procedure in terms the patient can understand.	The patient has the right to know what is being done and the right to refuse care. Thorough explanations reduce anxiety and promote patient compliance.
Tuberculin syringe and 25-ga., 5/8-inch needle	6. Obtain patient consent for the procedure.	This is a legal requirement.
1% lidocaine	7. Gather all necessary equipment.	This serves to economize time and reduce patient anxiety.
Three alcohol swab sticks	8. Carry out proper hand hygiene.	Good hand hygiene is the single most important means of preventing the spread of infection.
Three 2% aqueous chlorhexidine gluconate or povidone-iodine swab sticks	9. Provide for privacy.	Prevents patient embarrassment.
	10. Apply a tourniquet to the patient's arm and assess the arm for an appropriate insertion site. Remove the tourniquet.	Using the proper site helps reduce the risk of infection and dislodgement of the device.
	11. Measure the amount of line that will be needed according to agency policy and write that number down.	Will ensure that an appropriately sized catheter is used so the procedure can be done properly the first time.
Two sterile 2 × 2-inch gauze pads	12. Wash the patient's arm with soap and water 6 inches above and below the insertion site; dry thoroughly.	A clean surface will prevent infection.
Two sterile 4 × 4-inch gauze pads	13. Position the patient flat with the arm extended at a 90-degree angle.	Straightens the veins for easy insertion.
(continues)	14. Carry out proper hand hygiene and open the PICC kit using sterile procedure. Any additional supplies should be dropped on the sterile field.	Prevents the introduction of microorganisms.
	15. Place the underdrape under the patient's arm and shoulder area.	Maintains the sterile field around the insertion site.

SKILL 12-10

Insertion of the Peripherally Inserted Central Catheter

Equipment Needed:

Six 10-ml syringes with needles or needleless blunt-tipped spikes

Two 10-ml vials of sterile normal saline for injection

10-ml vial of heparinized saline

Peripherally inserted central catheter

Sterile tape measure

Steri-Strips

Transparent semipermeable membrane dressing

Extension tubing (one for each lumen)

Injection cap (one for each lumen)

Face mask

Gown

Goggles

Implementation/Action	Rationale
16. Don a mask, sterile gloves, and a sterile gown. Put a mask on the patient.	**Prevents the introduction of microorganisms.**
17. Prepare three 10-ml syringes with normal saline.	**Equipment should be ready prior to beginning the procedure.**
18. Remove the catheter from the tray and examine it; be sure the guidewire is straight.	**Ensures there are no breaks in the line.**
19. Prime the catheter with normal saline and place the sterile measuring tape alongside the catheter.	**Assures patency of the line.**
20. For a closed-ended catheter, measure the distance from the tip of the catheter to where it will exit the body and mark it. For an open-ended catheter measure the distance from the exit site to where the tip of the catheter will lie in the vessel. Note this marking and allow for the distance of the catheter that will extend out of the arm. Retract the guidewire to where the catheter tip will be cut, cut the tip straight across, advance the guidewire to within $^1/_8$–$^1/_4$ inch of the tip, bend the guidewire at a 90-degree angle at the external end of the device.	**Correct measurement will ensure the correct length of the PICC for this patient.**
21. Prime the catheter connector.	**To remove air from the line and maintain patency.**
22. Prep the insertion site first using three alcohol and then three 2% aqueous chlorhexidine gluconate or iodophor swabsticks. Work outward in a concentric circle. Allow each solution to completely dry before proceeding to the next step (Figure 12-34).	**Prevents introduction of microorganisms.**

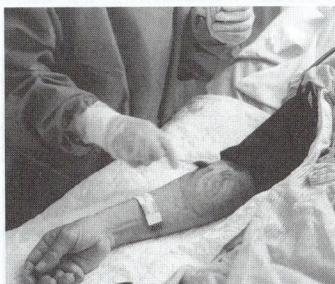

Figure 12-34 | Cleanse the injection site.

(continues)

SKILL 12-10

Insertion of the Peripherally Inserted Central Catheter (continued)

Implementation/Action	Rationale
23. Place sterile drapes around the insertion site (Figure 12-35).	Maintains a sterile field around the site.

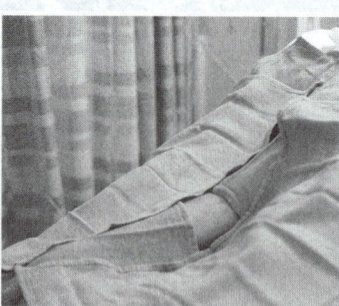

Figure 12-35 | Drape the injection site with sterile drapes.

Implementation/Action	Rationale
24. Apply the tourniquet; this should be above the elbow for most patients.	Allows for the dilation of veins.
25. Remove gloves used for preparation and apply second set of sterile gloves.	Prevents the spread of infection.
26. Anesthetize the insertion site (Figure 12-36).	Anesthetizes the insertion site for patient comfort.

1. Palpate and locate the distended vessel.

2. Anesthetize the venipuncture site (optional). Using the small needle attached to the syringe of the anesthetic, inject directly over the vein, bevel down. (If the vein is very superficial, do not inject over it so as to avoid inadvertent entry into the vessel with the anesthetic.) Inject on each side of the vein.

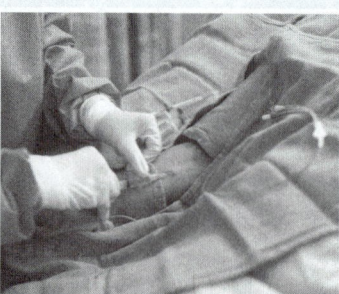

Figure 12-36 | Anesthetize the injection site.

The needle tip should first be placed on the skin, bevel down, while exerting pressure on the skin with the needle (to diminish pain sensation). The needle is then slipped beneath the epidermis, and a small amount is injected (0.1 to 0.5 ml) to produce an intradermal wheal and the initial numbing effect. The needle is then moved deeper into the tissue on each side of the vein and injected. The amount of NS injected depends on vein depth.

Implementation/Action	Rationale
27. Hold the skin below the insertion site taut.	Holds the vein in place during the venipuncture.
28. Perform the venipuncture holding the introducer needle at a shallow 15–30-degree angle with the bevel up. Go slow. Go low.	Prevents inserting the needle through both sides of the vein wall.
29. Look for a blood return in the flashback chamber and then slowly advance the introducer needle a fraction of an inch more so the sheath is in the vein.	Ensures the needle is in the vein.
30. Remove the tourniquet.	Prevents unnecessary trauma to tissue.

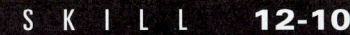

SKILL 12-10

Insertion of the Peripherally Inserted Central Catheter

Implementation/Action	**Rationale**
31. Maintain the stability of the introducer and advance it.	**Prevents trauma to the vein wall.**
32. Observe the pattern of blood flow.	**Ensures that a vein, not an artery, has been cannulated.**
33. Remove the needle from the introducer, leaving the introducer in place.	**Allows access to the vein for threading the PICC.**
34. Thread the PICC into the vein through the introducer to the depth determined by previous measurements (Figure 12-37). Use a steady, moderate rate of passage.	**Too rapid entry could cause venous spasm, too slow entry could cause catheter malposition.**

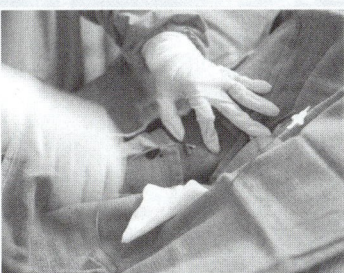

Figure 12-37 | Thread the catheter through the introducer needle.

35. Hold pressure over the insertion site until bleeding stops.	**Minimizes trauma to the site of the insertion.**
36. Cleanse the insertion site of all blood.	**Keeping the site clean prevents introduction of microorganisms, reducing the risk of infection.**
37. Remove the guidewire by spreading the fingers of one hand over the length of the catheter outside the insertion site and gently pressing down while grasping the hub of the guidewire with the opposite hand and pulling it parallel to the skin with a slow, steady motion.	**Allows removal of the guidewire only and not the catheter as well.**
38. Remove the introducer catheter from the PICC while applying pressure above the insertion site.	**Prevents removal of the catheter while introducer is being removed.**
39. Cut the PICC so that approximately 10 cm are left extending from the insertion site.	**Allows additional lines to be connected to the PICC line when infusion is necessary.**
40. Insert the connector into the catheter and apply a suture wing.	**Preps the line for the addition of other lines and securing the catheter in place.**

(continues)

SKILL 12-10

Insertion of the Peripherally Inserted Central Catheter (continued)

Implementation/Action	Rationale
41. Using a 10-ml syringe of saline aspirate to confirm placement of the catheter tip, flush using the pulsatile, push-pause method (Figure 12-38).	

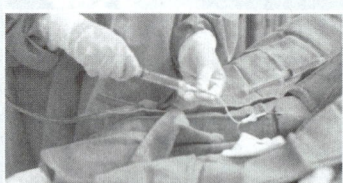

Figure 12-38 | Flush the line with normal saline.

42. Apply an injection cap.	**Allows the line to be accessed for medication delivery.**
43. Heparinize the injection cap.	**Maintains the patency of the line.**
44. Place a 2 × 2-inch folded gauze over the insertion site and place a transparent dressing over that for the first 24 hours (Figure 12-39).	**Controls bleeding, prevents introduction of microorganisms.**

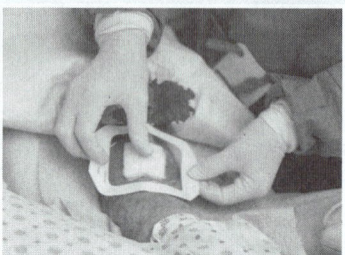

Figure 12-39 | Dress the site using a transparent semipermeable membrane dressing.

45. Label the insertion site with date, time, length, and gauge of catheter and your initials.	**Provides information for future care of the PICC.**
46. Remove gloves, gown, and mask and dispose of all materials in the proper waste receptacle.	**Prevents cross-contamination and the spread of microorganisms.**
47. Carry out proper hand hygiene.	**Prevents cross-contamination and infection.**
48. Document the procedure.	**Promotes legal protection and patient safety.**
49. Catheter placement must be verified with a chest x-ray.	**Ensures the catheter was placed properly.**
50. Dressing should be changed in 24 hours. Assess for swelling, drainage, and tenderness. Assess for migration of the catheter by checking the length of the catheter.	**Early identification of problems prevents further complications.**

Overcoming Problems with Threading of the PICC Line

Threading is often the most difficult aspect of PICC insertion. Never force insertion.

When there is a good blood return but the catheter will not advance to the premeasured length of the vein, consider the following:

- Cannulation of the wrong vessel
  Problem: When using the median cubital vein, there is a good blood return and the catheter seems to be threading straight up the middle of the arm, but then it meets with resistance or stops.
  Solution: First try flushing while threading.
  Problem: The brachial vein may have been inadvertently cannulated.
  Solution: Remove the catheter and cannulate another vein.

- Kinked Catheter Tip
  Problem: During threading, after getting a good blood return, the flexible catheter tip kinks over onto itself and usually won't pass beyond 10 to 15 cm.
  Solution: Pull back on the catheter and flush. Flushing indicates that the tip was kinked. If flushing is ineffective, another vein may need to be used. Never force a kinked guidewire, because it could puncture the catheter.

- Malpositioned Catheter Tip
  Problem: The catheter threads easily to the subclavian vein and then threading becomes difficult or cannot continue. It is possible to flush and (usually) difficult to draw blood. If it is possible to flush but not to draw blood, the catheter needs to be redirected.
  Solution: Always have the patient turn her head to the side, with the chin on the shoulder of the PICC insertion arm, to prevent malposition into the internal jugular vein.
  Solution: Flush-thread until reaching the insertion length. Pull the catheter back to a point where the tip is in the arm and reposition the patient and/or her arm and attempt to rethread. Have the patient lie flat or turn the patient on the side opposite to the arm in which the PICC is being placed.

Never force the catheter. The catheter may be curled in the arm or there may be blockage of the vessel. A chest x-ray may be necessary prior the repositioning attempts.

- Venous Occlusion
  Problem: Threading progresses to a point where the catheter abruptly stops. This may be due to a valve, vessel narrowing (stenosis), or a thrombus.
  Solution: Attempt to flush and thread past the valve or narrowing. Preinsertion history/evaluation is very important, as it may reveal a problem.

Never force the catheter.

- Venous Spasm
  Problem: During threading the vein clamps down.
  Solution: Flush to attempt to open the vein or wait up to 10 minutes while flushing intermittently.

PICC Dressing Protocol

For the first 24 hours following insertion, it is recommended that a gauze dressing be placed at the insertion site and covered with a transparent dressing, so bleeding can be assessed. Suturing is generally not recommended, although the suture wing is placed over the catheter to contribute added stability.

After the first 24 hours, a sterile transparent dressing is placed over the insertion site, catheter, and hub, and the site is cleansed according to dressing change protocols. A chevron formation piece of tape is placed under the connector where the transparent dressing ends and extends over its top to stabilize the catheter. A strip of tape is placed over the chevron and another strip is placed over any catheter extensions (Figure 12-40).

PICC Line Care and Maintenance Procedure

Once a PICC is inserted, there are protocols for care that must be meticulously followed. Proper assessment and maintenance are extremely important because the PICC, in most situations, serves as the patient's lifeline.

PICC Dressing Changes

PICC dressings are usually changed every seven days or when the dressing becomes loose, wet, or nonocclusive. More

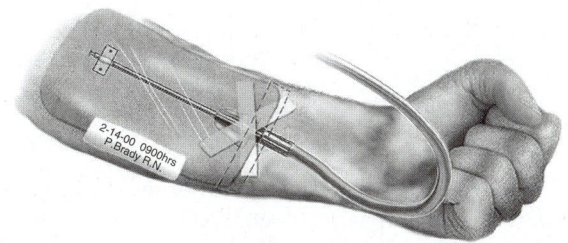

Figure 12-40 | Figure 12-40 | PICC Dressing

frequent changes may irritate the site, causing patient discomfort and increasing the chance of skin breakage, which predisposes the patient to infection. Should a skin tear occur, the usual treatment is to cover the breach with a transparent dressing and leave it in place until it deteriorates. *Note:* If moisture builds up under the dressing during normal day-to-day activities, it may be evaporated by using a blow dryer set on the low setting, held 6 to 8 inches from the site.

Before removing a dressing, always observe the way it was positioned so it can be replaced in the same manner. Know how much of the catheter should extend from the exit site to evaluate any possible change since insertion. If a change of more than 1 to 2 cm is noted, a chest x-ray may be indicated. Skill 12-11 summarizes the steps in dressing changes.

Injection Cap Change

Injection caps need to be routinely changed to prevent coring after repeated uses or when large-bore needles are used. Coring can allow a small segment of the cap material to enter the bloodstream, creating an embolus. Routine changes of the injection cap will help to eliminate this problem. Injection caps on PICCs are usually changed a minnimum of every seven days, more often if the line is frequently accessed. Caps are usually changed when changing the PICC dressing. When changing the caps on a multilumen line, all caps should be changed at the same time.

Injection caps are attached by a Luer-Lok connection. The connection needs to be checked frequently to ensure that it has not loosened and will not allow leakage and the indtroduction of microorganisms into the line.

SKILL 12-11

PICC Dressing Change and Site Care

Equipment Needed:	Implementation/Action	Rationale
Non-sterile gloves	1. Check the physician's order and institutional policy regarding a PICC dressing change.	A physician's order, and institutional guidelines, are legal requirements for infusion therapy.
Central line dressing change kit—usually contains a mask, sterile gloves, sterile drape, three alcohol swabs, three 2% aqueous chlorhexidine gluconate or povidone-iodine swabs, gauze 2 × 2s or 4 × 4s, antimicrobial ointment, transparent semipermeable dressing and tape	2. Introduce yourself to the patient.	By introducing yourself, you convey courtesy, establish/promote the nurse-patient relationship, instill patient trust, and thus alleviate patient anxiety.
	3. Identify the patient by checking the wrist band against the doctor's order and asking the patient, if conscious, to state his/her name.	Proper identification ensures that the procedure is being performed on the correct patient.
	4. Verify the allergy status of the patient.	This is a patient safety measure.
	5. Explain the proposed procedure, in terms the patient can understand.	The patient has the right to know what is being done and the right to refuse care. Thorough explanations reduce anxiety and promote patient compliance.
	6. Gather all necessary equipment.	This serves to economize time and reduce patient anxiety.
	7. Carry out proper hand hygiene.	Good hand hygiene is the single most important means of preventing the spread of infection.
	8. Provide for privacy.	Prevents patient embarrassment during the procedure.
	9. Put on the mask and assist the patient to put on a mask as well.	Prevents contamination of the insertion site by respiratory microorganisms.
	10. Apply non-sterile gloves.	Provides barrier to prevent spread of microorganisms.
	11. Instruct the patient to turn her head in the opposite direction of the insertion site and not move until the procedure is over.	Prevents the patient from breathing on the insertion site, lessening the chance of the introduction of microorganisms.

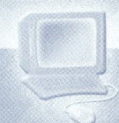

SKILL 12-11

PICC Dressing Change and Site Care

Implementation /Action	Rationale
12. Remove the old dressing using the stretch method, being careful not to dislodge the catheter. Note any abnormalities.	Careful assessment will note problems and allow for early interventions to prevent complications.
13. Remove gloves and carry out proper hand hygiene.	Sterile technique is required during the remainder of the procedure.
14. Open central line dressing pack, apply sterile gloves.	Sterile technique will lessen the chance for the introduction of microorganisms.
15. Pick up the sterile drape and drape the patient below the insertion site.	Provides a sterile field.
16. Cleanse the site with each of three alcohol swabs. Cleansing should occur in a circular motion, starting at the center of the insertion site and spiraling outward. Allow the alcohol to dry between swabs.	Cleanses body oils and any dirt that may have accumulated at the site.
17. Cleanse the site with each of three 2% CHG or povidone-iodine swabs. Cleansing should occur in a circular motion, starting at the center of the insertion site and spiraling outward. Allow the area to air dry.	Produces prolonged antimicrobial effect.
18. Apply either a transparent semipermeable dressing or gauze dressing over the site with the insertion site in the center. If a gauze dressing is used, tape over all the gauze and edges.	Prevents the introduction of microorganisms.
19. Note the date, time, the length of the catheter outside the insertion site, and the total length of catheter; then initial the dressing, being careful not to prevent visual inspection of the insertion site.	Allows for quick evaluation of site for the next dressing change.
20. Dispose of used equipment and carry out proper hand hygiene.	To prevent the spread of microorganisms.
21. Document the procedure.	To maintain patient safety and continuity of care.

NURSING ALERT

Preventing Air Embolism

The fluid level in the catheter drops when the catheter connector is held above the level of the patient's heart and opened to air. To prevent a drop in the fluid level and entry of air into the system while changing PICC injection caps, it is important to clamp and hold the connector below the level of the patient's heart before removing an injection cap.

The nurse should always refer to any specific information from the manufacturer before changing an injection cap. Skill 12-12 outlines the steps in changing injection caps on a PICC.

PICC Flushing

Flushing is an extremely important PICC maintenance measure. It must be done routinely, using 0.9% (normal) saline, followed by heparin (except for Groshong® tip catheters) based on agency policy guidelines regarding frequency and volume. Aseptic technique must be maintained.

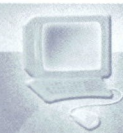

SKILL 12-12

PICC Injection Cap Changes

Equipment Needed:	Implementation/Action	Rationale
Injection cap	1. Check the physician's order and institutional policy regarding a PICC injection cap change.	A physician's order, and institutional guidelines, are legal requirements for infusion therapy.
Gloves	2. Check to be sure the cap needs to be changed.	Routine changes should be done to prevent complications.
Alcohol swap	3. Introduce yourself to the patient.	By introducing yourself, you convey courtesy, establish/promote the nurse-patient relationship, instill patient trust, and thus alleviate patient anxiety.
Syringe and needle or needleless blunt-tipped spike	4. Identify the patient by checking the wrist band against the doctor's order and asking the patient, if conscious, to state his/her name.	Proper identification ensures that the procedure is being performed on the correct patient.
1 cc normal saline for injection	5. Verify the allergy status of the patient.	This is a patient safety measure.
	6. Explain the proposed procedure in terms the patient can understand.	The patient has the right to know what is being done and the right to refuse care. Thorough explanations reduce anxiety and promote patient compliance.
	7. Obtain patient consent for the procedure.	This is a legal requirement.
	8. Gather all necessary equipment.	This serves to economize time and reduce patient anxiety.
	9. Carry out proper hand hygiene.	Good hand hygiene is the single most important means of preventing the spread of infection.
	10. Provide for privacy.	Prevents patient embarrassment.
	11. Draw up 1 cc of normal saline in the syringe. Flush all air out of the injection cap.	Helps prevent the introduction of air into the PICC.
	12. If the PICC cannot be clamped, place the patient in a supine position.	Helps to decrease the chance for introduction of air into the line during the procedure.
	13. Put on the gloves.	Prevents the spread of microorganisms.
	14. Cleanse the connection site between the injection cap and the PICC thoroughly with the alcohol swab. Allow the site to air dry.	Prevents the introduction of microorganisms into the PICC.
	15. Instruct the patient to turn her head away from the PICC during the procedure.	Helps to prevent the introduction of microorganisms by respiratory contamination.
	16. If not contraindicated, clamp the PICC. If clamping is contraindicated, instruct the patient to perform the Valsalva maneuver.	Helps to prevent the introduction of air into the PICC during the injection cap change.
	17. Remove the old injection cap by twisting the cap to the left.	Luer-Lok® connections are loosened by twisting.
	18. Add the new injection cap by twisting the cap to the right.	Luer-Lok® connections are tightened by twisting.

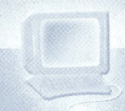

SKILL 12-12

PICC Injection Cap Changes

Implementation/Action	Rationale
19. Change all other caps, if present, following the same procedure.	All injection caps on a PICC should be changed at the same time.
20. Dispose of all used equipment and carry out proper hand hygiene.	To prevent the spread of microorganisms.
21. Document the procedure.	Provides for continuity of care.

Flushing is to be done at the following times:

- Whenever the line is locked
- After every blood draw—even attempts
- Following intermittent medication administration
- Following blood/blood product transfusion
- Following total or peripheral parenteral nutrition

1. Always flush with a 10-ml syringe or larger to maintain a psi of approximately 7 (well below the catheter burst pressure of 25 to 40 psi). *Important:* The psi exerted by a 1-ml syringe is greater than 300 psi and that exerted by a 3-ml syringe is over 25 psi.

2. The flushing volume is dictated by agency policy (Groshong® needs 5 ml NS). Open-ended PICC lines need to have the last 0.5 ml of heparin instilled using the end positive pressure method (simultaneously clamping) to prevent blood reflux.

3. The technique for flushing should be the pulsatile push-pause technique to remove residues and fibrin buildup.

4. Never force a flush. Some natural resistance should be felt because of the length (versus diameter) of a catheter. If the line cannot be flushed with a 10-ml syringe, the line is most likely occluded. (Refer to guidelines for clearing occluded catheters.)

Skill 12-13 outlines the steps involved in flushing the PICC.

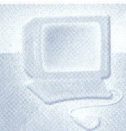

SKILL 12-13

Flushing the PICC

Equipment Needed:	Implementation/Action	Rationale
Gloves 70% isopropyl alcohol swabs 2% aqueous chlorhexidine gluconate or povidone-iodine swabs *(continues)*	1. Check the physician's order and institutional policy regarding PICC line flushes.	A physician's order, and institutional guidelines, are legal requirements for infusion therapy.
	2. Introduce yourself to the patient.	By introducing yourself, you convey courtesy, establish/promote the nurse-patient relationship, instill patient trust, and thus alleviate patient anxiety.
	3. Identify the patient by checking the wrist band against the doctor's order and asking the patient, if conscious, to state his/her name.	Proper identification ensures that the procedure is being performed on the correct patient.
	4. Verify the allergy status of the patient.	This is a patient safety measure.
	5. Explain the proposed procedure in terms the patient can understand.	The patient has the right to know what is being done and the right to refuse care. Thorough explanations reduce anxiety and promote patient compliance.

(continues)

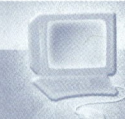

S K I L L   12-13

Flushing the PICC (continued)

Equipment Needed:	Implementation/Action	Rationale
10-ml syringe filled with sterile normal saline with appropriate needle or needleless adapter	6. Gather all necessary equipment.	This serves to economize time and reduce patient anxiety.
	7. Carry out proper hand hygiene.	Good hand hygiene is the single most important means of preventing the spread of infection.
	8. Provide for privacy.	Maintains patient dignity.
	9. Set up equipment.	Allows for the procedure to be completed quickly and efficiently.
	10. Put on gloves.	Prevents the spread of infection.
10-ml syringe with heparin (100 units/ mL) in the amount recommended by the manufacturer of the PICC or the amount dictated by agency policy	11. Cleanse the central venous catheter cap with 70% isopropyl alcohol followed by 2% CHG or povidone-iodine. Allow each solution to air dry.	Prevents the introduction of microorganisms into the system.
	12. Attach syringe containing normal saline to PICC.	To administer irrigation.
	13. Instruct the patient to perform the Valsalva maneuver and open the PICC clamp.	To prevent air embolism.
	14. Flush the line with normal saline. Use the pulsatile, push-pause method. Clamp the line.	Prevents a nidus for microbial growth, cleans the lumen of the PICC, and prevents occlusion of the line.
	15. Attach the syringe with the heparin.	To heparinize the line and prevent occlusion.
	16. Instruct the patient to perform the Valsalva maneuver and open the PICC clamp. Flush the line with the heparin. Clamp the line while infusing the last 0.5 ml of solution.	Prevents the IV from occluding.
	17. Dispose of all used equipment and carry out proper hand hygiene.	To prevent the spread of microorganisms.
	18. Document the procedure.	To provide continuity of care.

Blood Sampling

The ability to draw blood samples may depend on the catheter size. A 4 French 18 ga. is usually required for successful blood sampling. Skill 12-14 outlines the procedure for drawing blood from a PICC.

If it is not possible to draw blood, ask the patient to do the following:

- Turn her head toward the shoulder opposite the PICC arm.
- Raise the arm (with the PICC) straight out to the side, without hyperextending it.
- Turn from side to side.
- Sit up.
- Cough.

If it is still not possible to withdraw blood after trying these measures, flush the line vigorously with NS (push-pause). If the PICC flushes easily, but it is still not possible to draw blood, there may be a fibrin sheath/tail that prevents blood withdrawal. It may be necessary to declot, using the negative pressure method, with urokinase. (Refer to guidelines for clearing occluded CVCs described earlier in this chapter.)

Fluid, Medication, Blood/Blood Product, and TPN Administration

- Luer-Lok® connections should be used.
- For medication administration, check the product information. Be sure to check for medication-fluid compatibility to prevent precipitation of the infusate.

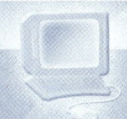

SKILL 12-14

Drawing Blood from the PICC

Equipment Needed:

2% aqueous chlorhexi- dine gluconate, 10% povidone- iodine or 2% iodine swabs

70% isopropyl alcohol swabs

Vacuum tube sleeve

Vacuum tube adapters for double- ended needles or single- ended needle (for puncture of collecting tubes) with reflux valve (for use with needleless systems)

Assorted blood collecting tubes or appropriate number of empty 10- to 20-ml syringes (if vacuum system is not used)

(continues)

Implementation/Action	Rationale
1. Check the physician's order and institutional policy regarding PICC line blood draws.	A physician's order, and institutional guidelines, are legal requirements for infusion therapy.
2. Check the orders for the lab work.	Different lab work requires different types of blood collection tubes.
3. Introduce yourself to the patient.	By introducing yourself, you convey courtesy, establish/promote the nurse-patient relationship, instill patient trust, and thus alleviate anxiety.
4. Identify the patient by checking the wrist band against the doctor's order and asking the patient, if conscious, to state his/her name.	Proper identification ensures that the procedure is being performed on the correct patient.
5. Verify the allergy status of the patient.	This is a patient safety measure.
6. Explain the proposed procedure in terms the patient can understand.	The patient has the right to know what is being done and the right to refuse care. Thorough explanations reduce anxiety and promote patient compliance.
7. Gather all necessary equipment.	This serves to economize time and reduce patient anxiety.
8. Carry out proper hand hygiene.	Good hand hygiene is the single most important means of preventing the spread of infection.
9. Provide for privacy.	Maintains patient dignity.
10. Set up equipment.	Allows for the procedure to be completed in an efficient and timely manner.
11. Put on gloves.	Prevents the spread of infection.
12. If an infusion is running, close the slide clamp. It is necessary to turn off all electrolyte and glucose-containing infusates that are infusing into other lumens for one full minute prior to the blood draw.	So the blood will be unaltered.
13. Instruct the patient to perform the Valsalva maneuver, and quickly disconnect the administration set tubing from the pigtail, cap the pigtail with the injection cap, and cap the distal end of the administration set with the sterile cap.	To prevent air entry and embolism and to maintain sterility of connection points.
14. Prep the injection cap of the pigtail with the alcohol followed by 2% CHG or iodophor.	To prevent contamination.
15. Attach a 10-ml saline-filled syringe. Open the slide clamp and ascertain placement and patency of the PICC, then vigorously flush with 10 ml of NS using the pulsatile, push-pause method. Clamp.	To prevent air embolism and ascertain patency of the line.

(continues)

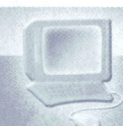

SKILL 12-14

Drawing Blood from the PICC (continued)

Equipment Needed:

Note: It is often difficult to obtain blood from a PICC line with vacuum tubes.

Two or three 10-ml syringes filled with sterile normal saline

30-ml syringe filled with 20 ml of sterile normal saline

10-ml syringe filled with 3 ml of heparin (100 units/ml)

Disposable gloves

Sterile injection cap (if applicable)

Normal saline for injection

Heparin 100 units/ml: 3 ml (or per agency guidelines) —none for Groshong® PICCS

Implementation/Action	Rationale
16. Attach the vacuum container or the empty 10- or 20-ml syringe to the injection cap. Unclamp.	To obtain the blood samples needed.
17. Draw 5 to 10 ml of blood into the discard tube.	So the blood will be unaltered.
18. Quickly insert and fill the required blood collection tube, then close the slide clamp on the pigtail and remove the vacuum container collecting device. Clamp.	To obtain the required specimen.
19. Prep the injection cap, open the slide clamp, and vigorously flush the line with at least 20 ml of NS to remove any residual blood. Clamp.	To clear the line and eliminate a site for microbial growth.
20. Reconnect the infusion line and unclamp so the infusion may run (or unclamp, heparin-lock the pigtail, and then clamp).	To resume the ordered infusate or to prevent occlusion of the PICC line.
21. Dispose of used equipment and carry out proper hand hygiene.	To prevent the spread of microorganisms.
22. Document the procedure.	To maintain continuity of care.
23. Deliver the sample to the laboratory as soon as the blood draw is complete and integrity of the PICC is ensured.	The blood will be delivered in a timely manner so that results can be obtained as soon as possible.

- For blood/blood product administration, remember that the flow rate depends on the catheter size. Blood should not be administered to an adult through less than a 20-ga. (2.8 to 3.0 French) catheter.
- TPN should be administered only if the tip of the PICC is positioned in the SVC. It should not be given if tip placement is midclavicular, because there is the potential for thrombosis.

Declotting

Determine the cause of the obstruction. If a fibrin sheath or clot is suspected, try the POP method. Use the same method to declot a PICC as described for a CVC, using the appropriate agent.

Catheter Repair

Preventing the need for catheter repair is a major consideration. To maintain the integrity of the catheter, it is important to do the following:

- Minimize catheter and catheter hub manipulation
- Use 10-ml barrel capacity syringes or larger to avoid overpressurization of the catheter
- Maintain dressings and tape to stabilize the catheter and any extensions

Catheter repair should be undertaken only if the appropriate repair kit is available and the manufacturer's guidelines are strictly followed. Never use a repair kit unless it is made by the manufacturer of the PICC being used.

PICC Exchange

A PICC exchange should be done only by a PICC certified nurse, following agency protocols. An exchange is often indicated when a catheter becomes irreversibly clotted, ruptured, or irreparable, and the patient may not have another viable vein to support a PICC. It is also useful when a PICC is inadvertently partially pulled out.

When an infection is suspected, and the PICC must be removed to culture its tip, an exchange can be made to maintain the line while waiting for the results of the culture. It is also a suitable procedure for conversion from a single- to multilumen catheter and vice versa.

When an exchange is done, it is considered the same as when a new PICC is inserted. The nurse is expected to follow the same postinsertion assessment/intervention parameters.

Seldinger Technique

A PICC exchange has traditionally been done using the Seldinger technique, where a guidewire is used to make the catheter exchange. It involves the entry of the guidewire into the vessel, with rethreading of the new catheter over the guidewire, followed by guidewire removal. This method demands expert practitioner skill in order to maneuver the guidewire and the catheter without traumatizing the insertion site and vessel. With guidewire exchange there is always the potential for serious complications, ranging from inflammation and phlebitis/thrombophlebitis to sepsis, vessel rupture, and pneumothorax. An easier and safer alternative to guidewire exchange is the sheath-catheter exchange method. Skill 12-15 outlines the sheath-catheter exchange for a PICC.

PICC Discontinuation and Removal Procedure

Once a PICC is no longer needed, it should be removed.

Sometimes, even though it is still needed, the PICC must be removed (usually due to infection or the client's inability to comply with the protocols for keeping it in place). Skill 12-16 outlines the steps in removing a PICC.

Risks and Complications Associated with PICC Lines

Many of the risks and complications associated with peripherally inserted catheters are the same as those of nontunneled and tunneled central venous catheters and can occur immediately following insertion or during their dwell time. The patient must be appropriately monitored so that complications can be handled with the relevant interventions. Some of the problems that are specific to PICCs include edema, bleeding, infusion pain, phlebitis, thrombophlebitis, retrograde leakage, catheter malposition, and a "stuck" catheter.

Arm Edema

The etiology of arm edema following PICC insertion is usually related to limited or absent range of motion (because of CVA, coma, restraints). Other causes of swelling include infection, retrograde catheter leakage, and thrombus. (Refer to these specific complications in the following paragraphs.) It is evidenced by generalized swelling, more so on the underside of the arm, with normal skin color. The edema is usually pitting. The primary nursing intervention involves the passive range of motion to the arm at least four times per day.

Bleeding

Minimal bleeding from a PICC insertion site is normal within 24 hours of placement. The physician must be notified if there is any excessive or persistent bleeding, which is usually caused by traumatic PICC insertion, patient coagulopathies, anticoagulation therapy, or vigorous physical activity.

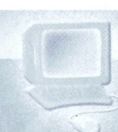

SKILL 12-15

PICC Exchange (Sheath-Catheter exchange)

Equipment Needed:	Implementation/Action	Rationale
Two pairs of sterile gloves	1. Check the physician's order and institutional policy regarding PICC exchange.	A physician's order, and institutional guidelines, are legal requirements for infusion therapy.
Two sterile drapes	2. Introduce yourself to the patient.	By introducting yourself, you convey courtesy, establish/promote the nurse-patient relationship, instill patient trust and, thus alleviate patient anxiety.
Sterile scissors	3. Identify the patient by checking the wrist band against the doctor's order and asking the patient, if conscious, to state his/her name.	Proper identification ensures that the procedure is being performed on the correct patient.
Tourniquet		
Tuberculin syringe and 25-ga., 5/8-inch needle	4. Verify the allergy status of the patient.	This is a patient safety measure.
	5. Explain the proposed procedure, in terms the patient can understand.	The patient has the right to know what is being done and the right to refuse care. Thorough explanations reduce anxiety and promote patient compliance.
1% lidocaine	6. Obtain patient consent for the procedure.	This is a legal requirement.
Three alcohol swab sticks	7. Gather all necessary equipment.	This serves to economize time and reduce patient anxiety.
Six 2% aqueous chlorhexi-dine gluconate or povidone-iodine swab sticks	8. Carry out proper hand hygiene.	Good hand hygiene is the single most important means of preventing the spread of infection.
	9. Provide privacy.	To maintain patient dignity.
	10. Elevate the bed level.	Conducive to successful access and alleviates back strain for the physician and nurse.
Two sterile 2 × 2-inch gauze pads	11. Secure all necessary supplies. The equipment and setup is the same as that for placing a new PICC, except for the use of an extra package of CHG or iodophor swabsticks.	To economize time and promote efficiency.
Two sterile 4 × 4-inch gauze pads	12. Place the patient comfortably in a semi-Fowler's position.	For proper access to the site and comfort of the patient.
Six 10-ml syringes with needles or needleless blunt-tipped spikes	13. Assess vital signs and level of consciousness and record.	To provide baseline physical and mental status.
	14. Remove the PICC dressing.	
	15. Following the procedure for inserting a new PICC, maintain a sterile field and drape the patient's arms appropriately.	A sterile field prevents introduction of microorganisms.
	16. Don sterile gloves.	Prevents the introduction of microorganisms.
Two 10-ml vials of sterile normal saline for injection	17. Cover the end of the PICC with a sterile 4 × 4-inch gauze and remove the PICC from the insertion site to expose at least 5 inches of the line.	
	18. Aseptically prepare the site, as for placement of a new PICC.	This is a sterile procedure.
(continues)	19. Cleanse the existing PICC, using the additional CHG or iodophor swabsticks.	To minimize entry of microorganisms.

(continues)

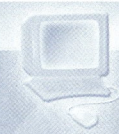

SKILL 12-15

PICC Exchange (continued)

Equipment Needed:	Implementation/Action	Rationale
10-ml vial of heparinized saline	20. Clamp the PICC 1 inch distal to its exit site from the body.	**To prevent air entry.**
Peripher-ally inserted central catheter	21. Cut the PICC 3 inches distal to the clamp. Discard the removed portion of the PICC off the sterile field.	**To prevent contamination of sterile supplies.**
	22. Remove the introducer needle from the plastic introducer sheath.	
	23. Thread the plastic introducer sheath over the end of the exposed PICC, advancing it up to the clamp.	**There should be an adequate length of the PICC extending from the introducer so that it can be folded beyond the end of the introducer.**
Two sterile tape measures	24. Fold the end of the PICC a short distance from the end of the introducer.	
Steri-Strips	25. While keeping the PICC doubled over, remove the clamp from its former position and place it between the introducer and the folded portion of the PICC.	**So air will not enter when the clamp is removed.**
Transpa-rent semiper-meable membrane dressing	26. Advance the introducer sheath over the PICC up to its exit site on the arm.	**To position it for advancement.**
Extension tubing (one for each lumen)	27. Apply normal saline around the PICC exit site and slowly advance the introducer into the site up to its hub.	**To ensure that the introducer enters the vein.**
Injection cap (one for each lumen)	28. Gently pull down on the existing PICC.	**To facilitate threading the introducer.**
	29. Pull the PICC out of the arm through the introducer.	**Successful placement of the introducer is evidenced by effortless removal of the PICC.**
Face mask	*Note:* Following removal there may or may not (more likely) be a retrograde flow of blood from the introducer. To stimulate a blood return, a tourniquet may be placed high on the upper arm.	
Gown		
Goggles		
	30. Introduce the new PICC into the introducer and advance it to its premeasured insertion length, following the usual insertion protocols.	**To ensure proper placement.**
	31. Withdraw the introducer sheath and retract it from the PICC.	**Once in place, the introducer is no longer needed.**
	32. Follow the same procedural guidelines for PICC placements, following advancement of the tip to its premeasured position.	**To assure proper tip location.**
	33. Lower bed to standard low position and raise rails.	**To promote safety and prevent falls.**
	34. Remove personal protective equipment and dispose of used materials in appropriate waste containers.	**Prevents cross-contamination and risk for infection.**
	35. Carry out proper hand hygiene.	**To prevent the spread of microorganisms.**
	36. Arrange for portable chest x-ray or transfer to radiology for x-ray.	**PICC placement in the superior vena cava can only be correctly verified with x-ray.**
	37. Document the procedure.	**To maintain continuity of care.**

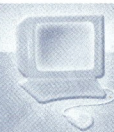

SKILL 12-16

PICC Removal

Equipment Needed:	Implementation/Action	Rationale
10–20 ml syringe filled with 0.9% (normal) saline	1. Check the physician's order and institutional policy regarding PICC removal.	A physician's order, and institutional guidelines, are legal requirements for infusion therapy.
	2. Introduce yourself to the patient.	By introducing yourself, you convey courtesy, establish/promote the nurse-patient relationship, instill patient trust and, thus alleviate patient anxiety.
Nonsterile gloves	3. Identify the patient by checking the wrist band against the doctor's order and asking the patient, if conscious, to state his/her name.	Proper identification ensures that the procedure is being performed on the correct patient.
Sterile 4 × 4-inch gauze	4. Verify the allergy status of the patient.	This is a patient safety measure.
Strip of adhesive tape or adhesive bandage strip	5. Explain the proposed procedure, in terms the patient can understand.	The patient has the right to know what is being done and the right to refuse care. Thorough explanations reduce anxiety and promote patient compliance.
	6. Obtain patient consent for the procedure.	This is a legal requirement.
Culture tube, if indicated	7. Gather all necessary equipment.	This serves to economize time and reduce patient anxiety.
Antiseptic swab-sticks, if a culture is ordered	8. Carry out proper hand hygiene.	Good hand hygiene is the single most important means of preventing the spread of infection.
	9. Provide privacy.	To maintain patient dignity.
	10. Elevate the bed level.	Conducive to successful access and alleviates back strain for the physician and nurse.
	11. Secure all necessary supplies.	To economize time and promote efficiency.
	12. Position the patient comfortably in a supine or semi-Fowler's position with arm extended at a 45- to 90-degree angle from the torso.	To facilitate removal.
	13. Flush the PICC with normal saline.	To ensure that there are no problems with the line.
	14. Don nonsterile gloves.	Protection of nurse against contamination from blood-borne pathogens.
	15. Remove the dressing (and sutures, if present).	
	16. If a culture is required, cleanse the PICC exit site.	To obtain an accurate culture, free skin of contaminants.
	17. Gently grasp the catheter at its exit site from the skin.	Grasping the catheter near its exit site on the skin gives better control along with the exertion of a more even force at the area of highest catheter resistance (which is usually the venotomy entry/exit area).

SKILL 12-16

PICC Removal (continued)

Implementation/Action	Rationale
18. Remove the catheter, pulling it straight out while maintaining gentle, constant traction and regrasping the catheter every few centimeters.	With this maneuver there is a decreased risk of catheter breakage in a subcutaneous area or in the length of catheter between the skin and the nurse's hand.
19. Measure the length of the removed catheter and compare it to the documented length that was inserted.	Ensures that the entire length of catheter has been removed.
20. Gently apply pressure with the 4 × 4-inch gauze.	To ensure hemostasis.
21. Fold the gauze over and apply a strip of tape or apply an adhesive bandage. Leave the dressing in place for 24 hours.	To maintain hemostasis.
22. Discard the catheter into the sharps container.	
23. Lower bed to standard low position and raise rails.	To promote safety and prevent falls.
24. Remove personal protective equipment and dispose of it in the appropriate container.	To prevent cross-contamination.
25. Carry out proper hand hygiene.	To prevent the spread of microorganisms.
26. Document the procedure.	For patient safety and as a legal document.

Infusion Pain

Infusion pain is seen more frequently in midarm, cephalic-vein placements and is usually caused by the chemical properties of the infusate. If the patient complains when infusions with high osmolarities or low pH are being administered, it may help to decrease the infusion rate and apply warm, moist compresses to the arm. If venospasm and phlebitis occur, it may be necessary to consider using a centrally placed catheter.

Sometimes infusion pain occurs because there is catheter damage. If this is suspected, the physician needs to be notified and an x-ray using a contrast medium may be necessary to rule out breaks or leaks in the catheter or to confirm that the catheter tip has not migrated out of the superior vena cava.

Mechanical Phlebitis

Mechanical (sterile) phlebitis, the most frequent complication (1.2% to 23%), is the noninfectious process of inflammation caused by the body's response to a foreign material inside a blood vessel. It occurs more often in females, due to their smaller veins, with a higher incidence in the left arm and with double-lumen catheters. It usually occurs within the first to tenth day, with the highest percentage by the fifth day. It is often referred to as postinsertion phlebitis (PIP).

The etiology of phlebitis may be the body's response to a foreign material; roughening or irritation of the vein wall during catheter insertion or by advancing the catheter too rapidly or forcefully into the vein; use of a large-bore catheter due to decreased blood flow; introduction of particulate matter such as glove powder or towel lint; or patient sensitivity to the catheter material. The signs and symptoms of phlebitis include tenderness and pain; redness and warmth; and induration, edema, and venous cording.

The major nursing intervention for phlebitis is prevention. A most important consideration is the skill of the person inserting the PICC. There is a clear correlation between the inserter's learning curve and the incidence of phlebitis, with more experience translating to a lower rate of phlebitis. Preventative measures include using powderless gloves; advancing the catheter slowly without forcing it; applying warm moist compresses, four times a day for 20 minutes during the first 24 to 48 hours postinsertion; encouraging mild arm exercise; and monitoring frequently during the first week.

Table 12-4 | Grading Scale for the Severity of Mechanical Phlebitis in the Patient with a PICC Line

Grade	Criteria
0	No pain, erythema, swelling, induration, or palpable venous cord at or around the IV site
1+	Pain at IV site; no erythema, swelling, induration, or palpable venous cord
2+	Some erythema or swelling at IV site; no induration or palpable venous cord
3+	Erythema and swelling at IV site; induration and palpable venous cord <3 inches above the site
4+	Erythema and swelling at IV site; induration and palpable venous cord >3 inches above the site

Courtesy of BARD Access Systems

Once phlebitis is evident, nursing interventions include application of dry or moist heat (depending on the policy of the agency) to the circumference of upper arm until phlebitis is resolved; elevation of the extremity; mild arm exercise to promote good circulation and venous return; administration of anti-inflammatory medication. Phlebitis must be assessed, reported, and documented (Table 12-4). Left untreated, phlebitis may progress to thrombophlebitis.

Thrombophlebitis

Thrombophlebitis associated with a PICC usually occurs when the tip of the catheter is not in the superior vena cava and a high osmolar infusate (e.g., TPN) is administered. The formation of intravascular clots is confirmed by a venogram. The incidence is extremely rare with proper tip placement and as high as 13% to 53% with improper placement. Thrombus formation begins within a few days of the initiation of TPN administration if it is infused into a vessel smaller than the SVC. Patients who are dehydrated (with increased blood viscosity) or who have reduced blood flow or hypercoagulopathy defects are at higher risk for the development of thrombophlebitis, as are those who have sustained injury to the intima of the vein due to sclerosing drugs or other factors.

The signs and symptoms associated with thrombophlebitis include the following:

- Swelling in the entire arm with edema that is firm and nonpitting due to capillary bed blockage and occlusion of the large vessel. The skin looks gray and pale.
- Swelling of the chest (unilateral), shoulder, neck, and face may be present.
- Discoloration of the arm and chest with the arm looking mottled. The fingertips are very pale and the arm takes on a gray cast with progression of the vessel obstruction.
- Arm pain that is described as pressure or an aching sensation.
- Distended arm or neck veins.

The interventions for thrombophlebitis include patient support with accurate status reports to the physician. Anticoagulant drugs are infused. The PICC must be removed or the thrombus will continue to grow.

Retrograde Leakage

Fluid drainage from the exit site of a catheter must be properly identified in order to determine its cause. Any unexplained, questionable drainage should be cultured to rule out catheter sepsis.

Drainage from the catheter site may occur in patients with decreased platelet counts or with platelet dysfunction. It can also occur in patients who have diminished skin integrity at the catheter insertion site.

Sometimes a fibrin sheath forms around the intravascular portion of the PICC. This may cause fluid to flow from the catheter tip, following the line of least resistance, back along the fibrin sheath down the catheter. The result is exit site leakage.

A PICC may have retrograde leaking if it is not properly placed or if the tip becomes displaced. Initially there is usually swelling at the insertion site that progresses to an infiltration of the tissue in the upper arm. An x-ray is needed to determine the problem. If the catheter is displaced after it has been in place for over 24 hours, it cannot be redirected or reinserted, so removal is necessary.

When there is swelling with redness and/or drainage from the insertion site within the first ten days of insertion, it is probably due to an infectious process. If this is the case, the PICC must be removed.

Retrograde leakage may be due to catheter rupture inside the vessel. If this is the case, retrograde leakage will increase when the infusion rate of the IV is increased. If this is suspected, the PICC must be pulled out to the area of rupture to determine the extent of damage. It may be necessary to remove the catheter or perform a catheter exchange.

Catheter Malposition

After it has been successfully placed, a PICC may become malpositioned within the veins of the arm or the larger vessels leading from them. If a PICC loops back on itself during insertion, it can be retracted and redirected.

Sometimes the catheter curls back on itself within the subclavian or superior vena cava. In this case, the infusion of fluid may straighten the catheter out or the line may need to be exchanged or removed. There have been instances where PICCs have formed loops in the upper arm. Blood returns were elicited and flushing was easy, so the lines were used to successfully complete the prescribed therapy regimens (Frey, 1995) in spite of malpositioning.

Catheter Occlusion

When there is difficulty flushing a PICC line or when flushing is not possible, the catheter may be occluded. Catheter occlusion may be caused by failure to flush following intermittent infusions, medication administration, or blood drawing; failure to perform scheduled flushes when the line is heparin or saline locked; failure to flush properly using the pulsatile push-pause method; or administration of incompatible infusates through the same port, causing precipitation formation.

It is important to determine the cause of the occlusion to treat it appropriately. When there is resistance to flushing, a fibrin accumulation or clot may be obstructing the line. When this is suspected, it is wise to try the POP method before using a declotting agent. The declotting agents (urokinase, hydrochloric acid, sodium bicarbonate, or ethanol 70%) and the methodologies used for clearing occluded PICC lines are the same as those described earlier for a central line.

When a precipitate has formed, it often cannot be removed. That is why it is so important to check for compatibility before administering combinations of infusates through the line. The most important reason for this is to prevent the discharge of precipitate particles into the circulation.

NURSING ALERT

Phenytoin

Dilute phenytoin (Dilantin) only with the special manufacturer-supplied diluent or preservative-free 0.9% normal saline. IV phenytoin will form a precipitate when mixed with anything else. Always flush IV lines thoroughly with *preservative-free NS* before and after intermittent injections of phenytoin. Due to the high alkalinity of the drug, diluting it with preservative-free NS and flushing thoroughly after administration are very important measures to avoid local irritation to the vein. Pain, inflammation, and necrosis may occur with infiltration into the subcutaneous or perivascular tissues. Never add phenytoin to a solution that is already infusing.

Stuck Catheter

Difficulty with PICC withdrawal is an uncommon but not infrequent problem, with resistance being encountered in 7% to 12% of removals (Lam, Scannell, Roessler, & Smith, 1994). Problems generally arise in the venous circulation of the medium-sized basilic and cephalic veins, not the larger, more central vessels that branch from them. The inability to remove a catheter usually occurs when it has been in place less than one week.

The most frequent cause of "stuck" catheters is venospasm (Marx, 1995), which is usually secondary to mechanical or chemical irritation. Spasm usually ensues after catheter removal has been initiated when the movement of the catheter irritates the intima of the vein. In response to the mechanical stimulation, the venous smooth muscle reacts with strong contraction. Other causes that hinder catheter removal are phlebitis, thrombophlebitis, valve inflammation, a knot in the catheter, or endothelialization of the catheter tip along the vein wall.

NURSING ALERT

"Stuck" Catheter

Never apply aggressive traction to a "stuck" catheter. The practice of stretching the catheter and taping it to the arm is not recommended. When the catheter is stretched, the resultant counter-resistance will cause either the catheter or the vein to break. Because of the thin-walled, small diameter of a PICC, forceful traction usually results in shearing of the catheter, commonly at the area of spasm.

Interventions for resistance to PICC removal include the following (asterisks* indicate interventions that require a physician's order):

- Release traction on the catheter and reattempt removal in 20 to 30 minutes.
- Gently massage the area of the upper arm over the PICC to relax the vein.
- Apply a warm, moist compress around the upper arm.
- Use mental relaxation exercises and distraction.
- Have the patient drink a warm beverage to increase vasomotor tone.
- Offer the patient an alcoholic beverage,* if not contraindicated or disagreeable to the patient.
- Ask the patient to open and close her hand and rotate the wrist to increase blood flow to the arm.

- Apply nitroglycerin paste to the arm over the vein where the PICC lies.*
- Start a peripheral IV distal to the PICC line and infuse warm normal saline to relax the vein and increase the flow/volume within the vein. In addition, administer a bolus of a vasodilator such as nitroglycerin.* The infusion of warm normal saline or nitroglycerin through the PICC is usually ineffective because the problem lies along the catheter shaft and is noncentral to the distal catheter port (Marx, 1995).
- The sublingual administration of smooth muscle relaxants, such as nitroglycerin or nifedapine, may be helpful.*
- Wait an additional 12 to 24 hours before attempting removal again. Spasm is not sustained indefinitely and the vessel eventually relaxes, even with the continued presence of the irritating stimulus (Marx, 1995). After 24 hours, part of the PICC may come out and another interval of time may be needed to remove the remainder of the line.

In the event that the PICC cannot be removed, the physician must be notified, because radiological removal using fluoroscopy, contrast media, and guidewire passage may be necessary.

MIDLINE CATHETERS

A midline catheter, or MLC, is any percutaneously inserted IV line that is placed between the antecubital fossa and the head of the clavicle. It is advanced into larger vessels below the axilla where there is good hemodilution. It is intended for intermediate-term therapy of one to six weeks for the delivery of nearly all infusion products except chemically caustic medications and total parenteral nutrition. Caustic medicine and TPN require dilution in the superior vena cava. The concept of an MLC is similar to that of a PICC. It may or may not require verification of tip placement by x-ray depending on agency policy, because it is inserted into the veins of the upper arm rather than those of the central venous system. In some agencies, the decision to insert an MLC lies with the nurse, negating the need for a physician's order.

A midline catheter is often used in home care situations where around-the-clock nursing care is not available and when repeated peripheral venipuncture would compromise venous access. It is a reliable delivery system for patients with osteomyelitis (often requiring four to six weeks of antibiotic therapy), pregnant women needing rehydration due to hyperemesis, and terminally ill patients in need of stable venous access for narcotic analgesia administration.

Placement

The three prominent veins of the arm in the antecubital region that are recommended for MLC placement are the basilic, cephalic, and median cubital. The ideal insertion site is one finger-breadth below or three finger-breadths above the bend of the arm.

The basilic vein is the preferred vessel because it is larger and follows a straighter path. At the level of the shoulder, it junctures with the deep brachial vein to form the beginning of the axillary vein (which continues on to become the subclavian). Because the basilic vein pierces the deep fascia above the antecubital fossa, it may not be possible to palpate it at this level.

The cephalic vein is usually smaller than the basilic, but is more superficial above and below the antecubital area, making it easier to palpate. As it moves upward on the lateral side of the forearm, its pathway continues over the biceps to the shoulder, crossing the shoulder, and terminating in the axillary vein, just distal to the clavicle. At the top of the shoulder area, where the tip of the catheter would reside, the cephalic vein usually narrows (owing to valves) as it merges with the axillary vein.

The median cubital vein connects the basilic with the cephalic vein. Because it is usually located where the arm bends at the elbow, direct insertion into this antecubital site may limit the patient's arm movement.

Patient Assessment and Premeasurement

Prior to placing an MLC, it is necessary to assess the anatomy of the patient's skin, subcutaneous tissues, and veins. There may be great variances, depending on age, weight, altered fluid volume or nutrition, disease processes, and history of vein use. Insertion is facilitated in a patient who is adequately hydrated. It is also important to assess the patient's activity level and the infusates she will be receiving, as well as the frequency of dosing. When choosing an insertion site, it is best to use the patient's nondominant arm, especially if she will be self-administering medications at home.

Owing to variations in patient size and vessel anatomy, it is always recommended that the arm be premeasured. For any MLC, the optimal catheter tip location is level with the axilla, just distal to the shoulder and deltoid muscle. Using a measuring tape, measure from the intended insertion site to this point and write down the distance.

Insertion and Management

The insertion and management protocols for a midline catheter follow the same principles and procedural guidelines described for a PICC line. As mentioned, TPN must not be administered through an MLC.

The arm must be assessed frequently and carefully as long as the catheter remains indwelling. Strick adherence to manufacturer's recommendations for admixing, diluting, and administering infusates must be followed.

Risks and Complications

As with any device, risks and unanticipated complications can occur at any given time during or following therapy with MLCs. Although the specific cause(s) of untoward events are sometimes hard to identify, there are several contributing factors. The most common cause of problems has to do with the medications being administered. The next most common cause of adverse events has to do with chemical or mechanical stimulation of the endothelial layer or nerves surrounding the vessels during insertion and therapy. Sensitivities to materials and solutions may exist as well. Nursing and medical management of the major complications associated with midline catheter use are essentially the same as for PICC lines.

IMPLANTABLE SUBCUTANEOUS VASCULAR ACCESS DEVICES

A subcutaneous vascular access device is an implantable port, sometimes called a vascular access port (VAP), that functions in much the same manner as a CVC, but is surgically inserted under the skin without any portion exiting the body. It consists of a single or double injection port with a self-sealing septum (partition) that is connected to a radiopaque catheter (Figure 12-41). The distal end is positioned in the superior vena cava. The catheter may be an open-ended system or a closed system (Groshong®). When used to deliver chemotherapy or other medications, the catheter tip may also be placed in various body cavities, such as the epidural space, the pleural cavity, and the peritoneum as well as arteries or vessels that lead into major organs, such as the liver or pancreas. The port sits in a surgically incised subcutaneous pocket that is centrally or peripherally located (Figure 12-42). The design allows for repeated entry into the vascular system, through percutaneous needle insertions, for the delivery of intravenous fluids, medications, blood or blood products, chemotherapy, and total parenteral nutrition, and for the withdrawal of blood samples. Figure 12-43 illustrates the placement of a port.

For most implantable VAPs on the market, only noncoring, nonbarbed needles are to be used, with the Huber™ point nee-

Portal Design	Material Composition
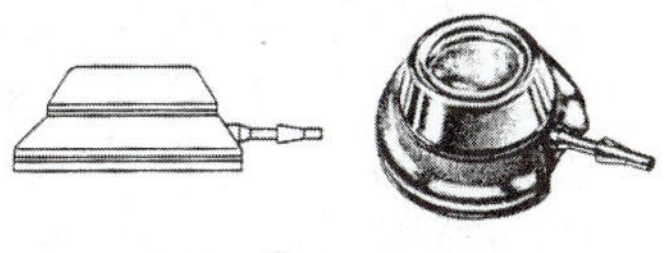 Hickman® Titanium Port	Titanium and Silicone
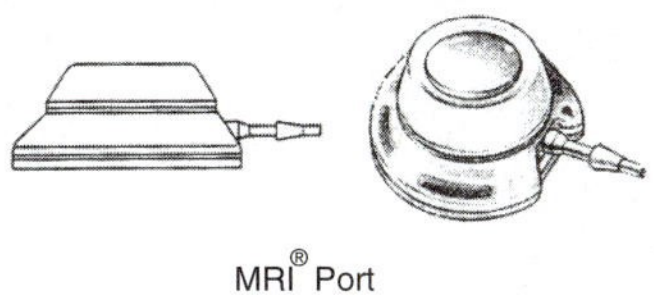 MRI® Port	Thermo Plastic and Silicone
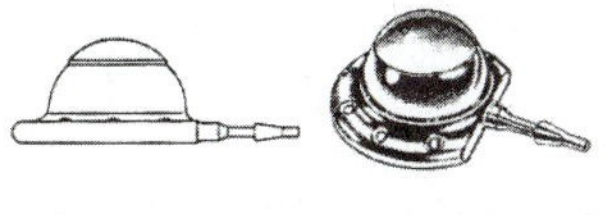 Dome™ Port	Titanium and Silicone
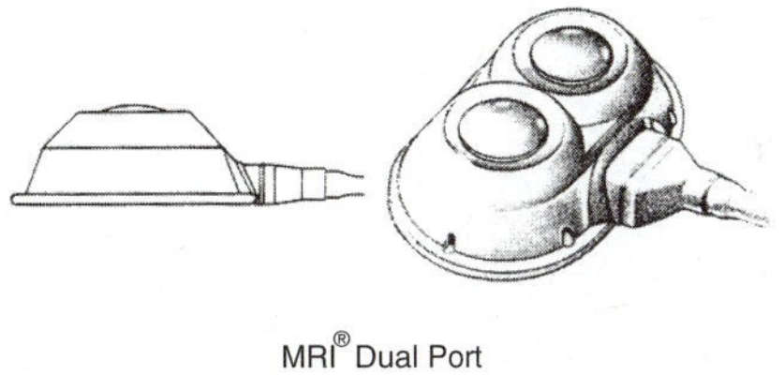 MRI® Dual Port	Thermo Plastic and Silicone

Figure 12-41 | Subcutaneously implanted vascular access systems *Courtesy of BARD Access Systems*

dle one of the most commonly used. Regular hypodermic needles, because of their design, will damage the portal septum, as will barbed (noncoring) types. Noncoring needles have a deflected point that helps avoid septal injury (Figure 12-44). The smallest gauge noncoring needle that can deliver the prescribed therapy should be used. VAP needles have metal or plastic hubs, come with or without Luer-Lok® extension tubings (Y-site or non-Y-site), and are either straight or have right-angle configurations. The straight needles are generally used only for bolus injections or blood sampling, while the right-angled ones are recommended for continuous or intermittent infusions, owing to their low profile and ease of securement. The Port-a-Cath® Gripper™ needle, a noncoring, nonsiliconized needle with a cushioned needle platform, has a removable contoured grip that controls placement and stabilizes the needle during insertion (Figure 12-45). It is compatible with ports made by most manufacturers. (The BARD CathLink™ implanted port, described in this chapter, is an exception to the rule of using noncoring needles. It is only to be used with over-the-needle catheters.)

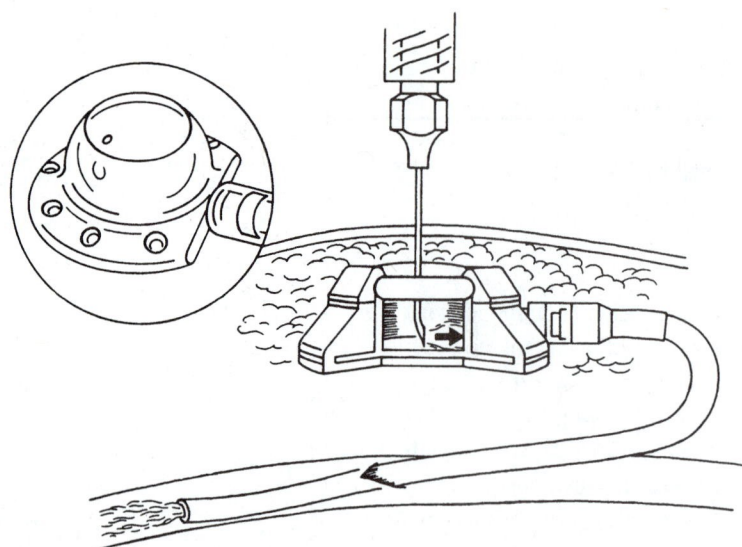

Figure 12-42 | Percutaneous needle entry into a vascular access port *Courtesy of BARD Access Systems*

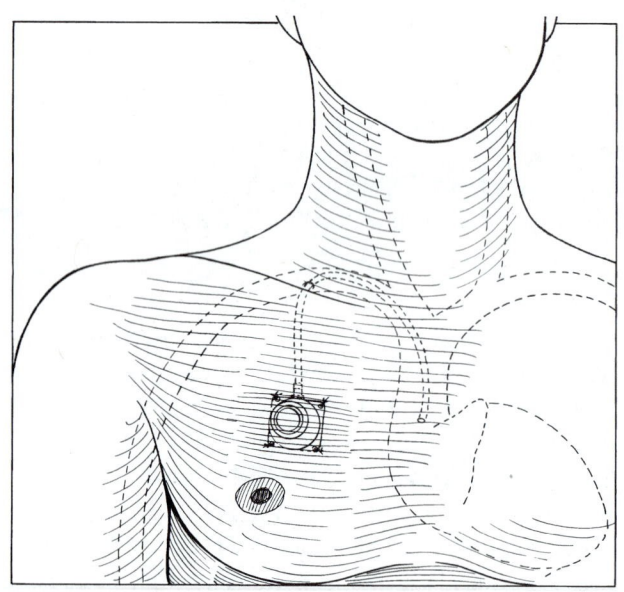

Figure 12-43 | Placement of subcutaneous implanted vascular access ports

Indications and Advantages

Implantable ports are indicated for patients who require vascular access for long-term infusion therapy but usually do not need to receive infusions or have blood samples drawn more frequently than every one to three weeks. They are indicated for all of the same reasons as tunneled and nontunneled CVCs. Since the ports are not externally exposed, they are cosmetically appealing, there is a reduced risk of infection, and patients can carry on virtually all activities without the need for exit site care or routine heparin or saline flushing, if the ports are not being used.

Contraindications, Precautions, and Complications

Implanted ports should not be used for patients who have a known or suspected infectious process, bacteremia, or septicemia. In addition, they should not be used if local tissue factors would prevent proper stabilization and venous access or if there were previous episodes of venous thrombosis at the prospective placement site. They cannot be used if the patient's body size is insufficient to accommodate the size of the implanted port. Table 12-5 lists the possible complications associated with implanted ports.

Only physicians qualified in the implantation of subcutaneous vascular access devices should insert them. Placement must be confirmed radiologically if insertion is not performed under fluoroscopy. When accessing these systems, only the manufacturer's recommended needles, following correct needle positioning guidelines, are to be used to maintain septal integrity and ensure proper infusate administration. Infusion pressures must never exceed 25 psi or catheter, blood vessel, or organ damage may occur.

Meticulous adherence to maintenance protocols is of major importance in the safe use and preservation of vascular access ports. Prior to administering any infusate through

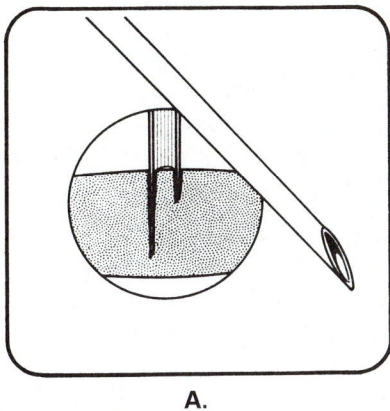

A.

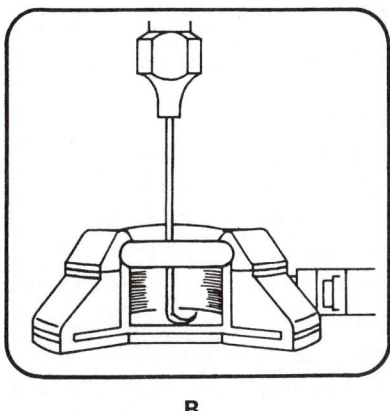

B.

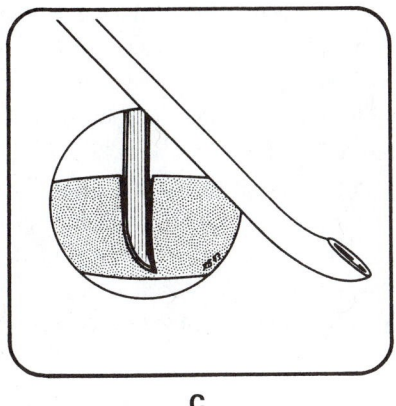

C.

Figure 12-44 | Needle tip comparisons: (A) hypodermic needle; (B) barbed needle; (C) noncoring needle
Courtesy of BARD Access Systems

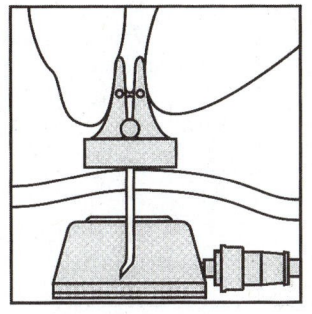

A. Insert the GRIPPER needle

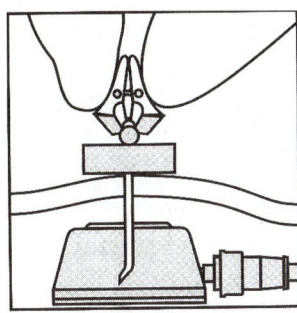

B. Peel back and remove tab

Figure 12-45 | The PORT-A-CATH® GRIPPER™ needle. (A) Hold the GRIPPER needle tab and insert the needle into the portal septum until the needle hits the base of the portal. The foam pad should be flush to the skin. (B) Remove the tab by grasping the top of the tab and squeezing firmly. Peel back, remove, and discard *Courtesy of SIMS Deltec, Inc.*

these devices, the nurse must be familiar with and observe all warnings, cautions, contraindications, and instructions as specified by the VAP's manufacturer. He must also follow the prescribed guidelines associated with the infusion of medications and other products. When accessing these devices, precautions must be taken to avoid air embolism.

The buildup of deposits, also known as residual sludge, is formed from blood products or drug precipitates that adhere to or reside in the internal pathway of subcutaneously implanted vascular access devices (Herbst, 1993). Residual sludge can serve as the nidus for infectious processes and thrombotic complications. The best way to prevent the buildup of residual sludge is through proper push-pause pulsatile flushing technique following the administration of medications, blood or blood products, and total parenteral nutrition. Should residual sludge and resulting catheter occlusion become a problem, the nurse must promptly institute the relevant clinical interventions, in accord with agency guidelines, to save the VAP. The problem is usually recognized by the ability to administer infusates through the port but the inability to aspirate a blood return when verifying catheter placement. Treatment is usually with a fibrinolytic agent or other declotting media (acids: hydrochloric acid; alkalines: sodium bicarbonate; lipids: 70% ethanol). The method is the same as for any CVC.

Table 12-5 | Possible Complications Associated with Implanted Subcutaneous Vascular Access Devices

• Air embolism	• Hemothorax
• Allergy to implant	• Hydrothorax
• Anesthesia-related complications	• Inflammation
• Bleeding	• Organ laceration
• Brachial plexus injury	• Pneumothorax
• Cardiac dysrhythmias	• Port erosion
• Cardiac tamponade	• Port malposition
• Catheter breakage	• Port migration
• Catheter damage	• Port occlusion
• Catheter embolism	• Scarring
• Catheter migration	• Sepsis
• Catheter pinch-off	• Skin necrosis over implant
• Device extrusion/rotation	• Surgery-related complications
• Endocarditis	• Thoracic duct injury
• Extravasation	• Thromboembolism
• Fibrin sheath formation	• Vessel erosion
• Hematoma	

NURSING TIP

Patient Teaching: Twiddler's Syndrome

The nurse must be instrumental in teaching patients and family members that the skin area over a subcutaneously implanted VAP should not be rubbed or manipulated in any way. There is a condition, known as Twiddler's syndrome, in which patients develop a habit of twiddling their ports. This can cause the internal catheter that is attached to the port to dislodge—a very serious situation—as the VAP may have to be surgically removed and replaced.

Insertion Protocols for Implanted Vascular Access Devices

There are many different single- and double-septa subcutaneous vascular access ports available. They all have similar physical structures and methods of access. It is the responsibility of the nurse to know and understand how the specific products used in his employing agency work.

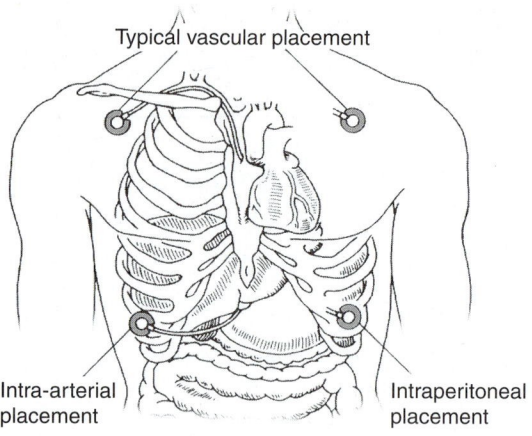

Figure 12-46 | Placement sites for vascular access ports *Courtesy of BARD Access Systems*

Catheter insertion may be accomplished by either standard cutdown technique through a small venotomy or by percutaneous technique. The catheter may be inserted into the vein directly through the pocket incision or via a subcutaneous tunnel to a remote venous entry site.

Placement should consider the amount of cutaneous tissue over the port septum. Excessive tissue will make it difficult to locate the septum and insert the needle, while too thin a layer may lead to port erosion. A tissue thickness of 0.5 cm to 2 cm is generally considered appropriate. Site selection should allow for port placement in an anatomic area that provides good port stability, does not interfere with patient mobility, does not create pressure points, and does not interfere with clothing.

Once the catheter is positioned in the superior vena cava, the physician surgically creates a subcutaneous pocket. It is secured by suturing it in place to the underlying fascia. Nonabsorbable sutures are used to reduce the risk of port migration and the possibility of it flipping over. The port is typically placed in the right infraclavicular fossa. The port is positioned so that it does not lie beneath the incision. A subcutaneous tunnel may be created for advancement of the catheter from the venous entry site to the port pocket.

For an intra-arterial port, the port is often placed over the lower ribs with the catheter inserted into the hepatic arterial system. For intraperitoneal implantation, the port is usually over the lower ribs with the catheter tip deep in the pelvis (Figure 12-46).

Use and Maintenance Procedures for Vascular Access Ports

Once the port is surgically implanted, the physician checks it for leaks and flow studies are conducted. Aspiration confirms the ability to draw blood. The catheter is flushed and heparin-locked. The incision site is closed and a dressing is applied. The implantation site should be inspected postoperatively for signs of swelling, infection, hematoma, seroma, and device rotation or erosion. Wound care and dressings should follow agency protocols. An implanted VAP may be used for bolus injections, continuous infusions, and blood sampling (intravenous ports only).

Note: Prior to any access, always instruct the patient to perform the Valsalva maneuver, as appropriate.

Site Preparation Prior to VAP Access

Inspection and aseptic preparation of the injection site should always be performed prior to accessing the port. Skill 12-17 outlines the steps in preparing the VAP access site.

Implanted Port Access

Port access is a sterile procedure requiring aseptic technique and sterile equipment. The use of sterile gloves and mask is recommended. Equipment will vary, depending on the procedure. Once the needle is in the septum, it must not be manipulated or the port may be damaged. Skill 12-18 identifies the necessary steps in accessing and deaccessing a VAP.

There is now available a one-handed Huber Loc extracting device that can be used to assist with the removal of a Huber needle. This device helps prevent needlestick injuries that can occur during standard removal, when the needle sometimes rebounds into the hand that is stabilizing the port. The device is plastic and disposable. One set of prongs on the device rests against the patient's skin to stabilize the port, while a second set pulls the needle out and stores it in the device. In addition to preventing needlestick injuries, the device lessens patient discomfort during needle removal and frees up the nurse's other hand to flush the port as the needle is being removed, thus reducing the patient's predisposition for clots and infection. Another device, the Doyle Extractor, also removes a Huber needle in a manner that is safer than manual extraction.

SKILL 12-17

Preparation of the VAP Access Site

Equipment Needed:	Implementation/Action	Rationale
Sterile gloves Three alcohol swab sticks Three 2% aqueous chlorhexidine gluconate or iodophor swab sticks Sterile 4 × 4-inch gauze Topical anesthetic, if indicated	1. Check the physician's order and institutional policy regarding VAP access. 2. Introduce yourself to the patient. 3. Identify the patient by checking the wrist band against the doctor's order and asking the patient, if conscious, to state his/her name. 4. Verify the allergy status of the patient. 5. Explain the proposed procedure, in terms the patient can understand. 6. Obtain patient consent for the procedure. 7. Gather all necessary equipment. 8. Carry out proper hand hygiene. 9. Provide privacy.	A physician's order, and institutional guidelines, are legal requirements for infusion therapy. By introducing yourself, you convey courtesy, establish/promote the nurse-patient relationship, instill patient trust and, thus alleviate patient anxiety. Proper identification ensures that the procedure is being performed on the correct patient. This is a patient safety measure. The patient has the right to know what is being done and the right to refuse care. Thorough explanations reduce anxiety and promote patient compliance. This is a legal requirement. This serves to economize time and reduce patient anxiety. Good hand hygiene is the single most important means of preventing the spread of infection. To maintain patient dignity. *(continues)*

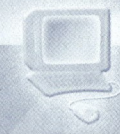

SKILL 12-17

Preparation of the VAP Access Site (continued)

Implementation/Action	Rationale
10. Elevate the bed level.	Conducive to successful access and alleviates back strain for the physician and nurse.
11. Secure all necessary supplies.	To economize time and promote efficiency.
12. Inspect the site.	To be sure the skin is free of abnormalities.
13. Wash insertion area with soap and rinse well with water and pat dry.	To remove any surface debris and oils from the skin and to promote asepsis.
14. Review the Valsalva maneuver with the patient.	To prevent air embolism.
15. Assess vital signs and LOC and record.	To provide baseline physical and mental status.
16. Set up the equipment in a sterile manner.	To maintain asepsis, promote efficiency, and economize time appropriately.
17. Expose the skin and palpate for the septum.	Ensures that the needle will be placed correctly.
18. Don gown, mask, and sterile gloves.	Prevents the spread of infection and prevents contamination of the nurse with chemotherapeutic agents/vesicants (if that is the therapy being initiated).
19. Instruct the patient to turn her head away from the VAP site.	Prevents the introduction of microorganisms.
20. Cleanse the septum site with each 70% isopropyl alcohol swab stick, starting at the intended puncture site and moving outward in a concentric circle 4 to 5 inches in diameter. Repeat for a total of three times. Allow the area to air dry.	Promotes asepsis and prevents the spread of infection.
21. Repeat the above steps, using the 2% CHG or iodophor swabsticks and allow the area to air dry after the third application.	Promotes asepsis by providing a prolonged antiseptic effect, thus preventing the spread of infection.
22. Gently wipe off any residue of the iodophor at the needle insertion site.	To prevent tracking any of the iodophor into the tissue upon needle insertion.

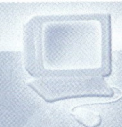

SKILL 12-18

Accessing and Deaccessing the VAP

Equipment Needed:	Implementation/Action	Rationale
Mask	1. Check the physician's order and institutional policy regarding VAP access.	A physician's order, and institutional guidelines, are legal requirements for infusion therapy.
Sterile gown	2. Introduce yourself to the patient.	By introducing yourself, you convey courtesy, establish/promote the nurse-patient relationship, instill patient trust and, thus alleviate patient anxiety.
Sterile gloves		
VAP access kit (containing antiseptic cleansing agents and needed sterile supplies)	3. Identify the patient by checking the wrist band against the doctor's order and asking the patient, if conscious, to state his/her name.	Proper identification ensures that the procedure is being performed on the correct patient.
	4. Verify the allergy status of the patient.	This is a patient safety measure.
	5. Explain the proposed procedure, in terms the patient can understand.	The patient has the right to know what is being done and the right to refuse care. Thorough explanations reduce anxiety and promote patient compliance.
Appropriate noncoring, nonbarbed needle	6. Obtain patient consent for the procedure.	This is a legal requirement.
	7. Gather all necessary equipment.	This serves to economize time and reduce patient anxiety.
Extension set with Luer-Lok® connector	8. Carry out proper hand hygiene. Prepare the site as outlined in Skill 12-17, steps 9–22.	Good hand hygiene is the single most important means of preventing the spread of infection.

Topical anesthetic, if used

Normal saline for injection

Two 10-ml sterile syringes filled with normal saline

10-ml syringe with appropriate volume of heparin solution for locking the system

Sterile 2 × 2-inch gauze

Single Port Access

23. Administer local anesthesia, if indicated, following agency protocols.	
24. Connect the needle with extension set to the 10-ml syringe filled with NS and clear the tubing of air, taking care not to contaminate the equipment, the site, or the nurse's gloved hands.	To prevent contamination and air embolism.
25. Locate the base of the port with the nondominant hand. Triangulate the port between the thumb and the first two fingers of the nondominant hand. Approximate the center of the port and aim for the center of these three fingers (Figure 12-47).	To locate the correct position of the septum of the port.

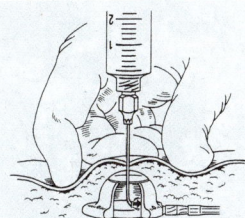

Figure 12-47 | Port access *Courtesy of BARD Access Systems*

(continues)

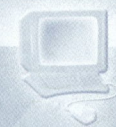

SKILL 12-18

Accessing and Deaccessing the VAP (continued)

Implementation/Action	Rationale
26. Instruct the patient to perform the Valsalva maneuver.	To prevent air embolism.
27. Insert the needle perpendicular to the port septum. Advance the needle through the skin and septum until reaching the bottom of the reservoir. Tell the patient to breathe normally.	To access the port correctly.
28. Aspirate for a blood return. Do not inject until placement is confirmed.	To verify correct needle placement.
29. Vigorously flush the line, using the push-pause, pulsatile method.	Maintains patency of the line.
30. Continue with procedure of administration of bolus injection, continuous/intermittent infusion, flushing, and heparin-locking, as indicated. Click here for a link to this skill.	

Dual Port Access

Prepare the site as outlined in Skill 12-17, steps 9–22.

Implementation/Action	Rationale
23. Administer local anesthesia, if indicated, following agency protocols.	
24. Connect the needle with extension set to the 10-ml syringe filled with NS and clear the tubing of air, taking care not to contaminate the equipment, the site, or the nurse's gloved hands.	To prevent contamination and air embolism.
25. Palpate to locate the port septum to be accessed.	To locate the correct position of the septum of the port.
i. Locate the base of the port with the nondominant hand.	
ii. Approximate the center of the dual port and place the index finger of the dominant hand to mark the spot.	
iii. Triangulate the right or left side of the dual port between the thumb and first two fingers of the dominant hand. Aim for the center point of these three fingers (Figure 12-48).	

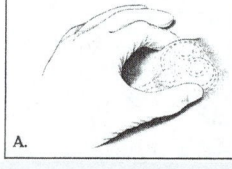
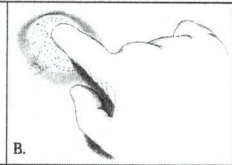
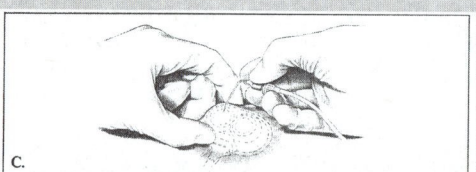

Figure 12-48 | Dual port access *Courtesy of BARD Access Systems*

Implementation/Action	Rationale
26. Instruct the patient to perform the Valsalva maneuver.	To prevent air embolism.

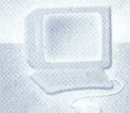

S K I L L 12-18

Accessing and Deaccessing the VAP

Implementation/Action	Rationale
27. Insert the needle perpendicular to the port septum. Advance the needle through the skin and septum until reaching the bottom of the reservoir. Tell the patient to breathe normally.	To access the port correctly.
28. Aspirate for a blood return. Do not inject until placement is confirmed.	To verify correct needle placement.
29. Vigorously flush the line, using the push-pause, pulsatile method.	To prevent buildup of residual sludge.
30. Each septum must be accessed separately and flushed with normal saline.	To access properly.
31. Continue with procedure of administration of bolus injection, continuous/intermittent infusion, flushing, and heparing-locking, as indicated.	

Deaccessing the VAP

Implementation/Action	Rationale
32. Stabilize the port with two fingers prior to withdrawal of the needle.	To prevent damage to the VAP and patient discomfort.
33. Instruct the patient to perform the Valsalva maneuver.	To prevent air embolism.
34. Slowly remove a noncoring needle while injecting the last 0.5 ml of infusate (Figure 12-49).	To maintain positive pressure in the system and reduce the potential for blood backflow into the catheter tip, which predisposes to residual sludge buildup.

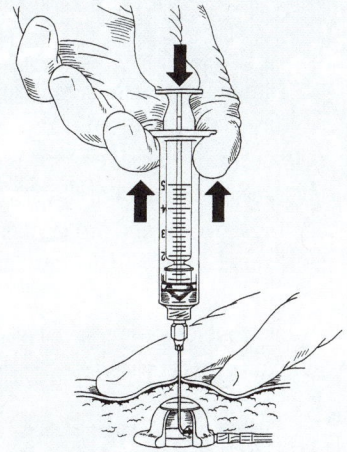

Figure 12-49 | Deaccessing a port
Courtesy of BARD Access Systems

Implementation/Action	Rationale
35. Dispose of used equipment and carry out proper hand hygiene.	To prevent the spread of microorganisms.
36. Document the procedure.	To maintain continuity of care.

Saline Lock Procedure for Port with Groshong® Tip Catheter

To help prevent clot formation and catheter blockage, a port with a Groshong® tip catheter should be filled with sterile normal saline after each use. If the port remains unused for long periods of time, the saline lock should be changed by flushing at least once every four weeks or per agency policy. The manufacturer-recommended (BARD Access Systems) volumes are as follows:

- For a port not in use, administer 5 ml of sterile normal saline.
- Following medication administration or TPN, administer 10 ml of sterile normal saline.
- After blood withdrawal, administer 20 ml of sterile normal saline.

1. Gather the following equipment:
   - 22-ga. noncoring needle
   - 10-ml syringe filled with the appropriate volume of NS
2. Explain the procedure to the patient and prepare the site aseptically.
3. Attach the syringe filled with NS to the needle or the extension set.
4. Have the patient perform the Valsalva maneuver.
5. Locate and access the port.
6. Flush the system using the push-pause pulsatile method. Stabilize the port with two fingers during needle withdrawal. Maintain positive pressure in the system by withdrawing the syringe and needle while injecting the last 0.5 ml.
7. Instruct the patient to breathe normally.

Heparin Lock Procedure for Ports with Open-Ended Catheters

To help prevent clot formation and catheter blockage, an implanted port with an open-ended catheter should be filled with sterile heparinized saline after each use. The manufacturer-recommended concentration of heparin is 100 units/ml. Other concentrations of heparinized saline (10 to 1,000 units/ml) have been found to be effective as well. The determination of the proper concentration and volume should be based on the patient's medical condition, laboratory tests, and prior experience. If the port remains unused for long periods of time, it should be heparinized at least every four weeks. The manufacturer-recommended flushing volumes are as follows:

- For a port not in use, administer 5 ml of sterile heparinized saline.
- Following medication administration or TPN administration, give 10 ml of sterile normal saline, followed by 5 ml of sterile heparinized saline.
- After blood withdrawal, administer 20 ml of sterile normal saline followed by 5 ml of sterile heparinized saline.

1. Gather the following equipment:
   - 22-ga. noncoring needle
   - 10-ml syringe filled with sterile heparinized saline (100 units/ml)
2. Explain the procedure to the patient and aseptically prepare the site. Have the patient perform the Valsalva maneuver.
3. Locate and access the port.
4. Attach a syringe filled with sterile heparinized saline to the needle.
5. Flush the system, using the push-pause pulsatile method. Stabilize the port with two fingers during needle withdrawal. Maintain positive pressure in the system by withdrawing the syringe and needle while injecting the last 0.5 ml. Tell the patient to breathe normally.

NURSING TIP

Preventing Occlusion

Proper flushing using the pulsatile, push-pause technique is one of the most important measures that can be used to prevent the buildup of sludge deposits in an implanted vascular port.

Additional procedures for working the VAPs are outlined in Skills 12-19 through 12-22.

Once a vascular access port is implanted, the most important aspect of maintaining its integrity and function is frequent assessment and proper maintenance, always following the manufacturer's guidelines and agency policy. Table 12-6 lists some of the preventive maintenance protocols and methods for troubleshooting problems associated with implanted vascular access ports.

The CathLink™ 20 Implanted Port

The CathLink™ 20 implanted port is a totally implantable vascular access device (Figure 12-50) designed to provide repeated access to the vascular system. It consists of two primary components: a titanium injection port featuring a multilayered silicone septum with a predetermined route of entry, and a radiopaque Chrono-Flex® polyurethane catheter. All materials are biocompatible and can be used with virtually all injectable solutions.

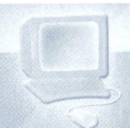

SKILL 12-19

Bolus Injection via the VAP

Equipment Needed:	Implementation/Action	Rationale
Mask	1. Check the physician's order and institutional policy regarding VAP access.	A physician's order, and institutional guidelines, are legal requirements for infusion therapy.
Sterile gown	2 Introduce yourself to the patient.	By introducting yourself, you convey courtesy, establish/promote the nurse-patient relationship, instill patient trust and, thus alleviate patient anxiety.
Sterile gloves		
VAP access kit (containing antiseptic cleansing agents and needed sterile supplies)	3. Identify the patient by checking the wrist band against the doctor's order and asking the patient, if conscious, to state his/her name.	Proper identification ensures that the procedure is being performed on the correct patient.
	4. Verify the allergy status of the patient.	This is a patient safety measure.
	5. Explain the proposed procedure, in terms the patient can understand.	The patient has the right to know what is being done and the right to refuse care. Thorough explanations reduce anxiety and promote patient compliance.
Extension set with Luer-Lok® connector	6. Gather all necessary equipment.	This serves to economize time and reduce patient anxiety.
Topical anesthetic, if used	7. Carry out proper hand hygiene.	Good hand hygiene is the single most important means of preventing the spread of infection.
Normal saline for injection	8. Provide privacy.	To maintain client dignity.
	9. Elevate the bed level.	Conducive to successful access and alleviates back strain for the physician and nurse.
Two 10-ml sterile syringes filled with normal saline (for an infusion, use one 10-ml syringe of NS and one 20-ml syringe of NS)	10. Secure all necessary supplies.	To economize time and promote efficiency.
	11. Inspect the site.	To be sure the skin is free of abnormalities.
	12. Wash insertion area with soap, rinse well with water, and pat dry.	To remove any surface debris and oils from the skin and to promote asepsis.
	13. Review the Valsalva maneuver with the patient.	To prevent air embolism.
	14. Assess vital signs and LOC and record.	To provide baseline physical and mental status.
	15. Set up the equipment in a sterile manner.	To maintain asepsis, promote efficiency, and economize time appropriately.
	16. Expose the skin and palpate for the septum.	Ensures that the needle will be placed correctly.
10-ml syringe with appropriate volume of heparin solution for locking the system	17. Don gown, mask, and sterile gloves.	Prevents the spread of infection and prevents contamination of the nurse with chemotherapeutic agents/vesicants (if that is the therapy being initiated).
	18. Instruct patient to turn her head away from the VAP site.	Prevents the introduction of microorganisms.
Sterile 2 × 2-inch gauze *(continues)*	19. Cleanse the septum site with each 70% isopropyl alcohol swab stick, starting at the intended puncture site and moving outward in a concentric circle 4 to 5 inches in diameter. Repeat for a total of three times. Allow the area to air dry.	Promotes asepsis and prevents the spread of infection.

(continues)

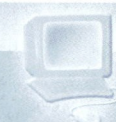

SKILL   12-19

Bolus Injection via the VAP (continued)

Equipment Needed:	Implementation/Action	Rationale
Extension set with slide clamp and Luer-Lok® connection	20. Repeat the preceding steps, using the 2% CHG or iodophor swabsticks, and allow the area to air dry after the third application.	Promotes asepsis by providing a prolonged antiseptic effect, thus preventing the spread of infection.
	21. Gently wipe off any residue of the iodophor at the needle insertion site.	To prevent tracking any of the iodophor into the tissue upon needle insertion.
One 22-ga. straight or right-angle noncoring, nonbarbed needle (for bolus injection)	22. Administer local anesthesia, if indicated, following agency protocols.	
	23. Connect the appropriate needle with extension set to the 10-ml syringe filled with NS and prime the tubing and needle to displace any air, taking care not to contaminate the equipment, the site, or the your gloved hands.	To prevent contamination and air embolism.
10-ml syringe containing ordered medication	24. Triangulate the port between the thumb and the first two fingers of the nondominant hand. Aim for the center point of these three fingers.	To locate the correct position of the septum of the port.
One 22-ga. right-angle noncoring, nonbarbed needle (for continuous infusion)	25. Instruct the patient to perform the Valsalva maneuver.	To prevent air embolism.
	26. Insert the needle perpendicular to the port septum. Advance the needle through the skin and septum until it reaches the bottom of the reservoir. Tell the patient to breathe normally.	To access the port correctly.
Paper tape	27. Aspirate for a blood return. Do not inject until placement is confirmed.	To verify correct needle placement.
	28. Vigorously flush the line, using the push-pause, pulsatile method.	To clear the line and prevent the buildup of residual sludge.
	29. Close the slide clamp on the extension tubing as the last 0.5 ml of NS is injected.	To maintain positive pressure and prevent bleed-back.
	30. Instruct the patient to perform the Valsalva maneuver.	To prevent air embolism.
	31. Disconnect the empty NS saline syringe and attach the 10-ml syringe containing the bolus medication.	To instill the medication into the line.
	32. Instruct the patient to breathe normally.	For patient comfort and compliance with the procedure.
	33. Open the slide clamp on the extension tubing.	To allow the medication to instill.
	34. Administer the drug, according to directions, while examining the injection site.	To assess for signs of extravasation.
	35. Clamp the extension set when the injection is complete.	To avoid leakage of infusate.
	36. Instruct the patient to perform the Valsalva maneuver and remove the syringe.	To prevent contamination with microorganisms.
	37. Attach the 10-ml syringe containing the NS.	To flush the line.

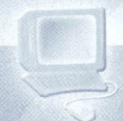

S K I L L 12-19

Bolus Injection via the VAP

Implementation/Action	Rationale
38. Instruct the patient to breathe normally and open the slide clamp on the extension tubing.	
39. Flush the line vigorously, using the pulsatile, push-pause method. Clamp the line as the last 0.5 ml is instilled.	**To maintain positive pressure in the line.**
40. Instruct the patient to perform the Valsalva maneuver and detach the empty NS syringe. If the VAP has a Groshong® tip, remove the needle at this time and do not flush with heparin.	**To prevent infection with microorganisms.**
41. Attach the 10-ml syringe containing the heparin flush.	
42. Instruct the patient to breathe normally and open the slide clamp on the extension tubing.	
43. Heparin-lock the port, closing the slide clamp as the last 0.5 ml is injected.	**To maintain positive pressure and patency of the line.**
44. Stabilize the port with two fingers, instruct the patient to perform the Valsalva maneuver, and remove the needle. Instruct the patient to breathe normally.	
45. Return the bed to the low position and raise the siderails.	**Patient safety must be maintained.**
46. Dispose of used equipment and carry out proper hand hygiene.	**To prevent the spread of microorganisms.**
47. Document the procedure.	**For patient safety and legal protection.**

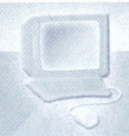

S K I L L 12-20

Continuous Infusion into the VAP

Equipment Needed:	Implementation/Action	Rationale
Mask **Sterile gown** **Sterile gloves** *(continues)*	1. Check the physician's order.	**A physician's order is a legal requirement for infusion therapy.**
	2. Introduce yourself to the patient.	**By introducting yourself, you convey courtesy, establish/promote the nurse-patient relationship, instill patient trust and, thus alleviate patient anxiety.**
	3. Identify the patient by checking the wrist band against the doctor's order and asking the patient, if conscious, to state his/her name.	**Proper identification ensures that the procedure is being performed on the correct patient.**
	4 Verify the allergy status of the patient.	**This is a patient safety measure.**

(continues)

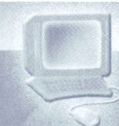

SKILL 12-20

Continuous Infusion into the VAP (continued)

Equipment Needed:	Implementation/Action	Rationale
VAP access kit (containing antiseptic cleansing agents and needed sterile supplies)	5. Explain the proposed procedure, in terms the patient can understand.	The patient has the right to know what is being done and the right to refuse care. Thorough explanations reduce anxiety and promote patient compliance.
	6. Gather all necessary equipment.	This serves to economize time and reduce patient anxiety.
	7. Carry out proper hand hygiene.	Good hand hygiene is the single most important means of preventing the spread of infection.
Extension set with Luer-Lok® connector	8. Provide privacy.	To maintain client dignity.
	9. Elevate the bed level.	Conducive to successful access and alleviates back strain for the physician and nurse.
Topical anesthetic, if used	10. Secure all necessary supplies.	To economize time and promote efficiency.
	11. Inspect the site.	To be sure the skin is free of abnormalities.
Normal saline for injection	12. Wash insertion area with soap, rinse well with water, and pat dry.	To remove any surface debris and oils from the skin and to promote asepsis.
	13. Review the Valsalva maneuver with the patient.	To prevent air embolism.
Two 10-ml sterile syringes filled with normal saline (for an infusion, use one 10-ml syringe of NS and one 20-ml syringe of NS)	14. Assess vital signs and LOC and record.	To provide baseline physical and mental status.
	15. Set up the equipment in a sterile manner.	To maintain asepsis, promote efficiency, and economize time appropriately.
	16. Expose the skin and palpate for the septum.	Ensures that the needle will be placed correctly.
	17. Don gown, mask, and sterile gloves.	Prevents the spread of infection and prevents contamination of the nurse with chemotherapeutic agents/vesicants (if that is the therapy being initiated).
Extension set with slide clamp and Luer-Lok® connection	18. Instruct the patient to turn her head away from the VAP site.	Prevents the introduction of microorganisms.
	19. Cleanse the septum site with each 70% isopropyl alcohol swab stick, starting at the intended puncture site and moving outward in a concentric circle 4 to 5 inches in diameter. Repeat for a total of three times. Allow the area to air dry.	Promotes asepsis and prevents the spread of infection.
22-ga. right-angle noncoring, nonbarbed needle	20. Repeat the preceding steps, using the 2% CHG or iodophor swab sticks, and allow the area to air dry after the third application.	Promotes asepsis by providing a prolonged antiseptic effect, thus preventing the spread of infection.
Ordered infusion attached to an infusion line that has been primed to remove air	21. Gently wipe off any residue of the iodophor at the needle insertion site.	To prevent tracking any of the iodophor into the tissue upon needle insertion.
	22. Administer local anesthesia, if indicated, following agency protocols.	

(continues)

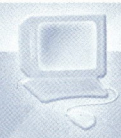

SKILL 12-20

Bolus Injection via the VAP

Implementation/Action	Rationale
23. Connect the appropriate needle with extension set to the 10-ml syringe filled with NS and prime the tubing and needle to displace any air, taking care not to contaminate the equipment, the site, or your gloved hands.	**To prevent contamination and air embolism.**
24. Triangulate the port between the thumb and the first two fingers of the nondominant hand. Aim for the center point of these three fingers.	**To locate the correct position of the septum of the port.**
25. Instruct the patient to perform the Valsalva maneuver.	**To prevent air embolism.**
26. Insert the needle perpendicular to the port septum. Advance the needle through the skin and septum until it reaches the bottom of the reservoir. Tell the patient to breathe normally.	**To access the port correctly.**
27. Aspirate for a blood return. Do not inject until placement is confirmed.	**To verify correct needle placement.**
28. Vigorously flush the line, using the push-pause, pulsatile method.	**To clear the line and prevent the buildup of residual sludge.**
29. Close the slide clamp on the extension tubing as the last 0.5 ml of NS is injected.	**To maintain positive pressure and prevent bleed-back.**
30. Place the 2 × 2-inch gauze (rolled up or folded in 4s) under the needle hub. Secure the needle and dressing in place with the transparent dressing.	**To prevent dislodgement of the needle from the VAP.**
31. Open the slide clamp and vigorously flush the line using the pulsatile, push-pause method.	**To maintain patency of the line.**
32. Clamp the line, have the patient perform the Valsalva maneuver, and disconnect the syringe.	**To prevent entry of microorganisms.**
33. Connect the fluid delivery system. Tell the patient to breathe normally.	**To allow infusion to run into the line.**
34. If an electronic infusion device is used, turn it on, open the slide clamp, and initiate the infusion.	**To begin the infusion and be sure it is run properly.**
35. Examine the site for signs of extravasation and initiate the appropriate interventions if needed.	**To maintain safety and skin integrity to the patient.**
36. Tape all tubing connections with the paper tape.	**To secure them in place while the infusion is running.**
37. When the infusion is complete, turn off the electronic infusion device (EID), clamp the extension set, have the patient perform the Valsalva maneuver, and disconnect the IV line from the extension tubing of the needle.	**To prevent contamination with microorganisms as the infusion is discontinued.**

(continues)

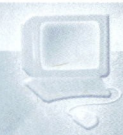

S K I L L 12-20

Continuous Infusion into the VAP (continued)

Implementation/Action	Rationale
38. Connect the 20-ml syringe containing the NS, have the patient breathe normally, open the slide clamp and flush vigorously, as before.	To maintain patency of the line.
39. Heparin-lock the port (unless it has a Groshong® tip), closing the slide clamp as the last 0.5 ml is injected.	To maintain positive pressure in the line.
40. Stabilize the port with two fingers, instruct the patient to perform the Valsalva maneuver, and remove the needle. Instruct the patient to breathe normally.	To prevent entry of microorganisms as the ine is deaccessed.
41. Return the bed to the low position and raise the siderails.	Patient safety must be maintained.
42. Dispose of used equipment and carry out proper hand hygiene.	To prevent the spread of microorganisms.
43. Document the procedure.	For patient protection and legal protection.

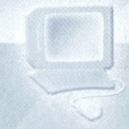

S K I L L 12-21

Blood Sampling from the VAP

Equipment Needed:	Implementation/Action	Rationale
Mask	1. Check the physician's order.	A physician's order, and institutional guidelines, are legal requirements for infusion therapy.
Sterile gown	2. Check the orders for lab work.	Different lab tests require different types of collection tubes.
Sterile gloves	3. Introduce yourself to the patient.	By introducing yourself, you convey courtesy, establish/promote the nurse-patient relationship, instill patient trust and, thus alleviate patient anxiety.
VAP access kit (containing antiseptic cleansing agents and needed sterile supplies)	4. Identify the patient by checking the wrist band against the doctor's order and asking the patient, if conscious, to state his/her name.	Proper identification ensures that the procedure is being performed on the correct patient.
	5. Verify the allergy status of the patient.	This is a patient safety measure.
Appropriate noncoring, nonbarbed needle	6. Explain the proposed procedure, in terms the patient can understand.	The patient has the right to know what is being done and the right to refuse care. Thorough explanations reduce anxiety and promote patient compliance.
(continues)	7. Gather all necessary equipment. Have all necessary heparin and saline drawn up prior to beginning the procedure.	This serves to economize time, reduce patient anxiety, and prevents interruptions during procedure.

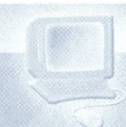

SKILL 12-21

Blood Sampling from the VAP

Equipment Needed:	Implementation/Action	Rationale
Extension set with Luer-Lok® connector	8. Carry out proper hand hygiene.	Good hand hygiene is the single most important means of preventing the spread of infection.
Topical anesthetic, if used	9. Provide for privacy.	Maintains patient dignity.
2-way stopcock or extension set	10. Set up equipment.	Allows for the procedure to be completed in an efficient manner.
19-ga. noncoring, nonbarbed needle	11. Put on gloves.	Prevents the spread of infection.
	12. Aseptically prepare the injection site (following the procedure for Accessing/Deaccessing a VAP).	To prevent the introduction of microorganisms.
10-ml syringe filled with 5 ml sterile normal saline	13. Flush the extension tubing, stopcock, and needle, maintaining sterility.	To prevent air from entering the VAP.
	14. Insert the needle, aspirate for a blood return, and vigorously flush the port with 5 ml of NS.	To ensure proper placement of the needle.
20-ml empty sterile syringe	15. Withdraw at least 5 ml of blood and discard the syringe into the sharps container.	So the blood will be unaltered.
20-ml syringe filled with sterile NS	16. Aspirate the desired blood volume into the 20-ml syringe and transfer it to the appropriate blood sample tube (or use a Vacutainer® per the manufacturer's protocols).	To obtain the required specimen.
1-ml syringe filled with appropriate volume of heparin flush solution (for open-ended catheters)	17. Flush the system vigorously with 20 ml of sterile NS, using the push-pause, pulsatile method.	To clear the line and eliminate a site for microbial growth.
	18. Heparin-lock the system (for ports with open-ended catheters).	To maintain patency and positive pressure in the line.
	19. Label the blood tubes and deliver the sample to the laboratory as soon as the blood draw is complete and integrity of the VAP is ensured.	The blood will be delivered in a timely manner so that results can be obtained as soon as possible.
	20. Dispose of used equipment and carry out proper hand hygiene.	To prevent the spread of microorganisms.
	21. Document the procedure.	To maintain continuity of care.

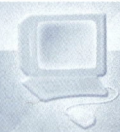

SKILL 12-22

Clearing a Blocked VAP

Equipment Needed:	Implementation/Action	Rationale
Mask	1. Check the physician's order.	A physician's order, and institutional guidelines, are legal requirements for infusion therapy.
Sterile gown	2. Introduce yourself to the patient.	By introducing yourself, you convey courtesy, establish/promote the nurse-patient relationship, instill patient trust and, thus alleviate patient anxiety.
Sterile gloves	3. Identify the patient by checking the wrist band against the doctor's order and asking the patient, if conscious, to state his/her name.	Proper identification ensures that the procedure is being performed on the correct patient.
VAP access kit (containing antiseptic cleansing agents and needed sterile supplies)	4. Verify the allergy status of the patient.	This is a patient safety measure.
	5. Explain the proposed procedure, in terms the patient can understand.	The patient has the right to know what is being done and the right to refuse care. Thorough explanations reduce anxiety and promote patient compliance.
Topical anesthetic, if used	6. Gather all necessary equipment.	This serves to economize time and reduce patient anxiety.
Appropriate noncoring, nonbarbed needle (usually a 22-ga.)	7. Carry out proper hand hygiene.	Good hand hygiene is the single most important means of preventing the spread of infection.
Extension set with Luer-Lok® connector and slide clamp	8. Access the port.	
	9. Using the 35-ml syringe, gently instill the declotting agent. Use a gentle pull-push action on the syringe to maximize mixing of the solution within the port and catheter.	To loosen blockage.
35-ml sterile syringe filled with appropriate declotting agent	10. Leave the declotting agent in place for 15 minutes.	To dissolve the blockage.
	11. Attempt to aspirate the declotting solution and the clot.	To remove the blockage.
10-ml syringe filled with sterile NS	12. Once the blockage has been cleared, vigorously flush the catheter with at least 10 ml of NS, using the pulsatile, push-pause method.	To clear declotting solution from line and maintain patency of line.
10-ml syringe filled with heparin-lock solution	13. Heparin-lock the port (for open-ended catheters).	Maintains positive pressure in the line.

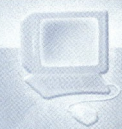

S K I L L   12-22

Clearing a Blocked VAP

Equipment Needed:

Mask

Sterile gown

Sterile gloves

VAP access kit (containing antiseptic cleansing agents and needed sterile supplies)

Topical anesthetic, if used

20-ml sterile syringe containing the appropriate declotting agent

Empty, sterile 20-ml syringe

Two 22-ga. noncoring, nonbarbed needles

Two Luer-Lok® extension sets with slide clamps

Alternate (Two-Needle) Declotting Method

An alternate method of declotting a VAP involves the use of two noncoring access needles. This method is especially useful when the blockage is in the port itself. It can be done by one nurse, but is more easily accomplished when done by two (with one maneuvering the syringe containing the declotting agent and the other pulling back on the empty syringe).

Implementation/Action	Rationale
1. Check the physician's order.	A physician's order, and institutional guidelines, are legal requirements for infusion therapy.
2. Introduce yourself to the patient.	By introducing yourself, you convey courtesy, establish/promote the nurse-patient relationship, instill patient trust and, thus alleviate patient anxiety.
3. Identify the patient by checking the wrist band against the doctor's order and asking the patient, if conscious, to state his/her name.	Proper identification ensures that the procedure is being performed on the correct patient.
4. Verify the allergy status of the patient.	This is a patient safety measure.
5. Explain the proposed procedure, in terms the patient can understand.	The patient has the right to know what is being done and the right to refuse care. Thorough explanations reduce anxiety and promote patient compliance.
6. Carry out proper hand hygiene.	Good hand hygiene is the single most important means of preventing the spread of infection.
7. Connect the extension sets to each needle and syringe. Purge the air from the extension set and needle connected to the syringe containing the declotting agent.	To prevent air from entering the VAP.
8. Access the port with both needles.	
9. Using the empty syringe, try the POP method to dislodge the clot. If this doesn't work, proceed to the next step.	To attempt to remove the clot.
10. Gently instill a small volume of the declotting agent into the port, then pull back on the plunger of the empty syringe. Continue to gently push and pull until all the declotting agent has been instilled.	To attempt to loosen the clot.

(continues)

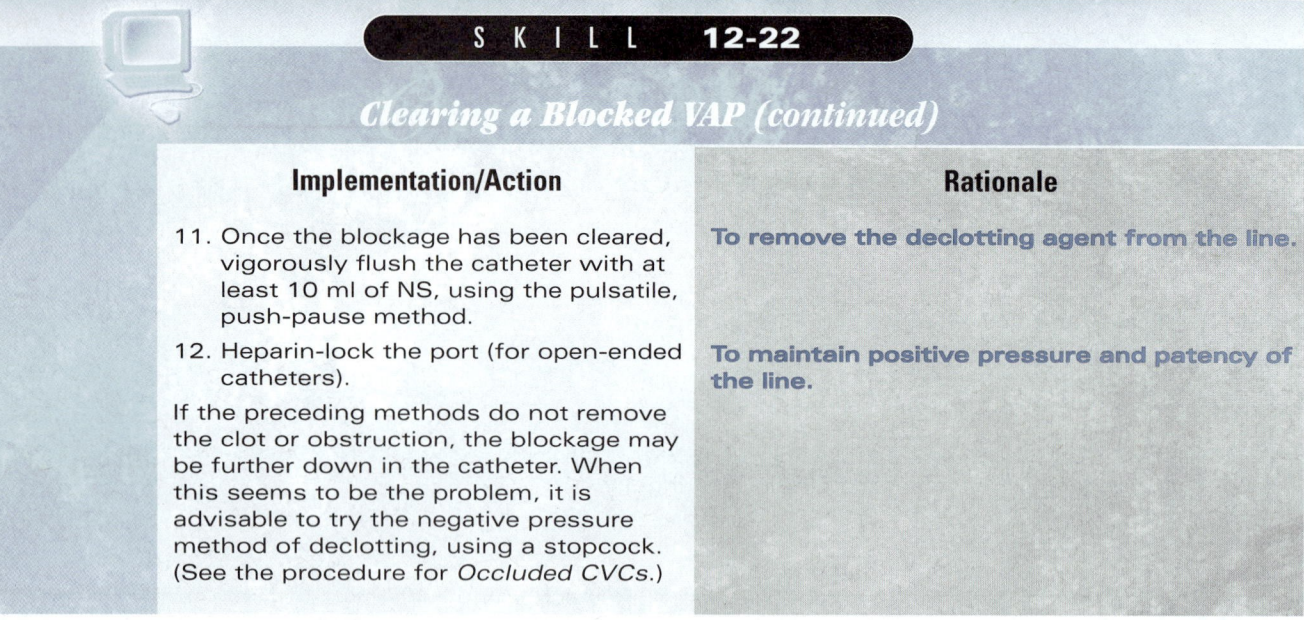

SKILL 12-22

Clearing a Blocked VAP (continued)

Implementation/Action	Rationale
11. Once the blockage has been cleared, vigorously flush the catheter with at least 10 ml of NS, using the pulsatile, push-pause method.	To remove the declotting agent from the line.
12. Heparin-lock the port (for open-ended catheters).	To maintain positive pressure and patency of the line.
If the preceding methods do not remove the clot or obstruction, the blockage may be further down in the catheter. When this seems to be the problem, it is advisable to try the negative pressure method of declotting, using a stopcock. (See the procedure for *Occluded CVCs*.)	

Table 12-6 | Implanted Ports: Preventive Maintenance Protocols and Troubleshooting Problems

Problem	Possible Cause	Nursing Intervention
Erythema	Infected incision or port pocket, poor healing postoperatively	Assess daily for redness/drainage. Notify physician. Antibiotic per physician's order.
Inability to flush or withdraw from system	Kinked IV tubing	Check tubing.
	Pump malfunction	Check equipment.
	Catheter lodged against the vein wall	Reposition patient by moving upper torso and arms.
	Incorrect needle placement	Reposition needle and advance tip to the bottom of the reservoir. Verify correct positioning by blood aspiration.
	Fibrin sheath formation	Flush with 3 ml of sterile normal saline and repeat if necessary. Increase frequency of flushing as prevention. use a fibrinolytic agent such as urokinase per physician's order.
	Occlusion (clots)	Use a fibrinolytic agent such as urokinase per physician's order.
	Catheter "pinch-off" (clavicle-first rib compression) catheter malposition, catheter kinked in the body, port rotation	Notify physician to evaluate patient for catheter or port replacement.
Burning sensation in subcutaneous tissue	Dislodgement of needle into subcutaneous tissue	Do not remove needle. Stop infusion and immediately notify a physician.
Swollen neck and/or arm	Large clot formation in superior vena cava	Notify a physician immediately

Reprinted with permission of BARD Access Systems

The CathLink™ 20 port is connected to an open-ended catheter. Access is performed by percutaneous insertion of a 20-ga. over-the-needle IV catheter (ONC), with a minimum length of 1¾ in. The funnel-shaped entrance to the port guides the ONC into the angled access pathway to the needle stop. The design is such that the needle cannot pass beyond the needle stop area. The flexible catheter tip, however, passes further through the access pathway. The layered septum seals around the flexible catheter tip once it has been advanced and the needle has been removed. Noncoring needles should not be used with this type of port.

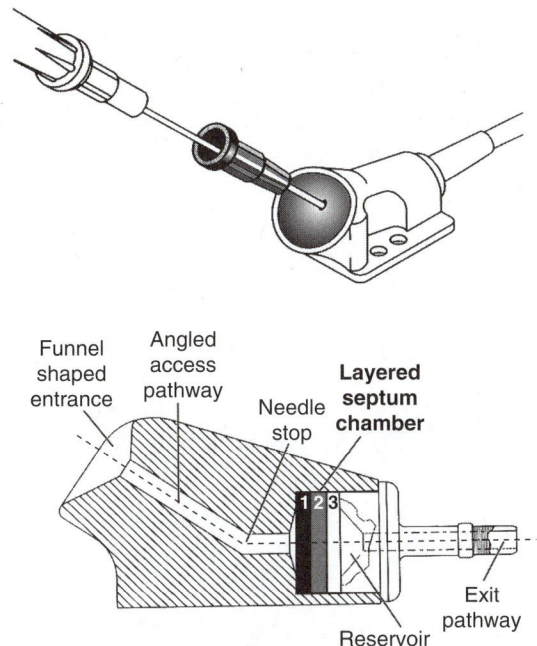

Figure 12-50 | The CathLink™ 20 vascular access port *Courtesy of BARD Access Systems*

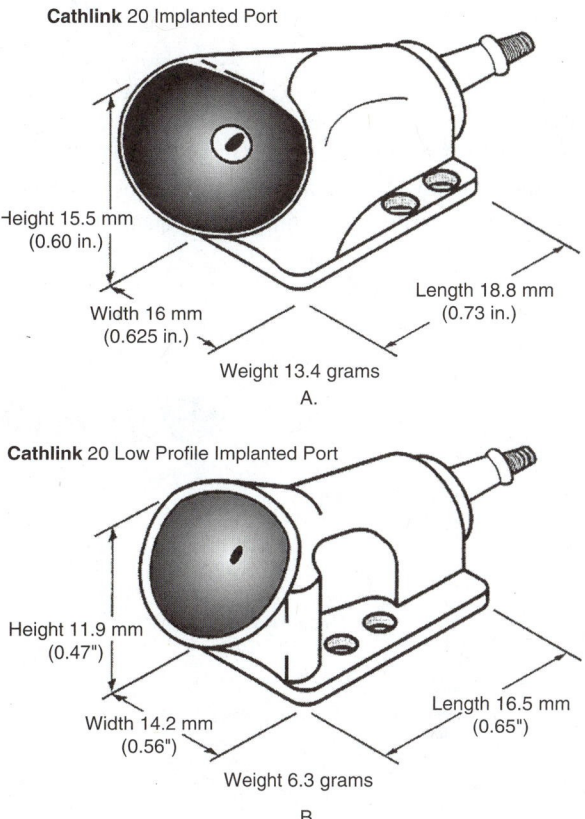

Figure 12-51 | CathLink™ 20 standard and low-profile ports *Courtesy of BARD Access Systems*

The CathLink™ 20 is available with standard and low-profile ports (Figure 12-51). The standard profile has an increased target area and larger base size that is ideal for chest placement. Its priming volume is 0.04 ml for the port and 1.2 ml for the catheter. (Catheter priming volumes are calculated at full catheter lengths [60 cm].) The smaller low-profile model is ideal for upper arm placement or for chest placement. Its priming volume is 0.02 ml for the port and 0.8 ml for the catheter.

Indications and Contraindications

The CathLink™ 20 implanted port is indicated for patient therapy requiring repeated access to the vascular system. It is used to deliver intravenous fluids, medications, and parenteral nutrition products. It is also used to draw blood samples and administer blood and blood products.

The CathLink™ 20 is contraindicated for patient therapy whenever the following is true:

- The presence of infection, bacteremia, or septicemia is known or suspected
- The patient's body size is insufficient to accommodate the size of the implanted port or catheter
- The patient is known or suspected to be allergic to the materials contained in the device or has exhibited prior intolerance to implanted devices
- Local tissue factors prevent proper device stabilization and/or access

- Previous episodes of venous thrombosis occurred at the prospective placement site
- Severe chronic obstructive lung disease interferes with percutaneous subclavian placement

Insertion and Placement of the CathLink™ 20

The tip of the CathLink™ 20 is the same as for any vascular access port: in the superior vena cava above the junction of the SVC and the right atrium. Catheter insertion is via percutaneous insertion into the subclavian vein (as described previously) with port placement in the infraclavicular fossa or via the brachial or basilic vein with port implantation in the upper arm.

Use and Maintenance of the CathLink™ 20

With the exception of the method of access, the general parameters of care associated with site asepsis (prior to access), the administration of infusates, blood sampling, flushing, locking, and declotting are the same as those described for standard implanted vascular access ports. The nurse is expected to follow the manufacturer's (BARD Access Systems) guidelines when using the CathLink™ 20.

Skill 12-23 outlines the steps used to access the Cath-Link™ 20.

Preventive Maintenance and Troubleshooting Problems for the CathLink™ 20 Implanted Port

Once the CathLink™ 20 is implanted, it is the responsibility of the nurse to maintain its integrity. Frequent assessment and adherence to maintenance protocols, following the manufacturer's guidelines and agency policy, are extremely important. For information about problems that may be associated with the device and how to prevent them or intervene, the nurse must follow BARD Access Systems' troubleshooting guide.

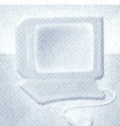

SKILL 12-23

Accessing and Deaccessing the CathLink™ 20 Implanted Port

Equipment Needed:	Implementation/Action	Rationale
Site antisepsis supplies	1. Check the physician's order.	A physician's order, and institutional guidelines, are legal requirements for infusion therapy.
Sterile gloves	2. Introduce yourself to the patient.	By introducting yourself, you convey courtesy, establish/promote the nurse-patient relationship, instill patient trust and, thus alleviate patient anxiety.
20-ga. ONC, with a minimum length of 1 3/4 in.	3. Identify the patient by checking the wrist band against the doctor's order and asking the patient, if conscious, to state his/her name.	Proper identification ensures that the procedure is being performed on the correct patient.
Two 10-ml syringes filled with sterile NS	4. Verify the allergy status of the patient. Assess for allergies, especially to iodine.	This is a patient safety measure. Decreases the risk of sensitivity reaction and maintains patient safety.
Extension set with clamp	5. Explain the proposed procedure, in terms the patient can understand.	The patient has the right to know what is being done and the right to refuse care. Thorough explanations reduce anxiety and promote patient compliance.
Supplies for infusion	6. Gather all necessary equipment.	This serves to economize time and reduce patient anxiety.
Heparin flush solution in 10-ml syringe	7. Carry out proper hand hygiene.	Good hand hygiene is the single most important means of preventing the spread of infection.
	8. Provide privacy.	To maintain client dignity.
	9. Elevate the bed level.	Conducive to successful access and alleviates back strain for the physician and nurse.
	10. Secure all necessary supplies.	To economize time and promote efficiency.
	11. Inspect the site.	To be sure the skin is free of abnormalities.
	12. Wash the insertion area with soap, rinse well with water, and pat dry.	To remove any surface debris and oils from the skin and to promote asepsis.
	13. Review the Valsalva maneuver with the patient.	To prevent air embolism.
	14. Assess vital signs and LOC and record.	To provide baseline physical and mental status.
	15. Set up the equipment in a sterile manner.	To maintain asepsis, promote efficiency, and economize time appropriately.

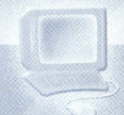

SKILL 12-23

Accessing and Deaccessing the CathLink™20 Implanted Port

Implementation/Action	Rationale
16. Cleanse the septum site with each 70% isopropyl alcohol swab stick, starting at the intended puncture site and moving outward in a concentric circle 4 to 5 inches in diameter. Repeat for a total of three times. Allow the area to air dry.	**Promotes asepsis and prevents the spread of infection.**
17. Repeat the preceding steps, using the 2% CHG or iodophor swab sticks, and allow the area to air dry after the third application.	**Promotes asepsis by providing a prolonged antiseptic effect, thus preventing the spread of infection.**
18. Attach a 10-ml syringe filled with sterile NS to the extension set. Expel air and close the clamp.	**To purge the line of air and prevent air embolism.**
19. Using a sterile gloved hand, locate the CathLink™ 20 implanted port and identify the funnel-shaped entrance by palpation.	
20. Stabilize the port by "holding" it between the thumb and forefinger of the nondominant hand (Figure 12-52).	**To stabilize the port and enhance access.**

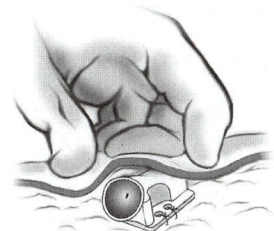

Figure 12-52 | Locating the CathLink™ 20 port *Courtesy of BARD Access Systems*

21. Aim for the funnel-shaped entrance (between two fingers) and insert the ONC into the port's funnel-shaped entrance until resistance is felt.	**To ensure proper access of the port.**
22. Ask the patient to perform the Valsalva maneuver.	**To prevent air embolism.**
23. Using the thumb and forefinger of the dominant hand, advance the ONC completely into the port by grasping and advancing the catheter hub only, while simultaneously withdrawing the needle (Figure 12-53). (This can also be accomplished by advancing the ONC with one hand and withdrawing the needle with the other.) The IV catheter should be advanced a minimum of 1 cm.	**To ensure adequate passage through the septum.**

(continues)

S K I L L   **12-23**

Accessing and Deaccessing the CathLink™20 Implanted Port (continued)

Implementation/Action	Rationale

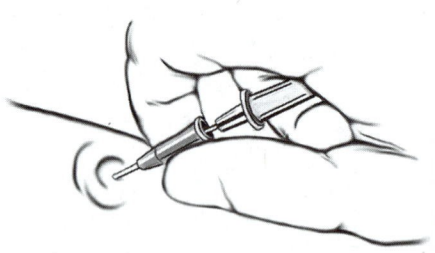

Figure 12-53 | Accessing the CathLink™ 20 port *Courtesy of BARD Access Systems*

24. Place a gloved finger over the IV catheter hub until a secondary device can be attached.

To prevent air entry.

25 Immediately attach the syringe or extension set to the ONC and tell the patient to breathe normally.

26. Dispose of the needle/stylet in the sharps container.

To prevent needlestick injury.

27. Aspirate for a blood return.

To verify placement of the cannula in the line.

28. Flush with NS.

To clear the heparin from line.

29. Proceed with the infusion protocol.

30. Following injection of medication/ infusion, the port is to be flushed with normal saline.

To clear the line of medication/infusate.

31. Heparin-lock the port.

To prevent the line from clotting.

32. To deaccess the port, stabilize the CathLink™ 20 with two fingers (Figure 12-54).

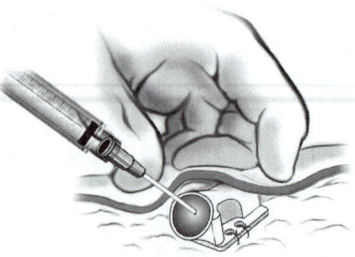

Figure 12-54 | Deaccessing the CathLink™ 20 port *Courtesy of BARD Access Systems*

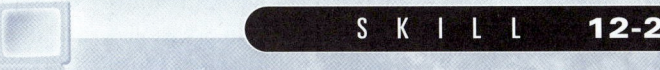

SKILL 12-23

Accessing and Deaccessing the CathLink™20 Implanted Port

Implementation/Action	Rationale
33. Remove the ONC slowly while injecting the last 0.5 ml of infusate.	To maintain positive pressure in the system and reduce the potential for blood backflow into the catheter tip, which predisposes to residual sludge buildup.
34. Return the bed to the low position and raise the siderails.	To ensure patient safety.
35. Dispose of used equipment and carry out proper hand hygiene.	To prevent the spread of microorganisms.
36. Document the procedure.	To maintain continuity of care.

HEMODYNAMIC MONITORING

The nurse is often involved in the assessment of a patient's cardiac functioning, using various techniques of hemodynamic monitoring. Hemodynamic testing is performed using various types of centrally inserted central venous catheters. Thermodilution catheters, in which temperature changes are recorded in the cardiopulmonary circulation, are often a component of such testing and are used to assess cardiac output.

Central Venous Pressure Monitoring

The central venous pressure (CVP) is the force of venous blood return within the junction of the superior vena cava and right atrium. It is an important indicator of a person's circulatory and fluid status since right atrial pressure is controlled by the heart's proficiency in pumping blood out of the right atrium and the competence with which peripheral blood flows back to the heart. Normal right atrial pressure is about equal to atmospheric pressure, or 0 to 4 mm Hg under normal circumstances. A normal CVP range when the CVC tip resides in the superior vena cava 3 to 4 cm above the right atrial-SVC junction is 2 to 8 mm Hg or 3 to 11 cm H_2O. The normal range varies among people, with actual pressures reflecting individual circulatory volume adequacy. Adequate circulatory volume depends on individual blood volume, myocardial status, and vascular tone.

The CVP can be estimated by observing the cervical neck veins or dorsal venous network of the hands when they are level with the heart. If they appear full, the pressure is normal. If they are flat (or collapsed), the pressure is low, indicative of diminished right ventricular function or the need for fluid replacement. If they are distended or engorged, the pressure is abnormally high, indicating the presence of circulatory overload.

In situations of cardiorespiratory compromise or following cardiovascular or thoracic surgery, CVP readings are done routinely. A transducer (which converts pressure to an electrical impulse) or a water-filled manometer is attached to a regular central venous catheter to obtain routine right atrial pressures. If a special thermodilution multilumen CVC is used, which is passed into the pulmonary circulation, the proximal lumen (which resides in the right atrium) is used for CVP readings.

The most accurate CVP readings (within 1 mm Hg of actual right atrial pressure) are obtained when the CVC tip is positioned 3 to 4 cm superior to the right atrial superior vena caval junction and the patient is in a supine position. If the patient cannot tolerate lying flat, the position that he is able to assume must be used for all CVP readings to ensure accuracy and consistency. In addition, if a water manometer is used, the zero marking must always be at the level of the right atrium (midaxillary region at the fourth intercostal space). The patient must also be quiet and in the same respiratory-cycle phase (inspiration, expiration, or the period between) when readings are taken. A patient on a positive-pressure ventilator usually has an elevated CVP (3- to 4-cm increase).

Pulmonary Artery Monitoring

Pulmonary artery monitoring is used to directly measure right intracardiac ventricular function and pulmonary circulation. Left ventricular filling pressure is indirectly evaluated when the pulmonary artery and pulmonary artery wedge pressures are measured. This is a vital assessment tool in diagnosing cardiac output, vascular tone, and circulatory status. CVP readings cannot measure left ventricular function or record left heart pressure gradients or cardiac output.

A pulmonary artery catheter is a flow-directed, balloon-tipped catheter (2 to 5 lumens), with a transducer that transmits a wavelike image to an oscilloscope screen. The catheter is inserted by a physician, using the same type of maneuver associated with CVC placement. The catheter is threaded into the right atrium (placement is gauged by an indicative waveform shown on the oscilloscope), at which time the balloon is inflated to float the catheter with the blood flow and into the right ventricle, through the pulmonary valve, and on to the pulmonary artery. Blood flow carries the catheter tip into the pulmonary artery and one of its smaller branches. The vessel eventually narrows to a point where the balloon becomes wedged. When the balloon is inflated and, therefore, wedged, it records the pulmonary capillary wedge pressure (PCWP), which reflects left atrial and left ventricular pressures. When the balloon is deflated and is floating freely in the pulmonary artery, it records pulmonary artery diastolic (PADP) and systolic (PASP) pressures. PADP reflects left ventricular pressures, specifically end-diastolic pressures, and PASP reflects right ventricular function and the force of pulmonary circulation.

NURSING TIP

Changing Catheters

The American Association of Critical-Care Nurses recommends changing pulmonary artery catheters and introducers at least every five days. It also advises that flush solutions, infusion tubing, stopcocks, and disposable transducers be changed every 72 hours (Moore, 1999).

A typical five-lumen pulmonary artery catheter (Figure 12-55) consists of a catheter stem, the tip of which is encased in a clear plastic cylinder for visualization of the balloon during pre-insertion testing. The five color-coded pigtails (usually labeled) are as follows:

1. A balloon-inflation lumen (with the inflation capacity imprinted on the pigtail) that exits in one of the pulmonary artery branches and, if it does not terminate in a "dead-end" lumen, may be used for blood sampling
2. A proximal lumen that exits in the right atrium and is used for CVP measurements
3. A lumen that exits in the superior vena cava and is used for the administration of infusates

4. A distal lumen that exits in the pulmonary artery and attaches to a pressure transducer for PAP measurements and PCWP measurements (during balloon inflation)
5. A lumen with a connector for thermoregulation electrodes used for cardiac output monitoring

ADVANCED MEDICATION DELIVERY SYSTEMS

The following nonvenous, intravascular access sites that are briefly discussed here are presented to give the nurse an overview of their indications and uses. Although they are not classified, per se, as peripheral or central intravenous delivery routes, the outcome of therapy is the same: to parenterally administer, for local, regional, or systemic delivery, the prescribed fluid or medication for therapeutic, prophylactic, or palliative reasons, in a safe manner that will meet the individual needs of each patient. For the most part, these techniques are used in medical-nursing specialty areas within the acute care setting, hospices, or in home health nursing in the community. Any nurse who is employed in these areas is professionally responsible for fully understanding all aspects of their use and administration, in accord with state licensure mandates and the policies and procedures of his employer.

Epidural and Intrathecal Administration

Epidural and intrathecal routes are accessed only by physicians (usually anesthesiologists) and, in some areas, by nurse anesthetists. Administration of medications by RNs must be in accordance with the state Nurse Practice Act. These routes are utilized when local concentrations of medication need to be delivered and absorbed directly to the tissues and vessels of the central nervous system. Such delivery cannot always be achieved with other routes because the blood-brain barrier, which selectively limits the passage of substances from the blood to the brain tissue, prevents the medication from reaching the CNS in adequate amounts, thus altering the needed dosage. Another advantage is that, when large concentrations of medication are required, the systemic side effects are minimized because there is direct delivery to the CNS. Pain control, using these routes, provides a better quality of analgesia, producing longer periods of relief between doses, while alleviating many of the side effects associated with pain medications, such as respiratory depression, drowsiness, depressed mental functioning, or nausea and vomiting. Because the drugs do not have to circulate through the liver, where they would normally be metabolized, smaller doses are needed for the alleviation of pain.

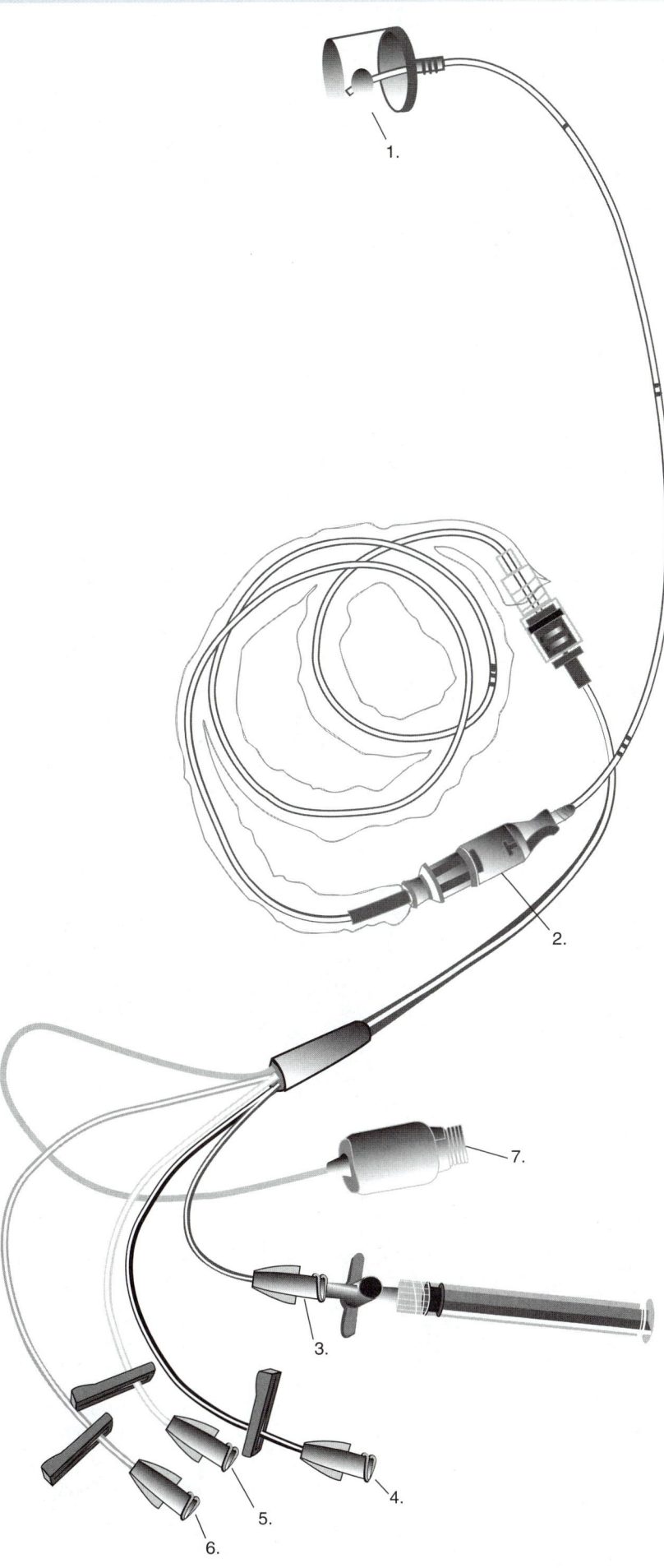

Figure 12-55 | Five-lumen pulmonary artery thermodilution catheter: (1) catheter stem with tip encased in clear plastic cylinder for visualization during balloon-tip inflation testing; (2) locking hub on distal end of the Cath-Gard™ to prevent catheter movement after it is locked to the catheter hub; (3) balloon-inflation and blood-sampling lumen; (4) proximal lumen for CVP measurements; (5) infusion lumen for fluid administration; (6) distal lumen for PAP and PCWP measurements; (7) connector lumen for electrodes used for cardiac-monitoring modalities *Courtesy of ARROW* ® *International, Inc.*

Epidural administration consists of injecting medication between two vertebral spines (usually L 2 and 3, L 3 and 4, or L 4 and 5) directly into the extradural space, the area outside and surrounding the dura mater of the brain and spinal cord (Figure 12-56). For lumbar puncture, a rigid spinal needle encased by a flexible intravascular catheter is inserted. Once in place, the needle is withdrawn and an intermittent infusion plug is attached to the hub of the catheter. The external portion of the catheter is usually taped to the back, directly over the spine. When needed for periods of more than a week, the catheter may be tunneled under the skin and exited in a more comfortable location for easier access, such as the shoulder area or abdomen. It can be used for intermittent medication or connected to an ambulatory infusion pump. Sometimes an epidural port is implanted subcutaneously, leaving the patient independent of external devices and less prone to the risk of infection, especially when long-term use is anticipated. An implantable port can be accessed intermittently using a special needle, it can be connected to an ambulatory infusion pump, or it may be connected to a subcutaneously implanted pump (Figure 12-57).

The epidural route is frequently used for regional anesthesia during childbirth or for surgical procedures when general anesthesia is contraindicated. Epidural delivery is the route of choice in treating acute CNS infections. It is usually employed for analgesia of the severe, unrelenting pain associated with degenerative joint disease (DJD), terminal cancer, or spinal trauma. Medications delivered by this route diffuse from the epidural space through the dura mater into the CSF in the intrathecal space. A single dose of morphine administered epidurally can relieve pain within 15 to 45 minutes, with analgesia lasting up to 24 hours (Table 12-7). This occurs because the medication is delivered to the

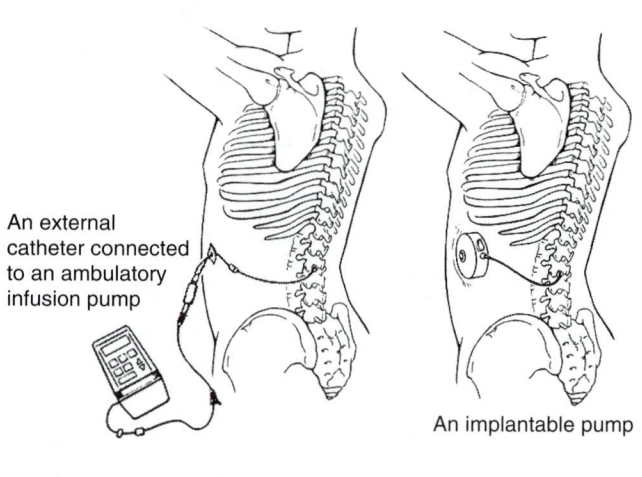

An external catheter connected to an ambulatory infusion pump

An implantable pump

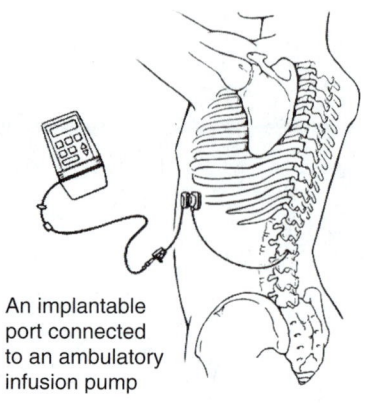

An implantable port connected to an ambulatory infusion pump

Figure 12-57 | Methods of epidural administration

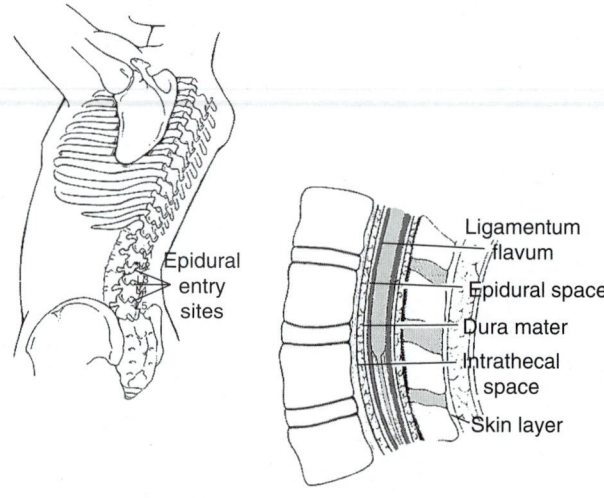

Epidural entry sites

Ligamentum flavum

Epidural space

Dura mater

Intrathecal space

Skin layer

Figure 12-56 | Epidural administration route

Table 12-7 | Comparison of Morphine HCl: Route versus Dosage for Analgesia

Route	Dose
Oral	10–30 mg q4h
Rectal	10–20 mg q4h
Intramuscular; Subcutaneous	5–20 mg/70 kg q4h
IV push	2.5–15 mg (in 4–5 ml water)/70 kg q4h
Continuous IV infusion	0.1–1.0 mg/ml in D5W by controlled-infusion pump
Epidural injection	5 mg/day and 1–2 mg additional mg not to exceed 10 mg/day
Continuous epidural infusion	2–4 mg/day and additional 1–2 mg if needed
Intrathecal	0.2–1 mg as a single daily injection

NURSING ALERT

Medication Delivered via Epidural

"Medication infused via an epidural device must be preservative-free. Alcohol is contraindicated for site preparation, cleansing the catheter hub, or dressing changes due to its potential deleterious effect as a neurotoxin" (INS, 2000, Standarrd 67, S62)

CSF and binds with opiate receptors in the spinal cord to impede the patient's sensation of pain. For home use, the catheter may be attached to a preprogrammed infusion pump containing a medication cassette that requires replacing on a weekly basis.

Intrathecal administration refers to the delivery of medication (antibiotics, antineoplastics, analgesics, and anesthetics) directly into the cerebrospinal fluid (Figure 12-58). This avenue of administration is also referred to as the intraspinal, subdural, or subarachnoid route. The CSF is usually accessed epidurally or via a ventricular reservoir, with the tip of the catheter residing in the intrathecal sac. It can be attached to an implanted port or tunneled to the exterior of the

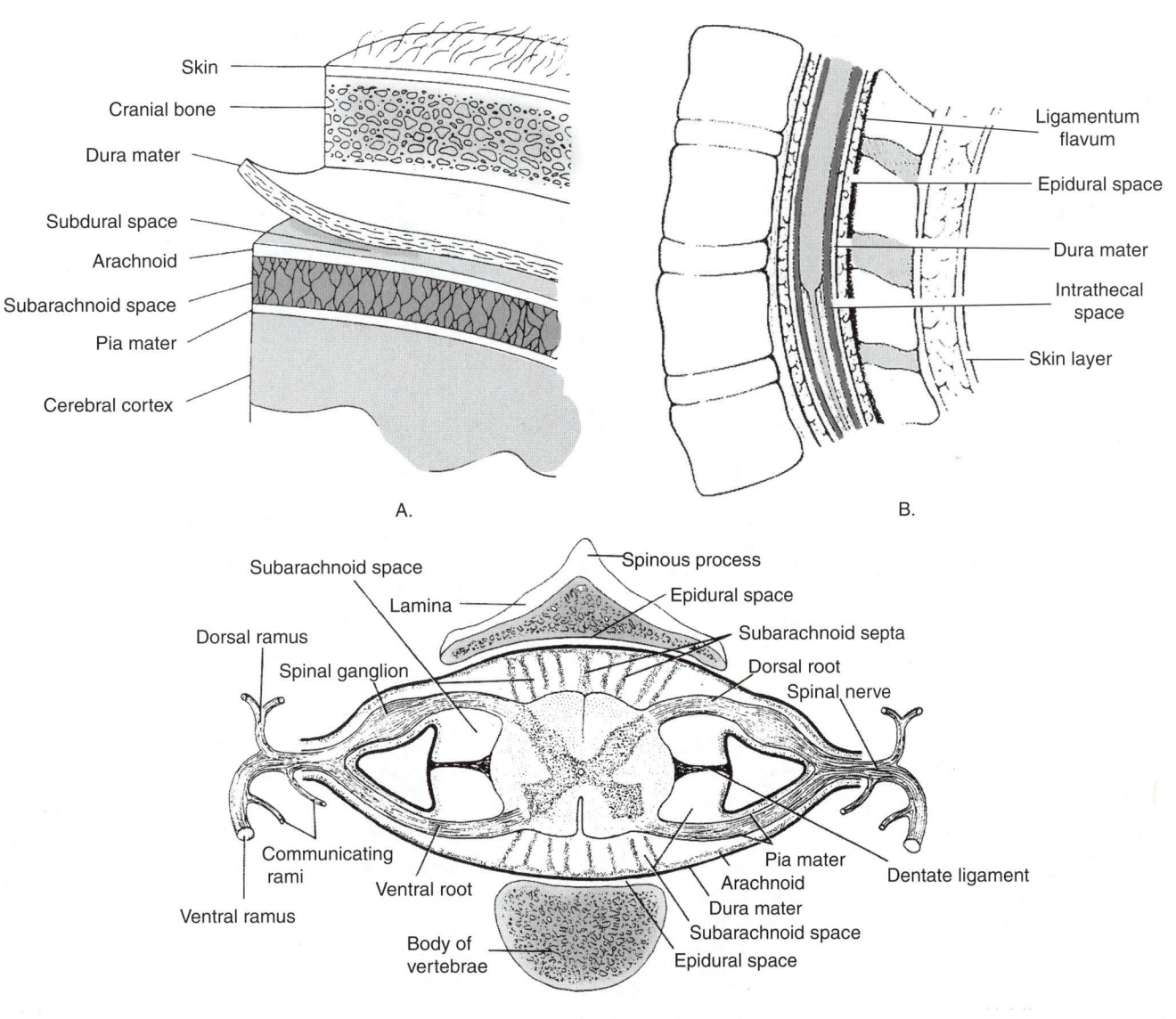

Figure 12-58 | Epidural, subdural, and subarachnoid spaces. (A) cross-section of the cranium; (B) Lateral view of the spinal cavity; (C) cross-section of vertebra and spinal cord

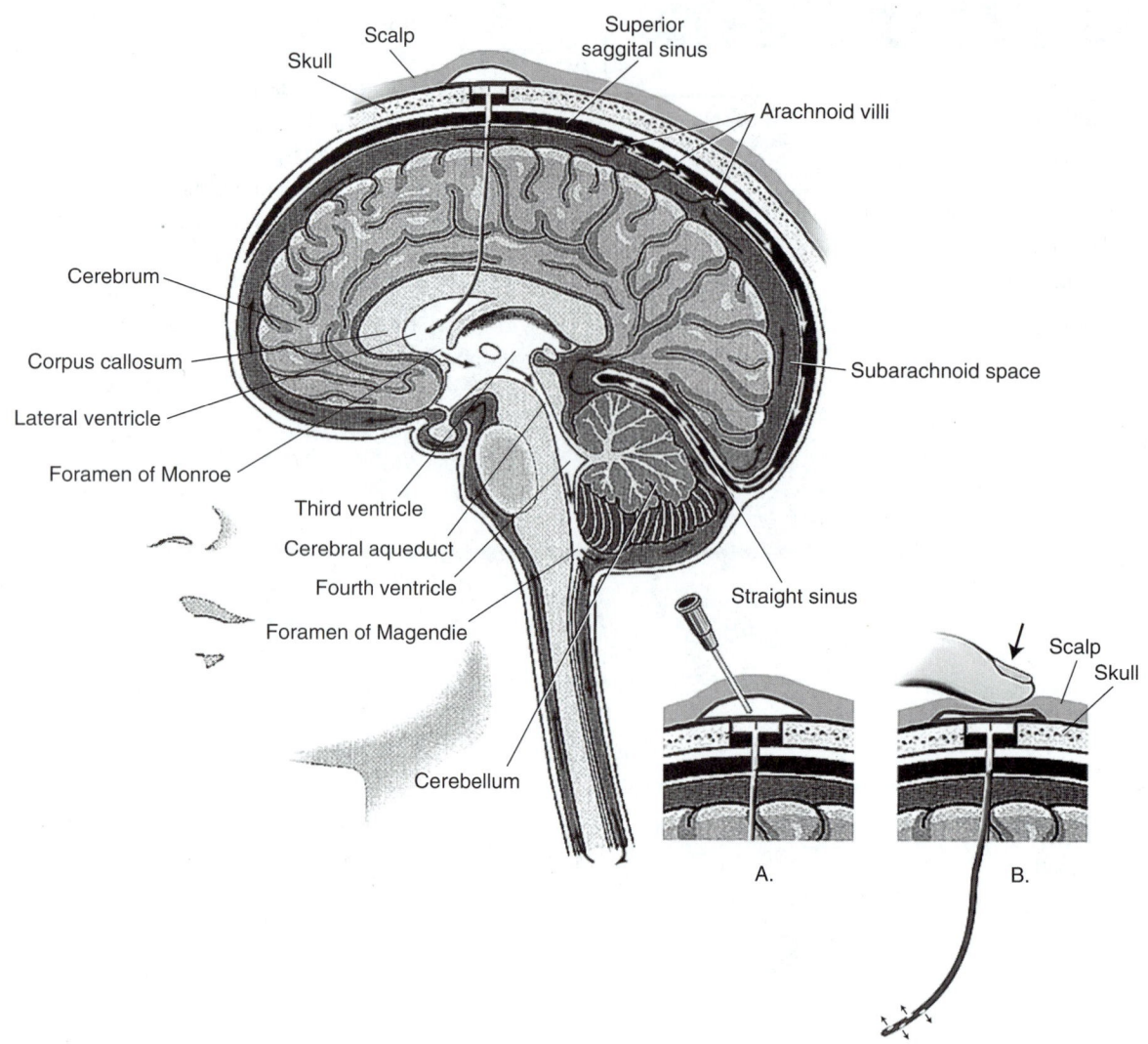

Figure 12-59 | Administration of medication into the dome of the Ommaya ventricular reservoir. Once injected, (A) gentle pressure is applied, (B) which infuses the medication through the port and into the lateral ventricle.

body and capped with an intermittent infusion plug. The ventricular reservoir is implanted subcutaneously in the scalp and allows for intermittent injections of medication. This device eliminates the need for repeated lumbar punctures to administer intrathecal medication.

The Ommaya reservoir, for intrathecal administration, is a mushroom-shaped, self-sealing silicone storage dome with an attached catheter that is surgically inserted through a burr hole in the cranium and threaded down into the lateral ventricle. Medications can be injected into the dome-shaped reservoir with a syringe, followed by gentle, manual compression of the dome, which mixes the drug with the CSF. The Ommaya reservoir, which can function for years, is used to deliver analgesics, antibiotics, and chemotherapy into the

subarachnoid space and the CSF (Figure 12-59). It is the route of choice for the chemotherapeutic treatment of leukemia and meningeal carcinomatoses, where the leptomeninges of the brain are infiltrated with cancer. It is also used to obtain samples of CSF for laboratory analysis, cystic tumor drainage, and ventricular drainage, and to measure cerebrospinal fluid pressure (Figure 12-60).

Intra-Arterial Administration

Intra-arterial routes are accessed for diagnostic angiography (by physicians) for the evaluation of the shape and size of various arteries and veins that perfuse the major organs and tissues of the body. This route of cannulation is also implemented,

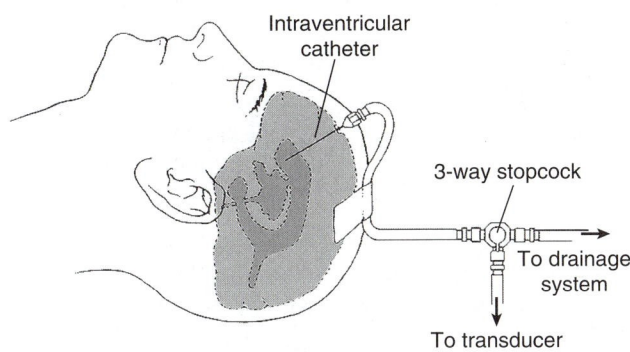

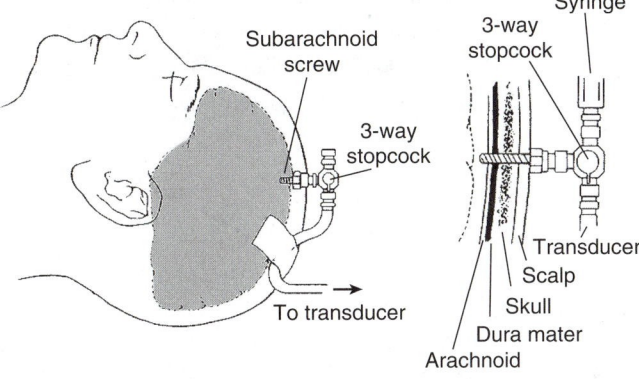

Figure 12-60 | Cerebrospinal pressure measurement

to avoid frequent punctures, when arterial blood gases need to be continually evaluated or when measurements of pressure and cardiac output are required. Arterial access and drug delivery by nurses and other trained personnel depend on individual state laws and professional practice acts.

When a tumor is unresponsive to chemotherapy dosages that can be safely administered via the systemic intravenous circulation, it is often necessary to introduce a cannula into the artery that supplies blood to the area of the tumor so higher concentrations can be administered. This is known as regional chemotherapy. Regional chemotherapy can be accomplished in one of two ways: by vessel isolation and extracorporeal exchange or by continuous infusion via a percutaneously inserted cannula or surgically implanted drug delivery device.

In the first method of regional therapy, a catheter is inserted into an artery that delivers blood to a large region, such as a limb. The artery is attached to a pump oxygenator that provides auxiliary **extracorporeal** exchange, outside of the body, so its blood will not perfuse the general circulation. By doing this, the dose of chemotherapy can be increased to ten times the dose that could safely be tolerated if delivered into the systemic circulation.

The second method of regional chemotherapy also involves the insertion of a cannula into the branch of the artery leading to the tumor. It may be percutaneously threaded into the artery and connected to an IV infusion or to an ambulatory infusion pump. This is usually used for short-term therapy. For long-term chemotherapy or pain management, an arterial cannula attached to an implanted infusion pump is surgically inserted into the subcutaneous tissue under anesthesia during a laparotomy. This allows for a continuous delivery of medication (Figure 12-61), which is refilled approximately every two weeks. There are no external components, so the pump is accessed subcutaneously, using a special needle inserted into an inlet septum. It has a permanent indigenous power supply derived from an inexhaustible charging fluid sealed in the pump during manufacture, so it can be left in place indefinitely.

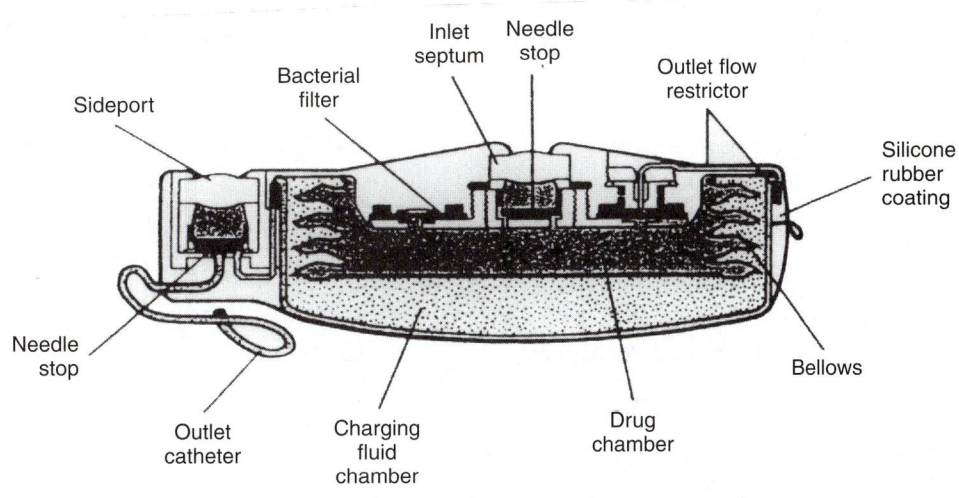

Figure 12-61 | Infusaid® Delivery System *Courtesy of Infusaid Corporation*

Intraperitoneal Administration

As with other modalities of treatment that are not delivered intravenously because of systemic intolerance and toxicity, the intraperitoneal route allows for higher concentrations of drug delivery directly into the peritoneal cavity. Doses up to 1,000 times greater than could be tolerated if infused by the IV route into the systemic circulation can be given intraperitoneally. Medications administered intraperitoneally are metabolized in the liver and removed through the portal circulation, so only minute concentrations are available to the systemic circulation, therefore reducing side effects. The semipermeable peritoneal membrane permits prolonged exposure of the malignant cells to the chemotherapy, while restricting passage of the drug out of the peritoneum. This route is often employed for the delivery of chemotherapy for colon cancer, where metastasis often occurs in the liver, and for ovarian cancer, where the peritoneal cavity is usually the site of tumor involvement. It is also used for malignant ascites associated with lymphatic and gastrointestinal tumor processes.

A Tenckhoff peritoneal catheter, usually employed in peritoneal dialysis, is used to administer chemotherapy. It is inserted under local anesthesia (by a physician), through the anterior abdominal wall into the peritoneal cavity, then tunneled subcutaneously to exit the skin. (The procedure is performed in the operating room as a precautionary measure because of the potential for bowel perforation associated with the maneuver.) The catheter has a Dacron® cuff that propagates fibroblast formation in the exit channel. During the healing process, the fibroblasts form a seal around the catheter, thus preventing contaminants from entering the abdominal cavity.

Chemotherapy, supplied in an IV bag or bottle, is delivered (by the nurse, patient, or trained family member in the home) to the peritoneal cavity via IV tubing attached to the Tenckhoff catheter. Once infused, the IV tubing is clamped and the beta clamp on the Tenckhoff catheter is closed, keeping the medication in the cavity for the prescribed time period. The cavity is then drained by gravity and patient positioning by lowering the infusate container, releasing the tubing clamp and the beta clamp, and allowing the backflow into the original container. Some physicians, however, prefer that the chemotherapy solution remain in the peritoneum for longer exposure to the tumor cells. The solution gradually reabsorbs into the system. With this method, though, the patient experiences more of the side effects of the chemotherapy.

Intraosseous Administration

The **intraosseous** (IO) route accesses the vasculature of the bones and provides an emergency route for the rapid delivery of infusates. It should be used when IV access is not possible and the patient's situation is such that her life is in danger. It is to be considered a short-term procedure, being required for 24 hours or less. It is indicated for children as well as adults. The long bones of the distal femur or the distal and proximal tibia are utilized in children; when intraosseous access is indicated for an adult, the preferred sites are the iliac crest and the sternum. "Intraosseous access should not be attempted on sites where intraosseous access has been previously attempted, a fractured or traumatized leg, areas of infected burns or cellulitis, or patients with osteoporosis." (INS, 2000, Standard 68, S64). The internal bone structure (marrow, medulla) provides a dense vascular network of venous sinuses that form a conduit with the venous circulation (Figure 12-62). (See Chapter 15 for pediatric use of the intraosseous route.)

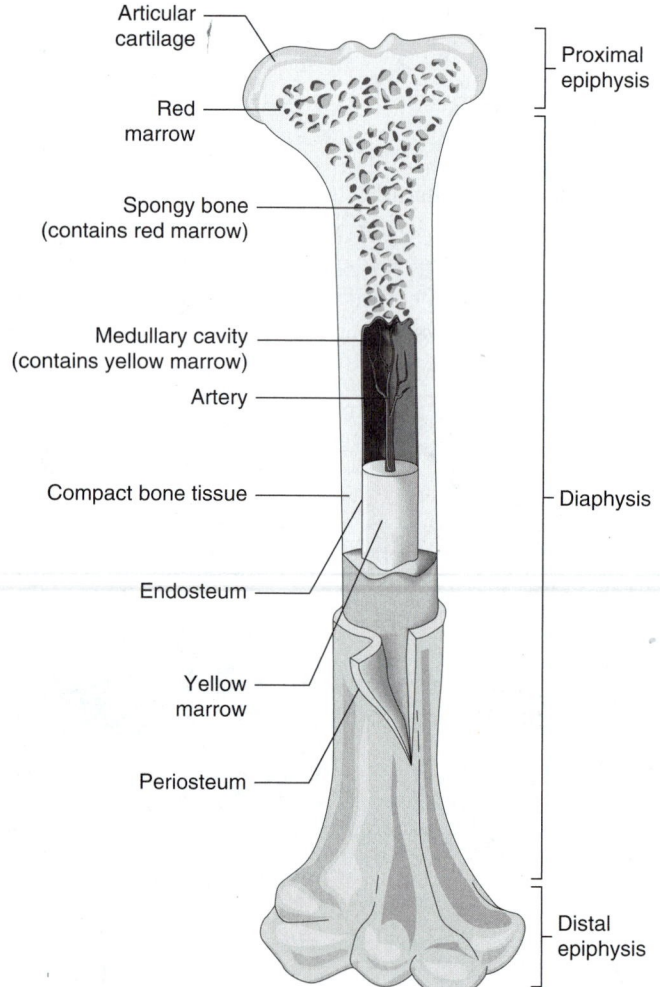

Figure 12-62 │ Intraosseous vascular network

Key Concepts

- Central venous access routes are established in order to deliver fluids, medications, blood or blood products, chemotherapy, and total parenteral nutrition, and to withdraw blood samples in patients requiring frequent or long-term infusion therapy.

- The nurse must know the insertion, use, and maintenance protocols for centrally and peripherally inserted central venous catheters, midline catheters, and subcutaneously implanted vascular access devices.

- The usual sites of insertion for centrally placed central venous catheters are the subclavian vein or the internal and external jugulars, with the right subclavian the preferred vein.

- The usual insertion sites for peripherally inserted central catheters are the basilic (preferred), cephalic, and median cubital veins.

- The tip of any central venous catheter should reside in the superior vena cava within 3 to 4 cm of the right atrial-superior vena caval junction. It must be free-floating and lie parallel to the vessel wall without any looping or kinking.

- Proper positioning of a CVC provides optimum dilution of infusates, large or rapid infusate administration, accurate CVP monitoring, and the least risk of vascular or cardiac trauma.

- The immediate complications associated with CVCs are usually related to problems involving insertion of the device, whereas problems associated with long-term CVC use are often the result of inadequate catheter care or the patient's clinical situation.

- The nurse must remember that air embolism is a major, preventable complication that can occur at any time during central line therapy, including the 24-hour period following removal. The nurse must instruct the patient how to perform the Valsalva maneuver so it can be used during catheter insertion, injection cap changes, and removal.

- The nurse must know the signs and symptoms of air embolism so that immediate emergency measures can be instituted should it occur. In the event of an air embolism, the patient must be positioned in the left lateral Trendelenburg position and given oxygen by mask.

- Syringes with capacities of less than 10 cc should never be used to access or irrigate central lines as excessive pressure can damage or break the CVC, resulting in catheter embolism or traumatized vessels.

- In dealing with any central venous access device, the nurse must be trained in its use, follow manufacturer guidelines, comply with agency protocols and policies, and be fully competent in the assessment, planning, intervention, and evaluation of a patient who has one in place.

- Epidural and intrathecal administrations are initiated when large concentrations of medication need to be delivered and absorbed directly into the tissues and vessels of the CNS. Other routes cannot be used because of the blood-brain barrier, which selectively limits the passage of substances from the blood to the brain tissue, or because the dosage needed would cause severe side effects. Using these routes, pain control is of a superior quality, requiring small dosages, and producing longer periods of relief between doses, while preventing many side effects.

- Intra-arterial infusions are administered for diagnostic evaluation and for the delivery of regional chemotherapy.

- The intraperitoneal route is used when high concentrations of medication need to be delivered directly into the peritoneal cavity. A Tenckhoff peritoneal dialysis catheter is generally used, or a port is subcutaneously implanted.

- The intraosseous route accesses the vasculature of the bones and provides an emergency route for the rapid administration of fluids and medications when other sites are unavailable. This route is generally reserved for children under 6 years of age and should be used no longer than 24 hours.

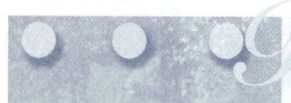

Review Questions

1. List the CDC guidelines regarding the following procedures associated with central venous access devices:

   (a) Barrier precautions during catheter insertion and site care

   (b) Cutaneous antiseptics and antimicrobial ointments

   (c) Dressing materials

   (d) Catheter site dressing changes

   (e) The routine use of filters

2. List the nursing interventions associated with preparing a patient for the insertion of a central venous catheter, assisting the physician with catheter placement, and caring for the patient immediately following the procedure.

3. What would you do in the following situation?

   As you are leaving the nursing unit at the end of your shift, you see a patient who is ambulating in the hall pull out his central venous catheter.

   List, in order of priority, the steps you would take to rectify this situation, stating the rationale behind each intervention.

4. Based on the following case study, write a nursing care plan focusing on how the care of the central venous catheter will relate to the other problems the patient is experiencing.

   Mr. Lundy is a 54-year-old Caucasian male admitted to the hospital complaining of abdominal pain, nausea, chills, pleuritic pain, and shortness of breath. He has a 30+ year history of chronic alcohol abuse and smokes 2 packs of cigarettes a day. He has had chronic pancreatitis for over 5 years and exhibits signs of malnourishment from malabsorption. He is 6'1" tall and weighs 140 lbs. He is now experiencing acute pancreatitis.

   Assessment Data:

   Temp. 101.2°F

   WBC: 22,000/mm3

   Serum glucose: 196 mg/dl

   Serum albumin: 3.0 g/dl

   BUN: 55 mg/dl

   Arterial PO2 54 mm Hg

   Ultrasound of abdomen: pancreatic abscesses; calcification of pancreatic ducts

   Treatment:

   Surgical drainage of pancreatic abscesses

   Insertion of quad-lumen ARROW® CVC by percutaneous insertion into SVC via Rt. subclavian entry

   Nasogastric tube insertion for suctioning

   Jejunostomy for nutritional support

   Continuous hemodynamic and blood gas monitoring

   Medications:

   Antipyretics

   Histamine H2-receptor antagonists

   Insulin

   Narcotic analgesics

5. List one indication for using each of the following vascular access routes:

   (a) Epidural

   (b) Intrathecal

   (c) Intra-arterial

   (d) Intraperitoneal

   (e) Intraosseous

Chapter 13

Intravenous Nutritional Support

COMPETENCIES

Upon completion of this chapter, the reader should be able to:

* Examine the indications for intravenous parenteral nutritional support.

* Diagram and explain the metabolic pathways of energy use in the body.

* Review the role of proteins, fats, and carbohydrates in the maintenance of homeostasis.

* Identify the components of parenteral nutrition.

* Differentiate between total parenteral nutrition and peripheral parenteral nutrition.

* Describe the risks and complications associated with the administration of parenteral nutrition.

* Discuss the major nursing assessment data and interventions related to monitoring the patient receiving parenteral nutrition.

Intravenous nutritional products are complex admixtures that provide a partial or complete source of nourishment for patients who are unable to ingest or utilize sufficient calories and nutrients to sustain metabolic functions. They are composed of water, carbohydrates (dextrose), proteins (amino acids), fats (lipid emulsions), electrolytes, multivitamins, and trace elements, and are formulated to meet individual patient needs and comply with restrictions imposed by fluid balance and various disease processes. Formulations that supply a complete source of sustenance for nutritionally depleted patients and are administered via a central venous catheter into the superior vena cava are classified as total parenteral nutrition (TPN). Formulations that provide a complete source of nutrients but are not sufficient for nutritionally depleted individuals and are administered through peripheral veins are classified as peripheral parenteral nutrition (PPN).

INDICATIONS FOR INTRAVENOUS NUTRITION

In order to survive, the body needs calories and nutrients to provide the energy to carry out vital functions during rest and activity. When stress or disease alters the ability to take in food or use food energy sources, the body compensates by using its own stores of energy (Figure 13-1). A state of negative nitrogen balance occurs if compensatory mechanisms fail or nutritional interventions are not initiated. Parenteral nutrition supplies the nutrients (in excess of those required for energy expenditure) to promote anabolism, in much the same ratio of those in a regular diet for a healthy person.

Parenteral nutrition is indicated for patients who are malnourished or in danger of becoming malnourished and who require continuous or intermittent intravenous nutritional support for periods of one to three weeks or longer (in the acute care setting or the home). In general, such patients have high metabolic needs that require high caloric intake, nitrogen balance restoration, and electrolyte, mineral, vitamin, and trace element replacement. Table 13-1 lists the major indications for parenteral nutrition therapy and Table 13-2 lists the contraindications.

Traumatic Stress and Nutritional Depletion

Stressful events such as burns, surgical intervention, infection, and trauma create a tremendous need in the nutritional status of the body and increase calorie and protein requirements. The neuroendocrine-mediated changes occurring in response to stress greatly increase energy expenditure (Figure 13-2). Under normal conditions the moderately

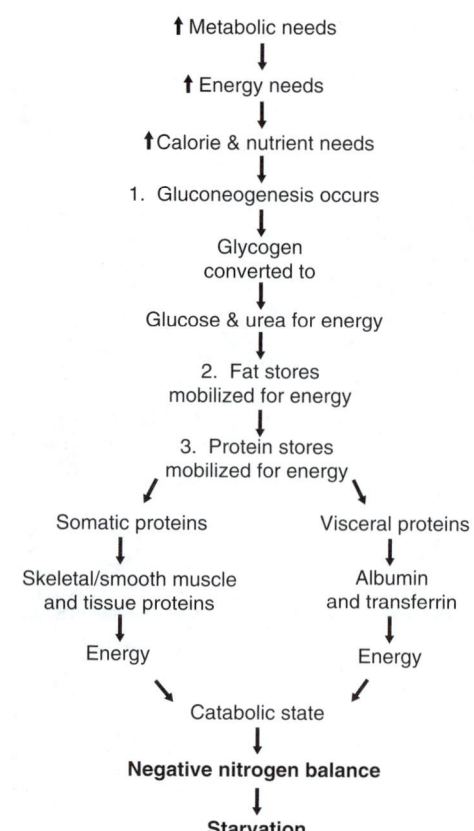

Figure 13-1 | Metabolic pathways of stored energy used by the body

active, 150-lb. healthy adult requires approximately 2,200 cal (32 cal/kg) and 50 g of protein (0.74 g/kg) per day. That same person on complete bed rest who becomes septic may require 3,400 cal (50 cal/kg) and 170 g of protein (2.5 g/kg) just to maintain nitrogen equilibrium. The stress of burns can elevate protein needs to 225 g and caloric requirements to 10,000 cal in some patients.

COMPOSITION OF PARENTERAL NUTRITION PRODUCTS

Parenteral nutrition products provide an intravenous approach to deliver the calories, dextrose, amino acids, lipids, and other essential elements needed for the health-sustaining functions of growth, convalescence, immunocompetence, tissue repair, wound healing, and other purposes. The preparations are similar in terms of their basic components but may vary considerably regarding the proportions of the ingredients. Each prescription is patient-specific, taking into consideration nutritional and metabolic status, stress factors, liver function, and renal competency.

Table 13-1 | Indications for Parenteral Nutritional Support

PARENTERAL NUTRITION	
Indication	**Problem**
Bowel surgery	Short-bowel syndrome
	Massive resection
Chronic weight loss (even with adequate oral intake)	
Coma	
Conditions requiring bowel rest	Acute pancreatis
	Bowel fistulas
	Inflammatory bowel disease
	Obstruction
	Paralytic ileus
	Peritonitis
Excessive nitrogen loss	Abscesses
	Fistulas
	Infections
	Wounds
Hepatic or renal failure	
Hypermetabolic states	Burns
	Critical illness
Malabsorption of enteral therapy	
Malnutrition	Anorexia nervosa
	Anorexia of cancer
	Cancer malabsorption syndrome
	Chronic vomiting or diarrhea
	10% of pre-illness weight loss
Multiple trauma	
Serum albumin below 3.5 g/dl	

Table 13-2 | Contraindications to Parenteral Nutrition Support

- Catheter-related complications (such as displacement, migration, or occlusion)
- Coagulopathies
- Local and systemic complications associated with central line placement and use
- Patient noncompliance or refusal to eat
- Patients with gastrointestinal tracts that should resume normal functioning patterns within 7 to 10 days
- Patients with functional gastrointestinal tracts
- Poor prognosis
- Superior vena cava thrombosis
- Terminal illness when all therapy has been discontinued

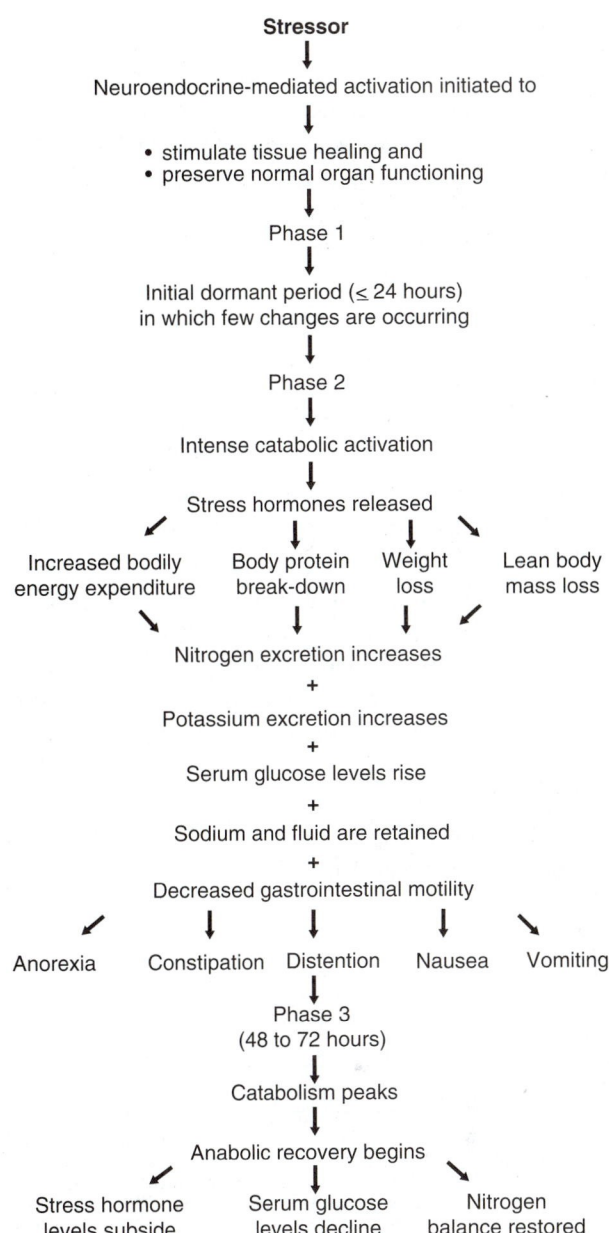

Figure 13-2 | Phases of the body's response to stress

Standard Parenteral Nutrition Components

In general, parenteral nutrition products contain three major nutrients: amino acids, dextrose, and fat emulsions. These components, which make up the bulk of most parenteral nutrition formulations, are referred to as macronutrients. Electrolytes, trace elements, and minerals are added, and the volume is adjusted with the addition of sterile water. Two-in-one TPN solutions contain protein and dextrose in base solution, with lipids usually being administered separately, while 3-in-1 solutions contain protein, dextrose, and fat in a base solution.

Amino Acids

Proteins are nitrogenous compounds that form an integral part of the protoplasm of every cell and produce heat and energy through the process of oxidation, providing 4 cal/g. Amino acids, which are essential for human growth and repair, are the building blocks of proteins and are composed of carbon, hydrogen, nitrogen, and oxygen. They contain a basic amino group, NH_2, and an acidic carboxylic group, COOH, both attached to a carbon atom stem that makes them capable of acting as neutralizing buffers for either acids or bases. In order for amino acids to be used as energy sources (when protein-sparing calorie intake from carbohydrates and fats is inadequate) or stored, the amino group has to be removed from the carbon stem. The NH_2 is used either to synthesize other compounds or is converted to urea in the liver and then excreted via the urine. The carbon stem is converted either to an intermediary for energy use by peripheral tissues, to glucose or fat for immediate energy use, or to fat and stored in adipose tissue.

Proteins are dietary necessities required to produce adequate supplies of amino acids for the synthesis of body proteins. The body cannot function without proteins (Table 13-3). There are over 80 known amino acids in nature with 23 needed by the human body (Table 13-4). Nine are known as essential amino acids because they cannot be synthesized by the body and must be (essentially) supplied in the diet. The other fourteen are nonessential (in terms of dietary intake) because they can be manufactured in the body from carbohydrates, fats, or nitrogen. (In infants, arginine, which is not synthesized in adequate amounts during periods of rapid growth, is considered an essential amino acid.)

Dietary proteins are classified as complete or high quality if they contribute all the essential amino acids needed by the body. They are incomplete or low quality if they are deficient in one or more of the essential amino acids.

The biologic value of amino acids refers to the percentage of absorbed nitrogen (from ingested amino acids) retained by the body. If dietary proteins provide essential amino acids with high proportions of nitrogen, they have significant biologic value. Proteins with biologic values above 70% are deemed high biologic value (HBV) proteins. These have the ability, when calorie intake is sufficient, to support growth and repair.

Table 13-3 | Functions of Proteins in the Body

Antibody formation	Proteins form the immuglobins that help the body resist disease and infection.
Body framework	Protein forms the structure of blood vessels, bones, hair and nails, muscles, and skin.
Detoxification	Foreign substances can be inactivated by proteins.
Energy production	Proteins supply 4 kcal/g (but are not as efficiently burned as carbohydrates).
Fluid balance	Plasma proteins, especially albumin, help maintain oncotic pressure.
Growth	Proteins promote tissue synthesis.
Repair	Proteins rebuild tissue that breaks down due to normal use.
Specific amino acid functions	Tryptophan is a precursor of niacin. Tyrosine is a precursor of the pigment melanin.
Synthesis of compounds	Proteins synthesize opsin, the visual pigment, and thrombin, the clotting protein.

Synthesis of fluids and secretions	Proteins synthesize essential bodily fluids and secretions:
	    Bile acids
	    Breast milk
	    Enzymes
	    Histamine
	    Hormones (epinephrine, insulin,
	        thyroxine)
	    Neurotransmitters (acetylcholine,
	        serotonin)
	    Plasma proteins (albumin, hemoglobin)

Transport	Albumin transports bilirubin, free fatty acids, and many drugs in the blood. Lipoproteins transport cholesterol, fat-soluble vitamins, phospholipids, and triglycerides in the blood. Protein-bound iodine transports iodine in the blood. Transferrin transports iron in the blood.

Table 13-4 | Amino Acids

Essential Amino Acids	Nonessential Amino Acids
Histidine	Alanine
Isoleucine	Arginine
Leucine	Aspartic Acid
Lysine	Citrulline
Methionine	Cystine
Phenylalanine	Glutamic Acid
Threonine	Glutamine
Tryptophan	Glycine
Valine	Hydroxyproline
	Hydroxylysine
	Norleucine
	Proline
	Serine
	Tyrosine

Parenteral Amino Acids

The base ingredient of any parenteral nutrition infusate is an amino acid solution, usually a crystalline preparation, that contains from 3.5% to 15% synthetic amino acids (essential and nonessential) without peptides (e.g., Aminosyn® and Travasol®). It is indicated as an adjunct in the off-setting of nitrogen loss or in the treatment of negative nitrogen balance. It promotes protein anabolism and prevents protein catabolism while acting as a buffer in intracellular and extracellular fluid environments.

Any parenteral amino acid formulation is concurrently administered with dextrose (providing 100 g to 150 g of carbohydrate in concentrations of 10% to 70%) so that the amino acids are retained by the body and utilized for protein synthesis. Fat emulsions are usually mixed into the preparation (or administered simultaneously) to prevent fatty acid deficiency. The osmolality can be adjusted, using dilution variances, to allow for central or peripheral intravenous administration. Protein amino acid formulations are available for general use, renal failure, hepatic failure or encephalopathy, and metabolic stress.

The amount of amino acid solution administered over a 24-hour period is determined by the patient's metabolic requirement and clinical response. The determination of nitrogen balance and accurate daily body weights, corrected for fluid balance, are presumably the best means of assessing individual nitrogen requirements. As a general rule, daily amino acid doses of approximately 1.0 to 1.5 g/kg, with adequate calories, are generally sufficient to satisfy protein needs and promote positive nitrogen balance.

Carbohydrates

Carbohydrates (CHOs) are a group of chemicals composed of carbon, hydrogen, and oxygen, that include sugars, glycogen, starches, dextrins, and celluloses. They provide a basic source of energy (glucose) that can be stored in almost all body tissues (as glycogen), but mainly in the liver and muscles, and be mobilized for use at any time. They provide approximately 4 cal/g (except cellulose, which is calorie-free because it cannot be digested).

Dietary carbohydrate intake must be sufficient to provide the needed calories for energy expenditure while sparing protein and preventing gluconeogenesis. In addition, carbohydrates are needed to completely oxidize fat, so that it is not broken down into ketones. In the normal healthy adult, approximately 50 g to 100 g of carbohydrate are needed daily to prevent ketoacidosis, gluconeogenesis, sodium depletion, and dehydration.

Parenteral Carbohydrates

Dextrose is utilized as the principal source of non-protein oxidative energy substrate in U.S.-formulated hydrous dextrose and is the principal source of carbohydrate in parenteral nutrition formulations. It is derived from corn sugar and provides water and calories (1 g of IV dextrose provides 3.4 kcal). It depresses gluconeogenesis and its nitrogen-sparing effect is of benefit in reducing protein catabolism and the utilization of protein as an energy source. Glycerol, used primarily in peripherally administered solutions, provides 4.3 kcal/g. Dextrose increases the body's metabolic rate, which, in turn, raises ventilatory requirements—thus the reason that lipids are added to the TPN regimen to reduce respiratory demands.

NURSING ALERT

Problems Associated with Rapid Infusion of Dextrose

Rapid infusion of a hypertonic dextrose injection may result in diuresis, hyperglycemia, glycosuria, or hyperosmolar coma. Careful clinical monitoring of the patient is mandatory in order to identify and initiate measures to avert or counteract these problems. This is an important aspect of patient-family teaching for home-bound patients receiving TPN/PPN.

NURSING TIP

Lipid-Containing Solutions

Complete the infusion of lipid-containing solutions (e.g., 3-in-1 solutions) within 24 hours of hanging the solution and complete the infusion of lipid emulsions alone within 12 hours of hanging the emulsion. If volume considerations require more time, the infusion should be completed within 24 hours (CDC, 2002a).

Invert sugar (for patients allergic to corn derivatives), alcohol, or fructose may be used in place of dextrose. Fructose and alcohol do not require insulin for peripheral utilization, but have potentially dangerous side effects that are not associated with dextrose use.

The number of dextrose calories in a parenteral preparation may vary considerably, depending on the needs of the patient. The range may be from 400 to 5,000 cal/day and depends upon the age, weight, clinical status of the patient, and laboratory determinations. For peripheral infusions, the dextrose concentration must be maintained at an isotonic or mildly hypertonic osmolality (not to exceed 10%) to avert vein irritation, damage to the vein, or thrombosis. Hypertonic concentrations must be administered through a CVC, the tip of which resides in the distal portion of the superior vena cava, above the right atrium.

Fats

Fats, or lipids, are chemical substances that are composed of one glycerol and three fatty acid molecules that are water-insoluble. Glycerol is a 3-carbon stem with alcohol groups attached to each carbon atom. It is an end product of fat digestion that is absorbed directly into the portal vein. Fatty acids are made up of straight chains of carbon atoms with a hydrogen atom attached and an acid group at one end. They have varying carbon-chain lengths and varying degrees of saturation (depending on the number of double bonds between carbon atoms), making them either saturated, monounsaturated, or polyunsaturated.

Fats oxidize to produce energy, carbon dioxide, and water and provide 9 cal/g, making them the most concentrated source of energy in the body. Fats are used as an energy source for all body tissues except the central nervous system (which is fueled by glucose) and have multiple functions (Table 13-5). The three major dietary classes of lipids are the fats and oils (in the form of triglycerides), the phospholipids, and the sterols. The first group comprises 95% of fat intake, while the other two make up the remaining 5%. Fat con-

Table 13-5 | Functions of Fat in the Body

Absorption of vitamins	Fat aids in the absorption of vitamins A, D, E, K.
Body structure	Phospholipids make up plasma membranes and myelin sheaths.
Delays gastric emptying	Fat, by remaining in the stomach 3 to 4 hr after eating, provides satiety and delays the return of hunger. When in the duodenum, fat stimulates the release of a gastric hormone that inhibits hunger.
Essential fatty acids (EFAs)	Fat provides linoleic and linolenic acid, long-chain polyunsaturated essential fatty acids that cannot be synthesized in the body. They are precursors of arachidonic acid. EFAs: 1. Metabolize cholesterol (along with other unsaturated fatty acids) and lower serum cholesterol levels 2. Maintain the function and structure of capillaries and cell membranes 3. Are precursors of prostaglandins and other hormonelike substances
Oxidation	Fats are oxidized to produce energy, carbon dioxide, and water.
Storage	Fat is stored as adipose tissue in two forms: White fat, the most abundant type, is stored under the skin, mainly in the abdominal cavity, to produce energy when needed, insulate and protect, and support the internal organs and protect them from injury. Brown fat, most abundant during infancy, is stored mostly around the neck and chest and generates heat to protect against cold.

sumed in excess of dietary requirements is stored as adipose tissue.

Parenteral Lipids

Parenteral lipids are administered to provide essential fatty acids and supply a non-carbohydrate, non-protein energy source, thus causing an increase in heat production, a decrease in respiratory quotient, and an increase in oxygen consumption. They are derived from safflower or soybean oil to contribute a blend of neutral triglycerides and unsaturated fatty acids to the nutrient intake to prevent or correct essential fatty acid deficiency (EFAD). (10% concentrations = 1.1 cal/ml; 20% = 2 cal/ml.)

Since lipids are isotonic, they may be delivered by either a peripheral or central venous line. They can be admixed with amino acid and dextrose preparations, but only if proper combining protocols are followed to minimize pH-related problems associated with combining typically acidic dextrose solutions with lipid emulsions. (The prime destabilizers of lipid emulsions are excessive acidity and inappropriate electrolyte content.) Because conventional administration sets and parenteral nutrition bags contain PVC that have DEHP as a plasticizer (which lipids extract), separate administration sets, glass infusate containers, or special non-PVC bags are generally recommended (with the lipids infused via a Y-connector or separate catheter lumen). Regular 0.2-μm porosity filters must not be used with fat emulsions, since the size of the fat particles is approximately 0.4 to 0.5 μm and would impede filter flow. When filters are used, a 1.2-μm size is generally employed.

NURSING ALERT

Inspecting Fat Emulsions

It is very important to carefully inspect fat emulsions for "breaking-out" or "oiling out," which is the separation of an emulsion visually identifiable by a yellowish streaking or the accumulation of yellow droplets in the admixed emulsion. Should this occur, or if any particulate matter is visible, the infusate must not be used and is to be discarded.

The usual adult dosage of parenteral lipids should not exceed 2.5 g/kg, with carbohydrate and amino acids comprising the remaining caloric input. Overdosage must be avoided. The patient's ability to eliminate the infused fat from the circulation must be carefully monitored with routine serum triglyceride evaluations and liver function tests. Caution should be used when administering fat

---

NURSING TIP

Rates for Lipid Infusions

The initial rate of lipid infusion should be 1 ml/min for the first 15 to 30 minutes of infusion. The rate may then be increased to 2 ml/min. No more than 500 ml should be administered to an adult in the first 24 hr of therapy. Thereafter, the rate should not exceed 2.5 g/kg/day.

NURSING TIP

Electrolyte Deficiencies

It is critical that the nurse know what the signs and symptoms of specific electrolyte deficiencies are so that problems can be detected as soon as they become evident.

---

emulsions to patients with anemia, coagulopathies, or severe liver damage, or when there is any danger of fat embolism.

Electrolytes

When patients are receiving parenteral nutrition it is critical that serum electrolyte levels be closely monitored. Those that require routine evaluation are the cations magnesium, potassium, and sodium and the anions of acetate, bicarbonate, chloride, and phosphate.

In general, electrolytes are added to parenteral nutrition admixtures at the start of therapy and adjusted on a routine basis, depending on the patient's clinical status and actual serum levels. Single and multiple electrolyte solutions are available for addition to the TPN. Single ingredient electrolyte solutions include potassium chloride, calcium gluconate, magnesium sulfate, sodium phosphate, and others. Multiple electrolyte solutions, which are intended to simplify compounding and standardize the electrolyte component of parenteral nutrition solutions, contain fixed combinations of electrolytes in a specific volume. Some commercial preparations have electrolytes combined with the amino acid infusate.

Minerals and Trace Elements

Minerals are inorganic elements occurring in nature that are not of animal or plant origin. They are found in all body fluids and tissues either in the form of salts or combined with organic compounds. Those that are found in the body in quantities greater than 5 g and are needed by the body in amounts of 100 mg or more are considered macrominerals (Dudek, 2001). All others normally found in very small amounts are considered microminerals or trace elements.

Minerals are essential for acid-base balance, blood volume regulation, bone, nail, and tooth structure, capillary and cell-membrane permeability, enzymatic and glandular secretory activity, neuromuscular excitability, osmotic regulation, and water metabolism. Mineral salts and water are excreted from the body on a daily basis and must be replaced by regular dietary intake.

For TPN, there are available single trace element solutions (with single-entity products such as copper sulfate, zinc sulfate, etc.) and multiple trace element solutions, which are offered in a variety of combinations with fixed quantities per given volume. The quantity of trace elements contained in these solutions vary from product to product and manufacturer to manufacturer. Common examples include MTE-4 and MTE-5, among others. Mixed electrolyte and trace element formulations, which are prepared to facilitate the ease of solution admixture, are made to be added to maintenance parenteral nutrition formulas for use in stable patients.

Vitamins

Vitamins are organic substances composed of carbon, hydrogen, oxygen, nitrogen (sometimes), and other elements. Most of them work by uniting with a protein (apoenzyme) to form a coenzyme that promotes an enzymatic effect. They are needed in very small quantities yet are essential in the regulation of body processes and chemical reactions. In general, they cannot be synthesized by the body and, when they are, there are inadequate quantities, so they must be obtained through dietary or synthetic supplementation.

NURSING TIP

Minerals in Parenteral Nutrition Therapy

Minerals are taken for granted in the average healthy person with normal dietary patterns, but must be evaluated in all patients undergoing parenteral nutrition therapy. The nurse must be aware of the normal values of these constituents as well as the signs and symptomatology of deficiencies (Table 13-6). With the exception of iron, which cannot be mixed with other drugs or infusates, minerals are usually admixed individually with parenteral nutrition preparations or in pre-mixed formulations.

Table 13-6 | Mineral Deficiencies

MACROMINERALS		
Element	Normal Value	Evidence of Deficiency
Calcium	4.5–5.3 mEq/L (9–11 mg/dl)	Convulsion, muscle cramps, seizures, tetany
Magnesium	1.8–3.0 mg/dl	CNS and neuromuscular irritability leading to loss of control, convulsions, disorientation, positive Chvostek's and Trousseau's signs, tetany, tremors
Phosphorus	2.5–4.8 mg/dl	Anorexia, circumoral paresthesia, hyperventilation, weakness
Sulfur	Unknown	No known deficiency symptoms
MICROMINERALS (TRACE ELEMENTS)		
Element	Normal Value	Evidence of Deficiency
Chromium	1–5 µg/L	Ataxia, confusion, impaired glucose tolerance, neuropathy
Cobalt	Unknown	Vitamin B_{12} deficiency (Cobalt is an essential constituent of vitamin B_{12}.)
Copper	80–163 µg/dl	Decrease in RBCs & WBCs, defective tissue growth, hair and skeletal abnormalities, hypercholesterolemia
Fluorine	>1.0 mg/dl	Dental caries, osteoporosis
Iodine	0.5–1.5 µg/dl	Cretinism, goiter, impaired thyroid functioning
Iron	60–180 µg/dl	Anorexia, fatigue, glossitis and stomatitis, headaches, pallor, vertigo, weakness
Manganese	6–12 µg/l	CNS alterations, nausea, vomiting, skin rash, weight loss
Molybdenum	Unknown	Coma, disorientation, edema, headache, hypouricemia, malaise, nausea, vomiting, tachycardia, tachypnea
Selenium	10–37 µg/dl	Cardiomyopathy, myalgia, kwashiorkor
Zinc	±100 µg/dl	Anemia, anorexia, depression, diarrhea, optic lesions, impaired wound healing, hepatosplenomegaly, malaise, nausea, taste alterations, vomiting

As a general rule, the patient who is undergoing parenteral nutrition therapy is in need of vitamin supplementation. It is usually the policy, unless the patient has cardiac, hepatic, or renal complications, to admix the fat-soluble vitamins A and D and the water-solubles B and C directly into the formulation or add multivitamin infusions (MVI) to the preparation.

CRITICAL THINKING

Assessing Your Own Nutritional Intake

Becoming more aware of your own nutritional intake and needs will help you better understand and evaluate a patient's nutritional requirements. This is especially helpful when evaluating a patient's need for IV parenteral nutrition.

Think about your food and beverage consumption over the past week and try to identify the nutritional value of what you ate and drank. Make a note of the effect, positive or negative, that each of these items has had on your body.

Total Nutrient Admixture Formulas

A total nutrient admixture (TNA) is a parenteral preparation that contains a 24-hour supply of nutrients in one non-PVC administration bag. It is often called a 3-in-1 system because the three main components—amino acids, dextrose, and lipids—are combined in one bag along with all of the other needed elements. Because all of the ingredients are combined, the tonicity of the end-product is decreased, making it a more tolerable infusion for many patients.

In general TNAs are used for relatively stable patients in whom it can be predicted that components of the admixture will not have to be altered within a 24-hour period. Because only one bag is used, there is less handling and manipulation, thus reducing the potential for contamination that may be associated with bag changes every 8 hours. Obviously, this system is more time-efficient for the nurse. This is an ideal system for home-bound patients receiving continuous parenteral nutrition.

Standardized Solutions and Order Forms

Many hospitals and home care infusion agencies have one or more standard base parenteral nutrition formulas that are commonly ordered by the physicians who practice there. The physicians usually prescribe one of the standard solutions, then tailor them to meet individual patient needs, with the addition of specific electrolytes. Many times agencies also have parenteral nutrition order forms that must be used by physicians when prescribing nutrient solutions. Examples of standard amino acid formulations include Aminosyn® and Travasol,® among others.

Standardization ensures that all nutritional elements are provided to the patient, affording less chance for omissions. The intent of the prescribing physician is made clear, thereby decreasing the possibility of error. In addition, the response time to new TPN or PPN orders by the pharmacy is improved because the base solutions are prepared in batches.

Specific Parenteral Nutrition Components

Formulations are specifically suited to accommodate individual patient needs. When certain disease processes or underlying conditions are present, some patients cannot tolerate some of the standard parenteral nutrition preparations.

Hepatic Formulas

Patients who have liver disease, such as cirrhosis or hepatitis, or manifest symptoms of hepatic encephalopathy and coma have low levels of branched chain amino acids and high levels of aromatic amino acids. Because of this, they are intolerant of crystalline amino acid preparations. These patients, when they require parenteral nutrition supplementation, are given amino acids with high levels of branched chain amino acids such as leucine, isoleucine, and valine. For patients with encephalopathy, these solutions bring about enhanced mental status and improved electroencephalography (EEG) patterns. Such preparations include BranchAmin,® HepatAmine,® and Novamine® 15% with 4% BCAA (branched chain amino acids). These are contraindicated if the patient is anuric.

CRITICAL THINKING

Hepatic Parenteral Nutrition Considerations

Why would the administration of a hepatic parenteral nutrition preparation be contraindicated in the anuric patient? What might happen if such a formulation were mistakenly administered to a patient with impaired renal function?

Renal Formulas

In patients with uremia and renal failure, who are in need of parenteral nutrition, minimal quantities of essential amino acids enhance urea utilization, promote protein synthesis, and improve cellular metabolic balance. Therefore, the administration of nonessential amino acids should be curtailed. Standard crystalline amino acid solutions contain both essential and nonessential amino acids. Amino acid formulations for renal failure contain only essential amino acids. Histidine is especially essential for uremic patients. Renal preparations decrease the rate of blood urea nitrogen formation and minimize deterioration of serum potassium, magnesium, and phosphorus in patients with impaired renal function. Such products include Aminess® 5.2%, Aminosyn-RF® 5.2% or 5.4%, and NephrAmine.® These are contraindicated in the presence of severe, uncorrected acid-base and electrolyte imbalances, decreased (subcritical) circulating blood volume, and hyperammonemia.

Stress Formulas

Patients faced with stressors such as infection, sepsis, and the trauma of burns, surgery, shock, and blunt or penetrating injuries often suffer acute metabolic consequences and become hypercatabolic. In these situations there is increased nitrogen excretion owing to altered protein metabolism. Severely stressed patients need more protein (with proportional increases in nonprotein calories) than conventional solutions can deliver. To meet increased nutritional needs, high metabolic stress formulas, which are similar to hepatic formulations, contain mixtures of essential and nonessential amino acids with high amounts of branched chain amino acids. Such products include Aminosyn-HBC,® 4% BranchAmin,® FreAmine HBC,® and Novamine™ 15%. Use of these products is contraindicated in anuria, severe uncorrected acid-base and electrolyte imbalances, and hepatic coma.

TOTAL PARENTERAL NUTRITION

Total parenteral nutrition (TPN) is the intravenous administration of hypertonic glucose (20% to 70%) and amino acids (3.5% to 15%), along with all the additional components required for complete nutritional support. It is indicated for long-term therapy to reverse the effects of severe weight loss (10% or more) and starvation, to promote normal metabolic function, and to support tissue repair and synthesis. It may be administered continuously over a 24-hour period or cyclically. With cyclic administration, the patient receives the bulk of his calories from the TPN during the evening and night hours. The

Patient ID:	123456	Created: 02-12-00
Patient name:	Doe, John	Updated: 02-15-00
Physician:	J. Luna, M.D.	Pharmacist: L. Clark, Pharm.D.
Order #:	5	

Infusion volume ordered:	3000 ml (3120 ml)
Infusion rate ordered:	125 ml/hr (130 ml/hr)
Infusion period ordered:	24.0 ordered
Overfill volume:	50 ml
Delivery time to patient:	On (mm/dd/yy): 02-16-03
	At (hh:mm) : 1600
Notes on bag label:	Protect from light
	Do not shake

Solution & Final Container Summaries (per liter)

Base solution totals:

Amino acids	10%	500 ml
Dextrose	70%	500 ml

Additive totals:

TPN electrolytes	20 ml
Multivitamins	10 ml
Folic acid	1 ml
Potassium phosphate	4 ml

Analysis:

Protein equivalent	50 g/L
Nitrogen	7.85 g/L
Calcium	4.5 mEq
Chloride	35 mEq
Magnesium	5 mEq
Potassium	40 mEq
Sodium	35 mEq
Phosphorus	12 nM
Total calories	1390 kcal/L
*Total volume	1040/8 hr

Figure 13-3 | Typical TPN formulation

remainder of the nutrients are taken in orally during the day. Cyclic therapy is usually reserved for relatively stable homebound patients. Figure 13-3 shows what a typical TPN formulation looks like.

Various formulas are used to determine individual requirements for TPN and weight-gain goals. When patients are malnourished, their ideal body weight is generally used to compute dietary requirements. Calories are estimated with the usual goal for the patient to achieve a steady weight increase of 0.5 to 1.0 kg (1.1 to 2.2 lbs.) per week. The Harris-Benedict equation is a reliable, easy-to-use calculation for estimating caloric needs and nutritional requirements (Figure 13-4). It takes into consideration the patient's age, gender, height, and weight. Calorimetry, which measures heat loss or gain and determines oxygen expenditure and carbon dioxide production, is also used to estimate calorie needs.

Administration Guidelines

Because of the hypertonic nature of TPN, it must be administered through a central venous catheter into the superior vena cava. All of the risks and precautions associated with a

Basal energy expenditure (BEE) formula:

Females: 65.5 + (9.6 x weight in kg)
+ (1.7 x height in cm)
- (4.7 x age)
= BEE
BEE x stress factor = total calories

Males: 66.0 + (13.7 x weight in kg)
+ (5.0 x height in cm)
- (6.8 x age)
= BEE
BEE x stress factor = total calories

Calorie needs are estimated by multiplying the BEE by a stress factor, using a stress factor scale.

Stress Factor Scale:
(Example)

1.1 : Lowest	1.6 : Lower limit of high
1.2 : (e.g., hospitalization)	1.7 :
1.3 :	1.8 :
1.4 :	1.9 :
1.5 : Upper limit of low	2.0 :
	2.1 :
	2.2 :
	2.3 :
	2.4 :
	2.5 : Highest stress factor level (such as severe burns or multiple trauma)

Figure 13-4 | The Harris-Benedict equation for estimating basal energy expenditure and caloric requirements

NURSING ALERT

Rapid Infusions of TPN

The rapid infusion of total parenteral nutrition can precipitate hyperosmolar diuresis, seizures, coma, and death.

NURSING TIP

Microbial Growth in TPN

Because of the high dextrose content in TPN, it is an ideal medium for microbial growth. For this reason, the CDC recommends that parenteral nutrition catheters not be used for anything other than the infusion of TPN (CDC, 2002).

Table 13-7 | Guidelines for the Administration of TPN

1.	The TPN catheter or CVC lumen is not to be used for anything other than the delivery of parenteral nutrition.
2.	Verify that the ordered infusate is correct for the patient. Check the expiration date and time.
3.	A container of TPN must not infuse beyond a 24-hour period. Be sure the next container is ready to hang before the previous one infuses. Should the next one not be ready, a 10% dextrose infusion to which 50% dextrose is added must be hung to prevent rebound hypoglycemia. Refrigerated TPN admixtures should be removed from refrigeration one hour before administration.
4.	When TPN is initiated, the infusion is to be introduced at a relatively slow rate (approximately 50 ml/hr) to preclude hyperglycemia. It is advisable to increase the rate in 25 ml/hr increments until the desired rate is established.
5.	The infusion must be maintained at the prescribed rate. Should it get behind schedule, do not "catch up," as this may precipitate hyperglycemia and metabolic complications. The infusion may be adjusted within no more than a 10% margin (up or down) of the original rate to compensate for any deviation in the infusion schedule. The rapid infusion of TPN can cause hyperosmolar diuresis, seizures, coma, and even death.
6.	TPN should be administered using an electronic infusion pump.
7.	The flow rate should be monitored at 30- to 60-minute intervals even if an EID is used.
8.	Vital signs should be monitored every 4 hours or more frequently.
9.	The patient needs to be weighed on a daily basis with strict intake and output monitoring. This is especially important in assessing for electrolyte imbalances and fluid overload.
10.	Adequate oral or enteral intake must be assessed prior to discontinuing TPN.
11.	Patients must be weaned off TPN once it is discontinued to prevent rebound hypoglycemia. This is usually done over a 24- to 48-hour period by gradually decreasing the volume of TPN while monitoring patient response.

central line pertain to the administration of TPN. Likewise, all the dressing change protocols and intricacies of care are applicable (see Chapter 12). The nurse who administers TPN is responsible for reviewing the patient's height, weight, nutritional status, diagnosis, and current laboratory values prior to administration. Table 13-7 lists several important nursing guidelines that must be followed when administering TPN. Although the TPN solutions are susceptible to microbial growth because of their high dextrose content, most infections that occur during TPN administration result from catheter contamination (CDC, 2002).

PERIPHERAL PARENTERAL NUTRITION

Peripheral parenteral nutrition (PPN) consists of a 2% to 5% crystalline amino acid preparation with 5% to 10% dextrose mixed with electrolytes and micronutrients. Fat emulsions (10% to 20%) are usually combined, but may be given separately.

PPN is usually indicated for patients who need a complete nutrient source but are not depleted nor need to gain weight. It is generally used for fairly stable patients needing short-term therapy lasting less than three to four weeks. It is most commonly used for fairly stable patients whose normal gastrointestinal functioning will soon be reestablished. Such patients must also be able to tolerate the relatively high fluid volume that allows for the delivery of about 2,000 cal/day.

PREPARATION OF PARENTERAL NUTRITION

Rigorous asepsis in the care of the patient, catheter, and catheter site has been shown to reduce greatly the incidence of parenteral nutrition-related infections. The centralized preparation of TPN and PPN using a laminar air flow hood has generally been regarded as the safest method of preparation. Laminar flow hoods are designed to decrease the risk of airborne contamination during infusate admixing by supplying an ultraclean environment. The CDC recommends that the admixture of all routine parenteral fluids be done in the pharmacy with a laminar flow hood using aseptic technique (CDC, 2002).

The major advantage of using a laminar air flow hood is its high-efficiency, bacteria-retentive filter commonly called a HEPA (high-efficiency particulate air) filter (Figure 13-5).

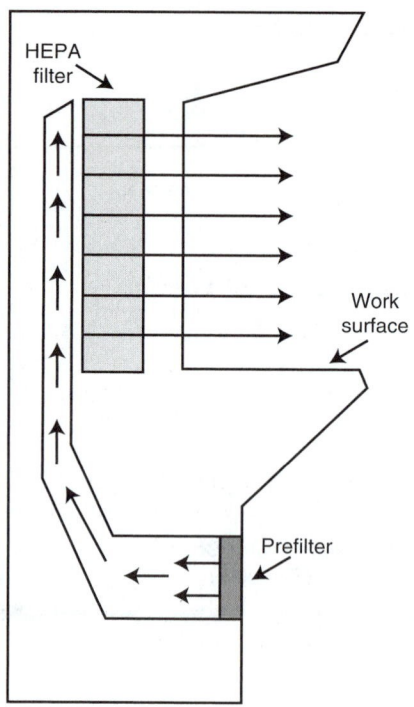

Figure 13-5 | Laminar air flow hood (side view) and high-efficiency particulate air (HEPA) filter.

Room air is taken into the unit and passed through a prefilter to remove relatively large contaminants such as dust and lint. The air is then compressed and channeled up, behind, and through the HEPA filter, where virtually all bacteria are removed. The purified air then flows out over the entire work surface area in parallel lines at a uniform velocity. The laminar flow hood promotes an environment that is practically devoid of airborne contaminants.

COMPOUNDING PARENTERAL NUTRITION FORMULAS

The compounding of parenteral nutrition products is a complex operation involving the preparation and admixing of base solutions and numerous additives. Extensive calculations are involved to determine the combination of the macronutrients and micronutrients. In addition, it must be remembered that some electrolytes may be incompatible when combined in high concentrations. Certain electrolytes, such as calcium or magnesium, when combined with phosphate must be maximally diluted and thoroughly mixed before adding them to base solutions or precipitation may occur. The order of mixing is extremely important when preparing parenteral nutrition admixtures that contain fat emulsions. The dextrose and fat emulsion should never be

Who Is Legally Responsible?

As a nurse you know that it is your professional responsibility to administer drugs and parenteral nutrition preparations in a safe manner, following correct and appropriate medical orders and institutional protocols. You must know what you are giving to a patient and follow the Five Rights of medication administration in all circumstances.

You also know that parenteral nutrition formulations are compounded by registered pharmacists. What is your legal status if you unknowingly administer an IV nutrition formula that a pharmacist labels as correct for your patient but, in fact, is incorrect and your patient suffers untoward effects? Who is to blame? You? The pharmacist? Is it a shared liability? Think about it. You need to know the answer to this dilemma.

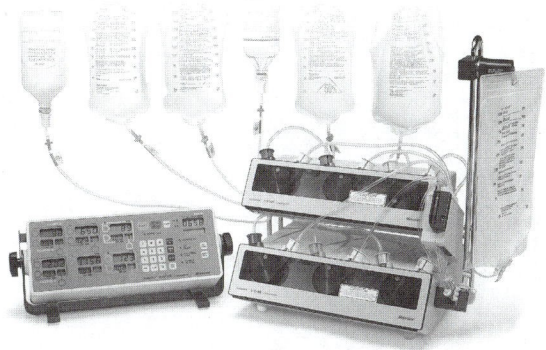

Figure 13-6 | The Accusource Monitoring System
Courtesy of the Baxter Healthcare Corporation

directly combined. The order of mixing should be to add the amino acid to the fat, then to add the dextrose. Two methods are used to compound parenteral nutrition admixtures. One is the gravity method and the other is automated mixing.

Gravity Method of Compounding Parenteral Admixtures

In the gravity method of compounding admixtures a special empty plastic bag with a pre-attached multiple-lead Y-type transfer set is used. Each lead of the transfer set is connected to a different macronutrient, and the required volume of each enters the bag, using the control flow clamp on each lead. After the specified volume of solution is transferred from each of the macronutrient containers, the clamps are closed and the transfer tubings are sealed with a special metal clamping device.

Automated Method of Compounding Parenteral Admixtures

In agencies where the pharmacy prepares large volumes of parenteral admixtures on a regular basis, high-speed compounders are often used. These computerized systems are able to efficiently process complex nutrition support preparations accurately and safely. An example of such a system is

the Accusource Monitoring System, which is designed for use under a laminar flow hood and consists of two principal parts, the pump module and the control module. The pump has six hangers for six source containers, pump rotors that sequentially pump solution from the source containers to the final container, and a hanger for the final solution container (Figure 13-6).

Some pharmacies have incorporated the use of a quality assurance feature into their automated compounding system to verify that the correct source solution container is attached to the correct lead of the transfer set. The lead of the transfer set and the source solution container both have small bar code labels attached that can be scanned with a hand-held laser. Whenever the system detects a mismatch, it sounds an audible alarm, displays an on-screen warning message, and locks up until a supervisory level password is entered. Scanning operations are logged with user identification, time, and date and can be viewed on-screen or uploaded to a personal computer.

In addition to automated macronutrient compounders, which mix base solutions, some now add electrolytes, trace elements, and drug additives. These machines save the pharmacist significant time and eliminate the need to prepare each drug additive in a syringe and have it checked by a pharmacist before adding it to the solution. They enhance safety and speed while eliminating the chance that syringes will get mixed up during preparation. They also minimize the potential for precipitate formation by automatically programming in a rinse between incompatible additives. The Micromix® Compounder is an example of such a device (Figure 13-7). It is capable of transferring to a final container selected volumes between 0.3 ml and 650 ml from up to 10 source containers.

RISKS AND COMPLICATIONS ASSOCIATED WITH PARENTERAL NUTRITION ADMINISTRATION

In addition to all of the risks and complications associated with the placement of peripheral or central venous access devices, there are special problems specific to parenteral nutrition. These include metabolic alterations; electrolyte, mineral, and vitamin imbalances; nutritional deficiencies; and abnormalities in hepatic and pulmonary function (Table 13-8). Most of the complications are usually avoidable or manageable if they are recognized promptly.

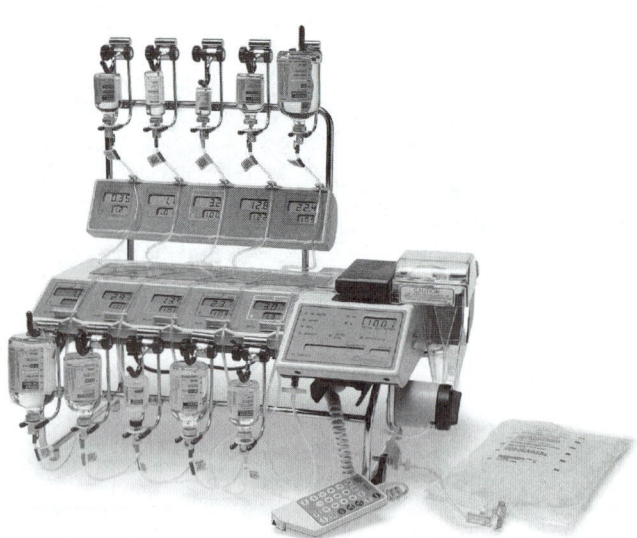

Figure 13-7 | The Micromix Compounder
Courtesy of the Baxter Healthcare Corporation

N U R S I N G   A L E R T

Administration of Parenteral Nutrition

It is critical that the nurse know and understand the potential complications regarding the administration of parenteral nutrition formulations so that she can assess for them and intervene in an appropriate and timely manner should they occur.

Table 13-8 | Risks and Complications Associated with Parenteral Nutrition Administration

I. Altered Metabolism

A. Acid-Base Imbalances

1. Metabolic Acidosis

Etiology: $\downarrow$ pH & $\downarrow$ plasma bicarbonate concentration from ketoacidosis in diabetes, lactic acidosis due to tissue hypoxia, uremia

Defining Characteristics: Confusion, headache, $\uparrow$ respiratory rate & depth, N/V, warm & flushed skin, $\downarrow$ pH, $\downarrow$ HCO$_3$, $\uparrow$ serum chloride, $\uparrow$ serum bicarbonate

Interventions: $\downarrow$ acetate in TPN, treat ketoacidosis

Evaluation (Prevention): Accurate I & O, specific gravity, CO$_2$, Na, & K

2. Metabolic Alkalosis

Etiology: Hypokalemia, vomiting or gastric suction, respiratory acidosis with inadequate ventilation and low renal compensation, Cushing's syndrome, hyperaldosteronism

Defining Characteristics: Circumoral paresthesia, carpopedal spasm, muscle hypertonia, depressed respirations, hypokalemia, vertigo, hypercapnia, $\downarrow$ serum chloride (relatively lower than Na level), $\uparrow$ serum bicarbonate level

Interventions: $\downarrow$ acetate, administer NH$_4$Cl, improve ventilation with bronchodilators, antibiotics, hydration

Evaluation (Prevention): Monitor CO$_2$, Cl, & K

B. Altered Glucose Metabolism

1. Hypoglycemia (rebound)

Etiology: abrupt cessation of TPN

Defining Characteristics: Diaphoresis, irritability, nervousness, shakiness

Interventions: Administer dextrose or decrease insulin; maintain IV at constant rate

Evaluation (Prevention): Maintain steady rate of infusion, wean gradually when discontinuing

2. Hyperglycemia

Etiology: CHO intolerance, insulin resistance, rapid TPN delivery, diabetes, sepsis, traumatic stress

Defining Characteristics: $\uparrow$ serum glucose, acetone (fruity) breath odor, anxiety, confusion, dehydration, polydipsia, polyuria, malaise

Table 13-8 | (continued)

Interventions: ↓ dextrose TPN concentration or ↓ rate, administer insulin per sliding scale

Evaluation (Prevention): Accurate glucose monitoring, gradual TPN rate increase, & stable TPN infusion rate

3. **Hyperglycemic Hyperosmolar Nonketotic Coma**

Etiology: Rapid TPN administration

Defining Characteristics: Confusion, coma, dehydration, ↑ serum glucose, lethargy, seizures, hypokalemia (which decreases insulin release), hypophosphatemia and thiamine or B_6 deficiency

Interventions: d.c. dextrose; give insulin & 0.45% NaCl

Evaluation (Prevention): Monitor serum chemistry, electrolytes, glucose, osmolarity

C. **Altered Hydration**

1. **Dehydration**

Etiology: Excessive fluid loss or inadequate fluid intake

Defining Characteristics: Dry, hot, flushed skin, intense thirst, confusion, oliguria or anuria, N/V

Interventions: Fluid administration

Evaluation (Prevention): Accurate assessment of skin turgor, accurate I & O, sodium, BUN, & hematocrit levels

2. **Overhydration**

Etiology: Excessive fluid intake

Defining Characteristics: Weight gain, increased sodium load, dyspnea, neck vein distention

Interventions: Diuretics, reduce fluid intake

Evaluation (Prevention): Accurate I & O, daily weights, daily BUN, serum sodium, & hematocrit levels

D. **Serum Ammonia Elevations**

Etiology: Liver disease where ammonia is shunted past the liver and accumulates in the blood

Defining Characteristics: Asterixis (flapping tremor), lethargy, neurologic changes, altered EKG, vomiting, coma

Interventions: Limit protein intake, enemas, and antibiotics to prevent growth of ammonia-producing bacteria in intestines

Evaluation (Prevention): Accurate monitoring of serum ammonia levels, protein limitation

E. **Serum Urea Elevations**

Etiology: Renal insufficiency, circulation disturbances, fluid imbalances, or altered protein metabolism (where there is retention of nitrogenous substances normally excreted by the kidneys)

Defining Characteristics: ↑ serum urea levels, vertigo, headache, N/V, convulsions, coma, odor of urine on breath and skin, uremic frost, dry skin, tachycardia, ↑ BP, oliguria (with albumin casts), anuria

Interventions: Decrease protein intake, cation exchange resins to increase potassium excretion from the bowel, calcium gluconate, sodium bicarbonate, dialysis

Evaluation (Prevention): Accurate monitoring of BUN and serum chemistry levels, restrict protein intake

II. **Altered Electrolyte Balance**

A. **Calcium**

1. **Hypocalcemia**

Etiology: Vitamin D deficiency, insufficient calcium or magnesium intake, malabsorption, hyperphosphatemia, malnutrition, hypoparathyroidism, pancreatitis

Defining Characteristics: CNS irritability, confusion, circumoral tingling/numbness, muscle cramps in extremities, abdominal muscle spasms, laryngeal spasm, serum Ca levels ↓ 8.5 mg/dl, dehydration, hyperglycemia, glucosuria, polydipsia, polyuria, positive Chvostek's & Trousseau's signs, seizures, tetany

Interventions: Supplement TPN with calcium or IV calcium supplementation, correct magnesium & phosphate deficiencies

Evaluation (Prevention): Accurate serum chemistry levels, avoidance of calcium-depleting medications, maintain adequate calcium & vitamin D intake

2. **Hypercalcemia**

Etiology: Excessive replacement, inactivity, prolonged immobility, hyperparathyroidism, pancreatic disease, neoplasia, stress

Defining Characteristics: Anorexia, constipation, itching, reduced neuromuscular excitability, N/V, polydipsia, polyuria, reduced sense of pain and vibration

Interventions: Reduce replacement in TPN, isotonic saline to dilute serum calcium and promote renal excretion, furosemide, calcitonin, corticosteroids, mobilization, inorganic phosphate administration

Evaluation (Prevention): Prevention

(continues)

Table 13-8 | (continued)

B. Potassium

  1. Hypokalemia

    Etiology: Alkalosis (due to the temporary shift of K into the cells), GI losses, diuretic therapy, TPN, hyperaldosteronism, steroid administration, osmotic diuresis, heavy diaphoresis, anorexia, alcoholism, debilitation

    Defining Characteristics: Serum K ↓ 3.5 mEq/L, ↓ serum osmolality, slight serum glucose elevation (due to insulin suppression), anorexia, fatigue, muscle weakness, decreased gastric motility, postural hypotension, PACs & PVCs, EKG changes, polydipsia, polyuria, increased sensitivity to digitalis

    Interventions: TPN supplementation, replace GI losses

    Evaluation (Prevention): Prevention is the best treatment since hypokalemia can be life threatening; monitor serum electrolyte levels, strict I & O, and assess for digitalis toxicity

  2. Hyperkalemia

    Etiology: Renal impairment, iatrogenic-induced, TPN, metabolic & respiratory acidosis where K shifts out of the cells, tissue damage (burns, crushing injuries), malignant cell lysis following chemotherapy

    Defining Characteristics: Serum K levels ↑ 5.5 mEq/L, acidosis, EKG changes, ventricular dysrhythmias, cardiac arrest, muscular weakness, flaccid muscular paralysis, paresthesia of face, mouth, hands, and feet, nausea, intestinal colic/diarrhea

    Interventions: Reduce TPN volume of K, cation exchange resins, dialysis

    Evaluation (Prevention): Accurate monitoring of serum K & Na levels, accurate I & O

C. Sodium

  1. Hyponatremia

    Etiology: Decreased intake, excessive dextrose/water administration during periods of stress, GI losses, excessive diaphoresis, adrenal insufficiency, osmotic diuresis, head trauma, stroke, pulmonary disorders, syndrome of inappropriate antidiuretic hormone (SIADH)

    Defining Characteristics: Serum Na ↓ 135 mEq/L, urine Na ↓ 10 mEq/L, ↓ specific gravity, anorexia, confusion and dulling of sensorium, muscle cramps, exertion-induced dyspnea, lethargy, ataxia, hemiparesis, Babinski's sign, seizures, coma

    Interventions: Sodium administration, increasing gradually

    Evaluation (Prevention): Monitor serum electrolytes, urine specific gravity, and I & O, assess for CNS alterations

  2. Hypernatremia

    Etiology: Water deprivation or loss (especially insensible losses), excessive TPN administration, profuse diaphoresis, diabetes insipidus, vomiting, diarrhea

    Defining Characteristics: Serum Na ↑ 145 mEq/L, urine specific gravity ↑ 1.015, serum osmolality ↑ 295 mOsm/kg, thirst, elevated temperature, dry, swollen tongue with sticky mucous membranes, lethargic when undisturbed but hyper-reactive when stimulated, disorientation, hallucinations

    Interventions: Gradually decrease serum sodium levels to prevent cerebral edema (as rapid reduction results in temporary plasma hyposmolality [to the cerebral fluid because of the blood-brain barrier] allowing water to osmose into the brain tissue

    Evaluation (Prevention): Monitor serum electrolytes, I & O, assess for insensitive water losses

D. Magnesium

  1. Hypomagnesemia

    Etiology: Alcohol withdrawal, GI losses, refeeding after starvation, drug-induced osmotic diuresis, diabetic ketoacidosis, renal disease, pancreatitis

    Defining Characteristics: Apprehension, depression, apathy, neuromuscular hyperexcitability with muscular weakness, tremors, and athetoid movements, PVCs, supraventricular tachycardia, ventricular fibrillation

    Interventions: Parenteral supplementation

    Evaluation (Prevention): Monitor serum electrolytes and assess neuromuscular status, as deficiencies of magnesium are largely confined to the neuromuscular system. *Note:* Hypomagnesemia is a common imbalance in critically ill and less acutely ill patients. It is often overlooked or is confused with potassium deficits.

  2. Hypermagnesemia

    Etiology: Excessive administration, renal failure (most common cause), ECF volume depletion, untreated diabetic ketoacidosis

    Defining Characteristics: If mild, there are no symptoms; serum Mg levels between 3 and 5 mEq/L; assess for mild hypotention, facial flushing, N/V; serum Mg levels between 5 and 7: assess for drowsiness, dysarthria, lethargy; serum Mg levels ↑ 7 mEq/L; assess for neuromuscular blockade, respiratory depression, apnea, coma, cardiac arrest

    Interventions: Prevention, dialysis with a magnesium-free dialysate

    Evaluation (Prevention): Monitor serum electrolytes and BP

E. Phosphorus

  1. Hypophosphatemia

    Etiology: TPN supplementation without adequate phosphorus replacement, burns, malabsorptive states and starvation, hypomagnesemia, glucose administration, calorie administration in patients with severe protein-calorie malnutrition, respiratory alkalosis, alcohol withdrawal, diabetic ketoacidosis

Table 13-8 | (continued)

Defining Characteristics: Signs and symptoms result from inadequate ATP (for cellular energy) and/or 2,3-DPG (for tissue O_2 transport). There may be apprehension, irritability, paresthesias, seizures, congestive cardiomyopathy, ↓ RBCs, muscle weakness, respiratory depression, insulin resistance.

Interventions: IV supplementation in the TPN

Evaluation (Prevention): Monitor serum magnesium levels

   2. Hyperphosphatemia

   Etiology: Excessive amounts in TPN, renal disease, chemotherapy for neoplasia, muscle necrosis, excessive vitamin D supplementation, hypoparathyroidism

   Defining Characteristics: Minimal symptomatology until long-term increases are sustained, at which time soft tissue calcification, hypocalcemia, and tetany may be present. If short-term effects occur, there may be numbness and tingling of the mouth and fingers and muscle spasms.

   Interventions: TPN restriction and treatment of underlying disorder

   Evaluation (Prevention): Monitor serum levels, do not administer to renal failure patients, monitor for symptoms of tingling around mouth and fingertips, and assess for muscle cramping

III. Altered Nutrition

   A. Essential Fatty Acid Deficiency (EFAD)

   Etiology: Deficient intake

   Defining Characteristics: ↑ BUN, alopecia, dry, cracked skin with dermatitis, CNS aberrations, pulmonary dysfunction

   Interventions: Fat emulsion supplementation in TPN or with intermittent infusions

   Evaluation (Prevention): Accurate calculation of protein, fat, and CHO ratios to maintain positive nitrogen balance

   B. Refeeding Syndrome

   Refeeding syndrome is a complication that can occur during the initial phases of parenteral nutrition administration. It occurs because the body, during its bout with starvation, has adapted somewhat to nutritional deprivation (compensating by decreasing basal energy requirements). The initiation of nutritional support, especially if it is undertaken too aggressively, can result in an electrolyte shift from the plasma to the intracellular fluid. This can be very dangerous, even fatal, due to cardiorespiratory complications. The result of refeeding syndrome may be manifested as follows:

   1. **Edema** because the process of rehydration causes a dilution of serum albumin, thus reducing the oncotic pulling force that the hemoconcentrated albumin has been providing

   2. **Hypernatremia** due to the release of sodium into the ECF to counteract extracellular ion losses

   3. **Hypokalemia** because potassium is shifted into the ICF (which may be further intensified with insulin administration), which enhances potassium and phosphate shifting

   4. **Hypomagnesemia**, shifted into the ICF (like phosphorus and potassium) during TPN

   5. **Hypophosphatemia** because, as protein synthesis begins, phosphate is shifted into the ICF as a component of ATP (which is needed for cellular energy)

   Once the body has reestablished normal albumin and electrolyte balances, the refeeding processes are reversed. Refeeding syndrome can often be averted by initiating TPN slowly, and gradually increasing the rate, while carefully monitoring the patient's response and serum electrolyte levels.

IV. Altered Mineral Balance (Deficiencies)

   Imbalances are usually the result of deficiencies, the etiologies being malnourishment/starvation and insufficient supplementation in the parenteral nutrition source. Treatment interventions are directed at supplying adequate supplementation.

   A. Chromium Deficiency

   Defining Characteristics: Elevated serum lipid levels, insulin resistance, glucose intolerance

   B. Copper Deficiency

   Defining Characteristics: Hypochromic microcytic anemia, neutropenia, loss of skin pigmentation

   C. Iron Deficiency

   Defining Characteristics: Fatigue, glossitis, stomatitis, hypochromic microcytic anemia

   D. Manganese Deficiency

   Defining Characteristics: CNS aberrations

   E. Selenium Deficiency

   Defining Characteristics: Cardiomyopathies

   F. Zinc Deficiency

   Defining Characteristics: Alopecia, apathy, confusion, depression, diarrhea, altered wound healing, taste aberrations

V. Altered Vitamin Balance (Deficiencies)

   Disease processes can alter vitamin requirements, and parenteral nutrition must supply the needed fat-soluble and water-soluble vitamin supplements. During illness, vitamin deficiencies can produce serious consequences for which the nurse must assess.

(continues)

Table 13-8 | (continued)

A. Fat-Soluble Vitamin Deficiencies

1. **Vitamin A:** Dry, scaly, rough, cracked skin with hardened mucous membranes, decreased saliva secretion and anorexia, impaired digestion and absorption; diarrhea

2. **Vitamin D:** $\downarrow$ serum calcium and/or phosphorus levels, $\uparrow$ alkaline phosphatase, relaxation of abdominal muscles and protrusion of the abdomen, involuntary spasms and twitching

3. **Vitamin E:** RBC hemolysis

4. **Vitamin K:** Delayed clotting and hemorrhage

B. Water-Soluble Vitamin Deficiencies

1. **Vitamin B_1 (thiamine):** $\uparrow$ serum and urine lactate/pyruvate levels, anorexia, confusion, edema, fatigue, muscle weakness, painful calf muscles, cardiomegaly, heart failure

2. **Vitamin B_2 (riboflavin):** Cheilosis, glossitis, stomatitis, dermatitis, photophobia, corneal redness

3. **Vitamin B_3 (niacin):** Dermatitis, glossitis, diarrhea, dementia

4. **Vitamin B_6 (pyridoxine):** Abnormal EEG, anemia, carpal-tunnel syndrome aggravation, cheilosis, glossitis, dermatitis, convulsions

5. **Vitamin B_{12} (cobalamin):** Anorexia, ataxia, depression, dyspnea, irritability, memory lapses, glossitis, diarrhea or constipation, pallor, paresthesias of hands/feet, delirium, hallucinations

6. **Folic Acid:** Macrocytic anemia, diarrhea, glossitis

7. **Vitamin C:** Anemia, bleeding gums, petechiae, depression

VI. Altered Hepatic Function

Indicators of hepatic problems are detected with elevated serum bilirubin, lactate dehydrogenase, and transaminase levels. When such problems present themselves, it is usually advisable to use hepatic parenteral nutrition formulations. Fatty liver may develop if surplus carbohydrates are administered in excess of the liver's ability to handle them.

Key Concepts

✳ Intravenous nutritional products are complex admixtures that provide a partial or complete source of nourishment for patients who are unable to ingest or utilize sufficient calories and nutrients to sustain metabolic functions.

✳ Parenteral nutrition is composed of water, carbohydrates, dextrose, amino acids, lipids, electrolytes, multivitamins, and minerals, all formulated to meet individual patient needs and to comply with restrictions imposed by fluid balance and various disease processes.

✳ The indications for parenteral nutrition support include the following:

– Catabolic states

– Chronic weight loss (even with adequate oral intake)

– Conditions requiring bowel rest

– Excessive nitrogen loss

– Hepatic or renal failure

– Hypermetabolic states

– Malabsorptive states

– Malnutrition

– Multiple trauma

– Serum albumin levels below 3.5 g/dl

✳ Parenteral nutrition is contraindicated in patients who have the following:

– Catheter-related complications

– Coagulopathies

– Local and systemic complications associated with central line placement

– Gastrointestinal tracts that should resume normal functioning patterns within 7 to 10 days

– Functional gastrointestinal tracts

- – A poor prognosis

- – Superior vena cava thrombosis

- – Terminal illness when all therapy has been discontinued

✳ Stressors, such as burns, surgical interventions, infection, and trauma, have a tremendous influence on the nutritional status of the body and can greatly increase caloric and nutritional requirements. Stressors induce neuroendocrine-mediated changes in the body that serve as life-preserving mechanisms in an attempt to return the body to a state of homeostasis. When the stressors are great enough, the body cannot compensate on its own, and parenteral nutrition is often indicated.

✳ The nurse must have a basic understanding of the nutritional requirements of the body in health and disease.

✳ Total parenteral nutrition (TPN) is the intravenous administration of hypertonic glucose (20% to 70%) and amino acids (3.5% to 15%), along with all the additional components required for complete nutri-tional support and is delivered through a central venous catheter situated in the superior vena cava. It is delivered continuously or cyclically.

✳ Peripheral parenteral nutrition (PPN), indicated for patients who need a complete nutrient source (but are not depleted), consists of a 2% to 5% crystalline amino acid preparation with 5% to 10% dextrose mixed with electrolytes and micronutrients. Fat emulsions of 10% to 20% may be combined or administered separately. Since it is only mildly hypertonic it may be administered via a large peripheral vein rather than a central vessel.

✳ Parenteral nutrition preparations should be compounded in a contaminant-free aseptic environment such as that provided by a laminar air flow hood.

✳ The nurse must have a full understanding of the risks and complications associated with the administration of parenteral nutrition so that untoward occurrences can be prevented or promptly identified should they develop. These include catheter-related and infection or sepsis problems, as well as those associated with metabolic, electrolyte, and nutritional imbalances.

Review Questions and Activities

Develop an ongoing nursing care plan using the following information.

1. Mr. Van Kirk is a 67-year-old retired mail carrier (40+ years) who has been receiving TPN via a triple-lumen Hickman® CVC for 4 days following a partial bowel resection for colon cancer (metastatic prostate malignancy). He is NPO with a Salem sump in place for gastric decompression. He has a Foley catheter in place and has a transverse colostomy.

2. Based on the preceding information and a pre-illness height of 5'10" and a weight of 186 lbs. calculate what might be an appropriate TPN replacement regimen for this patient postoperatively.

3. On the sixth postoperative day, Mr. Van Kirk develops fever and hyperglycemia with serum glucose levels ranging between 400 and 700 mg/dl. His BUN is 60 mg/dl. He is polyuric and polydipsic. Skin and mucous membranes are dry and he is experiencing fatigue and muscular weakness.

4. Within 24 hours, Mr. Van Kirk becomes septic. He becomes hypotensive and confused. He develops tachycardia and is hyperventilating. How will this influence his care and TPN requirements?

Blood and Blood Product Administration

Upon completion of this chapter, the reader should be able to:

✳ Review the basic concepts of immunology in terms of antigens, antibodies, and the immune response.

✳ Explain the basic components of immunohematology as they relate to blood grouping, the Rh factor, and the histocompatibility antigens.

✳ Identify the indications for and the administration protocols for the following blood and blood components:

– Whole blood

– Red blood cells

– Platelets

– Granulocytes

– Fresh frozen plasma

– Cryoprecipitate

– Colloid infusions, albumin, and plasma protein fraction

– Immune globulins

✳ Differentiate among the volume expanders available and their indications for use.

✳ Discuss the transfusion and blood salvaging options available to patients.

✳ Categorize the signs and symptoms of transfusion reactions as they relate to each body system for both the conscious and unconscious patient.

✳ Outline the signs and symptoms for the acute transfusion reactions that can occur and the appropriate treatment for each.

– Acute hemolytic

– Anaphylactic

– Circulatory overload

– Febrile, non-hemolytic

– Mild allergic

– Sepsis

✳ Outline the signs and symptoms for the delayed transfusion reactions that can occur and the treatment for each.

– Delayed hemolytic

– Graft versus host disease

– Hepatitis B

– Hepatitis C

– HIV-1 (AIDS virus) infection

– Iron overload

– Others that may occur

✳ Describe the nursing protocols involved in the administration, maintenance, and monitoring of transfusions.

✳ Review the documentation used by the nurse when administering transfusions.

KEY TERMS

acute normovolemic hemodilution	centrifuging	immunogen
agglutination	constant portion	indirect homologous donation
agglutinin	crossmatching	isoantigen
agglutinogen	epitope	leukopenia
allele	filtration	lyophilization
alloimmunization	freezing	major crossmatching
antibody	genotype	minor crossmatching
antigen	hemostasis	polymorphonuclear
antigenic determinant	histocompatibility	universal donor
autologous	homologous	universal recipient
autologous blood	homologous blood	variable portion
blood salvage	humor	washing
blood typing	immune response	
buffy coat	immunity	

Transfusion therapy is a major multidisciplinary health care responsibility with a myriad of significant implications. Such therapy is initiated, maintained, monitored, and discontinued by the RN, who is expected to be fully competent in all aspects of its protocols and care. Transfusion therapy is the injection of blood or blood products into the bloodstream.

BASIC IMMUNOLOGY

The human immune system is composed of all the cells, tissues, organs, and physiologic processes used to protect the body from harm by invading organisms. **Immunity** is the state or condition in which an individual is protected from disease. The **immune response** is the ability of the immune system to recognize and respond to foreign invaders and prevent damage by either neutralizing or eliminating them. For this to occur, the body must be able to recognize self from nonself. An **antigen** or **immunogen** is a molecular agent that is able to elicit an immune response by combining with an antibody. An **antibody** is an immunoglobulin (Ig) molecule that develops in response to an antigen that enters the system and combines with it. When an immune response occurs, an antibody does not attack the entire molecule, but combines with a portion of the antigen called an **epitope** or **antigenic determinant**.

Within the cell surfaces of the human body are various protein and glycoprotein properties that are genetically determined. With the exception of monozygotic twins, these surface substances are genetically different in all human beings. This is why when the cells of one person are introduced into the body of another (such as with blood and tissue grafts and transplanted organs) incompatibilities exist and rejection can occur.

BASIC IMMUNOHEMATOLOGY

Within each human being there is a unique combination of genes called a **genotype**. This determines a person's propensity for certain traits. The genetic differences among people occur because of the variations in cell surface composition. This concept forms the basis for blood compatibility between humans. The nurse "should have knowledge and understanding of immunohematology, blood grouping, blood and its components. . . ." (INS, 2000, Standard 75, *S*71).

Red Blood Cells

An **isoantigen** (alloantigen) is a substance that can stimulate antibody production when introduced into members of the same species. Blood groups are based on the isoantigens that are present on the surfaces of human red blood cells (RBCs). Although there are many isoantigen groups (as many as 30 common ones and hundreds of rarer ones have been identified), the two most significant are the ABO system and the Rh system. These groups are, more than any others, likely to precipitate blood transfusion reactions because of their cell surface composition (Figure 14-1).

Blood Groups

In a large percentage of the human population, two related antigens, A and B, occur on the surface of RBCs. Some people have only A antigens, some only B, some have both A and B, and some don't have either one. Those individuals with only A antigens are blood type A (41%) and those with only B antigens are blood type B (12%). If both antigens are present, the blood type is AB (3%). If neither A nor B antigens exists on the RBC surface, the person is blood type O (44%).

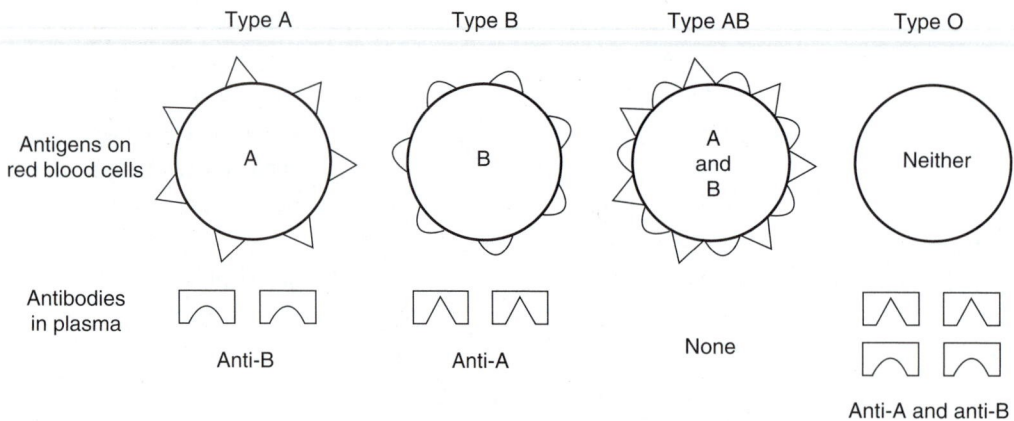

Figure 14-1 | ABO blood types.

Gene O does not have the genetic information needed to make any antigenic combination.

Individuals whose RBCs have neither A nor B antigens usually have in their plasma antibodies that react specifically with the A or B antigen on the surface of RBCs. This antigen-antibody response causes **agglutination**, or the clumping together of the solid antigen and the soluble antibody. For this reason, A and B antigens are categorized as **agglutinogens**. The plasma of the person who does not have A or B antigens has strong plasma antibodies that react with A or B antigens and are responsible for agglutination. Such antibodies are called **agglutinins**. Agglutinins are gamma globulin molecules (usually IgG or IgM). They attach to antigens on RBCs, causing them to agglutinate. Agglutinins are minimally present during fetal development but form almost entirely during postnatal life. They are genetically determined, so they don't require exposure to an antigen to be created.

Anti-A agglutinins form in the plasma of an individual when type A agglutinogens are not present on the surface of his RBCs. Likewise, anti-B agglutinins develop in the plasma of someone whose RBC surfaces do not have type B agglutinogens attached to them. The person with blood type O has both anti-A and anti-B agglutinins, even though he has no A or B agglutinogens. It is theorized that this occurs because sometime after birth, A and B antigens are introduced into the body in food, bacteria, or other unknown ways, and initiate the formation of anti-A and anti-B agglutinins. Blood type A has A agglutinogens and anti-B agglutinins, type B has B agglutinogens and anti-A agglutinins, and type AB has A and B agglutinogens, but no agglutinins (Table 14-1).

The major difference between the ABO and Rh systems is that, in the ABO system, the agglutinins that precipitate a transfusion reaction can develop spontaneously, whereas in the Rh system, the person must have a massive exposure to the Rh antigen before enough agglutinins will cause a significant reaction.

Every person has two genes (genotypes) that decide his blood type. These pairs determine one of four blood types, A,

Table 14-2 | Blood Types Determined by Genotypes

Genotype	Blood Type
AA	A
AO	A
BB	B
BO	B
AB	AB
OO	O

B, AB, or O. Because of this pairing, the genotypes may be AA, AO, BB, BO, AB, or OO. AA and AO genotypes produce type A blood, BB and BO generate type B blood, AB propagates type AB blood, and genotype OO produces type O blood (Table 14-2).

Rh Factor (Factor D)

The Rh (D) antigen is a component of the Rh blood groups and is made up of numerous complex antigens. When the Rh factor is present on the surface of RBCs, a person is designated as Rh^+ (Rh-positive). If it is not present, the person is Rh^- (Rh-negative). In African-Americans, approximately 95% are Rh^+ with the rest Rh^-, Native Africans are virtually 100% Rh^+. About 85% of all Caucasians are Rh^+, with the remaining 15% Rh^- (Guyton & Hall, 2000). Rh (D) is a powerful antigen, even though it is much less profuse on the RBC surface than A or B antigens. Antibodies (agglutinins) are not present in the plasma of Rh^+ or Rh^- blood. An Rh^- person must only be transfused with Rh^- blood, to avoid the formation of antibodies to Rh^+ blood. The Rh^+ patient may receive either Rh^+ or Rh^- blood.

When an Rh^- person receives Rh^+ blood for the first time, there is usually no reaction, but antibodies slowly begin to develop (over a two-week to four-month period). If he receives another transfusion, the Rh antibodies (agglutinins) will agglutinate (clump with the Rh antigens [agglutinogens] of the blood being transfused).

Table 14-1 | Blood Types and the Corresponding Agglutinogens and Agglutinins

Blood Type	Agglutino-gens	Aggluti-nins
A	A	Anti-B
B	B	Anti-A
AB	A & B	None
O	None	Anti-A Anti-B

NURSING ALERT

ABO Incompatibility

ABO incompatibility is the major immediate cause of fatal transfusion reactions because of antibody formation against the missing A antigen, B antigen, or both.

NURSING TIP

Antibody Production

Under normal circumstances, there must be exposure to red blood cell antigens (agglutinogens) via transfusion or pregnancy in order for antibodies (agglutinins) to be produced. This is not the case with A and B antigens, because some proteins in the environment are structurally similar to the A and B antigens.

Histocompatibility Antigens

Histocompatibility is the condition in which the tissue of a donor is compatible with that of the recipient. Histocompatibility antigens are present on most cell surfaces, the most potent ones being the major histocompatibility antigens and the weaker ones being the minor histocompatibility antigens.

The major histocompatibility antigens are the human leukocyte antigens (HLA) that are genetically controlled clusters of genes found on chromosome 6. This HLA cluster of genes, called the major histocompatibility complex (MHC), is distributed over six sites (loci) on chromosome 6, with three MHC on each pair (and each with a different code). They are HLA-A, HLA-B, HLA-C, HLA-DP, HLA-DQ, and HLA-DR. Each site has many **alleles,** forms of the gene. Of the known alleles at the six loci, over 200 million genotypes are conceivable. For this reason it is unlikely that any two individuals (except for monozygote identical twins) would be histocompatible. The HLA-A, HLA-B, and HLA-C clusters are classified as 1 HLA because they are found on all nucleated cells and platelets in the body. They play a vital role in tissue transplantation.

BLOOD TYPING AND CROSSMATCHING

Before a transfusion can be administered, it is critical to ascertain and correctly match compatibility between the blood types of the donor and the recipient. This process is referred to as blood typing and crossmatching (T & C). **Blood typing** is the test run on a person's blood, according to specified protocols, to determine what her blood type is. **Crossmatching** is the process in which compatibility between the blood of donor and the recipient is determined. **Minor crossmatching** tests for compatibility by mixing the donor's serum and the recipient's blood. **Major crossmatching** consists of mixing the donor's RBCs and the recipient's serum. Blood is typed, crossmatched,

---

NURSING ALERT

Donor–Recipient Compatibility

Donor-recipient blood compatibility is critical for transfusion. If an incompatibility exists, agglutination will obstruct blood vessels, which will obstruct circulation, and death will ensue.

---

and stored in a blood bank or blood processing service prior to transfusion administration.

It is extremely important for every individual to know his blood type, in case the need for surgery or an emergency should arise that would necessitate a transfusion. If the blood of a donor and recipient are incompatible, agglutination obstructs blood vessels, which obstructs circulatory flow and precipitates death.

Individuals with type A blood should receive only type A blood and those with type B blood should receive only type B blood. In emergency situations, blood type O can be transfused to persons with any of the four blood types, since type O blood contains no A or B antigens. A person with type O blood is considered a **universal donor**. Persons with type AB blood are able to receive, in emergency situations, all four types of blood, since they have no A or B antibodies. A person with type AB blood is considered a **universal recipient**. In spite of the fact that a person is a universal donor or recipient, unless an emergency exists, blood compatibility, in terms of typing, should be done to avoid any type of transfusion reaction. Table 14-3 illustrates blood types and their compatibilities with other blood types.

In addition to Rh determination, typing, and crossmatching, blood is tested for unexpected antibodies (under most circumstances). Donors who have been pregnant or who have had previous transfusions are routinely tested for unexpected antibodies. Blood is also tested for transmittable diseases, including HIV, hepatitis viruses, the human T-cell lymphotrophic virus (HTLV), and serologic tests for syphilis (STS).

BLOOD AND BLOOD COMPONENTS

The blood and its components are life-sustaining constituents. The registered nurse is responsible for administering and monitoring the transfusion of these products, based on the physician's order and the patient's condition. A high degree of knowledge and skill is fundamental to proper administration and management. Table 14-4 summarizes the administration guidelines for the blood and blood components covered in the following pages.

Table 14-3 | Blood Compatibilities

Type	RBC Antigen	Plasma Antibody	Recipient Status	Donor Status
A	A	B	A or O	A or AB
B	B	A	B or O	B or AB
AB	A & B	None	A, B, AB, O	AB
O	None	A & B	O	A, B, AB, O

Table 14-4 | Blood Product Administration Guidelines

Product	Rate of Administration	Cannula Size	Filter Size	Compatibility
Whole blood	IV: as fast as patient can tolerate, not to exceed 4 hr.	16–20 gauge	170 micron	0.9% NS
Packed RBCs	IV: as fast as tolerated 1– 3 hr, not to exceed 4 hr	16–20 gauge	170 micron	0.9% NS
Platelets	IV: Determined by volume tolerance, not to exceed 4 hr	16–20 gauge	170 micron	0.9% NS
Granulocytes	IV: slowly, over a 4-hr period, based on 200-ml volume	16–20 gauge	170 micron	0.9% NS
Fresh Frozen Plasma (FFP)	IV: 200 ml/hr, or as determined by clinical status	16–20 gauge	170 micron	0.9% NS
Antihemophilic Factor VIII	IV push, with a plastic (not glass) syringe at 2–10 ml/min	20–23 gauge	Filter needle	Use only diluent provided
Anti-inhibitor Coagulant Complex	IV push or IV drip at 50–100 U/kg/hr, not to exceed 200 U/kg/d	20–23 gauge	Filter needle	Use only diluent provided
Factor IX	IV push or IV drip: dosage is dependent on severity of bleeding, weight, and factor requirements (1 U/kg × weight [kg] × desired increase)	20–23 gauge	Filter needle	Use diluent provided or sterile water
Cryoprecipitate	IV push or drip 1–2 ml/min, infused within 15–20 min or determined by plasma volume	16–20 gauge	170 micron	0.9% NS
Albumin (colloid)	IV drip for volume expansion; for shock, 500 ml administered as rapidly as tolerated: 5%: 1–10 ml/min 25%: 0.2–0.4 ml/min	16–20 gauge	Depends on manufacturer	0.9% NS or 5% dextrose
Plasma Protein Fraction (PPF)	IV drip for volume expansion; for shock, up to 10 ml/min; for hypoproteinemia, up to 8 ml/min	16–20 gauge	Depends on manufacturer	Comes diluted; none other required, 0.9% NS or 5% dextrose
Immune Serum Globulins (for IV use)	IV or IV drip for treatment of acquired immune deficiencies to supply passive immune protection. Rate depends on product used and patient's condition.	16–20 gauge	Depends on manufacturer For single IV dose, use filter needle to draw up; for drip infusion, use filter attached to tubing	None

"The gauge of the cannula should be appropriate for accommodating the blood and/or blood components," INS, 2000, Standard 75, S71. Blood and its components are to be filtered.

Whole Blood

Whole blood consists of red and white blood cells, platelets, electrolytes, plasma (plasma proteins, globulins, antibodies, water, and waste products), and stable clotting factors. One unit (500 ml) of whole blood for transfusion has approximately 35% RBCs, 3% plasma, and 12% anticoagulant mixed with preservatives.

Indications

Whole blood is indicated for the treatment of acute, massive blood loss (greater than 25% to 30% of a person's total volume) for which both the blood volume expansion from the plasma and the oxygen-carrying attributes of the RBCs are needed. Whole blood that is less than five days old is also used for neonatal exchange transfusions.

> ### NURSING TIP
>
> #### Whole Blood Transfusion
>
> The signs and symptoms associated with the need for whole blood transfusion are related to massive blood loss, as evidenced by the following:
>
> - Decreased hematocrit
> - Decreased hemoglobin
> - Dyspnea (shortness of breath)
> - Hypotension
> - Pallor

Once active bleeding has ceased, one unit of whole blood raises the hematocrit by 3% to 4% and the hemoglobin by 1 g/dl. If the patient continues to bleed, the hemoglobin and hematocrit (H & H) will vary, depending on the rapid fluid shifts associated with the loss of volume.

The administration of whole blood has been largely replaced with the use of blood components, which supply only the specific constituents needed. With this change, the contents of one unit of whole blood can be separated into RBCs, plasma, and platelets, and used to treat several different patients. Another advantage is that the ABO incompatibility between blood groups is eliminated. Colloidal and crystalloid infusions can often be used when up to one-third of an adult's blood volume is lost.

Administration Protocols

Whole blood, which must be ABO and Rh specific, should be administered as rapidly as an adult patient can tolerate it (or as determined by clinical status) to restore red blood cell mass and hemodynamic indices. The nurse must always keep in mind that, for patients who are unable to tolerate excess fluid expansion, the plasma volume of whole blood can precipitate fluid volume overload.

Since the loss of potassium from the RBCs (into plasma) increases proportionately to the length of time whole blood is stored, such a transfusion can be contraindicated for some patients, especially those with cardiac problems. Nothing except 0.9% normal saline can be mixed with whole blood.

> ### NURSING ALERT
>
> #### Whole Blood Mixing
>
> NEVER add, piggyback, or mix anything with whole blood except 0.9% normal saline, not even medications intended for intravenous administration.

> ### NURSING ALERT
>
> #### Blood Storage
>
> Blood must be stored in a monitored blood bank refrigerator (or approved blood transportation refrigeration system). It must not be removed from such areas more than 30 minutes prior to the start of a transfusion. NEVER store blood in a nursing unit refrigerator. If there is a delay in starting a transfusion, return the blood to the blood bank for storage.

Whole blood can be stored under refrigeration in a blood bank for up to 35 days, depending on the preservative used. It must not be removed from a monitored refrigerator more than 30 minutes before beginning the transfusion.

For adults, a large-gauge cannula (16 to 20 ga.) must be used to administer blood. A standard or Y-type blood administration infusion set with a 170-μm filter (to eliminate cellular

> ### NURSING TIP
>
> #### Blood Administration
>
> As a general rule, blood should be administered as rapidly as the patient can tolerate it, and never exceed 4 hours.

debris) primed with 0.9% normal saline is required. Blood should not be infused over a period of time greater than 4 hours because of the potential for microbial growth, and because RBCs begin to deteriorate after 2 hours at room temperature.If it is anticipated that the infusion will take longer, the blood service should be contacted to divide the unit into smaller aliquots. Filters should not be used more than 4 hours.

It is extremely important that baseline vital signs be taken and recorded immediately prior to the initiation of a transfusion of whole blood. Once the blood is started, the rate should not exceed 50 ml in the first 15 minutes, in order to assess for a transfusion reaction. The reason for this is that the earlier a reaction occurs, the more severe it is apt to be. Once the transfusion begins, vital signs should be taken three times at 5-minute intervals, again at 30 minutes, and every 30 minutes for the duration of the transfusion. For the safety and protection of the patient, it is very important for the nurse to understand the transfusion protocols of her employing agency and follow them judiciously.

NURSING TIP

Vital Sign Recording

Vital signs must be taken and recorded, for a baseline point of reference, immediately prior to the start of a transfusion. Once the transfusion begins, vital signs should be taken at three 5-minute consecutive intervals, again at 30 minutes, and every 30 minutes until the transfusion is complete. The earlier a transfusion reaction occurs, the more serious it is likely to be. For this reason, unless an emergency exists, the rate of administration should not exceed 50 ml during the first 15 minutes of a transfusion, during which time the patient must be closely monitored by the nurse.

Packed Red Blood Cells

Packed red blood cells provide the same quantity of RBCs as whole blood, but have 80% of the plasma removed. They are available as one of two types of infusions: RBCs with CPDA-1 solution, having a hematocrit no higher than 80%, or RBCs with additive solutions (AS) with a hematocrit no higher than 55%–60%.

CPDA-1 solution is an anticoagulant-preservative additive that gives the red blood cells a shelf-life of 35 days. This RBC solution is available in 250 to 300 ml/unit containers and has a final hematocrit that is no higher than 80%. Because

of the viscosity of such an infusion, it may require dilution with 0.9% normal saline.

Red blood cells with added solution (AS-1, AS-3, or AS-5) have 90% of the plasma removed and contain 100 ml of a special additive solution (preservative) that increases shelf-life to 42 days and decreases viscosity. RBCs may be frozen for up to 10 years. The preservative in these solutions provides higher volume and lower hematocrit, so they do not have to be diluted prior to transfusion. These are available in 300 to 350 ml/unit with a final hematocrit of 55%–60%.

Indications

The administration of packed RBCs is indicated for anemic patients who do not need fluid volume expansion, such as those with renal failure or cardiac problems, yet need to increase the oxygen-carrying ability of their blood. One unit of packed RBCs and one unit of whole blood have the same number of red blood cells and raise the hematocrit of a non-bleeding adult by 3% and the hemoglobin by 1g/dl. The oxygen-carrying ability of the blood is usually adequate when the hemoglobin is 7 g/dl (Hct. of 21%) but can be even less if the intravascular volume is high enough to promote satisfactory perfusion.

A major advantage of packed RBCs over whole blood is the reduction of anti-A or anti-B agglutinins with the removal of the plasma. Therefore, in life-threatening situations where typing and crossmatching is not feasible, type O RBCs can be administered. It is still, however, best to give the ABO group and the Rh type that is specific to the patient.

NURSING TIP

RBC Transfusion

The signs and symptoms associated with the need for red blood cell transfusion owing to acute or chronic blood loss include the following:
- Decreased hematocrit
- Decreased hemoglobin
- Dyspnea (shortness of breath)
- Fatigue
- Pallor
- Tachycardia

Administration Protocols

Prior to the administration of RBCs, it is extremely important to evaluate the cause and severity of a patient's anemia. If the anemia can be resolved with the hematinic use of vitamin

B_{12}, folate, and iron, it should be considered prior to transfusion therapy. Another consideration is the evaluation of the patient's age, hemodynamic reliability, and the presence (or extent of severity) of cardiopulmonary or vascular problems. Unfortunately, the transfusion of RBCs is sometimes used for volume expansion when crystalloid or nonblood colloid infusions would be better utilized.

N U R S I N G   A L E R T

When NOT to Transfuse RBCs

RBCs should not be transfused for the following purpose:
- Fluid volume expansion
- Hematinic substitution
- Enhanced wound healing
- Improved general well-being

One unit of packed red blood cells should be administered as rapidly as the patient can tolerate it over a one- to three-hour period and should never exceed 4 hours. A large-gauge (16- to 20-ga.) cannula should be used for delivery, using a standard straight or Y-type blood administration set with a 170-μm filter primed with 0.9% normal saline. A larger surface-area filter is sometimes used to augment the transfusion rate. Vital signs should be monitored in the same manner as for whole blood administration.

Modified Blood Products

Modified blood products are produced either by removing certain components from whole blood, as with leukocyte-poor RBCs, or through the exposure of portions of the blood to specified degrees of radiation.

Leukocyte-Poor Red Blood Cells

Leukocytes are formed partially in the bone marrow and partially in the lymph tissue, after which they are transported to the blood so they can circulate to areas of inflammation and provide protection against infection. In the adult, there are about 7,000 WBCs/μL of whole blood. Three types of WBCs, the neutrophils, the eosinophils, and the basophils, are **polymorphonuclear**, meaning that they have nuclei made up of several parts, or lobes. These three types of cells (referred to as "polys") have a rough, granular appearance and are, therefore, categorized as granulocytes.

The other three types of WBCs are the monocytes, lymphocytes, and the plasma cells. The granulocytes and mono-

cytes ingest invading organisms by the process of phagocytosis, whereas the lymphocytes and plasma cells work in conjunction with the immune system. Lymphocytes are divided into two categories: (1) those that provide cell-mediated immunity (T lymphocytes) and (2) those that form antibodies (B lymphocytes) and are responsible for humoral immunity. (**Humor** is any fluid substance in the body.) B lymphocytes, when activated by a specific antigen, enlarge to form lymphoblasts, some of which form plasmablasts, the precursors of plasma cells. Mature plasma cells rapidly propagate gamma globulin antibodies, which are secreted into lymph and transported to the blood.

Leukocyte-poor RBCs are grouped in a category referred to as modified blood products. Such products are the result of removing the number of leukocytes in whole blood to 5×10^8, while retaining approximately 80% of the RBCs. ABO compatibility is the same as for packed RBCs. The leukocytes are removed according to several approved techniques: In order of increasing competency, they are centrifuging, filtration, washing, or freezing.

Centrifuging is the process by which whole, unclotted blood is placed in a tube in a centrifuge and spun at high speed to separate the constituents. The centrifugal force causes the components to separate according to their weight, with the heaviest going to the bottom of the tube and the lightest rising to the top. In whole blood, the RBCs are heaviest and sink to the bottom; the plasma, being the lightest, floats to the top. WBCs are lighter than RBCs, but heavier than plasma. When they are centrifuged, they form a thin layer between the RBCs and the plasma known as the **buffy coat**. Centrifuged blood components are layered from heaviest to lightest in the following order: RBCs, WBCs (buffy coat), platelets, lymphocytes, monocytes, granulocytes, reticulocytes, and plasma.

Filtration is the process of removing 70% to 99.9% of WBCs with a leukocyte depletion filter. Various types of filtration systems enable WBC removal to be accomplished prior to or during a transfusion.

Washing is the process in which 80% to 90% of the WBCs and almost all of the plasma are removed from the blood.

Freezing is the process in which blood is frozen; all of the plasma and 99% of the WBCs are eliminated when thawing takes place and the nontransferable cryoprotectant (glycerol) is removed. Freezing must be done within six days of collection and is then usable for up to 10 years. Once thawed, it must be transfused within 24 hours.

Indications

Leukocyte-poor red blood cells are indicated for the prevention of febrile, nonhemolytic transfusion reactions that are precipitated by the introduction of leukocytes and foreign proteins in patients who have had previous nonhemolytic transfusion reactions. Such reactions are produced when the donor's WBC agglutinogens (antigens) react with the transfusion recipient's WBC agglutinins (antibodies). Leukocyte-poor WBCs are also indicated for patients with disease processes in which multiple transfusions may be anticipated, such as leukemia or hemophilia. The removal of most of the leukocytes also reduces the chance of isogenic exposure and transmission of the cytomegalovirus (CMV) and malaria.

Administration Protocols

The administration protocols are the same as those for whole blood and packed red blood cell transfusions.

Irradiated Blood Products

When blood products are exposed to a controlled measure of radiation, it causes the donor lymphocytes to become incapable of replication. The process of irradiation is performed in a blood collection center or distribution center just prior to blood release for transfusion. Products such as cryopre-cipitate or fresh frozen plasma, which do not contain viable leukocytes, do not need to be irradiated. Irradiated blood products do not pose a radiation risk to the patient, blood bank personnel, or the nurse who administers them.

Indications

Irradiated blood products are used to prevent graft-versus-host (GVHD) reactions in patients receiving blood transfusions that contain viable leukocytes. They are usually indicated for patients with acute leukemia and lymphoma (Hodgkin's disease and non-Hodgkin's disease), bone marrow or stem cell transplant recipients, patients with immunodeficiency disorders that are congenital in nature, prenatal intrauterine transfusions, and for transfusion of neonates with low birth weights.

Administration Protocols

A label marked *irradiated* must be placed on the bag containing the product for transfusion. The protocols for administration are the same as for nonirradiated products.

Platelet Concentrates for Transfusion

Platelets are fragments of megacaryocytes, which are particles of a seventh type of leukocyte found in the bone marrow. They are responsible for **hemostasis**, the prevention of blood loss through the arrest of bleeding, which is accomplished through the process of platelet plug formation. Platelets, which live up to 12 days in the blood, do not have nuclei and are unable to reproduce. They contain no hemoglobin.

The cell membrane of platelets is coated with glycoproteins and phospholipids. The glycoproteins cause the platelets to adhere to injured areas of vessels while avoiding adherence to normal endothelial surfaces. The phospholipids, which contain platelet factor 3, exert their effect at numerous points in the process of blood clotting, but primarily in the conversion of prothrombin to thrombin. Platelets number 150,000 to 300,000/μL of whole blood.

Platelet concentrates are derived from random donors or single donors whose antigens are similar to those of the recipients. They are retrieved from whole blood or plasma, after which they are suspended in a specified volume of the original plasma.

Random Donor Platelets

Platelets are retrieved by separating the platelet-rich plasma from fresh whole blood obtained from random donors. One unit contains 50 to 70 ml and has a minimum of 5.5×10^{10} platelets and should raise the peripheral platelet count in a 70 kg adult by about 5,000/μL if the underlying cause of bleeding is controlled or resolved.

NURSING TIP

The Who and How of Blood Irradiation

Candidates for irradiated leukocytes include the following:

- **Patients who have previously had a febrile nonhemolytic transfusion reaction**
- **Patients who may need multiple transfusions in the future and need to avoid platelet alloimmunization**
- **Patients who have compromised immune systems and are at risk for transfusion-related graft-versus-host (GVH) reactions**
- **Patients who have Hodgkin's disease**
- **Patients who may be hematopoietic stem cell donors and require blood prior to stem cell harvesting**
- **Patients who have had (or may need) a bone marrow or stem cell transplant**

Whole blood, red blood cells, platelets, or granulocytes can be irradiated. Cryoprecipitate and fresh frozen plasma, which do not contain lymphocytes, do not require irradiation. The blood products, after being placed in a container, are put into a special canister. Gamma radiation, in the amount of 2,500 rads, is applied to inactivate the lymphocytes.

Indications

Random donor platelet concentrate is indicated for the prophylaxis or control of bleeding disorders associated with deficiencies in the number or function of platelets. As a preventive measure, platelets are administered when counts are in the 10,000 to 20,000/μL range, and spontaneous bleeding is not a problem. They are given to control active bleeding for counts <50,000/μL.

N U R S I N G   T I P

Platelet Transfusion

The signs and symptoms associated with the need for platelet transfusion are as follows:
- Blood in the stool
- Ecchymoses
- Gum bleeding
- Hematuria
- Petechiae
- Platelet counts <20,000/μL

In patients with a medical history of nonhemolytic, febrile reactions, leukocyte-poor platelets should be used. They are also indicated to reduce the risk of **alloimmunization** (lymphocytic response to specific antigens on the cell surfaces of transfused blood) and transmission of CMV infection. Leukocyte-depletion filters, which are designed specifically for platelet administration, should always be used when giving leukocyte-poor platelets.

Prior to the transfusion of platelet concentrates, which contain negligible RBCs, testing for ABO-compatibility is not required. By using ABO compatible blood, however, the recovery and survival of platelets is enhanced.

N U R S I N G   A L E R T

Platelet Administration

Platelets should not be administered in the following situations:
- As a prophylactic measure following cardiopulmonary bypass surgery
- As a prophylactic measure with massive blood transfusion
- To patients with immune thrombocytopenia purpura, unless the bleeding presents a life-threatening situation

---

In women of childbearing age who are Rh⁻, it is advisable to transfuse platelets from Rh⁻ donors, to prevent the development of antibodies. If this is not possible, the woman should be given Rh immune globulin prior to transfusion.

Administration Protocols

Platelets are stored, while undergoing gentle agitation, in a blood bank at room temperature for a maximum of five days. If replacement needs are great, the units are often pooled into one container. Once the container is opened, for any reason, the platelets must be used within four hours.

The rate of infusion for platelets is determined by the clinical situation and the patient's fluid volume tolerance. A large-gauge cannula (16 to 19 ga.) must be used for delivery. A blood component administration set with a 170-μm filter primed with 0.9% normal saline is to be used. Platelets must be transfused within four hours.

Apheresis Platelets

Apheresis platelets are collected from single rather than multiple donors and retrieved with automated cell separation devices. Each container contains 200 to 400 ml and contains a minimum of 3.0×10^{11} platelets. This volume approximates 5 to 6 units of pooled random donor platelets.

Indications

As with random donor platelets, apheresis platelets are also indicated for the control or prevention of bleeding affiliated with deficiencies in the number or function of platelets. The use of single-donor platelets, however, may diminish the risks associated with diseases transmitted via transfusion. There is also a reduction in HLA antibody formation because of fewer donor exposures.

Administration Protocols

Administration protocols for apheresis platelets approximate those for any platelet concentrate.

Human-Leukocyte Antigen Matched Platelets

HLA-matched platelets are collected, by apheresis, from a donor whose human leukocyte antigens are similar to those of the recipient. This is a very costly procedure that requires advance scheduling. It is extremely rare to find identical HLA-matched platelets from unrelated individuals. When HLA antibodies are the fundamental cause of platelet destruction, however, a less-than-perfect match may be adequate. Siblings or family members of a patient provide the most acceptable matches.

Leukopenia, the abnormal decrease in leukocytes (usually below 5,000/mm^3), makes it difficult to determine HLA typing. For patients for whom immunosuppressive treatment may be required, blood samples for HLA typing should be collected prior to the onset of leukopenia.

Indications

HLA-matched platelets are indicated to minimize the premature destruction of donor platelets by HLA antibodies in the transfusion recipient. They are only effective when HLA antibodies are the main cause of platelet eradication. Several causes contribute to the loss of platelets (in addition to platelet-specific antibodies), such as disseminated intravascular coagulation (DIC), fever, infection, hemorrhage, and splenomegaly.

Administration Protocols

Administration protocols for HLA-matched platelets are the same as those for any platelet concentrate transfusion.

NURSING TIP

Platelet Count Timeframe

It is vital that platelet counts, ordered following all types of platelet administration, be performed within an hour of the completion of the transfusion in order to accurately assess the therapeutic effect.

Granulocytes

Granulocytes are polymorphonuclear leukocytes (basophils, eosinophils, and neutrophils) that destroy invading organisms by the process of phagocytosis. They are obtained for transfusion by the process of granulocytapheresis. One unit of platelet-poor product contains at least 1.0×10^{10} granulocytes, less than 10% lymphocytes, 30 to 50 ml of RBCs, and 100 to 400 ml of plasma. When platelets are added, the amount is usually 6 to 10 units.

Indications

The administration of granulocytes is indicated for patients with congenital WBC (granulocyte) dysfunction or acquired neutropenia. They are also used to treat patients with severe infections that are unresponsive to conventional antibiotic treatment.

Administration Protocols

In the United States, granulocytes are not licensed by the FDA, and continue to be evaluated, as they have not been used enough to determine their long-term benefits. Granulocyte therapy provides only temporary results. When used, pretransfusion testing for ABO and Rh compatibility is the same as for RBCs.

Granulocyte transfusions are accompanied by a high frequency of nonhemolytic, febrile reactions. It is often necessary to prophylactically medicate patients with acetaminophen, antihistamines, and steroids. If granulocytes are infused slowly, over a one- to four-hour period for a 200-ml volume, there is less chance of reaction formation. Infusing slowly enables the early detection of reactions.

NURSING ALERT

Granulocyte Infusions

Infuse granulocytes slowly, while closely monitoring the patient for nonhemolytic, febrile transfusion reactions.

Granulocyte concentrates are administered with a large-gauge (16- to 20-ga.) cannula, using a standard blood infusion set and a 170-μm filter primed with 0.9% normal saline. Depth-type microaggregate or leukocyte depletion filters must never be used because they trap the granulocytes. Granulocyte concentrates are stored in a blood bank at room temperature and have a very short survival time (less than 24 hours), so they must be transfused as soon as possible after collection (within 6 hours) for best results.

The usual protocol, for effective resolution or treatment of infection, is to administer one unit (1×10^{10} granulocytes) daily for several consecutive days. The only way the efficacy of therapy can be evaluated is by the clinical picture the patient presents. In adults, the serum WBC count usually does not demonstrate an increase in number following granulocyte transfusion.

NURSING ALERT

Preventing Pulmonary Insufficiency Complications

To prevent complications of pulmonary insufficiency, NEVER administer granulocytes within four hours of amphotericin B infusions.

Plasma and Plasma Derivatives

Plasma and Fresh Frozen Plasma

Plasma is the liquid portion of the blood and lymph in which nutrients are carried to body tissues and wastes are transported to areas of excretion. It is a colorless, thin, aqueous solution (91% water) that contains chemicals (bile pigments, bilirubin, electrolytes, enzymes, fats, and hormones), protein (7%, consisting of albumin, antibodies, clotting factors, and globulins), carbohydrate (2%), and serum, along with dissolved gases and solutes. Plasma does not contain RBCs.

Fresh frozen plasma (FFP) is the amount of liquid retrieved from one unit of whole blood that has been centrifuged, separated, and then frozen. The process of freezing, which must be done within six hours of collection, preserves all of the clotting factors. The usual volume for transfusion is 200 to 250 ml.

Indications

Liquid plasma is indicated to replace plasma proteins lost from a burn injury. Because it is not frozen, but stored under refrigeration, it does not provide the clotting factors that are needed for patients with coagulation deficiencies.

FFP is indicated for patients with a demonstrated deficiency of those clotting factors that are not commercially available for transfusion. The deficiency is usually a complication secondary to another disease process, such as DIC or liver impairment. In DIC, the extensive amount of clotting diminishes the number of procoagulants, thus preventing hemostasis, which results in massive bleeding. The liver, under normal circumstances, synthesizes the following clotting factors: Factor I (fibrinogen), Factor II (prothrombin), Factor V (proaccelerin, accelerator globulin, Ac-globulin, labile factor), Factor VII (proconvertin, autoprothrombin I, serum prothrombin conversion activator, stable factor), Factor IX (plasma thromboplastin component, antihemophillic factor B), Factor X (Stuart-Prower factor), and, possibly, Factor XI (plasma thromboplastin antecedent, antihemophilic factor C). The synthesis of these factors cannot occur with liver disease.

FFP contains, in addition to liquid plasma, all of the major and minor protein clotting factors (glycoproteins). Clotting factors are inactive forms of proteolytic enzymes that become activated when the clotting process is initiated. Once activated, some of the factors act as enzymes to activate other factors. The freezing process preserves all of the clotting components: Factor I (fibrinogen) is preserved in abundance, with 200 to 400 mg/unit, Factor V (proaccelerin; labile factor; Ac-globulin) and Factor XI (plasma thromboplastin antecedent [PTA], antihemophilic factor C), which are not commercially available in concentrates.

Administration Protocols

Since there are no RBCs in plasma, Rh crossmatching is not necessary. ABO compatibility must be ascertained, however. AB plasma can be given to all ABO groups when the blood group is not known (in emergency situations), since it does not have anti-A or anti-B agglutinins. If only volume expansion is needed, crystalloid or colloids should be used, rather than plasma to avoid the risk of disease transmission. If the prothrombin time (PT) and partial thromboplastin time (PTT) are less than 1.5 times the normal, FFP transfusion is not indicated.

Plasma is administered according to the patient's clinical status and underlying disease processes. The usual rate of infusion is 200 ml/hr, unless there is a potential for fluid volume overload. A large-gauge cannula (16 to 20 ga.) is to be used, and a blood component recipient set with 170-μm filter primed with 0.9% normal saline is required. Medications and diluents must never be added to plasma.

NURSING TIP

Monitor Patient for Fluid Volume Overload

Because plasma is an isotonic volume expander, the patient must be carefully monitored for fluid volume overload.

FFP is thawed in the blood bank. Once it is in a liquid state, it must be administered within 24 hours or labile clotting factors (V and VIII) will be lost. To preserve these factors, FFP must be used within a year of the freezing process. Once thawed, plasma can be stored under refrigeration (33 to 50°F) for up to four years and used for noncoagulation purposes. The effectiveness of plasma transfusion therapy using FFP is evaluated with coagulation studies or factor-specific assays. Diluents or medications must never be added to plasma.

Coagulation Factor Concentrates

Coagulation factor concentrates are used to treat factor-specific deficiencies. They are prepared from large pools of

---

NURSING TIP

FFP Contraindications

FP is not indicated for the following:
- Fluid volume expansion, since it carries with it the same risk for disease transmission as whole blood (with the exception of CMV)
- Nutritional supplementation
- Prophylaxis following cardiopulmonary bypass
- Prophylaxis with massive blood transfusion

donor plasma using a process known as lyophilization. **Lyophilization** is the procedure in which a product is rapidly frozen at an extremely low temperature, then dehydrated in a high vacuum. It is the same as freeze-drying. Because of the mechanisms used to produce factor concentrates, heat, solvent-detergent treatments, or both, there is minimal risk of viral disease transmission.

Hemophilia is an inherited bleeding tendency. The genetic trait is carried in women and passed on almost exclusively to their male offspring with an occurrence of approximately 1 in 10,000. Eighty-five percent have classic hemophilia A, and 15% have hemophilia B (Guyton & Hall, 2000). Coagulation factor concentrates include Factor VIII, anti-inhibitor coagulant complex, Factor IX, and cryoprecipitate.

Factor VIII

Classic hemophilia, or hemophilia A, is caused by a genetic deficiency in Factor VIII. Factor VIII is made up of two components, a smaller one with a molecular weight in the hundred thousands, and a larger one with a molecular weight in the millions. The smaller component is important in the intrinsic clotting pathway. A deficiency of this part causes hemophilia A. The larger component, when deficient, or missing, results in von Willebrand's disease (vWD).

Indications

Factor VIII is an antihemophilic element used for systemic hemostasis in the treatment of severe hemophilia A and for the treatment of some types of von Willebrand's disease. Milder forms may be responsive to treatment with desmopressin acetate (DDAVP), a synthetic antidiuretic without oxytocic and vasopressor effects, which increases Factor VIII and von Willebrand's factor. When Factor VIII is used, coagulant activity at levels of 30% to 50% is usually the desired outcome. One unit of Factor VIII correctional activity is defined as "the quantity of activated prothrombin complex which, when added to an equal volume of Factor VIII-deficient or inhibitor plasma, will correct the clotting time to normal (i.e., 35 sec)" (Sprath & Woods, 2003).

The parenteral administration of purified Factor VIII is the only effective therapy for a patient with (classic) hemophilia A. Because it is obtained from human blood in very small amounts, it is very costly to retrieve. Since the amount needed to achieve a therapeutic dose must come from numerous donors, the chance for viral transmission is always a possibility, though minimal with newer extraction techniques.

Administration Protocols

The dosage of purified Factor VIII is based on body weight and the level of deficiency determined by laboratory assays. It is available in vials, with varying numbers of units (stated on the label) for reconstitution with a prescribed, accompanying diluent and instructions. It may be administered IV push through a 170-μm filter needle or given by IV drip, using a blood component recipient set.

Anti-Inhibitor Coagulant Complex

Anti-inhibitor coagulant complex is an antihemophilic product derived from pooled human plasma. It contains both precursor and activated clotting factors.

Indications

Anti-inhibitor coagulant complex is primarily useful for hemophiliacs with Factor VIII inhibitors (documented by laboratory assay) greater than 10 Bethesda units (the standard of measure), or whose inhibitor levels do not rise satisfactorily following treatment with antihemophilic factor. It is also used in patients with incidents of minor bleeding, in order to keep the inhibitor at low levels.

Administration Protocols

Anti-inhibitor coagulant complex is administered intravenously in the same manner as Factor VIII concentrate. For soft tissue hemorrhage, 100 U/kg is administered every 12 hours, and should not exceed 200 U/kg/day. With joint hemorrhage, 50 to 100 U/kg is administered every 12 hours and continued until swelling, pain, and immobility have subsided.

Factor IX Concentrate

Factor IX, known as plasma thromboplastin component (PTC) or Christmas factor, is a systemic hemostatic that is vital to the coagulation process. A deficiency of this coagulation component is usually genetic in nature, but can also be caused by a deficiency of vitamin K. Vitamin K, a fat-soluble vitamin, is necessary to promote the development of the four major clotting factors, Factor II (prothrombin), Factor VII, Factor IX, and Factor X. In liver impairment (either from disease or obstruction), where bile is not secreted into the intestinal tract, there is inadequate fat digestion and absorption which, in turn, results in depressed vitamin K absorption and synthesis.

Indications

Factor IX concentrate is indicated in the treatment of bleeding associated with hemophilia B or Christmas disease. It acts to promote hemostasis by increasing factor IX activity. It is also used in the treatment of congenital Factor VII and X deficiencies and to treat hemophiliacs with Factor VIII inhibitors. It may be indicated to reverse coumarin-induced hemorrhage.

Administration Protocols

Dosage is based on the patient's weight and the need for hemostasis, based on Factor IX laboratory assays. The infusion protocols are the same as for Factor VIII.

Cryoprecipitate

Cryoprecipitate is the cold-insoluble component of plasma that is obtained after the thawing of fresh frozen plasma. It contains approximately 80 to 120 units of Factor VIII (antihemophilic factor or AHF), which is about 50% of the amount present in the original unit of whole blood. It also contains von Willebrand's factor, 250 mg of Factor I (fibrinogen), and 20% to 30% of the Factor XIII (fibrin-stabilizing factor) present in the original unit. Depending on the method of preparation, cryoprecipitate is available in 5 to 10 ml/unit volumes or 10 to 20 ml/unit volumes, with 80 to 120 units of Factor VIII in each bag. A hemostatic dose (2 g of fibrinogen) is supplied with 8 to 10 bags.

Indications

Cryoprecipitate is indicated to correct deficiencies of Factor I, Factor VIII, von Willebrand's factor, and Factor XIII. It is sometimes used in uremic patients to control bleeding.

Cryoprecipitate does not have RBCs and only a very small volume of plasma. Plasma compatibility testing is not required, but is preferred.

Administration Protocols

Cryoprecipitate dosages depend on the patient's plasma volume. The National Blood Resource Education Program Office of Prevention, Education, and Control of the National Heart, Lung, and Blood Institute provides a method to calculate the adult requirements for Factor VIII transfusions, based on a patient's plasma volume (Figure 14-2). To calculate a patient's plasma volume, the following formula is used:

Blood volume (ml) = weight (kg) × 70 ml/kg.

Plasma volume (ml) = blood volume (ml) × 1.0, minus the hematocrit.

To calculate a patient's need for units of Factor VIII for transfusion, the following formula is used:

Plasma volume (ml) × desired Factor VIII level (U/ml) minus the initial Factor VIII level in U/ml.

Bags of cryoprecipitate = units of Factor VIII

To achieve a therapeutic level of Factor VIII, the established dose often needs to be given again in 8 to 12 hours.

Individual units of cryoprecipitate are usually suspended in 10 to 20 ml of residual plasma. Some transfusion services or blood banks prepare it with a minimal amount of plasma. If this is the case, it is usually necessary to dilute the product

---

1 unit (available in 5–20 ml/unit bags) of cryoprecipitate supplies:

    80–120 units of Factor VII and 250 mg of fibrinogen

    2 g fibrinogen = hemostatic dose (8–10 units)

Formula:

1. Blood volume (ml) = Weight (kg) × 70 ml/kg
2. Plasma volume (ml) = Blood volume (ml) × (1.0 − Hct)
3. Units Factor VIII required = Plasma volume (ml) × (desired Factor VIII level U/ml - initial Factor VIII level U/ml)
4. Bags of cryoprecipitate = Units of Factor VIII/100.

(National Blood Resource Education Program Office of Prevention, Education, and Control, National Heart, Lung, and Blood Institute)

Example 1:   143 lb. patient (65 kg);

    Hct = 36% (0.36);

    initial Factor VIII level = 0 U/ml;

    desired Factor VIII level = 0.5 U/ml.

1. 65 kg × 70 ml/kg = 4,550 ml (blood volume)
2. 4,550 ml × (1.0 - 0.36) = 2,912 ml (plasma volume)
3. 2,912 ml × (0.5 - 0) = 1,456 units
4. 1,456 units/100 = 14.56 (15 bags) of cryoprecipitate

Example 2:   198 lb. patient (90 kg);

    Hct = 44% (0.44);

    initial Factor VIII level = 0 U/ml;

    desired Factor VIII level = 0.7 U/ml.

1. 90 kg × 70 ml/kg = 6,300 ml (blood volume)
2. 6,300 ml × (1.0 - 0.44) = 3,528 ml (plasma volume)
3. 3,528 ml × (0.7 - 0) = 2,469.60 units
4. 2,499.60/100 = 24.69 (25 bags) of cryoprecipitate

Figure 14-2 | Calculation of cryoprecipitate units needed to supply hemostatic dose of factor VIII (antihemophilic factor—AHF)

---

with 5 to 10 ml of 0.9% normal saline in order to administer the full dosage. Individual units of cryoprecipitate must be transfused within 6 hours of thawing.

Because of the quantity of cryoprecipitate usually needed by a patient, individual units are often pooled into one large container by the blood bank or transfusion center. Pooled units must be transfused within 4 hours of thawing.

The rate of administration is 1 to 2 ml/min. As with other plasma derivatives, a large-gauge cannula (16 to 20 ga.) should be used for delivery of cryoprecipitate. A standard blood component administration set, with a standard 170-μm filter primed with 0.9% normal saline is to be used.

Blood-Product Volume Expanders

Colloid Solutions

Colloid solutions are indicated to provide volume expansion and to maintain satisfactory blood pressure. They are used as volume expanders in cases where crystalloid solutions cannot provide adequate support, as seen in massive hemorrhage, plasma exchange, and shock. They are also indicated for the treatment of acute liver failure, burns, and neonatal hemolytic disease. Because there are no ABO blood group antibodies, compatibility does not have to be taken into consideration for administration. They are pasteurized, which destroys the hepatitis and human immunodeficiency viruses. They do not contain clotting factors, so they are not used in place of liquid plasma.

Normal Human Serum Albumin

Albumin, classified as a blood volume expander, contains 96% albumin and 4% globulins and other proteins. It is prepared from plasma, whole blood, or placenta. It is available as a 5% solution, which is isotonic and isosmotic with normal human plasma, or as a 25%, salt-poor solution, in which 50 ml is osmotically equal to 250 ml of citrated plasma. The 5% solution is available in 250 ml and 500 ml containers and the 25% solution is available in 50 ml and 100 ml containers.

Indications

Albumin is mainly indicated for fluid volume expansion to correct shock associated with burns, hemorrhage, surgical losses, and trauma. It is also used to treat hypoproteinemia, adult respiratory distress syndrome (ARDS), and acute hepatic failure, and is administered as a presurgical blood diluent for cardiopulmonary bypass surgery.

Administration Protocols

The dosage is dependent on the clinical situation. The rate of administration for the 5% solution when used to treat shock is 500 ml infused as rapidly as the patient can tolerate it, and repeated at 30-minute intervals, depending on the response. Once the plasma volume is near normal, the rate should not exceed 2 to 4 ml/min. For hypoproteinemia, the rate should not exceed 5 to 10 ml/min. When used in the treatment of burns, it must be infused to maintain the plasma albumin level at 2 to 3 g/100 ml, with the total serum protein level at about 5.2 g/100 ml.

The 25% solution dose, when used to treat shock, is dependent on the patient's condition. For massive volume depletion, it must be given as rapidly as possible. Once the plasma volume is near normal, the rate should not exceed 1 ml/min. For hypoproteinemia, the adult dosage is 50 to 75 g/day, at a rate not to exceed 2 ml/min. Burn treatment is dependent on the extent of damage. The infusion should be adjusted to maintain plasma albumin levels at 2 to 3 g/100 ml, keeping the plasma oncotic pressure at 20 mm Hg.

Albumin is administered with a large-gauge cannula (16 to 20 ga.), using a standard IV infusion set. If a filter is required, the manufacturer usually supplies one, or the package insert describes the type to be used.

Plasma Protein Fraction

Plasma protein fraction (PPF), classified as a blood volume expander, contains 83% albumin and 17% globulins extracted from plasma. It is not as pure as albumin, having a higher concentration of other plasma proteins. It is available as a 5% solution of human plasma proteins suspended in sodium chloride. It is prepared in 250-ml and 500-ml containers. As with albumin, ABO compatibility is not a consideration for administration, and pasteurization destroys the HIV and hepatitis viruses.

Indications

PPF is indicated for the treatment of shock related to fluid volume depletion. It is also used in the treatment of hypoproteinemia.

Administration Protocols

The rate of infusion is based on the patient's condition. For hypovolemic shock, plasma protein fraction is administered intravenously at an initial rate of 250 to 500 ml/hr, not to exceed 10 ml/min, with subsequent doses dependent on the patient's response to treatment. For the treatment of hypoproteinemia, 1 to 1.5 L is given (50 to 75 g protein) at a rate not to exceed 5 to 8 ml/min. The equipment for administration is the same as for albumin. It is very important to read the manufacturer's product insert to correctly set up and administer colloidal infusions.

Plasma protein fraction must be used within 4 hours of opening the vial. It must never be administered through the same set as alcohol, amino acids, or protein hydrolysates, because the proteins are likely to precipitate.

Serum Globulins

Immune Serum Globulins

Immune serum globulins (ISG), which comprise about 20% of all plasma proteins in the blood, are gamma globulins called immunoglobulins (Ig) (antibodies). The ability of a person to resist infection correlates with his concentration of these proteins. Although scientific researchers are certain that all antibodies are immunoglobulins, they are not sure that all immunoglobulins function as antibodies.

The immunoglobulins in the human body are categorized in five classes: IgA, IgD, IgE, IgG, and IgM. Each has several subclasses. They are identified by the configuration of their base structure. Each immunoglobulin has four polypeptide chains. Two are identical, have a high molecular weight, and are called H (for heavy) chains. The other two are lower-weight chains and are called L (for light) chains. Although the L chain is the same in all Ig classes, the H chain is different, thereby differentiating one Ig class from the other. Table 14-5 lists the five classes of immunoglobulins and identifies their locations and functions in the body. All Igs have the two heavy and light chain pairs. Some Igs, however, have additional sets, thereby rendering them larger and heavier. On the end of each light and heavy chain is a **constant portion**, which characterizes the properties of the antibody in terms of its ability to diffuse in tissues, adhere to certain substances, and pass through membranes. Also present is the **variable portion**, which gives the Ig its specificity in attaching to a particular antigen. The segment where it attaches is called an antigen-binding site.

Immunoglobulins G (IgG) are concentrated aqueous solutions of gamma globulin with high antibody titers (greater than 90% IgG). They may be nonspecific or specific in nature. The nonspecific gamma globulin products for IV administration consist of polyvalent antibodies obtained from a large pool of random human donors. The specific IgG products are procured from donors with high levels of antibodies to specifically known antigens.

Immune serum globulins are indicated for the treatment of congenital or acquired immune deficiencies. They are administered to supply passive immune protection when the body is immunocompromised and unable to generate antibodies, or to treat hypogammaglobulinemia resulting from other disease processes. Treatment with ISG does not cure the underlying diseases or conditions, but only diverts the deficiencies associated with them.

Nonspecific Immune Serum Globulins

There are several nonspecific ISG preparations available for intravenous use: Gammimune N, Gammogard, Gammar-IV, IGIV, Iveegam, Sandoglobulin, Venoglobulin-1, and Venoglobulin-S; and IGIM, Gamostan, and Gammar for intramuscular use. Before administering a nonspecific ISG prepara-

Table 14-5	Human Immunoglobulins		
Name	**Location in the Body**	**Functions and Indications**
IgA	IgA is present in the following exocrine secretions (and referred to as *secretory IgA*): colostrum breast milk saliva tears secretions of the respiratory tract secretions of the gastrointestinal tract A different form of IgA is present in the blood.	IgA provides the neonate with immunity and protects mucosal surfaces from bacterial, viral, and yeast invasions.
IgD (Rho or D Ig)	IgD comprises a very small percentage of the total immunoglobulins in the body. It is present in the plasma of individuals with high levels of Rh antibodies. It is present on the surface of B cells, especially during the prenatal and early neonatal periods. IgD crosses the placenta.	It is hypothesized that IgD contributes to the development of maturation of an individual's immunocompetence. IgD is administered to the Rh⁻ mother during pregnancy, after amniocentesis, and following the abortion or delivery of her first Rh⁺ offspring, to provide isoimmunization and prevent hemolytic disease of the fetus or neonate in subsequent pregnancies.
IgE	IgE attaches to mast cells in the respiratory and gastrointestinal tracts and is present, in small amounts, in exocrine secretions.	IgE plays a major role in allergic reactions and in the formation of reagin (IgGE) in the blood of individuals with atopic hypersensitivity.
IgG	IgG is the principle immunoglobulin in human serum, but is also present, in small quantities, in exocrine secretions. IgG crosses the placenta.	IgG is the major antibody for antitoxins, bacteria, viruses, fungi, and yeasts. It also activates complement and serves as an opsonin.
IgM	IgM, the largest of the immunoglobulins, is a component of an immune response and formed in the early period of a reaction. IgM does not cross the placenta.	IgM controls the ABO blood group antibody responses and stimulates complement activity.

tion, it is very important to read the manufacturer's packaging information to ascertain that the one being used is appropriate for the patient and his condition.

Indications

These products are formulated using a cold fractionation process and are approved for use in treating congenitally acquired gamma globulin deficiency (or absence), combined immunodeficiency syndromes, and primary immunodeficiency disorders. Some are also indicated for the treatment of acute and chronic idiopathic thrombocytopenia purpura (ITP) and chronic lymphocytic (B-cell) leukemia.

If nonspecific ISG is prepared using the Cohn fractionation of pooled plasma process, there is the possibility of exposure and transmission of non-A and non-B hepatitis (Hepatitis C). Hepatitis B and HIV are not transmitted by immune serum globulins.

Administration Protocols

Patients who have a history of severe allergic reactions to plasma must not be given nonspecific ISG. The dosage of immune globulins varies among ISG products. It is important to read the package insert that accompanies any product for dosage recommendations and administration protocols.

Nonspecific ISG should only be administered intravenously. All preparations require reconstitution with a diluent and filtration. For single-unit IV doses, a filter needle must be used to draw up the product. For infusion, the appropriate filter must be attached to the administration tubing. Other than the recommended diluents, any other solution or medication is considered incompatible with ISG. To prevent foaming, it is important to gently rotate or agitate, not shake, vials of immune globulins when dissolving. Once diluted, ISG must be used within 2 hours or discarded.

Specific Immune Serum Globulins

Indications

These preparations are administered to provide passive immunity prior to or following exposure to disease-specific antigens. Immunoglobulin research, it is hoped, will lead to the development of treatments for such devastating diseases as cancer and AIDS.

Administration Protocols

The majority of the specific ISGs are administered by intramuscular (IM) injection, with a few available as intravenous preparations. As with all products, it is important to read the package directions in order to administer the ISG by the correct route. An intramuscular preparation given intravenously can result in anaphylaxis. The specific ISGs should be administered prior to or as soon as possible after exposure. The IM injections are usually painful and cause local irritation, so use of z-track technique into a large muscle and the application of warm compresses to the injection site is recommended.

Cytomegalovirus Immune Globulin

Cytomegalovirus immune globulin intravenous (CMV-IGIV) is obtained from the pooled plasma of adults with high antibody titers for cytomegalovirus. It is highly purified using special processing.

Indications

CMV-IGIV is given to raise the CMV antibodies in recipients and, therefore, lessen or reduce the symptoms associated with CMV disease. It is almost always used to weaken primary CMV that accompanies kidney transplantation. It must be given to transplant recipients who are seronegative for CMV when the donor is seropositive.

Administration Protocols

The cytomegalovirus immune globulin injection is given as a single 150 mg/kg dose by IV infusion (at 15 mg/kg/hr, for the first 30 minutes, to assess for adverse reactions) and must be administered within 72 hours of transplant. The rate must not exceed 75 ml/hr. It is repeated at 100 mg/kg doses at 2-week intervals for 8 weeks, then given at 12 and 16 weeks at 50 mg/kg. Once reconstituted, the infusion must be started within 6 hours and used within 12 hours. Filters are not to be used. It is best to administer CMV-IGIV through a separate line, but if this is not feasible, it may be piggy-backed in dextrose and normal saline solutions.

Hepatitis B Immune Globulin

Indications

HBIG (H-BIG®, Hep-B-Gammagee®, HyperHep®) has high titers of hepatitis B antibody to the hepatitis B surface antigen. It provides passive immunity to hepatitis B virus (HBV), following exposure. It is also given to babies born to HBsAg-positive mothers.

Administration Protocols

The hepatitis B immune globulin is administered intramuscularly and should be given within 7 days of exposure to the virus, but preferably within 24 hours. The dose is 0.06 mg/kg, with the adult dosage volume ranging between 3 to 5 ml (in divided doses). It must not be given intravenously. The HBIG is not the same as the hepatitis B vaccine (Energix, Heptavax, Recombivax HB), the standard immunization administered to prevent HBV.

Lymphocyte Immune Globulin

Indications

Lymphocyte immune globulin (antithymocyte globulin [equine], or Atgam) is a lymphocyte-selective immunosuppressant used in the management of allograft rejection in renal transplant patients. It reduces the number of thymus-dependent lymphocytes. It is used prophylactically to prevent rejection and to treat rejection, once it has started.

Administration Protocols

The usual dosage for lymphocyte immune globulin is between 10 to 30 mg/kg/day administered in equal amounts over a minimum of 4-hour increments. It is given intravenously into a central vein or high-flow vascular shunt, as it will cause phlebitis if injected into peripheral veins. Before use of lymphocyte immune globulin can be initiated, an intradermal skin test is required to determine sensitivity. Even with a negative skin test, anaphylaxis is always a possibility.

The length of treatment is dependent on the patient's condition and propensity for allograft rejection. It is usually administered with other forms of immunosuppressive therapy. Lymphocyte immune globulin is stored under refrigeration before and after dilution. Once reconstituted, the solution must be used within 12 hours, or discarded. It is incompatible with anything other than 0.9% or 0.45% saline.

Rh Immune Globulin

Indications

Rh immune globulin (RhIG) (Gamulin Rh, HypRho-D, RhoGAM) has high titers of Rh (D) antibody and is given to Rh⁻ patients who have been exposed to Rh(D) antigens through pregnancy or blood transfusion accident. When given to women following the abortion or delivery of an Rh⁺ infant, it prevents hemolytic disease of the Rh⁺ neonate of subsequent pregnancies.

Administration Protocols

For protection, Rh immune globulin must be given within 72 hours of exposure. It is given at 28 weeks gestation, following amniocentesis or abortion, and as soon as possible after delivery (3 hours optimum, but within 72 hours). It is also given following the transfusion of incompatible blood or packed cells and in the treatment of immune thrombocytopenia purpura (ITP). It is given intravenously or intramuscularly, depending on the product, strictly following manufacturer's guidelines for reconstitution and administration. RhoGam must be given intramuscularly, never intravenously. The IV route is required for treatment of ITP and transfusion accidents.

Immediately following abortion or amniocentesis, 600 IU (120 mcg) is given. For threatened abortion, 1,500 IU (300 μg) must be given as soon as possible. During pregnancy, the pre-delivery dose is 1,500 IU (300 μg) at 28 weeks gestation, and the post-delivery dose is 600 IU (120 μg). Following a transfusion of incompatible blood (or massive fetal hemorrhage), 3,000 IU (600 μg) is administered every 8 hours until the total dose is given. The total dose for Rh⁺ blood is 45 IU (9 μg)/ml of blood infused and the dose for Rh⁺ RBCs is 90 IU (18 μg)/ml of cells infused. For ITP, 250 IU (50 μg)/kg of body weight is given initially, with a maintenance dose of 125 to 300 IU (25 to 60 μg)/kg given according to the patient's clinical response.

Varicella-Zoster Immune Globulin

Indications

The varicella-zoster immune globulin is indicated to provide passive immunity for immunocompromised patients who have been exposed to the varicella (chickenpox) virus. It is not the same as the Varivax vaccine, which is used as an immunization in the prevention of chickenpox.

Administration Protocols

The varicella-zoster immune globulin is administered IM, preferably in the deltoid muscle, and must never be given IV. It has to be given within 72 hours of exposure to the chickenpox virus to achieve optimal effect.

NONBLOOD-PRODUCT VOLUME EXPANDERS

Many clinical situations indicate the need for replacement or volume expansion from nonblood products. Such preparations are complex carbohydrates with molecular weights similar to albumin. Because of their large molecular size, they cannot pass out of the capillaries or vascular walls. Being confined to the vascular space, they increase colloid osmotic pressure, thus generating osmotic forces that draw fluid from the interstitial spaces into the blood.

Dextran

Dextran is a plasma volume expander (or replacement) made from water-soluble synthetic polysaccharide polymers. It is not considered a substitute for whole blood or its fractions. It is available in assorted molecular weights.

Because of the chemical makeup, the administration of dextran can lead to an anaphylactic reaction from a polysaccharide-reacting antibody and polysaccharide antigen reaction. To prevent such a response, dextran 1 (Promit), a dextran adjunct, is given intravenously prior to dextran infusions. It inhibits the formation of immune complexes that arise from the polyvalent dextrans. Dextran 1, a monovalent hapten, binds to one of the sites on the dextran-reacting antibody.

Dextran 40

Dextran 40 is a low molecular weight, hypertonic colloidal solution. It creates an immediate (up to double the volume within minutes) but brief (up to 12 hours depending on renal clearance) intravascular expansion. Seventy-five percent of the product is excreted unchanged by the kidneys within 24 hours of administration.

Indications

Dextran 40 (10% LMD, 10% Gentran® 40 in 0.9% NaCl, 10% Gentran® in dextrose, Rheomacrodex®) is a low molecular weight, preservative-free solution indicated for fluid replacement and the treatment of shock resulting from the volume deficits of burns, hemorrhage, surgical losses, or other trauma. It is sometimes used prophylactically in high-risk surgical patients predisposed to acute thrombosis and pulmonary embolization. Dextran 40 greatly improves microcirculation by impeding RBC sludging and decreasing blood viscosity.

Administration Protocols

Dextran 40 is administered only by intravenous infusion. The solution must be clear. If there are any visible crystals, they must be dissolved by placing the container in a warm-water bath at 100°F for 15 minutes. Crystal or flake formation can be circumvented by storing unopened containers at a constant room temperature of 77°F. It is advised that a 0.22-μm filter be used because of the possibility of microcrystal formation.

For the treatment of shock, dextran 40 is administered at the rate of 2 g/kg (20 ml/kg/day), with the initial 10 ml infused rapidly. Thereafter, the dose should not exceed 1 g/kg (10 ml/kg/day), nor should treatment extend beyond five days. The dose for preoperative prophylaxis of thrombosis and pulmonary embolism is 1 g/kg (10 ml/kg) on the day of surgery and 50 to 100 g (500 ml/day) for 48 to 72 hours postoperatively. Thereafter, the dose is reduced to 500 to 1000 ml infused over 48 to 72 hours for up to 14 days.

Dextran is contraindicated in patients with cardiac, hepatic, or renal failure. It must not be used for patients undergoing corticosteroid therapy. For patients with decreased platelets and clotting factors, or in the presence of bleeding disorders, dextran should not be used.

High Molecular Weight Dextran

High molecular weight dextrans are polysaccharides with colloidal characteristics on a par with albumin. They generate plasma volume expansion in excess of the actual amount of dextran administered within an hour of treatment. They are slowly broken down into dextrose and evacuated from the body as carbon dioxide and water.

Indications

High molecular weight dextran is indicated for the emergency treatment of hypovolemic (actual or impending) shock from the fluid losses of burns, surgery, or trauma. It should be used only when whole blood or blood products are inaccessible or when the situation is so critical that time does not allow for the crossmatching of blood.

Administration Protocols

High molecular weight dextran is administered only by intravenous infusion at the rate of 1.2 g/kg or 20 ml/kg, for the first 24 hours. If needed, it is followed by 10 ml/kg/day. The contraindications and precautions are the same as those associated with dextran 40. The two, however, are not to be interchanged.

Hetastarch

Hetastarch or hydroxyethylstarch (HES) is a water-soluble synthetic polymer plasma volume expander-replacement solution. Approximately 90% of the product is composed of amylopectins, the insoluble constituents of starch. HES is similar, in terms of colloidal properties, to albumin. It is isotonic, with approximately 310 mOsm/L. While its actions are much the same as dextran, it does not produce as many allergic reactions. It also does not interfere with blood typing and crossmatching. As with dextran, hetastarch is not a substitute for blood or its components.

Indications

Hetastarch is indicated to expand plasma volume, in excess of the infused volume, for about 24 hours. HES dilutes the hematocrit and total serum protein values. It is used in the treatment of shock and hypovolemia from burns, hemorrhage, sepsis, surgery, or other trauma. It is also used to retrieve granulocytes more efficiently during the leukapheresis process.

Administration Protocols

Hetastarch is administered only by intravenous infusion, with the dose individualized to meet patient needs. For acute hemorrhage, the usual dose is up to 20 ml/kg/hr (1,500 ml maximum) with 500 to 1,000 ml (6% solution) given for plasma expansion. The rate is considerably slower for burns and septic shock.

HES is contraindicated in patients with cardiac, hepatic, and renal failure. It should not be given to those with severe bleeding disorders because it can diminish the coagulation proficiency of the circulating blood. It is incompatible with many drugs and should not be mixed with anything.

BLOOD AND BLOOD PRODUCT TRANSFUSION

Blood is essential in the transport and delivery of antibodies, electrolytes, hormones, nutrients, oxygen, and vitamins to all cells, tissues, and organs of the body. It also supports thermal and chemical regulation and carries carbon dioxide and waste products to the appropriate areas of excretion. It constitutes approximately 8% of the body's weight.

Blood Supply Safety

The U.S. Food and Drug Administration (FDA) is responsible for ensuring the safety of our nation's blood supply. The Center for Biologics Evaluation and Research (CBER) regulates the collection of blood and blood components used for transfusion or for the manufacture of pharmaceuticals derived from blood and blood components, such as clotting factors, and establishes standards for the products themselves. CBER also regulates related products such as cell separation devices, blood collection containers, and HIV screening tests that are used to prepare blood products or to ensure the safety of the blood supply. CBER develops and enforces quality standards, inspects blood establishments, and monitors reports of errors, accidents, and adverse clinical events. CBER works closely with other parts of the Public Health Service (PHS) to identify and respond to potential threats to blood safety, to develop safety and technical standards, to monitor blood supplies, and to help industry promote an adequate supply of blood and blood products. Although a blood supply with zero risk of transmitting infectious disease may not be possible, the blood supply in the United States is safer today than at any other time in recent history. Within the perspective of other harmful health-related occurrences, the risks from blood transfusion are minimal. The present safety level has evolved because of ongoing modifications and improvements in donor education and screening, serologic analysis, and by nucleic acid testing methods, as well as various treatment and inactivation procedures. All blood donations are routinely assessed for HIV, hepatitis B virus, hepatitis C virus, human T-lymphotropic virus, and syphilis. Use of nucleic acid testing (NAT) techniques has reduced the risk of HIV transmission to about one per million units of blood transfused.

Indications for Transfusion

The need for transfusion therapy is based on the clinical situation. The usual indications for blood and blood product administration are as follows:

- Blood volume maintenance
- Blood volume replacement
- Neonatal exchange (whole blood)
- Blood component maintenance
- Blood component replacement
- Coagulation component supplementation

In general, whole blood is transfused only in emergency situations where there is massive loss of volume, impending shock, and where it is necessary to replace vascular losses in order to restore the transport capabilities of the blood. When blood loss is such that the vascular compartment volume is depleted, cardiac output declines and arterial blood pressure plummets. The systemic result is diminished tissue perfusion of oxygen and nutrients.

Approximately 10% of a person's normal blood volume can be removed without serious sequelae. The rate at which blood loss occurs is a major factor in the maintenance of homeostasis because of the time needed for physiologic compensatory mechanisms to mobilize (Figure 14-3). For this reason, a rapid depletion of volume is far more precarious than a relatively slow loss. It is also more serious in terms of the time needed to procure replacement therapy.

For severe volume deprivation, losses must be restored (when compensatory mechanisms fail to sustain the patient), or death will ensue. Once the cascade of events in uncompensated progressive shock from hypovolemia occurs and progresses to the point of myocardial deterioration and protracted tissue damage, transfusion administration cannot reverse the situation even if the blood pressure and cardiac output are returned to normal (Figure 14-4). It is critical, therefore, that replacement measures be initiated as soon as possible in hypovolemic crises (when arterial pressure falls below 70 mm Hg).

Oxygen transport depletion not related to volume loss is restored by transfusion therapy with blood constituents. Component replacement is preferable to whole blood in preventing exposure to nonessential blood elements and in the prevention of fluid volume excess in normovolemic individuals or exacerbation of overload in hypervolemic patients.

Transfusion Options

Two categories of blood transfusion, each having three methods of blood collection, are available. The systems presently used are **homologous** or allogenic (volunteer, designated [directed], or cadaver) and **autologous** (preoperative autologous blood donation [PABD], autotransfusion [via salvaged blood], and acute normovolemic hemodilution [ANH]). The decision to use either transfusion option depends on medical evaluation, the patient's clinical situation, and time constraints.

Homologous Transfusion

Homologous blood is blood collected from donors for allogenic transfusion to other human beings. It is also called **indirect homologous donation** because the blood is removed from a donor, stored under specified conditions, then

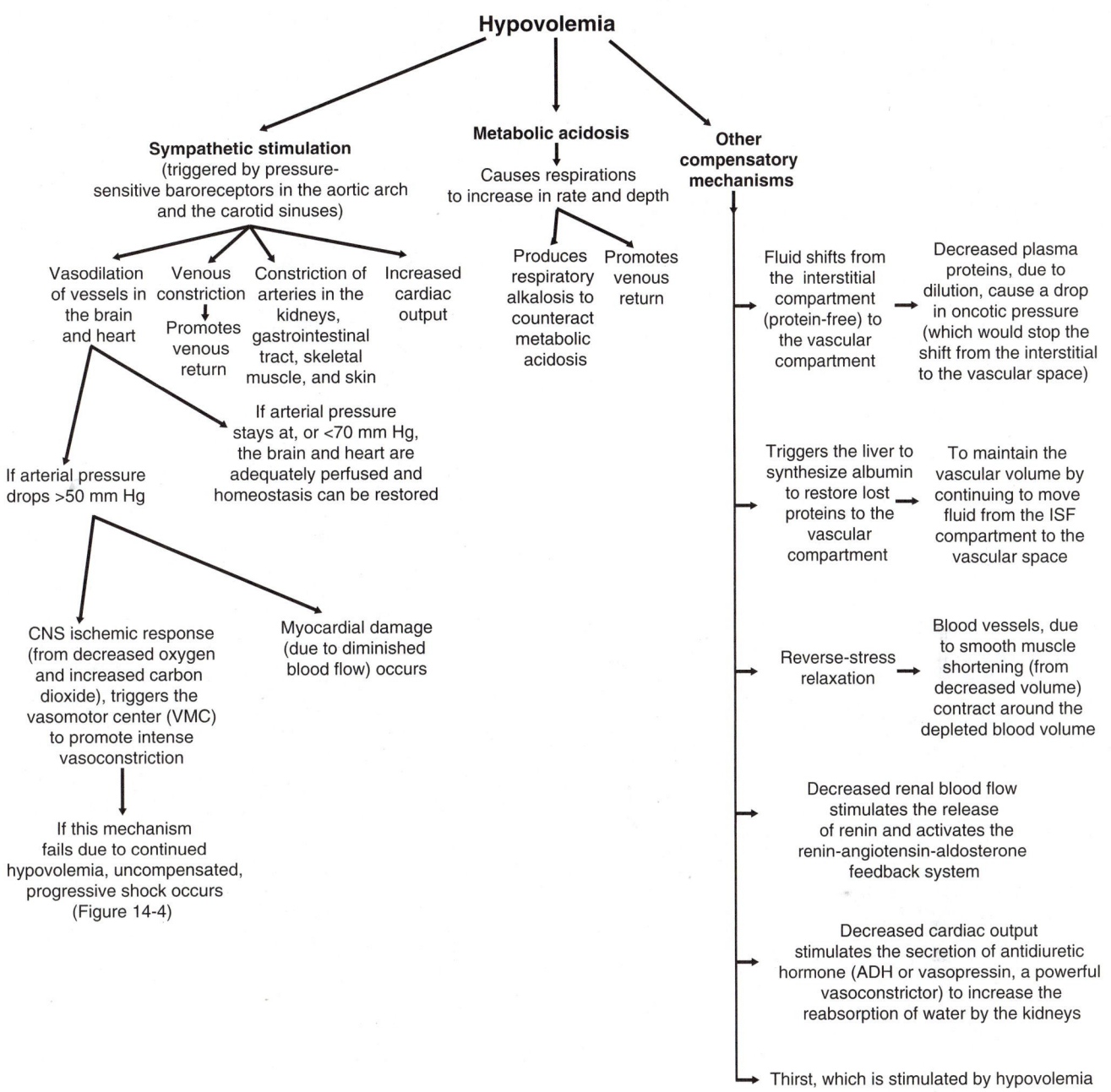

Figure 14-3 | Compensatory mechanisms in hypovolemia work to increase peripheral resistance and maintain blood pressure through vasoconstriction

administered to a recipient at a later date. These transfusions are derived from volunteer donations, designated donations, or cadaver blood. When volunteer donations are processed, the units must be labeled *volunteer donation*. In emergency situations, where the need for transfusion is unpredictable and immediate, homologous volunteer or cadaver blood and blood components are generally used. Blood from a cadaver is collected within a short time following death, usually with the body on artificial life support. Designated (directed) donation

is provided by one person or several persons chosen by the intended transfusion recipient.

In addition to FDA recommendations, the American Association of Blood Banks (AABB) Scientific Committee of the Joint Blood Council and Standards Committee has detailed the criteria that must be met for all homologous blood. These include the donor's medical, surgical, drug, and alcohol history, a qualifying physical examination to determine state of health, and laboratory studies to determine

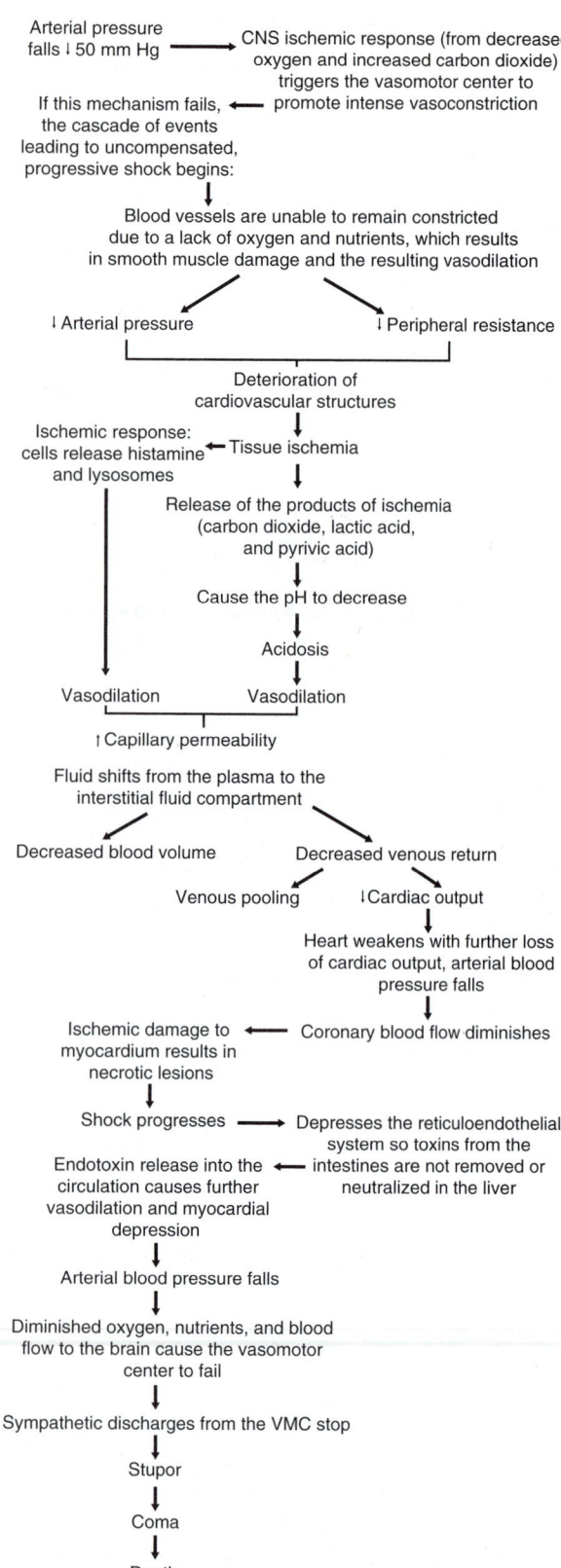

Figure 14-4 | Uncompensated progressive shock from prolonged hypovolemia

ABO group, Rh type, and screen for unanticipated antibodies and diseases that can be transmitted via blood transfusion. All of these criteria are necessary for the safety and protection of transfusion donors and recipients. After donor blood is drawn, ABO and Rh analysis is done, and assessments for any unexpected red blood cell antibodies (that may cause problems in the recipient) are completed, the following screening tests are performed:

- Cytomegalovirus (CMV)
- Hepatitis B surface antigen (HBsAg)
- Hepatitis B core antibody (anti-HBc)
- Hepatitis C virus antibody (anti-HCV)
- Human immunodeficiency virus (HIV-1 and HIV-2) antibodies (anti-HIV-1 and anti-HIV-2)
- Human immunodeficiency virus HIV p24 antigen
- Human T-cell lymphotropic virus (HTLV-I and HTLV-II) antibody (anti-HTLV-I and anti-HTLV-II)
- Nucleic acid amplification testing (NAT). (The FDA has licensed the first nucleic acid test systems for screening donors of whole blood and blood components, including fresh plasma, red cells and platelets. The semi-automated, highly sensitive systems can directly and rapidly recognize the genetic material of HCV and HIV, and thereby detect the infections before the appearance of their symptoms.)
- Serologic test for syphilis

In compliance with the FDA and the AABB, the minimum volunteer donor requirements are based on the following criteria:

- Age of 17 to 65 years
- Blood or plasma donation: none in previous eight weeks; no apheresis within 48 hours
- Laboratory data:
  - Male: Hgb: 13.5 g/dl, Hct: 41%
  - Female: Hgb: 12.5 g/dl, Hct: 38%
- Skin: lesion-free venipuncture site; no evidence of intravenous drug abuse
- Vital signs:
  - Blood pressure
    Systolic: 90–180 mm Hg
    Diastolic: 50–100 mm Hg
  - Pulse: 50 to 100/min and regular
  - Temperature, oral: not to exceed 99.6°F (37.5°C)
  - Weight: minimum of 110 lb (50 kg)
  - Normal liver function tests

Designated (Directed) Homologous Transfusion

Designated directed homologous blood is blood collected from a donor selected by the intended recipient. Such blood must meet all the specifications for homologous blood, including negative results for transfusion-transmitted disease markers.

Designated donation may be no safer than homologous blood collected from members of the community, because designated donors may be less likely to disclose risk behaviors.

Autologous Transfusion

Even with the stringent regulations established for the testing of homologous blood, the general public is still in fear of contracting AIDS or hepatitis from volunteer donor transfusions. For this reason, autologous donation is still used in some situations. The alternatives to homologous transfusion can be used alone or in conjunction with each other. The choice is based on the clinical situation. The three main alternatives are preoperative autologous blood donation (PABD), perioperative blood salvage, and acute normovolemic hemodilution (ANH). Each requires special handling under strict guidelines by trained phlebotomy personnel and carries stringent constraints regarding labeling, storage, and reinfusion. Because of these factors, autologous transfusion therapy is more expensive than homologous transfusion therapy.

Preoperative Donation

Autologous blood is blood collected from an individual for that individual's use in advance of its actual need and stored for reinfusion at a later time. Autologous donation is for selected patients who are likely to require blood transfusion during the perioperative period. Whenever preoperative medical orders include blood crossmatching, and the patient is relatively healthy, autologous donation is usually a choice.

The FDA recommends testing autologous blood for HBsAg, HCsAg, anti-HIV, and syphilis. Although not required, most blood services also test for anti-HTLV-1, ALT, and anti-HBcAg. If the blood is anti-HIV positive or HBsAg reactive, it can only be transfused with a written, signed medical order, but the FDA does not condone its use.

Orthopedic surgical procedures for hip replacement and scoliosis repair in patients free of osteomyelitis are ideal candidates for autologous donation. Patients who are free of infection and in need of surgery for congenital heart disease, stable coronary artery or vascular disease, aortic procedures, or leg revascularization can be donors as well. In these cases age is not a major factor. Children as young as 8 and the elderly can donate successfully. If they are under 110 lbs., the volume drawn (per donation) is proportionate to body weight.

The standard requirements usually include two or more weeks notice and a baseline hemoglobin of 11 g/dl and a hematocrit of 33%. The optimal donation period is four to six weeks prior to surgery, with the last donation no later than 72 hours before surgery. The usual donation interval is weekly, but it can be as frequent as every three days.

In recent years some controversy has developed over autologous blood donation. One reason is that the U.S. blood supply is now considered safer and, the other is that the cost of autologous blood is far more expensive than donor blood, with it often being discarded when not used. The findings of some investigations are leaning toward the decision that autologous donations are unnecessary in many circumstances. It seems that patients whose levels of hemoglobin are high, prior to donations, rebuild their blood levels rapidly and end up not needing the blood. Those who have high hemoglobin levels often don't lose enough intraoperative blood to trigger the production of more blood. Others, however, who have lower preoperative hemoglobin levels are more likely to need a transfusion intraoperatively or postoperatively. By donating blood ahead of time, their systems may not have the time/ability to satisfactorily rebuild their hemoglobin prior to surgery. As a result, they may end up needing their own blood along with that of a homologous donor. More research is needed in this area to determine updated guidelines regarding preoperative autologous donation.

Perioperative Blood Salvage

Perioperative **blood salvage** is the collection and reinfusion of blood lost during the intraoperative and early (4- to 12-hour) postoperative period. It is normally employed during major surgeries such as cardiovascular bypass, vascular procedures, orthopedic procedures, trauma (associated with major blood loss), splenectomy, and organ transplantation.

The greatest benefit associated with the use of salvaged blood is that exposure to homologous donor antigens is eliminated. In addition, the amount recovered is usually about 50% of that lost, so, if combined with other blood conservation measures, it is usually adequate to preclude homologous transfusion. Post-transfusion viability of recovered RBCs is comparable to that of homologous administration.

While perioperative blood salvage is a useful technique for the maintenance and replacement of surgical blood losses, it is not without risk. Table 14-6 lists the major drawbacks to blood salvage along with the associated implications.

Intraoperative Blood Salvage

When lost blood is collected under strictly sterile conditions, it can be safely reinfused at once or undergo a washing process prior to reinfusion. Unwashed blood is administered back into the patient with a standard blood filter using gravity. The suction systems used to salvage the blood do not traumatize the RBCs. During the washing process, the recovered blood is mixed with normal saline under sterile conditions and centrifuged until an adequate hemoconcentration is achieved and the plasma is clear. The main disadvantage associated with this method is that there is a considerable loss of coagulation factors, as well as platelets.

Intraoperative blood salvage is contraindicated if there is any likelihood of contamination, as seen in patients with

Table 14-6 | Risks Associated with Perioperative Blood Salvage

Risk	Implications
Dilutional Coagulopathy	There is a deficiency of coagulation factors and platelets in salvaged blood that may result in the following postoperative complications: – Fibrinogen deficiency – Prolonged PT and PTT – Thrombocytopenia This is the most common risk associated with perioperative blood salvage.
Disseminated Intravascular Coagulation (DIC)	Some research suggests that the presence of coagulation abnormalities, following salvaged RBC infusions, is an indication of DIC.
Anticoagulant Reinfusion	If heparin is used in the blood salvage container, and the blood is not washed prior to reinfusion, it may result in systemic anti-coagulation.
Renal Insufficiency	Some hemolysis occurs during the salvaging process, due to aspiration pressure and surface suctioning. The reinfusion of unwashed blood and hemolyzed cells may contribute to renal failure, especially in patients with compromised renal function.
Air Embolism	As with any intravenous infusion, air embolism is always a danger. There is minimal risk, however, with the use of modern blood salvaging equipment.
Contamination	Salvaged blood can contain body fluids, bone fragments, irrigating solutions, or topical agents, which may not be removed, even when the blood is washed before reinfusion.

peritonitis, intra-abdominal or thoracic abscesses, osteomyelitis, or when intestinal contents contaminate the sterile operative field. Washing and filtering do not eliminate bacteria. In surgical procedures that involve resection of malignancies, the blood is not salvaged because of the risk of seeding the malignant cells into the blood, which provides a means of transportation to other body locations.

Postoperative Blood Salvage
Following major surgery, mainly cardiovascular, thoracic, and (some) orthopedic procedures, blood is often retrieved. Even though it is dilute, it is sterile and contains RBCs. It is usually salvaged from chest and mediastinal drains, then reinfused without washing.

Acute Normovolemic Hemodilution
Acute normovolemic hemodilution is the preoperative removal of a patient's blood via an arterial or venous catheter with the concurrent infusion of cell-free solutions to maintain normal volume. The procedure, usually performed by the attending anesthesiologist, is done immediately before or after the induction of anesthesia. It is only indicated for patients who are physiologically able to tolerate a rapid extraction of several units of blood prior to intraoperative blood loss. The amount of blood withdrawn is determined by the physician and based on anticipated surgical losses, body size, and hematocrit.

Once removed, the blood can be stored for up to four hours at room temperature. The blood is usually reinfused at the completion of surgery when hemostasis is reestablished. If more than four hours elapse before reinfusion, the blood is to be refrigerated according to blood service protocols.

Researchers continue to study hemodilution to ascertain its safety and value because it is a fairly new procedure. Advocates of the process endorse its use because fresh autologous whole blood is available should it be needed. In addition, there is a decrease in the loss of RBCs during surgery because the circulating volume has a reduced hematocrit (which also augments tissue oxygenation). Hemodilution decreases the viscosity of the blood, which also enhances tissue perfusion.

BLOOD TRANSFUSION REACTIONS

The administration of blood or any of its components presents a significant risk of an adverse event called a transfusion reaction. It is important for the nurse to understand and recognize the signs and symptoms associated with a transfusion reaction and to comprehend the serious and potentially fatal sequelae that can occur if any of them are not immediately addressed. In addition, the nurse must know and be able to carry out the interventions necessary to avert or reverse the devastating effects of reaction.

It is important to keep in mind that an acute (immediate) reaction can occur within five minutes of the start of a transfusion or as late as 48 hours after its discontinuation. Delayed reactions may develop any time after 48 hours, extending to a period of up to six months. There are also reactions that occur in individuals requiring multiple transfusions because of the products used in the storage of blood components. Table 14-7 distinguishes the general signs and symptoms of transfusion reactions using a body systems approach.

General Nursing Interventions for All Transfusion Reactions

Should a transfusion reaction occur, it is the nurse's responsibility to terminate the transfusion and tubing, maintain patency of the cannula via an infusion of 0.9% normal saline, notify the physician and transfusion services, and

Table 14-7 | Systemic Identification of the General Signs and Symptoms of a Transfusion Reaction

Body System	Clinical Manifestations
General	Back pain Chest pain Chills* Headache Heat at infusion site and/or over vein* Muscle aches or pains Rise in temperature 1°C or 2°F above baseline*
Cardiovascular System	Circulatory status: 　Bleeding (generalized DIC; oozing from surgical site)* 　Cool/clammy skin* 　Cyanosis* 　Dry/flushed/hot skin* 　Edema* 　Facial flushing* Vital signs: 　BP: 　　Hypertension 　　Hypotension (VMI)* 　　Shock* 　Pulse: 　　Bradycardia (VMI)* 　　Tachycardia (VMI)* 　　Weak pulse* VMI = vasomotor instability
Gastrointestinal System	Abdominal cramping or pain Diarrhea (may be bloody)* Nausea Vomiting
Integumentary System	Diaphoresis* Edema* Hives (urticaria)* Itching Rashes* Skin color: 　Cyanosis* 　Facial flushing* Skin temperature: 　Cool/clammy* 　Dry/flushed/hot*
Musculoskeletal System	Abdominal cramping Back pain
Nervous System	Apprehension Fever* Headache Numbness Sense of impending doom Tingling
Renal System	Flank pain Urine color: 　Amber, brown, or red (indicative of RBCs [hematuria] or free hemoglobin [hemoblobinuria])* 　Concentrated, dark* Urine volume: 　Anuria* 　Oliguria* 　Renal failure*
Respiratory System	Apnea* Cough Dyspnea* Rales* Tachypnea* Wheezing

*Identifying factor in the unconscious or mentally handicapped patient.

implement other appropriate interventions. The nurse is accountable for written documentation and communication of relevant data to the physician and all health care providers concerned with the patient's care.

Acute (Immediate) Transfusion Reactions

Because of advances in blood screening, testing, and storage, as well as protocols for administration, acute reactions can usually be averted. The reactions that might develop are acute hemolysis, mild to serious allergic effects, circulatory overload, or sepsis. Should any reaction occur, the untoward effects can be deflected if they are immediately recognized, and the appropriate measures are taken to support the patient (Table 14-8).

NURSING TIP

Nursing Interventions for Transfusion Reactions

Should a transfusion reaction occur, the general (and immediate) nursing interventions include the following:
1. Stop the transfusion immediately, but do not discontinue the intravenous line.
2. Connect new IV tubing to the cannula hub and keep the line open with 0.9% normal saline.
3. Stay with the patient and monitor vital signs.
4. Notify the physician.
5. Follow medical orders regarding symptomatic treatment.
6. Notify the blood service.
7. Notify the lab to collect blood and urine samples specified by blood administration services.
8. Check the tags and numbers on the blood containers to verify correlation with the patient's blood identification bracelet and document this verification.
9. Send the blood bag with its administration set and all attached labels to the blood transfusion service.
10. Document all assessment data, nursing interventions, and patient responses in the medical record and fill out a transfusion reaction report.

Delayed Transfusion Reactions

Delayed reactions can occur up to six months after a patient has been transfused. Delayed transfusion reactions can be reduced with thorough pretransfusion testing of donor blood or with irradiation of blood products intended for adminis-

Table 14-8 | Acute (Immediate) Transfusion Reactions

REACTION AND ETIOLOGY	DEFINING CHARACTERISTICS, NURSING INTERVENTIONS, AND PREVENTION

Acute Hemolytic Transfusion Reaction

Etiology: Hemolysis occurs when antibodies in the recipient's plasma attach to antigens on the donor's RBCs. This is due to the infusion of ABO-incompatible blood: whole blood, RBCs, or components containing 10 ml or more RBCs.

Defining Characteristics. The clinical manifestations seen are usually a combination of any of the following:

Acute renal failure	Flushing	Tachycardia
Bleeding	Hemoglobinemia	Tachypnea
Cardiac arrest	Hemoglobinuria	Vascular collapse
Chills	Low back pain	
Death	Shock	

Nursing Interventions. The clinical management of an acute hemolytic reaction includes the following:

Treat shock, if present

Maintain BP with colloidal solutions

Administer ordered diuretics to maintain urine flow

Draw blood (removing slowly, to avert hemolysis), obtain urine sample, and send both to the lab along with any other samples required by the blood service

Monitor urine output hourly to assess for renal failure and the need for dialysis

Do not transfuse any RBC-containing components until the transfusion service has procured newly crossmatched units.

Preventive Measures. To prevent an acute hemolytic reaction, it is vital that donor-recipient blood be tested for compatibility, under strict guidelines, then verified prior to its transfusion into a patient.

Allergic Reaction (Mild)

Etiology: Mild allergic transfusion reactions occur when there is recipient sensitivity to the donor's foreign plasma proteins.

Defining Characteristics. The clinical manifestations of a mild allergic reaction usually include the following:

Facial flushing	Rash
Itching	Rhinorrhea
Ocular congestion with tearing	Urticaria (hives)

Nursing Interventions. The nursing management for a patient with an allergic reaction includes the following:

Antihistamine administration, as ordered

Restarting the transfusion, slowly, if the symptoms are mild and transient, with close monitoring of the patient

Never restart the transfusion if fever or any respiratory-pulmonary symptomatology exists.

Prevention. Mild allergic reactions are usually treated prophylactically with antihistamine administration.

Remember: A mild allergic reaction can always precede a severe allergic reaction that causes systemic anaphylaxis.

Anaphylactic Transfusion Reaction

Etiology: Anaphylaxis occurs when donor blood with IgA proteins is transfused into an IgA-deficient recipient who has developed IgA antibody.

Defining Characteristics. The defining characteristics of an anaphylactic reaction include the following:

Anxiety	Hypotension	Cardiac arrest
Urticaria	Gastrointestinal	Death
Wheezing	distress	
Cyanosis	Shock	

Table 14-8 | Acute (Immediate) Transfusion Reactions

REACTION AND ETIOLOGY	DEFINING CHARACTERISTICS, NURSING INTERVENTIONS, AND PREVENTION

Anaphylactic Transfusion Reaction

Etiology: Mild allergic transfusion reactions occur when there is recipient sensitivity to the donor's foreign plasma proteins.

Defining Characteristics. The clinical manifestations of a mild allergenic reaction usually include:

Facial flushing	Rash
Itching	Rhinorrhea
Ocular congestion with tearing	Urticaria (hives)

Nursing Interventions. The clinical management of anaphylaxis includes the following:
Discontinuing the transfusion and keeping the vein open with normal saline
CPR, if necessary
Following medical orders that may entail the administration of epinephrine subcutaneously or intravenously
Administration of steroids
IV fluid administration to maintain intravascular fluid volume
Maintaining blood pressure through the administration of drugs to counteract hypotension

Prevention. Anaphylaxis can be prevented by using blood from donors who are IgA deficient or by administering only well-washed RBCs in which all plasma has been extracted.

Circulatory Overload

Etiology: Circulatory overload occurs when blood is administered more rapidly than the circulatory system can adjust to it.

Defining Characteristics. Circulatory overload is identified by the following:

Cough	Hypertension	Pulmonary edema
Dyspnea	Neck vein distention	
Headache	Pulmonary congestion	

Nursing Interventions. If circulatory overload occurs, the nurse must do the following:
Stop the transfusion and KVO, very slowly, with normal saline
Raise the head of the bed and place the feet in a dependent position
Notify the physician and administer diuretics, oxygen, and other ordered medications
Carry out orders for a phlebotomy, if necessary

Prevention. Prophylaxis for circulatory overload includes the following:
Pretransfusion administration of diuretics
Use of packed RBCs rather than whole blood
Modification of infusion rate and volume to meet individual patient needs
Requesting the blood service to divide units into smaller alliquots to allow for longer intervals of administration

Sepsis

Etiology: Sepsis occurs when contaminated blood components are administered.

Defining Characteristics. Sepsis is evidenced by the following:

Chills, with rapid onset	Marked hypotension
Diarrhea	Nausea and vomiting
High fever, with rapid onset	Shock

Nursing Interventions. The clinical management includes the following:
Discontinuation of transfusion, KVO with normal saline, and return of tubing and container to blood services
Obtaining a blood culture
Treatment of septicemia, as medically ordered, which may entail antibiotic, fluid, steroid, and vasopressor administration

Prevention. Following the proper protocols for the collection, processing, storage, and transfusion (strict aseptic technique and infusion within a four-hour period) of blood products is necessary for the prevention of sepsis.

tration to immunocompromised individuals. Such reactions include delayed hemolytic responses, graft versus host disease, viral exposure (HBV, HBC, and HIV-1), and iron overload. They are infrequent, however (Table 14-9). In some cases, reactions cannot be predicted; therefore, they cannot be prevented.

Reactions as a Result of Multiple Transfusions

A third category of reactions (Table 14-10) results from frequent exposure to the hematologic or chemical products contained in stored blood. These are encountered in patients

Table 14-9 | Delayed Transfusion Reactions

REACTION AND ETIOLOGY	DEFINING CHARACTERISTICS, NURSING INTERVENTIONS, AND PREVENTION
Delayed Hemolytic Transfusion Reaction	
Etiology: Delayed hemolytic reactions are not due to ABO incompatibility, but occur as a consequence of the destruction of transfused RBCs by alloantibodies not discovered during the process of crossmatching.	**Defining Characteristics.** The clinical manifestations of a delayed hemolytic reaction are as follows: 　　Decreased hematocrit and hemoglobin 　　Fever (continual, low grade) 　　Jaundice (mild) 　　Malaise
	Nursing Interventions. There are no specific interventions, unless hemolysis is severe, in which case, further transfusions may be needed.
	Prevention. Strict attention to crossmatching protocols is the best prevention.
Graft-versus-Host Disease	
Etiology: Graft-vs-host disease occurs when donor lymphocytes from the graft propagate in the recipient	**Defining Characteristics:** When the recipient (host) manifests rejection, the following may result: 　　Diarrhea　　　Hepatitis 　　Fever　　　　Rash
	Nursing Interventions. Since there is no effective therapy, the nursing protocols revolve around the treatment of symptoms.
	Prevention. The primary preventive measure is the irradiation of all blood products used on immunocompromised patients.
Hepatitis B	
Etiology: Hepatitis B is viral in origin and spreads by blood and serum-derived fluids and by direct contact with body fluids.	**Defining Characteristics.** The clinical manifestations usually include the following: 　　Anorexia　　　　　Headache　　　Pharyngitis 　　Dark urine　　　　Jaundice　　　Photophobia 　　Elevated liver enzymes　Malaise　　　Vomiting 　　Fever　　　　　　Nausea
	Nursing Interventions. Since there is no specific treatment, nursing care revolves around symptomatic treatment. Teaching regarding the following is recommended: The disease process Signs and symptoms of complications The need for a balance between rest and activity The measures to be taken to prevent transmission to others
	Prevention. The major preventive measure is the hepatitis B vaccine. In addition, the pretransfusion testing of donor blood for HBsAg (surface hepatitis B) and anti-HBc (anti core hepatitis B) is available. Blood services do not accept donations from persons with a history of drug addiction, exposure to AIDS or viral hepatitis, or who have been tattooed within six months.

Table 14-9 | Delayed Transfusion Reactions

REACTION AND ETIOLOGY	DEFINING CHARACTERISTICS, NURSING INTERVENTIONS, AND PREVENTION
Hepatitis C	
Etiology: Hepatitis C, like hepatitis B, is viral in origin and spread by blood and serum-derived fluids and by direct contact with body fluids.	**Defining Characteristics.** The clinical manifestations are similar to hepatitis B.
	Nursing Interventions. The nursing care is the same as with hepatitis B.
	Prevention. There is not a vaccine for hepatitis C. The preventive measures include donor testing and the same protocols for blood donation that are required for hepatitis B.
HIV-1 (AIDS Virus) Infection	
Etiology: Infection is from the human immunodeficiency virus, transmitted via bodily secretions from an HIV-positive individual to another person through breaks in the mucous membranes or skin. HIV infection is known to occur through the following: 1. Sexual intercourse 2. Contaminated needles or blood 3. Placental transfer from mother to fetus	**Defining Characteristics.** Using the Walter Reed Classification System, there are 6 stages, each with clinical indicators: Stage 0 Exposure Stage 1 Infection, with antibodies to HIV in the blood (HIV+), flulike syndrome (fever, lymphadenopathy, malaise, and myalgias) Stage 2 Chronic lymphadenopathy Stage 3 T4 count <400 Stage 4 Lowered delayed hypersensitivity reaction to common allergies Stage 5 Total anergy with chronic fungal or viral infections to mucous membranes Stage 6 Acquired immune deficiency syndrome (AIDS), the combination of opportunistic infections where the virus attaches to the CD4 receptor on T4 lymphocytes causing their demise, with progressive destruction of immune function
	Nursing Interventions. Since there as yet is no cure, the treatment is symptomatic, with administration of drugs that may halt the progression of the disease. Care to all patients involves the use of CDC Standard Precautions and teaching to prevent infection and transmission of the HIV.
	Prevention. Public education is a major factor in the prevention of infection. Compliance measures regarding intimate sexual contact, needle sharing, and blood donation are vital.
Iron Overload (Hemosiderosis)	
Etiology: Iron overload usually occurs in patients with chronic anemia who have received in excess of 100 units of RBCs. Hemosiderin (iron pigment) accumulates in the liver and spleen with RBC destruction.	**Defining Characteristics.** With iron overload, the clinical manifestations include the following: Cardiac arrhythmias / Elevated plasma iron (>200 mg/dl) Cirrhosis / Endocrine dysfunction (diabetes mellitus, Congestive heart failure / impaired gonad and thyroid function)
	Nursing Interventions. Treatment for iron overload is essentially symptomatic. Administration of drugs, as medically ordered, to inactivate, neutralize, or remove accumulated iron (by way of renal excretion) may be indicated.
	Prevention. Do not administer blood unless absolutely essential.

receiving multiple transfusions and can include elevated blood ammonia titers, coagulation imbalances, decreased tissue oxygenation, hypocalcemia, and hyperkalemia.

TRANSFUSION ADMINISTRATION

In accord with the regulations set forth by governmental agencies, the AABB, the INS, the policies and procedures set forth by his employer, as well as the nurse practice act of the

Table 14-10 | Reactions Associated with Multiple Transfusions Caused by Products Contained in Stored Blood

REACTION AND ETIOLOGY	DEFINING CHARACTERISTICS, NURSING INTERVENTIONS, AND PREVENTION
Blood Ammonia Elevation	
Etiology: There is an increase in blood ammonia levels in stored blood formed by the decomposition of blood products.	**Defining Characteristics.** Under normal conditions, blood ammonia is present only in trace amounts. When elevated, the clinical picture includes the following: Altered consciousness Asterixis (liver tremor) Electroencephalogram (EEG) changes Neurological changes **Nursing Interventions.** The nursing care, in accord with medical orders, includes the following: Administration of enemas and antibiotics to prevent intestinal bacterial growth that produces ammonia Monitoring and reporting abnormal laboratory results Provision of safety **Prevention.** Preventive measures are mainly aimed at transfusing only the freshest blood or RBCs available, or the use of FFP.
Coagulation Imbalances	
Etiology: Dilutional thrombocytopenia and altered clotting is the result of transfusing stored blood in which there is a diminished platelet count.	**Defining Characteristics.** The main indication of coagulation disturbances is any abnormal bleeding, especially from surgical sites, IV insertion sites, or any breaches in the skin. **Nursing Interventions.** Care involves the following: Monitoring laboratory reports, coagulation studies, and platelet counts Patient protection from bruises, falls, or any trauma that might precipitate bleeding Platelet administration **Prevention.** Fresh blood that is less than a week old is best in preventing bleeding problems.
Decreased Tissue Oxygenation	
Etiology: There is an increase in the attraction of oxygen to hemoglobin in the blood, due to a decrease in 2,3-diphosphoglycerate in stored blood. This prevents the oxygen from leaving the blood and getting to the tissues, thus inducing hypoxia.	**Defining Characteristics.** The clinical picture is the same as it is in any hypoxic state as follows: Confusion Lethargy Cyanosis Respiratory depression (depth and rate) **Nursing Interventions.** Nursing care is mainly directed toward the following: Promotion of respiratory integrity Provision of respiratory support Monitoring and reporting abnormalities in arterial blood gases (ABGs) **Prevention.** The decreased levels of 2,3-diphosphoglycerate can be averted with the use of fresh blood or RBCs.
Hypocalcemia	
Etiology: Citrate, a preservative used in blood storage, can cause hypocalcemia, especially if it is infused rapidly. The citrate ion chemically binds with calcium, thus causing a deficiency of calcium.	**Defining Characteristics.** The patient with a calcium deficiency may present with any of the following: Cardiac dysrhythmias Nausea and vomiting Excessive bleeding Seizures Hyperirritability Tingling of the extremities Hypotension Tetany Muscle cramping Vomiting

Table 14-10 | Reactions Associated with Multiple Transfusions Caused by Products Contained in Stored Blood

REACTION AND ETIOLOGY	DEFINING CHARACTERISTICS, NURSING INTERVENTIONS, AND PREVENTION
Hypocalcemia	
	Nursing Interventions. When signs and symptoms of hypocalcemia occur, the nurse intercedes by doing the following: Slowing or stopping the transfusion Notifying the physician Administering calcium gluconate IV Protecting the patient from injury, especially if seizure activity or tetany occur
	Prevention. To prevent hypocalcemia do the following: Administer blood that is very fresh (less than two days old) Infuse the transfusion slowly Keep the patient warm (hypothermia intensifies a reaction) Monitor and report abnormal calcium and potassium levels. Patients with elevated potassium levels have more adverse reactions than those in the normal range.
Hyperkalemia	
Etiology: Potassium is released into stored blood during RBC destruction.	**Defining Characteristics.** The signs and symptoms of potassium excess can range from mild to severe, and may include the following: Asystole Diarrhea Oliguria, progressing Bradycardia Intestinal colic to anuria EKG deviations Muscle twitching Renal failure
	Nursing Interventions. In situations of potassium excess, the nurse must do the following: Slow, or stop, the transfusion Resuscitate, if necessary Monitor the EKG Notify the physician Administer polystyrene sulfonate orally or by enema
	Prevention. Hyperkalemia can be prevented in patients receiving massive transfusions by infusing only the freshest blood.

state in which he is licensed, the RN is responsible for the safety of the patient during all aspects of blood transfusion therapy. He is expected to continually assess, evaluate, and document the patient's responses in the period preceding administration, throughout the infusion, as it is discontinued, and during the post-transfusion period. The INS requires that the nurse must "have knowledge and understanding of immunohematology, blood grouping, blood and blood components, administration equipment and the techniques appropriate for each component, and transfusion reactions, as well as the potential risks to the patient and the nurse" (INS, 2000, Standard 75, S71). Blood or its constituents may be administered only with medical authorization and proper consent.

Patient Preparation, Explanations, and Teaching

As with all procedures, the patient has the right to know what is being done and why it is necessary. The physician who writes the order for the transfusion is responsible for disclosing the risks associated with the procedure. The nurse, however, plays a critical, collaborative role in verifying that the disclosure is signed, in clarifying and explaining any misunderstandings or concerns, and in answering the patient's questions. The patient must be apprised of any procedures involved, the expected duration of the transfusion, and anything she needs to do to assist in making the procedure progress uneventfully.

Once risk disclosure is verified, the patient must sign a consent for blood transfusion. Prior to signing this

NURSING TIP
Recognizing Transfusion Reaction Symptoms

The nurse must always remember that reactions from different causes can display similar symptoms. Once a transfusion begins, any sign, symptom, or complaint elicited from the patient should be regarded as a potentially significant indicator that a reaction may be occurring. It is also important that pretransfusion symptoms be assessed, documented, and reported so as not to mistake them for a reaction to the blood or its components.

NURSING TIP
Blood Warming

For patients in need of rapid or massive infusions of blood or fluid, the infusate should be warmed so as to prevent hypothermia from occurring. Whenever any fluid warmer is used it is important for the nurse to understand how to use it, following manufacturer's instructions and agency policy.

document, the nurse must reassess the patient's understanding of the ordered transfusion. It is important for the patient to know that, once the transfusion commences, anything unusual (physical, mental, or emotional) must be reported to the nurse immediately. Any symptom may be an indicator of a potential transfusion reaction.

Administration Equipment

The equipment required for the administration of blood or its components include the administration set, filter, needle or catheter, and priming solution. In addition, special regulation equipment, such as electronic infusion devices, pressure cuffs, or warmers might be required. (Caution must be taken when cuffs are used, as hemolysis may occur.) Table 14-11 delineates the equipment required for the administration of blood and its components.

Table 14-11 | Transfusion Administration Equipment

ITEM	INDICATION	FEATURES/RATIONALE
Administration Sets		
Y-type	RBC infusion	
Straight line	Used when blood or blood components are the only constituents to be infused	
Specialty Sets		
Component recipient set	To administer cryoprecipitate or platelets	Shorter line, smaller filter
Component infusion set	To administer a small amount of blood component	For direct IV push
Filters		
	Required to trap clots and other debris from all blood components, except albumin and IV immune globulin	Prevents contamination and emboli
In-line	Required to trap clots and other debris from all blood components, except albumin and IV immune globulin	Depending on institution policy, one filter may be used to infuse 4 units of blood. To avert problems of infection from bacterial contamination, hemolysis, or delayed infusion, a filter should only be used for 1 or 2 (at the most) units. 170-μ pore size
Specialty Filters		
Microaggregate	Used to remove fibrin and small clusters of debris when transfusing multiple units or when giving products stored over five days	20- to 40-μ pore size
Leukocyte depleting	Removes leukocytes for those with history of severe febrile reactions	

Table 14-11 | Transfusion Administration Equipment

ITEM	INDICATION	FEATURES/RATIONALE
Catheter or Needle		
16–20 gauge	Used for all blood and most components	Must be large enough for RBCs to pass through with out being damaged
Delivery Systems		
Electronic infusion devices	Serve as pump or controller to regulate infusion	Prevent too rapid or too slow infusion, but are only to be used in tested and approved blood transfusions
External pressure infusion cuffs	Used for rapid infusion	Use cuffs designed only for blood transfusion; do not use standard blood pressure cuff Use only with large-bore cannula Do not exceed 300 mm Hg when transfusing components with RBCs
Warmers	Used to warm blood when rapid transfusion of large amounts of blood is needed for patients with potent cold agglutinins, and for neonate exchange transfusions Use of warmers may slow transfusion rate	Rapid administration of large volume of cold blood can precipitate cardiac dysrhythmias and cardiac arrest Warm blood only in approved in-line warmers with a maximum temperature of 38°C Never immerse or hold blood container under hot tap water or place in a microwave oven Overheating damages RBCs
Priming Solution		
0.9% NaCl	Used to prime IV tubing and to precede and follow blood	Other solutions or medications must not be mixed with blood because they can cause agglutination, hemolysis, or other effects

Infusion Protocols and Procedures

The administration of blood or any of its components is a major nursing responsibility that carries with it a significant measure of accountability. Inherent in the implementation of any transfusion are essential nursing measures that include, but are not limited to, obtaining informed consent, positive patient identification, blood product inspection, verification of donor-recipient compatibility, and verification of product expiration date. In addition, the nurse is accountable for patient education, staying with the patient at the start of the infusion for a minimum of five minutes, careful monitoring during and after administration, and appropriate documentation. In the event of a transfusion reaction—immediate or delayed—the nurse must intervene for patient safety, then communicate to the physician and other health care providers involved with the patient's care all pertinent information. Written documentation of all information related to the incident must be anecdotal and thorough. The steps for initiating, maintaining, and monitoring the transfusion of any blood product are delineated in Skill 14-1.

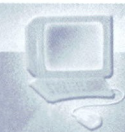

S K I L L   14-1

Transfusion of Blood Components

Equipment Needed:	Implementation/Action	Rationale
Blood administration set Filters Intravenous solution of 0.9% normal saline Disposable gloves Infusion pump, if compatible with blood product to be administered Tape Pressure bag—if needed (Caution must be taken when cuffs are used, as hemolysis may occur.) Blood warmer—if needed	1. Verify the prescriber's order. 2. Verify informed consent. Assess the patient's understanding of the procedure, then describe the procedure, and provide the patient with the opportunity to ask questions and ventilate concerns. Ask if she has ever had any type of transfusion in the past (including cryoprecipitate, FFP, platelets, and RBCs). Assess for symptoms that may be misinterpreted for a reaction during the transfusion. If possible, although not absolutely contraindicated, transfusion should be avoided in febrile (fever >38°C or 100.4°F) patients. 3. Verify the patient's identity. If conscious, ask the patient to state her full name. She must have an identification band as well as a blood administration I.D. bracelet (put on by the blood administration service when a blood sample was drawn for type and crossmatching). Validate that the name and numbers on both I.D. bands correlate with those on the patient's chart and on the laboratory forms for pretransfusion testing of the blood. 4. If the patient is ambulatory, it is recommend that she go to the bathroom and empty her bladder. If bedridden, provide a bedpan (or urinal). 5. Assemble all necessary equipment and start an infusion of 0.9% NaCl, if ordered, using the appropriate administration set, filter, and correct cannula size. *Never* piggyback blood into an existing IV line.	The administration of blood/blood components requires a physician's order or that of a prescriber authorized by the State Nurse Practice Act (INS, 2000, Standard 75, S71). The patient has the right to be informed and to give her permission for any procedure or treatment done for her. The patient who is well informed is better able to cope with her treatment regimen and becomes a partner in the decisions regarding her care. For a person who has had previous transfusions, premedication with antipyretics and antihistamines may be indicated to avert a febrile nonhemolytic reaction. Fever can conceal the symptoms of an untoward reaction, or it may diminish the intended effect(s) of the component(s). Identification and verification are necessary in the provision of patient safety. Never give any blood product unless donor-recipient compatibility are verified. The patient must have the proper identification bands on. (In critical situations when time is of the essence, type O blood may be administered on the order of a physician and with meticulous monitoring.) It is better for the patient to stay in one place for the duration of a transfusion, which may take several hours. An empty bladder promotes comfort. Normal saline is the only infusion that is compatible with blood components and can be used to precede or follow a transfusion or flush the line.

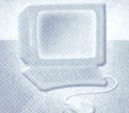

SKILL 14-1

Transfusion of Blood Components

Implementation/Action	Rationale
Obtain an extra set of tubing and a container of 0.9% NaCl, (neither of which are opened, nor charged to the patient) and leave them at the bedside. Locate the availability of emergency drugs.	Should a reaction occur, the transfusion must be stopped, the line disconnected from the hub of the cannula, new tubing attached, and a new container of normal saline started. Emergency drugs may be indicated to counteract a serious reaction.
6. Premedicate the patient with antihistamines, antipyretics, or diuretics, as ordered by the physician.	Premedication with antihistamines and antipyretics are prophylactic measures for febrile, nonhemolytic reactions. Diuretics are administered to patients at risk for fluid volume overload.
7. Obtain the blood component from the transfusion service just prior to its administration. Unless an emergency exists, only one unit per patient is released at a time.	The start of a transfusion must be initiated within 30 minutes of the component's release from the blood administration service. Once the product reaches room temperature, there is always the potential for the deterioration of its components and bacterial growth.
Blood components, other than plasma derivatives (albumin and FFP), which are stored at room temperature, must be stored only in refrigerators (or freezers) that are strictly controlled and monitored (1–6°C or 33.8–42.8°F for refrigeration). *Never store any component in an unmonitored refrigerator.*	If there is any delay in starting the transfusion, the blood product must be returned to the transfusion service for storage, under strictly monitored conditions.
8. Verification. Prior to the start of a transfusion, the nurse must meticulously adhere to the following protocols:	
Recheck the physician's order.	The administration of blood components requires a physician's order.
Obtain the component from the transfusion service and record the name of the person issuing it, as well as the date and time of issue. Record this information on the proper forms in the medical record, which become permanent parts of the chart.	All members of the health care team are accountable for the safety of the patient.
Inspect the blood component and its container for abnormalities:	Any abnormalities may indicate contamination.
Bubbles Clots Color aberrations Cloudiness Excessive air Leaks	
These must be documented in the medical record and the transfusion service must be notified.	
Compare the ABO group and Rh type on the blood label and the tag attached to it with the type and crossmatching information in the chart. Verify and record the findings. Make a note if the blood product is autologous or homologous.	The correct type and crossmatch establishes compatibility between a donor and a recipient. The transfusion of incompatible blood components can result in serious, or fatal, complications.

(continues)

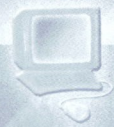

SKILL 14-1

Transfusion of Blood Components (continued)

Implementation/Action	Rationale
Read the instructions on the product label and check the date and time of expiration. (If the time is not specified, expiration occurs at 2400 hours on the date indicated.)	Failure to follow the instructions for administration can jeopardize the safety of the patient. Expired blood is not safe for administration due to the deterioration of its components and the possibility of bacterial contamination.
Identify the patient and verify the information in the chart regarding the blood component to be administered with another licensed nurse (or qualified individual approved by the employing agency). Together, the two personnel must do the following:	Most transfusion reactions occur as a result of errors made regarding patient or component confirmation.
Compare the name and I.D. number on the blood bag and its tag (which are not to be removed) with those on the patient's I.D. bands and with the transfusion forms to verify that they are the same.	There is less probability for error when two people verify the needed information. To be safe, one person should read all of the information to the other as the second person verifies it. The other person should then do the same.
Ask the patient to state her full name, if possible.	This further confirms identity.
Document the name of anyone who verifies the patient and the component to be transfused.	There is shared accountability and liability.
Do not continue with any aspects of a transfusion unless all comparisons are identical.	Notify the transfusion service immediately if there is *any* discrepancy.
9. Reassess the patient's condition and level of consciousness, ascertain vessel patency, take a full set of vital signs (temperature, pulse, respiration, and blood pressure), and document in the medical record.	A patent vessel is necessary for transfusion. Vital signs are taken and recorded in the medical record to serve as a baseline for the identification of changes that may transpire during the transfusion.
Abnormal vital signs require physician notification and documentation.	The physician may order premedication to correct vital sign abnormalities.
10. Initiation of the transfusion.	
Carry out proper hand hygiene.	
Apply gloves.	Gloves must be worn when handling blood components.
Spike the container, stop the normal saline, and initiate the transfusion at the rate of 5 ml/min or slower. No more than 50 ml should be administered within the first 15 minutes of a transfusion.	The signs and symptoms of a severe reaction are usually exhibited during the administration of the first 50 ml, or less, of the transfusion.
Observe the patient closely and take/record vital signs every 5 minutes for the first 15 minutes of a transfusion.	The patient must be monitored throughout the course of any transfusion, but special observation is warranted during the first 15 minutes.
Record on the medical record the time the transfusion is started and the patient's response.	

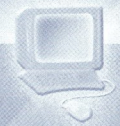

Transfusion of Blood Components

Implementation/Action	Rationale
If there are no signs of an untoward reaction, regulate the transfusion according to medical orders, the patient's condition, and the viscosity of the product being administered.	
Take vital signs again after the transfusion has been running for 30 minutes.	
Depending on the situation, electronic infusion devices, external pressure cuffs, or warmers may be required. If used, the nurse is responsible for their regulation and maintenance.	**The nurse is responsible for following institutional policy and manufacturer's guidelines when using any type of special administration device. He is expected to know and understand the types of equipment used in his employing agency, as well as their indications and conditions for use.**
Any blood that has been warmed but not used must be discarded.	**Once warmed, the potential for bacterial growth increases. After 30 minutes at room temperature, the components begin to deteriorate.**
11. Monitoring and maintenance.	
Monitor and document the patient's level of consciousness and vital signs every 30 minutes for the duration of the transfusion.	**Vital signs and level of consciousness are the primary indicators of a patient's condition.**
Do not use the same blood filter for more than 4 hours.	**Filters collect clots and debris that provide an ideal medium for the growth of bacteria. If used beyond the recommended period of time, contamination, hemolysis, and slowing of the transfusion rate can occur.**
Do not remove any identification attached to the blood container.	**In the event of a reaction, the attached information may be crucial in determining the cause.**
If multiple consecutive blood components are ordered, verify with the physician the order in which they are to be transfused.	**The order in which multiple blood components are administered is determined by the patient's clinical status.**
Should a transfusion reaction occur, the nurse must initiate the appropriate interventions and complete a blood transfusion reaction report required by the employing agency.	
12. Discontinuation.	
Once the blood product has infused, the line should be flushed with ≈50 ml of normal saline.	**Flushing clears any remaining blood product that is in the tubing. If additional blood components or other infusions are required, the line is cleared for their administration.**
The time the transfusion terminated and the amount infused must be documented in the medical record.	
The patient's response must be monitored and documented after the termination of the transfusion.	**Immediate reactions can occur within 2 hours after the completion of a transfusion. Delayed reactions can arise within days.**

(continues)

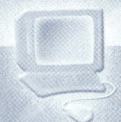

S K I L L 14-1

Transfusion of Blood Components (continued)

Implementation/Action	Rationale
If additional transfusions are required, the institution's policy regarding filters is to be followed.	The same filter may be used for up to 4 units, but many agencies require that the filter be changed with each unit.
Any additional transfusion must be handled, verified, and administered just as if it were the first one.	With every transfusion, there is the potential for serious sequelae if proper transfusion protocols are not followed.
Blood product containers and a completed transfusion report should be returned to the blood administration service within 24 hours of transfusion discontinuation, if it is a policy of the facility. If not required, the container is disposed of in properly lined containers for contaminated products.	In case of delayed transfusion reactions, these containers may provide the information needed to determine the cause.
Once a transfusion is completed, the blood administration set should be discarded, but the policies of some institutions allow for it to be used to infuse other fluids for up to 24 hours.	Following any transfusion there is always the possibility that some products and debris from the blood component may be retained in the blood administration set. These substances provide a perfect medium for the growth and proliferation of bacterial contaminants.
13. Documentation.	
Documentation is required throughout the course of any transfusion. All assessment data germane to the transfusion must be documented in the medical record, as required by the employing institution.	Documentation of all relevant data is required for the safety and protection of the patient, health care personnel, and the health care institution.

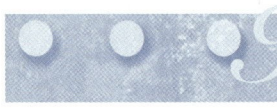

Key Concepts

* The human immune system is composed of all the cells, tissues, organs, and physiologic processes used to protect the body from harm caused by invading organisms. Immunity is the state of protection from disease that results from the interactions of antigens and antibodies.

* Genotypes, found on various cell surfaces, determine each person's propensity for certain traits. Blood groups are based on the isoantigens present on the cell surface of red blood cells. The two major isoantigen groups are the ABO and the Rh systems. These two groups, because of their cell surface composition, are the reason for blood transfusion reactions. Every human being has two genotypes that, when paired, determine one of four blood types (A, B, AB, or O). ABO incompatibility is the major cause of fatal transfusion reactions. The majority of people ([a]85%) have the Rh antigen, making them Rh^+. Those without it are Rh^-.

* Blood and its components are life-sustaining constituents. Different components are transfused to meet the patient's needs as determined from his clinical status.

* Volume expanders are indicated to increase the intravascular content. They fall into two categories: blood product and nonblood product expanders.

* Transfusion therapy is the safe and effective replacement of blood components administered according to patient needs. Such therapy is initiated, maintained, monitored, discontinued, and documented by the RN.

✳ Blood product transfusions are indicated for the following:
- Blood volume maintenance
- Blood volume replacement
- Neonatal exchange
- Blood component maintenance
- Blood component replacement
- Coagulation component supplementation

✳ Transfusion options include homologous (allogenic) and autologous donations.

✳ The administration of blood or any of its components carries with it the risk of transfusion reaction. The nurse must be able to recognize any of the reactions that might occur and to treat them appropriately.

✳ Governmental agencies, the AABB, the INS, employer policies, and state nurse practice acts dictate the responsibilities of the nurse in the safe administration of blood transfusions.

Review Questions and Activities

1. Outline the basic components of the human immune system.

2. Using a table format, parallel the ABO and Rh isoantigen groups, indicating which are compatible for transfusion with each other.

3. List the indications for transfusion of the following blood components:
   - Whole blood
   - Red blood cells
   - Platelets
   - Granulocytes
   - Fresh frozen plasma
   - Cryoprecipitate
   - Albumin
   - Plasma protein fraction
   - Immune globulins

4. For the components listed in the previous question, describe the protocols for administration in terms of the equipment needed and the rate of infusion.

5. Design a three-column table, listing each acute (immediate) transfusion reaction, its clinical indicators, and the nursing interventions appropriate to its management.

6. List two clinical manifestations of a transfusion reaction for each body system that would be observable in an unconscious patient.

7. Examine the advantages and disadvantages associated with autologous and homologous transfusions.

8. Demonstrate how, without using any medical terminology or clinical expressions, you would explain to a patient the methods presently used to screen volunteer donor blood that make it as safe as possible for transfusion.

9. Look up the protocols for blood transfusion therapy in your institution's procedure manual and compare them to those presented in this chapter.

10. Using the following case study, write a nursing care plan, with three to five appropriate nursing diagnoses (in prioritized order, beginning with the most important one). Describe the nursing interventions associated with caring for this patient, with emphasis on the transfusion-related management of his care.

Lyle McGregor is a 28-year-old male brought in to the emergency department (ED) of a county hospital in New Mexico complaining of "a bad cold, with fever and weakness." Don, his companion, says they had been driving cross-country for several days to visit friends. For the last several days, however, they have been unable to go on because Lyle "has been too sick."

Don tells the ED nurse that Lyle has been very weak and tires easily (for about four weeks). He has lost a lot of weight and hasn't felt like eating because of sores in his mouth. He's even stopped drinking his usual six-pack of beer a day. He's been taking aspirin for the fever and cold medicine for the cough, both about every four to six hours, but they're not helping. He's also been taking antacids for stomach burning. Don reveals that Lyle has been HIV-positive for over two years, but hasn't exhibited any symptoms of AIDS. Don asks the nurse if Lyle might have it now.

The nurse's initial assessment, on admission, reveals the following:

Vital signs: Temperature: 103.2. Apical pulse: 108 per minute, irregular and weak. Respirations: 28 per minute, shallow and labored, with decreased breath sounds in both lower lobes. Blood pressure: 96/70. The skin is pale and very dry, with diffuse patches of dermatitis. There is a dry, nonproductive cough and swollen cervical lymph nodes. The mucous membranes are dry and pale, with numerous white lesions in the mouth, and there is general abdominal tenderness. Lyle does not initiate conversation and responds to questions slowly, with slurred speech.

Additional data obtained reveal the following:

CBC: WBCs: 2,100, Hgb.: 6 g/dl, Hct.: 15%, platelets: 30,000.

Sed Rate: 28 mm/hr

BUN: 68 mEq/L

UA: bloody with numerous bacteria and WBCs

CXR: diffuse interstitial infusates

Medical orders given were:

Admit to Medical ICU.

Type and crossmatch stat.

Transfuse 2 U washed RBCs as soon as available.

Insert # 18 ga. ONC and start D5/0.45NS at 125 cc/hr until RBCs started.

Blood cultures ¥ 3, 15 min apart.

Throat C & S.

Consult with Dr. J. Moore for CVP line insertion.

O2 per mask. 6 L with nebulization.

Insert Foley.

Urine for C & S.

Will give further orders after transfer to MICU.

D. Cannaby, M.D.

Intravenous Infusion Needs of the Pediatric and Gerontologic Populations

Chapter 15

Intravenous Infusion Therapy for the Pediatric Patient

Martha Patricia Yee-Nevarez,
MSN, RN, C, Pediatric Nurse Practitioner

COMPETENCIES

Upon completion of this chapter, the reader should be able to:

* Identify the developmental differences between a child and an adult as related to fluid and electrolyte balance.

* State measures to address psychosocial issues in the nursing care of the pediatric patient.

* Outline the assessment and evaluation process for a child who has a potential fluid and electrolyte imbalance.

* Differentiate between isotonic, hypotonic, and hypertonic dehydration in the pediatric patient.

* List the clinical manifestations of mild, moderate, and severe dehydration in the child.

* Describe the principles of nursing management for the child with a fluid and electrolyte imbalance.

* Explain the pathophysiology of acute gastroenteritis.

* Examine the nursing interventions required for parenteral fluid therapy in the pediatric patient.

* Identify the intravenous access routes utilized in the administration of fluid and electrolyte therapy in the pediatric patient.

* Describe the signs and symptoms of overhydration as a complication of parenteral fluid therapy in the pediatric patient.

* List the nursing interventions for the prevention and treatment of overhydration.

* List the nursing interventions used for safe chemotherapy administration in a child.

KEY TERMS

band

chemotherapy

Child Life Specialist

comatose

dehydration

hypertonic dehydration

hypotonic dehydration

isotonic dehydration

obtunded

osteomyelitis

steatorrhea

The nurse who provides care to neonatal and pediatric patients must have a thorough understanding of anatomy, physiology, and growth and developmental patterns as they relate to this population. Intravenous therapy for pediatric patients requires that the nurse be familiar with several issues. These include (1) the physiologic concepts of fluid and electrolyte balance within the body, as a system; (2) the special considerations that provide the rationale for administering safe and effective intravenous therapy; (3) principles of growth and development; and (4) concepts required for making astute assessment and evaluation of the physiologic, cognitive, and psychosocial status of children.

BODY FLUIDS

The seriousness of body water and fluid and electrolytes in terms of losses and gains is proportionate to the size of the child, with the smaller child always at greater risk of imbalance. The fluid in the body is predominately water. In a premature infant up to 85% of body weight is water; in the full-term infant, about 70% of body weight is water. For a young adult body water comprises approximately 60% of body weight in males and 50% of body weight in females. The percentage of body weight that is water varies according to the amount of body fat that is present. This is because fat is essentially water-free; thus, the more fat the individual has, the smaller the amount of water in the body. This is an important fact to remember because this will aid in assessing the hydration status of a patient prior to calculating replacement fluid, such as fluid loss from dehydration and shock or fluid maintenance needs. (See Chapter 2 for the discussion of the pathophysiology of fluid balance.)

PHYSIOLOGIC DIFFERENCES: ADULT VERSUS PEDIATRIC PATIENTS

When changes in plasma volume and plasma osmolality occur, the body responds by activating mechanisms to regu-

late the retention and excretion of water. It is especially important to remember that *children are not small adults*! Their bodies function differently from adults. These differences, which are too often overlooked, must be considered when caring for children.

Basal Metabolic Rate

Because of the rapid growth of a child, his basal metabolic rate (BMR) is significantly higher than that of an adult. In the unstressed infant, the BMR is three times that of the adult. When illness occurs, which may be associated with stressors such as fever, hypoxia, dehydration, or burns, the BMR further increases. This higher metabolic rate in a child requires that enough water be present for the excretion of metabolic wastes.

Body Surface Area (BSA)

The body surface area (BSA) of an infant or young child is proportionately greater than that of the older child or adult. The relationship of surface area is found to be five times greater in the premature infant and two to three times greater in an infant compared with an adolescent or an adult. Because of this, the risk in an infant or young child for insensible water losses through the skin is greatly increased. A child normally has a higher respiratory rate than an adult, which contributes to the potential for water loss by way of the lungs. Furthermore, the surface area of the gastrointestinal tract of the younger child is also proportionately greater when compared with the older child or adult. The healthy child is able to reabsorb the fluids secreted into the intestinal tract, but the child with vomiting and diarrhea runs a great risk for rapid expenditure of body fluids.

Immature Renal Function

Because a child's kidneys are not able to concentrate urine as efficiently as those of an adult, more water is excreted with metabolic wastes. Nevertheless, under most circumstances, the kidneys of a child are able to meet his homeostatic requirements. Qualitatively, the physiologic ability of an infant's kidneys to dilute urine is the same as an adult's.

Psychosocial Needs

Infants and young children are not equipped with the verbal or the psychomotor skills needed to independently provide for their fluid needs. Older children with physical or mental delays may, in varying degrees, lack the communication tools needed to actively request fluids. For these reasons, they are highly dependent on their caregivers to provide for these and other needs. This area will be elaborated on in a later section of this chapter.

PRINCIPLES OF GROWTH AND DEVELOPMENT

The INS recommends that the "nurse shall have a knowledge and understanding of growth and development, including the psychological and behavioral development relevant to the patient's age group" (INS, 2000, Standard 2, S12). Throughout a lifespan, the human being progresses through several stages of growth and development. Many theories describe and explain these stages as well as the common behaviors that characterize each stage (Table 15-1). Theories are useful to nursing practice in that they provide insight into a child's thinking, abilities, and likely responses to a situation. By looking at them in depth, one is much less likely to stereotype a child and categorize him in the vastly different realm of the adult.

CONDITIONS CAUSING FLUID AND ELECTROLYTE IMBALANCES

The major cation in the extracellular fluid is sodium. Its most important function is to preserve the distribution of water within the fluid compartments of the body. Water balance is controlled by sodium through osmotic equilibrium between the intracellular and extracellular fluid. Because an imbalance of water will affect the balance of sodium, and an imbalance of sodium, in turn, affects the balance of water, the relationship between the two elements must always be considered in the child with a fluid and electrolyte deviation.

Dehydration

Dehydration is defined as a condition that results in excess body fluid loss. It is important to understand that a patient

with dehydration exhibits a deficiency in both fluid *and* electrolyte levels. Dehydration occurs when the total amount of fluid and electrolyte output exceeds the child's fluid intake — the result of either excessive fluid loss or insufficient fluid intake. Conditions that commonly result in dehydration are vomiting, diarrhea, burns, fever, diabetes, gastrointestinal surgery, gastric suctioning, and tachypnea.

Dehydration can be classified according to severity (expressed as a percentage of total body weight loss): mild (5%), moderate (10%), or severe (15%), as well as its effects on serum sodium and osmolality: isotonic (or isonatremic) dehydration, hypotonic (or hyponatremic) dehydration, and hypertonic (or hypernatremic) dehydration. With isotonic dehydration sodium and water are lost in equal amounts. Hypotonic dehydration occurs when there is a sodium loss greater than water loss. Hypertonic dehydration is evidenced when water loss exceeds sodium loss.

Types of Dehydration

Isotonic dehydration occurs when there is a loss of water and sodium in equal amounts. Serum sodium concentration and serum osmolality are not affected as the fluid loss is from intravascular fluid, and, consequently, a fluid shift does not exist. Serum sodium remains within normal limits, between 135 and 145 mEq/L.

Hypotonic dehydration occurs when sodium loss exceeds fluid loss or when the body retains water and serum sodium concentrations fall below 135 mEq/L. The lack of enough sodium to keep water from entering the cells causes shifting of water from the extracellular to the intracellular spaces. Causes of hypotonic dehydration include improper administration of plain water (e.g., when a child is playing in the hot sun, perspires excessively, and fluids are given in the form of electrolyte-free solutions, such as tap water), improper administration of intravenous fluids (e.g., D_5W or a hypotonic solution), or the administration of tap water enemas instead of saline enemas. Other causes of dehydration occur because of abnormal excretion of sodium (as in patients with cystic fibrosis).

Table 15-1 | Growth and Development Theories

STAGE	FREUD PSYCHOSOCIAL	ERIKSON PSYCHOSOCIAL	PIAGET COGNITIVE	NURSING INTERVENTIONS RELATED TO IV THERAPY
Infancy	Oral-Sensory Birth–12 mo	Trust v. Mistrust	Sensorimotor Birth–18 mo	Comfort through swaddling in blankets, rocking, holding, provide pacifier for sucking. Encourage parents to participate to decrease stranger anxiety (esp. the older infant). Do not feed before IV insertion as infant may vomit and aspirate.
Toddler	Anal-Urethral 1–3 yr	Autonomy v. Shame & Doubt	Preoperational (Preconceptual thought) Birth–18 mo	Expect little cooperation, restrain as needed during IV insertion, promote safety, allow parental participation to decrease stranger anxiety. Remember toddlers are curious. After IV started, use distraction and play with imitating behaviors such as house, mommy, kitchen. Establish trust with the child, be honest and do not make promises you cannot keep.
Preschooler	Phallic 3–6 yr	Initiative v. Guilt	Preoperational (Intuitive thought) 4–7 yr	Explain in simple terms. Allay fears, as preschoolers have great fear of pain, needles, and body mutilation. Provide bandage to cover "owie" or "boo-boo." Explain everything in simple terms as there is some ability to reason and understand cause and effect.
School-Age	Latency 6–12 yr	Industry v. Inferiority	Concrete Operations	Take time to answer all questions. These children enjoy learning about their bodies. Allow child to play with medical equipment before procedure and touch all that is not sterile. Allow child to watch as procedure is being completed as these children are concrete thinkers. Reward positive behavior.
Adolescent	Genital 13–19 yr	Identity v. Role Confusion	Formal Operations	Allow as much control as safely possible. Teens like to be treated as adults and are usually cooperative. They enjoy own clothing; secure IV to allow for this. Explain as much as patient desires. Usually comprehend anatomy, and procedures can be explained in detail.

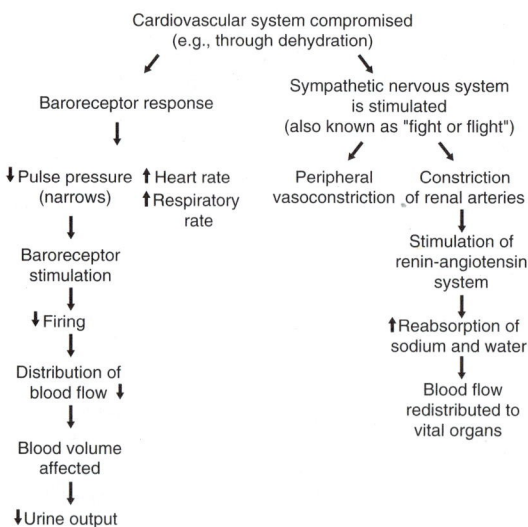

Figure 15-1 | Activation of compensatory mechanisms

Hypertonic dehydration occurs when fluid loss exceeds sodium loss or when there is a decreased intake of water or increased intake of sodium. In this condition, fluid shifts from the intracellular to the extracellular spaces owing to the increased osmotic pressure of the blood from the excess sodium. Consequently, shock is less apparent, but neurologic distress, such as seizures, are more likely to occur. Other signs of neurologic involvement may include change in level of consciousness, hyperirritability, lethargy, hyperreflexia, and hypersensitivity to external stimuli (auditory, tactile, and visual). Any clinical condition that depletes the body of water, such as insensible losses by way of the skin and respiratory tract from fever or hyperventilation, can lead to hypertonic dehydration. Other causes of this condition include the administration of hypertonic intravenous fluid (e.g., >0.9% normal saline) or gastric feedings with high sodium concentrations. Changes in circulatory status are rare because of the relative increase in vascular volume.

Compensatory Mechanisms

If interventions are not implemented and dehydration progresses to a severe state, intravascular volume, cardiac output, and systemic perfusion are compromised. Once systemic perfusion is compromised, compensatory mechanisms are activated. The goal of these compensatory mechanisms is to restore intravascular volume and to maintain perfusion of tissues and vital organs. If systemic perfusion is severely compromised, the patient may manifest metabolic acidosis and multisystem organ failure.

When the cardiovascular system is compromised, the sympathetic nervous system responds by inducing tachycardia, tachypnea, peripheral vasoconstriction, and constriction of the renal arteries. In turn, renal blood flow is diminished, thus stimulating the renin-angiotensin-aldosterone (RAA) system. Renin and aldosterone serve to increase the reabsorption of sodium and water. Angiotensin serves as a peripheral vasoconstrictor. When the renin-angiotensin-aldosterone system is activated, blood flow is redistributed to vital organs to an adequate level (Figure 15-1). However, if severe intravascular volume is lost and the volume loss progresses, hypovolemic shock ensues.

Clinical Manifestations

The child with dehydration presents with a history of poor oral intake or excessive loss of fluid from vomiting, diarrhea, or both. The child generally looks ill, is febrile, has dry conjunctivae and mucous membranes, and poor skin turgor. The infant will have sunken fontanels. There may be changes in vital signs, among other abnormal physical findings. Typically the severity of these changes is used to estimate the degree of dehydration, presuming that isotonic dehydration is present. Table 15-2 illustrates the relationship of signs and symptoms with severity of dehydration in children with isotonic dehydration.

Mild isotonic dehydration is evidenced by a weight loss of 5% or a fluid deficit of up to 50 ml/kg. The child's behavior can be normal or he may be irritable, the fontanels are flat or depressed, mucous membranes are dry, skin turgor is mildly decreased, skin temperature is warm with a natural color, capillary refill is ≤2 seconds, there is mild tachycardia, blood pressure is normal, peripheral pulses are normal on palpation, and there is slight oliguria.

With moderate isotonic dehydration there is a weight loss of 10% or a fluid deficit of up to 100 ml/kg. The child is irritable or lethargic, the fontanels are depressed, mucous membranes are very dry, skin turgor is moderately decreased, extremities are cool, skin color is pale, capillary refill is

Table 15-2 | Relationship of Signs and Symptoms with Severity of Dehydration

	MILD	MODERATE	SEVERE
Body Weight Loss	5% (50 ml/kg)	10% (100 ml/kg)	15% (150 ml/kg)
Sensorium	Normal or irritable	Irritable or lethargic	Unresponsive
Fontanel	Flat or depressed	Depressed	Significantly depressed
Mucous Membranes	Dry	Very dry	Parched
Skin Turgor	Fair to poor	Very poor, may have skin tenting	Skin tenting is evident
Skin Perfusion	Warm, natural color Capillary refill ≤2 sec	Extremities cool, pale Capillary refill 2–5 sec	Extremities cold, mottled, or gray Capillary refill >5 sec
Heart Rate (apical)	Mild tachycardia	Moderate tachycardia	Extreme tachycardia
Blood Pressure	Normal	Normal	Reduced
Peripheral Pulses	Normal to slightly increased	Diminished (esp. distal)	Weak, thready, or absent (distal may not be palpable)
Urine Output	Slight oliguria	Oliguria	Significant oliguria

between 2 and 5 seconds, the patient has moderate tachycardia, blood pressure is normal, peripheral pulses are diminished (especially the distal pulses), and oliguria is evident.

Severe isotonic dehydration is a potentially fatal condition and presents with a weight loss of 15% or greater or a fluid deficit of approximately 150 ml/kg. Usually the patient is unresponsive, the fontanels are significantly depressed, mucous membranes are parched, skin turgor is severely decreased, the extremities are cold, the skin is mottled or gray, capillary refill is >5 seconds, there is evidence of extreme tachycardia, blood pressure is decreased, pulses are difficult to find or absent (especially the distal pulses), and marked oliguria is present. The presence of these symptoms in combination present the clinical picture of shock. Because of fluid loss in the intravascular compartment, the patient has poor systemic perfusion, as manifested by the preceding signs and symptoms.

The classification of symptoms can be very subjective, according to the individual health care provider. Obtaining a serum sodium level provides more accuracy in calculating the severity of a child's dehydration. If hyponatremic dehydration is present, signs of hypovolemia and poor systemic perfusion will be evident even if the dehydration is mild. On the other hand, because there is an intracellular fluid loss and the intravascular volume is maintained, the patient with hypernatremic dehydration will not demonstrate signs of hypovolemia until dehydration is severe. Table 15-3 illustrates signs and symptoms of the various types of dehydration.

Management

The nurse must strive for several goals when treating dehydration. These include restoration and maintenance of

Table 15-3 | Clinical Manifestations of Dehydration

	ISO-TONIC	HYPO-TONIC	HYPER-TONIC
ECF Volume	Markedly ↓	Severely ↓	Decreased
ICF Volume	Maintained	Increased	Decreased
Skin Temperature	Cold	Cold	Cold or hot
Skin Turgor	Poor	Very poor	Fair
Skin Feel	Dry	Clammy	Thickened and doughy
Mucous Membranes	Dry	Dry	Parched and shriveled
Eyeballs	Sunken	Sunken	Sunken
Fontanel	Sunken	Sunken	Sunken
LOC	Lethargic	Coma	Hyperirritable
Pulse	Rapid	Rapid	Moderately rapid
BP	↓	↓	↓
Serum Sodium (mEq/L)	135–145	<135	>145

intravascular volume and systemic perfusion, correction of fluid and electrolyte imbalances, and the administration of maintenance fluid requirements. When a step-by-step approach is taken, the nurse is able to accurately evaluate the child's reaction to each intervention and can evaluate the response (Table 15-4). The child's systemic perfusion must be

Table 15-4 | Steps in Treating Dehydration with Signs of Shock or Poor Systemic Perfusion

1. *Treat shock and restore systemic perfusion*

   Use NS or LR at 20 ml/kg, may repeat until blood pressure, capillary refill, and temperature of extremities improve.

2. *Replace the deficit*

   Calculate in one of two ways:
   (a) based on present weight vs. pre-illness weight
       or
   (b) based on clinical presentation: mild, moderate, severe dehydration

   With isotonic and hypotonic dehydration, replace one-half of the deficit within the first 8 hours, the other half within the next 16 hours.

   With hypertonic dehydration, replace the deficit over the next 48 hours.

3. *Provide maintenance fluid*

4. *Provide supplemental nutrition as necessary*

If mild dehydration, may treat with oral, clear liquids and advance diet as tolerated.

assessed carefully, and, if present, shock must be corrected. While therapy is being administered to restore fluid and electrolyte balance, it is imperative that the child's response and neurologic status be continually assessed and evaluated.

The patient with mild dehydration may be rehydrated with oral fluids. Several types of liquids are offered in an attempt to promote oral intake and prevent further dehydration: clear fluids such as noncarbonated drinks, diluted fruit juices (no orange juice or apple juice if the patient is having diarrhea), sugar-free liquids, or solid gelatin, tea, popsicles or formulas containing electrolytes. Milk, ice cream, and other dairy products are not of benefit since they curdle once in contact with the gastric environment and may cause more vomiting and diarrhea. Generally the child feels ill and has a poor appetite, making it very important to be creative in getting the child to drink fluids. The parents must be educated regarding signs and symptoms of dehydration so they will seek medical attention immediately should the signs and symptoms present again in the future. Moreover, signs of improvement should also be discussed with the parent.

As a rule of thumb, infants who have been unable to take oral fluids for 12 to 16 hours and older children who have been unable to take oral fluids for 18 to 24 hours need parenteral fluid administration. Parenteral fluids are required for patients with more severe dehydrations, for those who are vomiting, have diarrhea, or have other ongoing losses. Fluid resuscitation is considered an emergency in patients with signs of severe dehydration (e.g., poor systemic perfusion) or

signs of shock. Fluid therapy is calculated in the same manner as medication dosages. The dose is determined independently by at least two people, then compared for accuracy as a precautionary measure to prevent errors. Strict fluid intake and output (I&O) must be maintained and urine output is tallied by weighing diapers after each voiding.

Reestablishment of adequate intravascular volume is typically accomplished through the insertion of a reliable intravenous (IV) access route. Preferably two large bore cannulas are inserted in order to have more access sites for rapid IV fluid administration. If peripheral IV access is not obtainable, fluid resuscitation can take place through the intraosseous (IO) route (covered later in this chapter).

Once IV access has been obtained, volume resuscitation from a shock state requires the rapid administration of isotonic fluid (either 0.9% normal saline or Ringer's lactate) at a dose of 20 ml/kg. This bolus therapy may be repeated until the patient demonstrates signs of improved systemic perfusion as indicated by warming of the skin and extremities, brisk capillary refill, a blood pressure that is appropriate for the child's age, and the presence of urine output. Other fluids such as colloids may be administered later during resuscitation (i.e., 10 ml/kg of 5% albumin). Fluid resuscitation is designed to replace fluid and electrolyte losses that occurred before the child was admitted for medical care. The goal of therapy is to return the child's intravascular volume and composition to a normal state.

A patient with hypotonic dehydration requires aggressive fluid resuscitation owing to the significant loss of intravascular volume. If the patient has hypertonic dehydration, rapid administration of fluid should only be provided if systemic perfusion is poor. Rapid fluid administration will cause the serum sodium concentration to fall abruptly, causing rapid fluid shifts and potential neurologic complications. In hypertonic dehydration, serum sodium should recover at a rate not greater than 10 mEq/L/24 /hr.

Once systemic perfusion has returned to normal and the clinical picture improves, the fluid deficit must be replaced.

NURSING ALERT

Serum Sodium Level Recovery Rate

When a child has hypertonic dehydration (a serum sodium greater than 145 mEq/L), his serum sodium level should be returned to normal levels at a rate not greater than 10 mEq/L in a 24-hour period. This is done to avoid a rapid fall in serum sodium, which in turn can cause cerebral edema or intracranial hemorrhage.

Fluid replacement therapy is based on the type and severity of dehydration. The ideal situation is to calculate the exact volume of fluid to be replaced based on the pre-illness weight and present weight of the child. If, however, the pre-illness weight is not known, the patient's clinical picture is the basis for calculating fluid replacement.

In isotonic and hypotonic dehydration, the fluid deficit is replaced over the first 24 hours. Normal maintenance fluids must be calculated along with replacement of the fluid deficit. Half of the fluid deficit is given within the first 8 hours and the other half is given within the next 16 hours. The patient's clinical status must be evaluated on an ongoing basis while rehydration is taking place.

In hypertonic dehydration, the fluid deficit is replaced over the first 48 hours, and fluid maintenance is calculated along with the replacement of the fluid deficit. Severe hyperosmolality may result in cerebral destruction, with widespread intracranial hemorrhages and permanent neurologic damage. During the period of dehydration, there is an increase in the sodium content of cerebral cells, which in turn results in an excessive movement of water into these cells during rehydration before excess sodium is extruded. A rapid fall in serum sodium and a consequent rise in sodium within the cerebral cells will cause cerebral edema and seizures. This may be prevented by correcting the hypernatremia slowly over a period of days (not more than 10 mEq/L/24 hr).

Once systemic perfusion has been restored and the fluid deficit is calculated, fluid maintenance must be initiated. Maintenance therapy replaces ongoing and abnormal fluid and electrolyte losses. The goal is to maintain patients in normal balance and prevent deficits. Several formulas are available to assist in calculating fluid maintenance for the pediatric patient. The most commonly used methods are (1) using the patient's weight and a formula to calculate his fluid needs (Table 15-5), or (2) using his body surface area and a formula to calculate his fluid needs (Table 15-6 and Figure 15-2). When a nomogram is not available, body surface area can be calculated by taking the square root of the following:

Table 15-6 | Using the Nomogram for Calculating Fluid Maintenance

1.	Obtain a nomogram (see Figure 15-2).
2.	Obtain the patient's height and weight (can be either in the metric or English system).
3.	Plot the patient's height and weight on the nomogram.
4.	Draw a line connecting the height and weight of the child.
5.	Read the number where the line crosses the surface area (SA) column.
6.	This number is the child's body surface area in square meters.
7.	Apply the formula: For fluid maintenance, give 1,500 ml/m2/24 hr.

$$\frac{Wt\ (kg) \times Ht\ (cm)}{3,600}$$

Example:

Patient Lilly V. weighs 20 kg and is 120 cm tall.
$20 \times 120 = 2,400$, divided by $3,600 = 0.67$, the square root of this $= 0.82$.
Lilly's BSA $= 0.82$.
$0.82 \times 1,500$ (maintenance fluid requirement) $= 1,230$ ml/24 hr

Replacement and maintenance fluids and electrolytes are calorically inadequate and will not sustain growth, making them inappropriate for prolonged use. When supplemental therapy is required, other types of fluids are considered.

The patient's physical, physiologic, and psychosocial conditions must be evaluated continually, with the patient's ventilatory and oxygenation status a priority. The patient must be positioned in such a manner so as to support airway patency, with supplemental oxygen administered as needed. Elective intubation, using strictly controlled safeguards, should be initiated *before* respiratory deterioration or arrest complicates the management of shock.

Table 15-5 | Formula for Calculating Fluid Maintenance Using Weight in Kilograms

1.	The child's weight must be broken down by tens in kilograms.
2.	For the first 10 kg (up to 10 kg), give 100 ml/kg/24 hr.
3.	For the second 10 kg (11–20 kg), give 50 ml/kg/24 hr.
4.	Any remaining weight (21–70 kg), give 20 ml/kg/24 hr.

NURSING TIP

The Value of the BSA Formula

The formula using BSA accounts for the patient's height and weight, thus making the BSA formula a more accurate method of calculating fluid maintenance needs for each individual child.

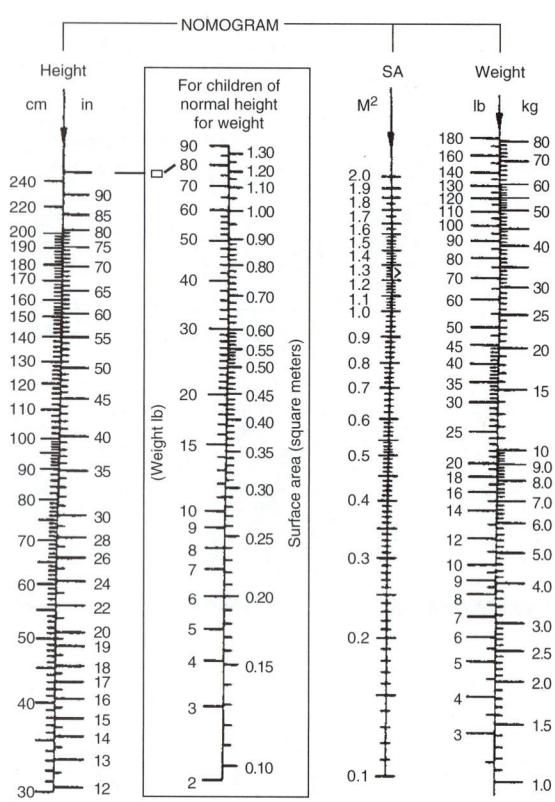

Directions for use: (1) Determine client height. (2) Determine client weight. (3) Draw a straight line to connect the height and weight. Where the line intersects on the SA line is the derived body surface area (M²).

Figure 15-2 │ Nomogram for estimating body surface area. *Reprinted with permission from Behrman, R. E., Kliegman, R., & Arvin, A. (Eds.) (1999). Nelson's textbook of pediatrics (16th ed.). Philadelphia, PA: Saunders.*

When an acid-base imbalance is present (i.e., metabolic acidosis with a pH of <7.15), the condition is treated with hyperventilation and restoration of effective systemic perfusion. Sodium bicarbonate is given only for severe, documented metabolic acidosis. The patient's glucose and temperature must be monitored closely, because a child who is under stress metabolizes glucose at a rapid rate, thus placing her at risk for hypoglycemia. Parenteral fluids should never be administered cold, since this predisposes to hypothermia. Overhead lights and blankets are used when working with the patient in order to keep him warm and comfortable, and to support normal body temperature.

A urinary catheter is inserted for strict intake and output, and an accurate weight is obtained as soon as possible, for this is the basis for calculation of fluid resuscitation and maintenance. The patient is weighed on the same scale every day, preferably at the same time, to ensure consistency and

CRITICAL THINKING

Dealing with Patient and Family Fears

Fifteen-month-old Parker presents to the hospital with a diagnosis of 10% dehydration secondary to vomiting and diarrhea. Lynne, his somewhat high-strung 20-year-old mother, appears exhausted and worried. Lynne explains that this is her first child, and she has tried everything she could think of to get Parker to keep fluids and food down. You explain to the mother that you will need to start an IV on Parker to get fluids into him immediately. Lynne becomes very upset; she is afraid of needles and does not want Parker to go through any "ordeal." Parker, sensing his mother's apprehension, cries and clings to her. It becomes evident to you that Lynne's presence may only make the situation worse. How would you handle the situation from here? What actions could you take to comfort both the mother and the child? What are the priorities for action in this situation?

Before beginning the procedure, the nurse must ensure that all the equipment necessary for starting an IV is set up. This includes the cannula to be used, IV start kit, tubing, volume control cylinder, and IV fluid. All materials that will be used for securing the IV site will also need to be ready for immediate use. Since the patient may be apprehensive, bringing a pacifier and a blanket to the treatment room may help the patient to feel more secure and comfortable. The nurse encourages Parker's parents to participate in comforting their child as much as possible. They should not assist in restraining the child as Parker may misinterpret this as a punishment from his parents. In performing the procedure, the nurse explains to the parents all that is happening, while they assist in consoling Parker. When accessing a peripheral vein for fluid therapy, the nurse must keep in mind that a child with dehydration may have poor peripheral perfusion. All measures to prevent complications must be initiated at this time. Parker's weight must be obtained prior to the procedure so that accurate dosing of maintenance fluid can be calculated.

accuracy of fluid replacement. Interventions are implemented with any increase or decrease in weight to prevent further imbalance of fluid and electrolyte levels.

If the child has diarrhea, he must be isolated according to institutional policy. The CDC guidelines recommend that all agencies place patients on Standard Precautions. Strict hand hygiene practice before and after caring for every patient and the wearing of gloves (when body substance exposure is possible) must be used to prevent cross-contamination. Caregivers must remember that any child with acute gastro-enteritis is usually harboring highly contagious pathogens.

As the patient's condition improves, he is weaned off parenteral fluid supplementation, and oral fluids are slowly increased until he can fully tolerate oral foods and fluids. Teaching the parents or significant others about the preventive measures regarding dehydration must begin early in the nurse-patient relationship.

Acute Gastroenteritis

Acute gastroenteritis (AGE) is the presence of an infectious organism in the gastrointestinal (GI) tract. AGE can be caused by bacteria, viruses, or parasites. It is primarily manifested by diarrhea, which eventually causes a decrease in the absorption of water, electrolytes, and nutrients.

Etiology

Most AGE is viral in origin, with 50% to 70% caused by a virus, whose sequelae include lactose malabsorption and monosaccharide intolerance.

The causative organisms leading to bacterial gastroenteritis depend on environmental factors. Organisms known to cause AGE are *Campylobacter*, *Yersinia*, *Shigella*, *Salmonella*, *Staphylococcus aureus*, and *Escherichia coli*. Parasitic pathogens affecting children are usually *Giardia lamblia* and *Dientamoeba fragilis*.

Pathophysiology

The pathophysiology of any viral infection is yet to be fully defined. It is known, however, that the viral agent damages or destroys the epithelial cells that line the intestinal tract. A viral infection is usually self-limiting and lasts 48 to 96 hours.

The pathophysiology of bacterial infections usually follows three pathways: (1) the production of an enterotoxin (Figure 15-3), (2) the invasion and destruction of the intestinal mucosa (Figure 15-4), or (3) the penetration of the intestinal wall with systemic invasion (Figure 15-5).

Clinical Manifestations

Regardless of the cause, the most common final pathway of AGE is dehydration. The signs and symptoms of dehydration in the pediatric patient usually include irritability or lethargy, sunken fontanels and sunken eyes, absence of tears with crying, dry mucous membranes, poor skin turgor, tachycardia, tachypnea, decreased urine output (<6 wet diapers/24 hr), and serum imbalances (hyponatremia or hypernatremia, hypokalemia, metabolic acidosis, increased hematocrit).

Transmission

Most AGE-causative organisms are spread by the fecal-oral route. Person-to-person contact usually transmits the disease. *Shigella*, *Giardia*, and *Campylobacter* are spread by direct contact. *Salmonella* is ingested with milk, meat, or eggs contaminated by the pathogen during preparation or storage.

Diagnosis

The diagnosis of AGE is primarily derived from the patient's history. There are generally a large number of watery stools that are usually green (from excretion of bile). If the AGE is bacterial in origin, the stools may contain pus and even blood. The nurse must obtain an accurate history: a vital tool in differentiating normal changes in stool (which vary with age and diet). An accurate nursing history, expediently gathered, also assists the physician in formulating an accurate medical diagnosis.

Typically a total white blood cell count (WBC) and differential reveal whether the WBC is normal, increased, or decreased.

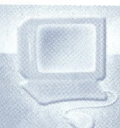

SKILL 15-1

Child with Acute Diarrhea

Case Presentation

Tommy is a 22-lb (10-kg) child who presents with the following clinical manifestations: His mom reports that Tommy has not wet his diapers very much today but has been having watery diarrhea since last night. His fontanels are sunken, the periorbital area is sunken, mucous membranes are dry, there is evidence of skin tenting, capillary refill is 5 seconds, and distal pulses are weak and thready. The serum sodium concentration is 131 mEq/L, but all other electrolytes are within normal limits.

Nursing Diagnosis

Fluid Volume Deficiency Related to Excessive GI Losses in Stool

Planning

Frequent vital and neurologic signs (every 15 to 30 minutes), careful assessment for changes in overall condition, concentrating on hydration status, which includes level of consciousness, vital signs, quality of pulses, capillary refill, skin assessment, color, and presence or absence of urine output, careful inspection of the IV site for signs of complications, strict hourly recording of intake and output, and monitoring laboratory values for recovery of normal sodium level.

Implementation/Action	Rationale
1. Institute systematic assessment, head to toe approach, basing the assessment on clinical findings, lab values, and other monitoring systems (e.g., cardiorespiratory monitor, pulse oximeter).	A systematic assessment assists organization of thoughts and prompt recognition of changes in the patient's clinical condition.
2. Keep the IV patent.	Intravenous access is of utmost importance in the treatment regimen of a child with acute diarrhea. Fluid losses (e.g., through GI tract, tachypnea, and fever) must be replaced, and fluid needs must be maintained by way of the IV route.
3. Do not offer any food or fluids.	Depending on the patient's level of consciousness, if his sensorium is diminished, offering foods or fluids may lead to aspiration. Further, if the patient already has diarrhea, stimulating the bowel with food or fluid may worsen the patient's condition.
4. Have oxygen and suction equipment at the bedside.	Equipment is readily available in case of an emergency.
5. Keep side rails up and the bed in low position.	Prevents the child from falling out of bed.

Evaluation

The nurse evaluates the child's response to therapy as evidenced by stabilization of vital signs, improvement in mental status, normalization of muscular status, presence of signs of adequate perfusion, presence of adequate urine output, absence of vomiting and diarrhea, and increasing appetite.

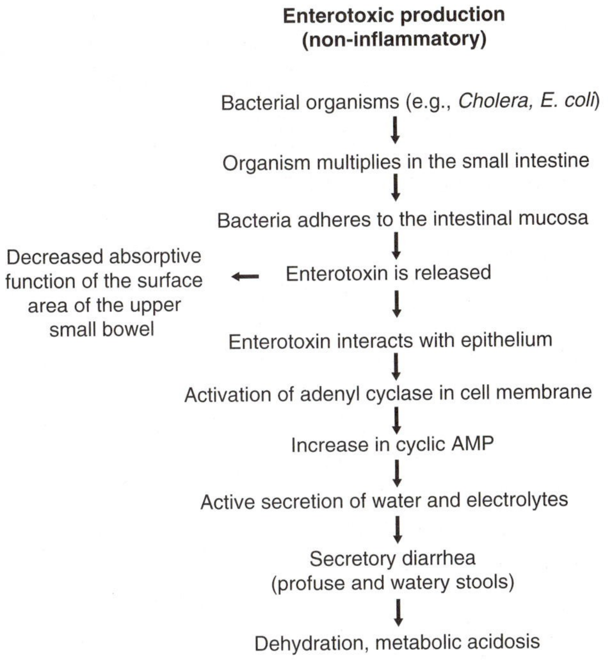

**Enterotoxic production
(non-inflammatory)**

Bacterial organisms (e.g., *Cholera, E. coli*)

↓

Organism multiplies in the small intestine

↓

Bacteria adheres to the intestinal mucosa

↓

Decreased absorptive   ← Enterotoxin is released
function of the surface
area of the upper
small bowel

↓

Enterotoxin interacts with epithelium

↓

Activation of adenyl cyclase in cell membrane

↓

Increase in cyclic AMP

↓

Active secretion of water and electrolytes

↓

Secretory diarrhea
(profuse and watery stools)

↓

Dehydration, metabolic acidosis

Figure 15-3 | Pathophysiology of acute gastroenteritis (AGE) secondary to enterotoxin production

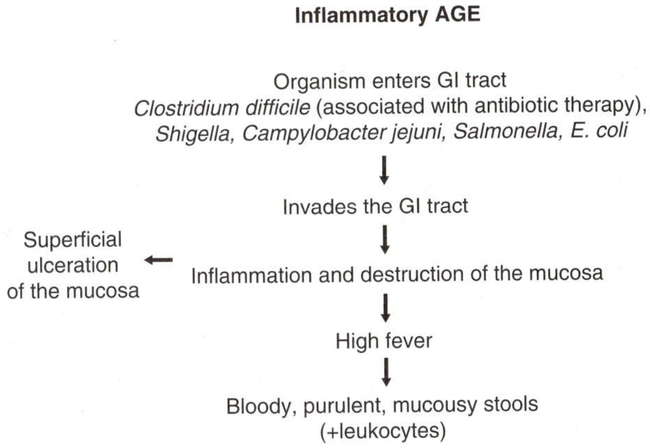

Inflammatory AGE

Organism enters GI tract
Clostridium difficile (associated with antibiotic therapy),
Shigella, Campylobacter jejuni, Salmonella, E. coli

↓

Invades the GI tract

↓

Superficial   ← Inflammation and destruction of the mucosa
ulceration
of the mucosa

↓

High fever

↓

Bloody, purulent, mucousy stools
(+leukocytes)

Figure 15-4 | Pathophysiology of inflammatory AGE

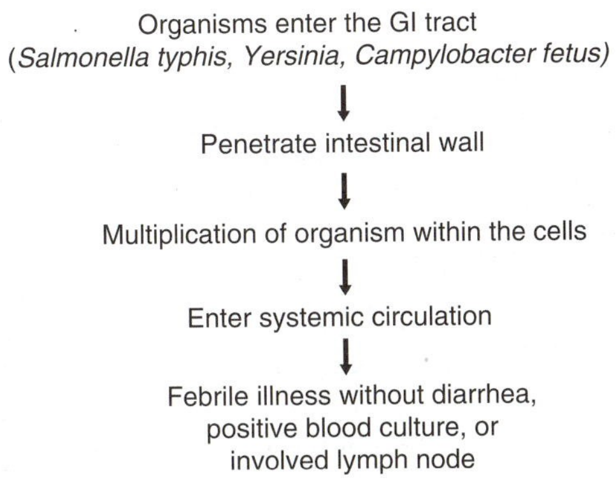

Organisms enter the GI tract
(*Salmonella typhis, Yersinia, Campylobacter fetus*)

↓

Penetrate intestinal wall

↓

Multiplication of organism within the cells

↓

Enter systemic circulation

↓

Febrile illness without diarrhea,
positive blood culture, or
involved lymph node

Figure 15-5 | Penetration of the intestinal wall with systemic invasion

More than 50% of all children with infectious diarrhea have an increased **band** (immature neutrophil) count, an important objective diagnostic tool for AGE. The nurse is responsible for the collection of fresh stool samples from the patient and expediting their transfer to the laboratory for testing. The stools are microscopically examined for leukocytes, occult blood (guaiac or hemoccult test), culture and sensitivity, stool virology, and tested for ova and parasites. The pH of the stools is also checked, along with the glucose content and fecal fat. A stool pH of ≤ 5.5 and a positive Clinitest ($\geq 0.5\%$ glucose) suggest alterations in utilization of carbohydrates, usually due to a noninfectious process such as lactase deficiency. The presence of fecal fat (**steatorrhea**) and leukocytes suggests an inflammatory process.

Management

The management of AGE involves three steps: (1) maintain or restore fluid and electrolyte balance, (2) restore the bowel to normal functioning, and (3) prevent the spread of the organism to others. A patient with a mild case of diarrhea usually does not need to be hospitalized. He is placed NPO for 2 to 6 hours, then oral fluid intake is increased gradually, beginning with clear liquids and advancing as tolerated to full liquids and bland soft foods. The child should not be offered any dairy products since this may cause the diarrhea to return.

The infant who is being breast fed can continue to nurse. The older infant and toddler may drink soy or lactose-free milk. The child's parents are educated regarding the signs and symptoms that indicate worsening of AGE and dehydration and are cautioned to seek medical attention if they reappear.

A child with more severe diarrhea requires hospitalization for observation and fluid and electrolyte replacement. Treatment includes resting of the bowel with parenteral rehydration and maintenance of fluid and electrolyte balance, as described in the dehydration section of this chapter. Once the patient's condition improves, oral fluids are advanced slowly.

Acid-Base Imbalances

Acid-base and electrolyte imbalances in children are manifested much the same as in adults. The reader is referred to Chapter 2 for details on this as well as electrolyte imbalances.

IMPLEMENTING THE NURSING PROCESS

The steps of the nursing process—assessment, analysis, planning, intervention, and evaluation—provide the foundation for administering to the needs of the patient and his family. The use of these steps promotes the safety and well-being of the patient and fosters the nurse-patient relationship. (See Chapter 1.)

Assessment

The nurse's assessment skills must continually be fine-tuned so she can quickly identify fluid and electrolyte imbalances and safely administer the interventions required to correct them. Assessment of a patient's hydration status involves a systematic approach. The nurse continues to utilize the nursing process so that all pertinent information is gathered, categorized, and prioritized.

History

When an imbalance of fluid and electrolytes is suspected, certain questions must be included in the nursing history. The nurse must make every attempt to establish rapport with the patient and his family. The child should be approached by calling him by his first name (or nickname) when speaking with him. The interview includes questions about any recent change in activity level or behavior, what foods or fluids the child has ingested since becoming ill, and the presence or absence of vomiting or diarrhea. (If the parents are present, ask them to describe the vomitus and stools.) It is important to find out what events led up to the vomiting or diarrhea, whether the child has been urinating as usual, and whether the child has had any significant weight loss or gain. If fever is present, inquire what the temperature range has been, how long it has lasted, and what has been done to to lower it. In addition it is important to find out if the child has been exposed to any communicable diseases, and what medications the child is receiving now or has received lately.

Vital Signs

Measurement of a child's temperature, pulse, respiratory rate, blood pressure, and pulse oximetry readings provide valuable information regarding his physiologic status. Table 15-7 illustrates the variances in vital signs that are manifested in volume depletion and contrasts early findings with late findings.

Temperature

When the body temperature is elevated in a child, fluid balance can be easily disrupted. Fever increases the patient's metabolic rate, which in turn increases the amount of metabolic wastes produced. For the effective excretion of such products, an increase in fluids is required. If extra fluids are not provided, dehydration will occur or an already existing dehydration will worsen. Moreover, water is lost through diaphoresis and hyperventilation, two conditions that com-

monly accompany fever, thus compounding the problem. In the early phase of volume depletion, the body temperature is elevated, whereas a low ($< 97.6°$ R) core body temperature is evident in the later stages of volume depletion.

Heart Rate and Pulse Quality

Heart rate and pulse characteristics are evaluated for number of beats per minute, quality, intensity, and rhythm. When fluid shifts from the intravascular compartment to the extravascular compartment, the pulse becomes rapid, weak, and thready. A bounding pulse is indicative of excess intravascular fluid volume, such as in hypertonic dehydration or an excess of total body fluid volume. An irregular pulse or even dysrhythmias can be seen with certain electrolyte abnormalities (e.g., hypokalemia or hyperkalemia). The heart rate is measured when a child is sleeping or calm. The heart rate must be counted apically for one full minute, since a child may normally exhibit an irregular rate, as in sinus arrhythmia. Evaluation of the pulse includes palpation (either radial or brachial) and differentiation of both central (e.g., carotid and femoral) and distal pulses (e.g., radial and pedal).

Respiratory Rate

The rate, effort, and quality of respirations also contributes information regarding the body's fluid and electrolyte status. Respirations may be affected by altered fluid volume and electrolyte imbalances. With dehydration, an increase in respiratory rate is due to a compensatory mechanism triggered by metabolic acidosis. A weakness or paralysis of respiratory muscles secondary to a potassium imbalance may cause shallow breathing. The respiratory rate can be counted either by observation or auscultation. As with the heart rate, respirations are measured when a child is calm and counted for one full minute, since an irregular rhythm is often seen in the infant and young child.

Table 15-7 | Vital Sign Findings in Volume Depletion: Early vs. Late Signs

	EARLY	LATE
Temperature	↑	↓ (<97.6°F rectally)
Heart Rate	↑	↓
Respiratory Rate	↑	↓
Blood Pressure	↑ or normal wide pulse pressure	↓ narrow pulse pressure
Pulse oximetry	"tall" waveform normal saturations	"short" waveform decreased saturations

Blood Pressure

The blood pressure of a child can be difficult to obtain because arterial pressure is normally low, and there is increased fatty tissue in the arms and legs (which decreases the intensity of Korotkoff sounds during auscultation of cuff pressures). An increase in blood pressure is seen in fluid volume excess or when anxiety or fear is present. A decrease in blood pressure is a late sign of physiologic compromise in a child and must be reported immediately. Interventions are implemented without delay. If a patient's condition permits, the nurse should not wait until hypotension is evident before implementing necessary interventions. In the early phases of hypovolemia, the pulse pressure (the difference between systolic and diastolic pressures) will widen, whereas in the later phases of hypovolemia, the pulse pressure narrows.

Weight

A child's weight provides important information about his hydration status. The degree of dehydration is based on the child's pre-illness and present weight. When a child's pre-illness weight cannot be obtained, the degree of dehydration will be based on the intensity of how bodily systems are affected. A child is weighed (daily), using the same scale, at the same time each day, without wearing any clothing or diapers. The nurse must account for any dressings or intravenous lines that alter the patient's weight. An increase in weight indicates fluid retention, whereas a decrease in weight can indicate loss of fluid (especially when other signs of dehydration accompany the drop). Any increase or decrease must be assessed and the hydration status evaluated.

Clinical Examination

A systematic assessment from head to toe will assist the nurse in determining the hydration status of a child. A child's sensorium will change when dehydration is present. Initially, the child will be irritable and restless, but as the severity of dehydration progresses, the child becomes obtunded and may even progress to coma. A child who is **obtunded** will have a limited physical and verbal response to his surroundings and is asleep unless stimulated either through noise or touch (McCance & Huether, 2001). A child who is in a **comatose** state does not have "motor or verbal response to the environment or to any stimuli even noxious stimuli such as deep pain or suctioning" (McCance & Huether, 2001). The nurse should be concerned when a child does not respond to the mother, father, or significant other, especially when the individual leaves the room. If a child responds by crying when a parent leaves the room, it is a sign that the child's sensorium is still intact. The fontanels of an infant are sunken or depressed with dehydration, but will bulge with fluid overload or meningitis. Normally, the fontanels are said to be normotensive and are usually level with the top of the head.

Typically, a child's periorbital area will appear sunken when he is experiencing dehydration, whereas they will appear puffy or swollen with overhydration. Mucous membranes and conjunctivae appear dry with dehydration. There may be an absence of tears when the child cries. However, tears often are not present with crying until after 1 to 3 months of age.

Skin turgor is another area to be assessed in determining the hydration status of a child. When skin on an area such as the abdomen is gently pinched (between the nurse's thumb and index fingers) for a few seconds then released, and the skin remains tented, it is usually a manifestation of dehydration. Another method to assess skin turgor is with decreased recoil, the amount of time in seconds the skin takes to settle back to its natural position. Normal skin turgor is evidenced by a brisk recoil. The sacral area of a pediatric patient is also assessed for signs of fluid retention.

Pulses should be assessed and compared bilaterally. Table 15-8 describes a method for quantifying pulses. Capillary refill will also indicate fluid imbalances. Normal capillary refill is 2 seconds or less. Moderate dehydration is manifested by a capillary refill of 3 to 5 seconds, and severe dehydration (or state of shock) is manifested by a capillary refill greater than 5 seconds. Both upper and lower extremities are compared for capillary refill to assist in determining the progression of shock.

Normal urine output for a child is from 0.5 to 2 ml/kg/hr. Any increase or decrease can indicate a fluid overload or dehydration and needs to be examined carefully. A specific gravity is obtained to assist in evaluating the concentration of the child's urine. Normally, a child's specific gravity is between 1.002 and 1.015. If the specific gravity is less than 1.002 or greater than 1.015, further evaluation and corresponding interventions must be implemented, and the specific gravity evaluated on a periodic basis.

Table 15-8 | Quantifying the Pulses

GRADE	0	1+	2+	3+	4+
	Not palpable	Weak, thready, easily obliterated with pressure	Difficult to palpate, easily obliterated even with slight pressure	Normal, easy to locate, easy to palpate, not obliterated with pressure	Bounding, forceful, not obliterated with pressure

NURSING TIP

Assessing Hydration Status

Remember, the presence or absence of any one of the following symptoms should not be used as a sole indicator of hydration status:

Irritability	May be an indicator that the child is sleepy or tired
Circumoral cyanosis	May indicate that the child is cold (e.g., a child who has been swimming or in a cold environment)
Tachycardia	May indicate that the patient is anxious, frightened, in pain, or febrile

In summary, all of the symptoms must be taken into consideration as a full picture, as opposed to one or two isolated symptoms.

Nursing Diagnosis

Once all pertinent data has been gathered and organized, the nursing diagnosis is made. This statement of the problem provides the basis for planning.

Planning

Planning provides the guidelines regarding what the health care team wants to achieve with fluid therapy. Although many institutions have standardized care plans, each patient's plan of care must be individualized based on his needs.

Interventions for Parenteral Fluid Therapy

The treatment of fluid and electrolyte imbalances involves the administration of solutions via the circulatory system. The nurse has an important role in the safe administration of IV fluid therapy. IV fluid therapy is used for various reasons in hospitals, ambulatory care settings, and the home. It is used in the treatment of emergency conditions, to maintain arterial blood pressure, to prevent or treat shock states, to replace blood components, to maintain fluid states, or to rehydrate and correct electrolyte imbalances, to assist with nutritional support, and to administer medications. (See Chapters 1, 5, 13, and 14.) For many medications, the IV route is the most effective method of administration, because most drugs are absorbed best when delivered directly into the circulatory system. It is also ideal because many children cannot tolerate oral medications when their illnesses encompass vomiting and diarrhea.

The management of pediatric patients with IV therapy is a major nursing responsibility. The nurse must be able to assess, monitor, and evaluate the effects of parenteral therapy. A strong knowledge of the principles of the physiologic, cognitive, and psychosocial needs of pediatric patients must accompany their nursing care. This section is devoted to the methodology for placement of lines and cannulas for intravenous access. The nurse must carefully examine the knowledge base and psychomotor skills of pediatric patients to ensure that safe and effective interventions are implemented.

Physiologic Principles

As stated earlier, children are not small adults! Although many principles apply to both adults and children, pediatric patients have special needs that are related to their size and body composition. The INS stresses that "the nurse providing infusion therapy for neonatal and pediatric patients shall have specific clinical knowledge and technical expertise with respect to this population" (INS, 2000, Standard 2, S12).

Principles of Cognitive Development

A patient's response to IV therapy depends largely on his age, previous experiences, education, and family background. A young child is not able to verbalize his needs and typically displays crying and demonstrations of anger as a means of communicating pain, fear, and discomfort.

The nurse must observe and be able to interpret such behavior. A child who is hospitalized will typically regress to an earlier developmental age; therefore, the nurse must provide care at the child's developmental level and not at his chronologic age. For example, a 2-year-old child who has suffered a burn injury cannot understand that his IV therapy is related to yesterday's accident. He cannot comprehend that he needs IV therapy for rehydration and pain management.

Psychosocial Considerations

The nurse caring for a patient receiving IV therapy must have knowledge of the psychosocial needs of the pediatric patient in order to form a basis for understanding the behavior and responses of the various age groups. A Child Life Specialist can be consulted to assist the family to better cope with the fears associated with IV therapy. A **Child Life Specialist** is a professional who organizes, plans, directs, and carries out a program of activities and services for hospitalized children. The planned activities are designed to decrease psychological trauma and minimize stress and anxiety. The goal of the activities is to ensure that a pediatric patient's hospitalization provides an environment that supports positive coping and adaptation skills. Through medical play and dialogue, a Child Life Specialist helps a pediatric patient and his family adjust to many of the stressors of illness and hospitalization.

Safety

Even though he may seem complacent or cooperative, a young child, as a rule, must be restrained during the insertion of an IV. Usually more than one person is required to carry out the procedure safely. Throughout the procedure, the child's status is assessed for signs of distress. A score sheet such as the one shown in Table 15-9 provides the nurse with a tool to quantify the progression or regression of the patient's condition. This score sheet allows for the assignment of points that reflect the patient's clinical picture and the number of attempts at cannulation. Because an infant may be at higher risk for rapid deterioration, the smaller the child, the higher the number of points allotted.

Instructions for completing the score card follow:

This score card is to be used with invasive procedures to assist the nurse in documenting the condition of the patient before, during, and after the invasive procedure. The score card is to be completed before beginning the procedure to obtain a baseline status of the patient's general condition. The score card is again completed at the end of the procedure. If the procedure lasts for 30 minutes or longer, the score card must be completed every 30 minutes. The last row on the score card allows for at least four scores: if more than four scores are obtained, the time and score can be documented in the area below this last row.

1. Obtain the patient's weight in kilograms and perform a head-to-toe assessment. Areas to concentrate on include the following:
   Area 1: Patient's weight
   Area 2: Patient's sensorium
   Area 3: Respiratory effort and status
   Area 4: Circulatory status and color
2. For each of the areas, place a check mark in the box that corresponds with the patient's clinical presentation. Only one box per area can be checked. Pay close attention to the number at the top of the column where each check mark has been placed. A column is vertical, a row is horizontal.
3. Add the number of points assigned for each of the columns and place the number in the bottom row of each column.
   Then add the numbers across the bottom row and place this number in the bottom row of the last column, marked "Total."

Table 15-9 | Score Card

CLINICAL CONDITION	0 POINTS	1 POINT	2 POINTS	
Weight in kg	>20 kg	10–20 kg	<10 kg	
Sensorium	Awake, alert, recognizes mother and/or significant other	Irritable, restless, still recognizes mother and/or significant other	Lethargic or unresponsive	
Respiratory Effort	Synchronized respirations, no retractions, no nasal flaring, no adventitious breath sounds	Lag on inspiration, mild retractions, minimal nasal flaring, adventitious breath sounds on auscultation	Labored respirations, moderate to severe retractions, marked nasal flaring, audible adventitious sounds	
Circulation/Color	Capillary refill <2 seconds, warm extremities, pink or natural color	Capillary refill 2–5 seconds, cool extremities, pale color	Capillary refill >5 seconds, cold extremities, mottled or cyanotic color	
Number of Attempts*	1–2	3–5	≥6	
Date/Time:	Points =	Points =	Points =	Total =
Date/Time:	Points =	Points =	Points =	Total =
Date/Time:	Points =	Points =	Points =	Total =
Date/Time:	Points =	Points =	Points =	Total =

*The next to the last row (number of attempts) is to be filled out only with the second and subsequent scores.

This is the total score of the patient. The higher the score, the worse the patient's condition. If the score is 4 or greater, interventions must be implemented; for example, offer blow-by oxygen; allow the patient to rest for a few minutes and then proceed; elevate the head of the bed; obtain a more detailed assessment, including O2 saturation and vital signs; call the physician. If the score increases each time the score card is completed, interventions must be taken to help improve the patient's clinical condition. If intravenous access is not obtained after four to six attempts by experienced clinicians, consider a central venous line or intraosseous access.

Infants

An infant is comforted through rocking, holding, and providing a pacifier for sucking. Restraints or even the adhesive tape used to secure an IV line may interfere with parent-infant bonding. The parent(s) must be assured that holding and cuddling the child will not cause any harm but will in fact help. The older infant (6 to 12 months) is at the peak of anxiety about strange people. Whenever possible, parents are encouraged to actively participate in comforting the child before, during, and after the procedure but should not be forced to do so, if they are uncomfortable about it.

Toddlers

A toddler also has stranger anxiety. A child in this age group typically regresses to a prior developmental level when faced with illness and hospitalization. A toddler is curious, has a short attention span, and dislikes restraints. Parental presence and a supportive environment will assist the child to better deal with uncomfortable situations. The nurse can usually expect minimal or no cooperation from a toddler, but must be supportive and reward his positive behavior.

Preschoolers

A preschooler has a vivid imagination. It is normal for a child in this age group to ask many questions and have a great fear of pain, needles, and body mutilation. The nurse must be honest about the degree of pain and must explain the equipment and the procedure in simple terms. The nurse must reassure the child and let him know that it is okay to cry. An IV line will not (and should not) slow a preschooler down. Play must be encouraged, and the child must be reminded that IV therapy is not punishment for bad behavior or negative thoughts, rather a way to give medicine to help the child feel better, or to make the "owie" or "boo-boo" go away.

School Age Children

The child in this age group is usually cooperative and aims to please others, even though he may be fearful. The nurse must acknowledge that it is okay to be scared. Structured group activities should be planned, especially between children of the same sex. The nurse strives to de-emphasize IV therapy and emphasize positive behavior and cooperation.

Adolescents

A teenager wants to be treated like an adult. The nurse should give an adolescent the option of whether or not he would like a parent or significant other to be present during IV therapy procedures. Because of a longer attention span in this age group, detailed explanations about IV therapy may be appropriate. An adolescent is extremely concerned with his body image and prefers to wear his own clothing rather than a hospital gown. The nurse must allow interaction with peers and provide privacy, as appropriate.

Therapeutic Play

Children of all ages may benefit from medical or therapeutic play. A Child Life Specialist can assist by providing dolls and other medical equipment throughout the phases of illness and IV therapy. Play activities can provide opportunities for the child to act out and express fears and anxieties.

Choosing the Right Solution

The IV solution to be used is based on the patient's clinical condition, serum electrolyte levels, and other laboratory values. IV solutions are classified according to their osmolality and electrolyte content. (See Chapter 6 for the discussion of types of solutions.)

Five percent dextrose in water (D_5W) is isotonic in the container. Because glucose is rapidly metabolized, once this infusate enters the body, the osmolality decreases, thereby making it hypotonic. D_5W is used only for mixing medications such as dopamine, dobutamine, and filgrastim and should not be used for the treatment of shock, rehydration, or IV fluid therapy.

Most children receive a solution with dextrose and sodium chloride. Glucose serves to prevent hypoglycemia, especially if the patient is NPO. Unless contraindicated by the patient's condition, all maintenance IVs should contain at least 0.2% normal saline because of the child's high risk for rapid fluid shifts.

Gathering the Equipment

Prior to beginning the actual venipuncture, the nurse must prepare all the equipment necessary for the venipuncture. An acutely ill child typically has compromised immune responses, making strict adherence to Standard Precautions extremely important. Furthermore, because "most intravenous complications in the pediatric patient are attributed to dosing, fluid administration, or both, the nurse administering IV therapy to the pediatric patient must "have an understanding of drug calculations with reference to age, height, weight, or body surface area, dosage, and volume limitations for neonatal and pediatric patients" (INS, 2000, Standard 2, S13).

The following steps are suggested:

1. Choose the correct solution. To prevent fluid overload and avoid unnecessary wasting of infusates, a child's IV bottles or bags should contain no more than 500 ml, except for a child £12 months, who should have a 250 ml bag/bottle. Label the container with the initials of the person opening the bag/bottle and the date and time it was hung. Be aware of hang times for infusates according to facility policy.

2. Obtain an IV tubing, a volume control cylinder (Soluset,® Buretrol®), and an extension set (T-connectors, K-48). Some IV tubings already come manufactured with this cylinder, others do not. Close all the clamps.

3. Connect the IV fluid to the volume control cylinder and the volume control cylinder to the IV tubing with the extension. Fill the cylinder with enough fluid to prime the tubing plus fluid for a maximum of 2 hours. (Volume in the volume control cylinder and the volume to be infused on the infusion machine is set to a maximum of 2 hours plus 5 to 10 ml.)

4. Prime the cylinder, the tubing, and the extension set.

5. Label the tubing with the initials of the person setting up the system and the date and time the tubing expires. For infection control, tubing is changed every 24 to 72 hours, depending on the situation. Tubing with fluids with a concentration of $>D_{10}W$ are usually changed every 24 hours.

6. Prepare to perform the venipuncture and insert the cannula. If the vessel is small in relation to the cannula (e.g., with poorly perfused children), the cannula may be advanced with the bevel down so that penetration of the vessel's opposite wall may be avoided. In some patients, the use of a tourniquet is discouraged as the veins may be so fragile that a tourniquet can cause an increased amount of pressure causing the vessel to rupture.

7. Once the vein is accessed, connect the extension set to the cannula and assess for flow by gravity. If the fluid does not flow freely, check for signs of infiltration.

8. Once venous access is assured, the cannula must be flushed with fluid and secured, and the extremity immobilized to prevent accidental dislodging. The cannula may require special attention and securement measures, depending on the site selected for venous access, the device used, and the patient's age and level of activity.

9. Connect the tubing to the infusion machine and adjust the settings as ordered.

IV Start Kits

Most institutions use packaged IV start kits. These IV start kits usually contain a tourniquet, antiseptic solution, sterile gauze, transparent dressing, adhesive tape, and a label with an area for date, time, type of cannula, size and length of cannula, and initials or signature of person who accessed the vein.

Cannulas and Needles

An over-the-needle cannula is preferred for peripheral IV access. These cannulas are available in various lengths and sizes (gauges) ranging from 27 ga. (⅝ inch) to 14 ga. (2½ inch). The size of the cannula is inversely proportional to the number. The cannula chosen should be the smallest size possible to administer the chosen fluid. For example, if IV access is needed for rehydration, a 27 ga. (⅝ inch) will suffice. Although blood and blood products can be administered via a small cannula, a larger gauge cannula is preferred.

Butterfly needles are also available when IV access is difficult. These needles are usually made of steel and come in sizes as small as 27 ga. Butterfly needles allow for rapid, temporary access of tiny veins until rehydration or peripheral circulation improves.

Electronic Infusion Devices

Several electronic infusion machines are available for administration of IV fluids. Most are easy to use and can be set to deliver in ml/hr, mcg/kg/min, and units/hr. Many models are available, and most machines detect air in the line, occlusions, and increasing resistance and alert the nurse to these conditions, such as when the IV fluid has or is about to run out.

Electronic infusion devices (EIDs) are recommended for pediatric IV therapy. Although convenient and practical, there are risks associated with their use. The nurse must be fully aware of the machine's capacities as well as its limitations prior to utilizing the equipment. Caution must be taken to use the EID to its maximum capacity while providing safe nursing care to the pediatric patient. An electronic infusion device is recommended for administration of pediatric infusions.

Evaluation

The final step of the nursing process is the evaluation phase. This is to be done concurrently with the other steps to determine that the appropriate assessment, analysis, planning, and intervention strategies are being used. When evaluation of a child's response to infusion therapy is carried out on an ongoing basis, the nurse is equipped with the information needed to identify whether changes need to be made and to intervene expediently.

Access Routes

Fluid therapy can be achieved through accessing the circulatory system via peripheral veins (Figure 15-6). In some instances, such as in emergency situations, the intraosseous route is used to administer fluid and medications (Figure 15-7). (See Chapter 12.)

When time permits, central venous cannulas can be surgically placed. The peripherally inserted central catheter (PICC) is used to administer parenteral fluids for long-term therapy. Access routes are summarized in Table 15-10. (See Chapter 12.)

Peripheral Access

The choice of site for administration of intravenous fluids varies according to the age, condition of the child, and acces-

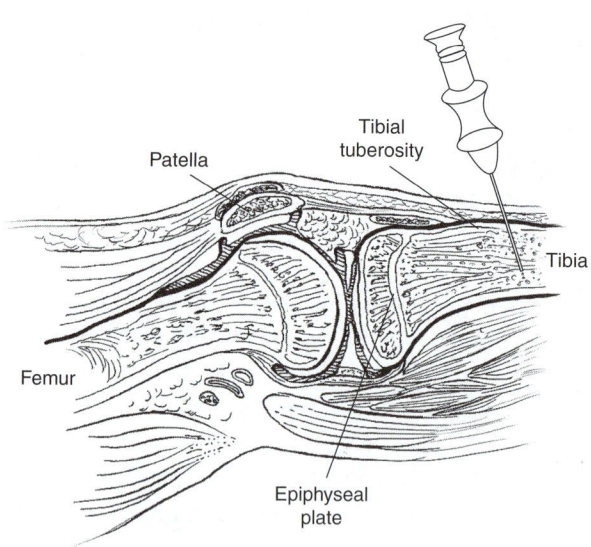

Figure 15-7 | Intraosseous landmarks with needle in place

sibility and integrity of his veins. The site selected should involve minimal risk and maximum efficiency, safety, and comfort. The first choice for administering intravenous fluids should always be peripheral access. Peripheral veins are found throughout the body but, in certain areas, peripheral veins are more prominent and are better choices for administering IV fluids. Intravenous cannulas may be placed in the veins of the scalp, hands, arms, lower legs, or feet.

Note: Cannulation of extremity veins in the neonate often presents a challenge. With small, fragile extremity veins, it is often difficult to locate suitable veins, thus making the scalp the only suitable site. The Venoscope II transilluminator can be easily inserted through the openings within an isolette. By placing the light beneath the extremity, the arms or feet are transilluminated, making it possible to visualize the veins from the top. Sometimes, the baby's arm is so fat that it cannot be transilluminated from beneath. In this situation, the Venoscope II light can be placed on the surface of the skin so the arm, leg, chest, scalp, and so on can be scanned until a dark line (the vein) between the dual arms is visualized. The vein can then be marked or can be held in place during venipuncture. The technique applies to children as well as obese adults.

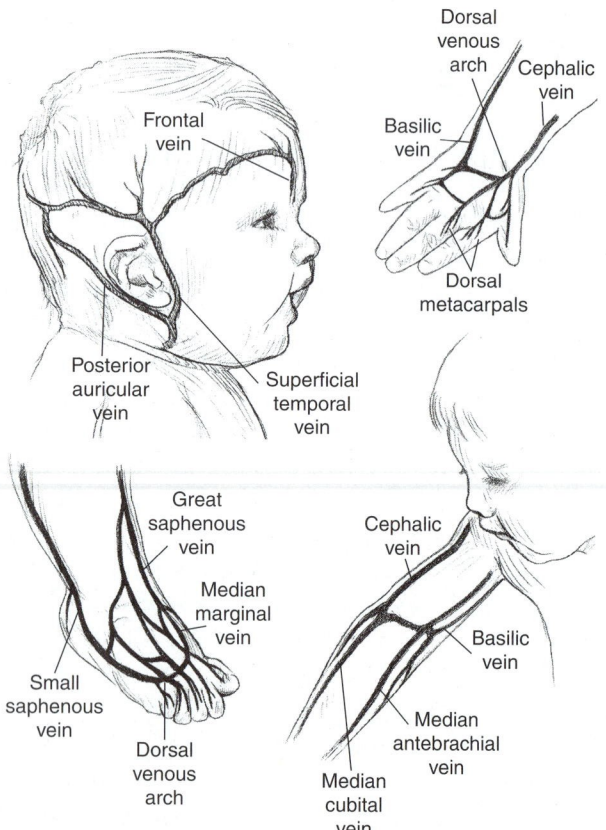

Figure 15-6 | Anatomy of peripheral veins in infants and children

> ## NURSING ALERT
>
> ### *Avoid Shaving the Scalp Area*
>
> Shaving of the hair in the scalp area is discouraged. It can lead to the introduction of microorganisms and infection through microabrasions.

Table 15-10 | Preferred Pediatric Access Sites

AGE OF CHILD	PREFERRED ACCESS SITE	RATIONALE
Infant	Scalp, dorsal hands or dorsal feet	These areas are readily visible even in the child with excess fat.
Toddler and preschooler	Dorsum or antecubital area of the nondominant hand/arm	This provides independence in mobility with feeding, comforting (i.e., thumb or pacifier sucking) and ambulation.
Older child and adolescent	Dorsum or antecubital area of the nondominant hand/arm	This provides independence in mobility with feeding, writing, playing, talking on the phone

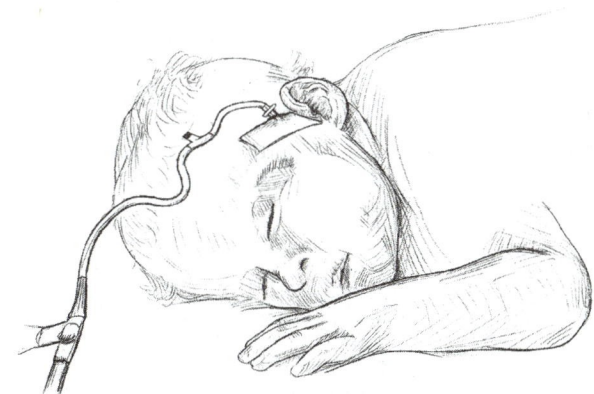

Figure 15-8 | Infant with scalp IV in place

When the scalp is used for intravenous access, the response of the child's parents and family is usually one of fear, anxiety, and concern. The parents and family of the patient must be informed prior to the procedure to help allay these feelings. A Child Life Specialist can assist in allowing the patient and his parents to alleviate their fears prior to and following the procedure.

Quite often scalp veins are used in children approximately one year and younger because these veins are more prominent than the peripheral veins of the extremities (Figure 15-8). The hair in the area of the chosen site may have to be clipped with scissors for visualization of the vein and for securing the cannula and tubing. For this reason and because the veins of the scalp directly communicate with dural sinuses, meticulous cleansing with a disinfecting solution is necessary prior to the venipuncture. If a povidone-iodine solution is used, the nurse must wait at least 30 to 60 seconds to allow the solution to dry, thus maximizing the antimicrobial effect.

A wide rubber band with an adhesive tag taped onto itself is placed around the infant's head to assist in distending the veins of the scalp. The adhesive tag facilitates quick grasping of the rubber band and allows for both easy and safe cutting of the rubber band once the vein is accessed. As scalp veins do not have valves, a cannula in the scalp can be inserted in either direction along the course of the vein. Scalp veins are not used in patients with confirmed or suspected hydrocephalus or infection in the head. Another precaution that must be taken is that prior to puncturing the vessel, the nurse must palpate for a pulse. The presence of a pulse indicates the vessel is an artery and must not be cannulated.

The technique for starting an IV in a child is similar to starting an IV line in an adult. However, safety is an even bigger issue with a child since he is usually not cooperative because of his inability to comprehend the need for a painful procedure. The procedure is carried out in a treatment room or in an area away from his assigned room. This will allow the child to think of his room as a "safe haven," and to be fairly certain that painful procedures will be carried out in the treatment room and not in his room. Prior to bringing the child into the treatment room or area where the IV will be started, all equipment must be set up and within the nurse's reach. All tubing must be primed and ready, and the tape that will be used to secure the IV site must be cut so it can be applied as soon as the vein is accessed.

When starting an infusion on a child, usually more than one person is needed. The child must be safely restrained and positive behavior must be continually rewarded either with words or through "contracting" with the child. For example, promising to give a coloring book after the completion of the procedure if the child stays still will promote cooperation from a preschooler. Remind the child that it is okay to cry, but he should try to remain as still as possible throughout the procedure. If the child does cry or move about, it is important not to instill feelings of guilt or shame. It is important to educate parents so that they do not use medical procedures or "shots and needles" as a threat to get the child to behave or to do what is necessary to help him get better.

Choosing an access site in a pediatric patient is similar to that of an adult patient. When using an area in the upper extremities, the nurse should choose an area in the non-dominant hand, starting distally to preserve the proximal veins for future use. The nurse must make every attempt to avoid veins of the lower extremities in an ambulatory child, as this restricts his freedom to roam about as he pleases.

Once the vein is accessed, the site is secured, preferably with a transparent dressing, so the site can be easily monitored. When applying the tape, the arm or foot is placed on an age- and size-appropriate board to assist with immobilization and prevent dislodgment of the cannula or needle. The adhesive tape is used to prevent the joint from moving. The areas distal and proximal to the insertion site are left uncovered for continuous visual and tactile assessment. Fingers and toes are assessed for circulation, mobility, and sensation (CMS), necessitating exposure of the tips of both appendages.

A label is placed directly on and to the side of the dressing (never over the insertion site) indicating the date, time, type of cannula, gauge, length and the person accessing the vein. To prevent infection and phlebitis, CDC guidelines recommend that IV cannulas and needles are to be changed every 72 to 96 hours (CDC, 2002a). If the site is obliterated by a dressing, the site is assessed as defined by facility policy. Dressings must be changed when they become loose, wet, or soiled (and not necessarily at specified intervals) (CDC, 2002). In any case, the nurse must follow institutional policy. Everyone involved in the care of the child must be aware of his condition, and meticulous care must be provided to prevent any potential problems.

Once the cannula is to be removed, the most painful part of the procedure is the removal of the tape. Whenever possible (such as with a cooperative patient or one who does not move very much), double-backed tape should be used to promote minimal contact of tape with the skin. When removing tape, adhesive tape remover can be used to promote comfort. The older child is usually allowed to assist with the procedure, which permits him an increased sense of control and (hopefully) decreases his fears.

Intraosseous

In emergency situations when a peripheral vein cannot be accessed, a needle or a cannula can be inserted into the medullary cavity of a bone to administer fluid and medications. Intraosseous access is a safe and reliable method for rapidly accessing a route for the administration of drugs, fluids, and blood products into a noncollapsible marrow venous plexus. Intraosseous cannulation is recommended in emergency situations for children who are six years of age or younger when intravenous access is difficult (AHA, 2002). This technique can be used in patients of all ages, ranging from premature neonates to adults. Long uninjured bones such as the distal tibia, distal radius, or distal ulna can be used. The superior iliac spine can also be used for insertion

of an intraosseous needle. The most commonly used site is the anterior tibia (1 to 3 cm below the tibial tuberosity). Physicians and other trained personnel can access the marrow for fluid or medication administration.

Needles used for bone marrow access are ideal for this technique; however, angiocaths and spinal needles with a stylet can also be used. The INS recommends the use of standard steel hypodermic spinal, trephine, sternal, and standard bone marrow needles (INS, 2000, Standard 68, S64). The needle is inserted after the area has been aseptically cleansed, since a major complication of this therapy is **osteomyelitis**, inflammation of bone marrow. Once the needle is inserted, the leg is assessed and monitored for circulatory status. Signs of infiltration are the same as for a peripheral line, and the line is removed when these and other signs of circulatory or neurovascular complications arise. All fluids, including vasopressors, blood and blood products, antibiotics, and sodium bicarbonate can be administered via the intraosseous route. In children, growth plates in the bone are to be avoided by leaning the intraosseous needle toward the center of the bone away from the growth plate.

Other complications of intraosseous infusion include cellulitis, damage to the epiphyseal plate, and embolus from fat dislodgment within the bone marrow, from tibial fractures, compartment syndrome, or skin necrosis. Although these complications are rare, their severity is greater than in peripheral vein cannulations. Only trained personnel should insert these lines, and the procedure must be reserved only for those children who are critically ill and for whom difficult access of peripheral veins will delay treatment.

NURSING TIP

Intraosseous Cannulations

The following are circumstances that ensure that the needle is in the bone marrow cavity.

1. The needle remains erect without support.
2. Bone marrow is aspirated (although its absence does not mean incorrect placement of the needle).
3. IV fluid flows easily without signs of infiltration (i.e., changes in circulatory status distal to the insertion site, edema, resistance when flushing).

PICC and CVC

The use of, precautions for, and maintenance of peripherally inserted central catheters (PICC) and central venous catheters (CVCs) is the same in children as it is in adults.

(See Chapter 12 for a detailed discussion of CVCs and PICC lines.)

When a catheter is used for withdrawing a blood sample from a child, the child's circulating blood volume as well as the tests to be performed must be taken into consideration. The infusion is stopped, the catheter is scrubbed with an antiseptic wipe, and enough blood is drawn for discard. Then the amount needed for testing is withdrawn. The catheter kit or package insert defines the priming volume of the catheter based on its size. It is recommended that serum drug levels not be drawn from silicone catheters as certain drugs, such as aminoglycosides, tend to stick to the walls of the catheter, resulting in falsely elevated results.

If the catheter becomes blocked, dye studies are performed to help confirm the problem. When resistance is met during an attempt to draw blood, several strategies are used: side-to-side positioning of the child, placing him in the reverse Trendelenburg position, raising his arms above the head, or inducing a Valsalva maneuver. If these measures fail to bring about a free flow within the catheter, the POP method (described in Chapter 12) or alteplase (tPA) is used to dissolve a clot. Never force a clot into the circulatory system.

Syringes no smaller than 10-ml capacity are to be used for flushing. When the plunger is advanced or retracted in the barrel of small syringes, excess pressure is exerted on the catheter, which may damage or rupture it. The stopcock technique is often used when declotting a catheter with a maximum of 3 ml of alteplase 1mg/ml (see Chapter 12). Although scant literature exists regarding the maximum times for retreatment in case the catheter continues clotted, the author recommends capping the total dosage at 5–10 mg.

When accessing subcutaneous ports or starting a peripheral IV line, topical anesthetics are available (such as EMLA, which is topical lidocaine 2.5% and prilocaine 2.5%, or Elamax, which is an over-the-counter medication containing 4% or 5% lidocaine) that can be used to numb the cannula insertion area prior to accessing the port. If applied well in advance of percutaneous puncture, according to manufacturer's directions, discomfort is greatly decreased for the patient.

COMPLICATIONS OF INFUSION THERAPY

As with the adult, IV therapy in the pediatric patient is associated with several risks. Nursing interventions, such as frequent and meticulous checks of the entire system, are needed

---

NURSING TIP

Changing IV Site Dressings

When changing dressings on any IV site, whether peripheral or central, the old dressing should be pulled *off* in the direction toward the tip of the catheter (Figure 15-9). Pulling the dressing *away* from the catheter insertion site can dislodge the catheter.

Have the patient turn his head away from the exposed catheter site to prevent contamination of the site with organisms transmitted via the respiratory or airborne route.

NURSING ALERT

Preventing a Clot from Entering the Circulatory System

Forcing a clot into the circulatory system can be fatal to a patient. Extra precautionary measures, such as those listed here, must be taken to prevent this from happening.

- Only use syringes 10 ml and larger.
- Never continue to flush a catheter when resistance is met.
- Try the POP method.
- Use the stopcock method for declotting catheters.

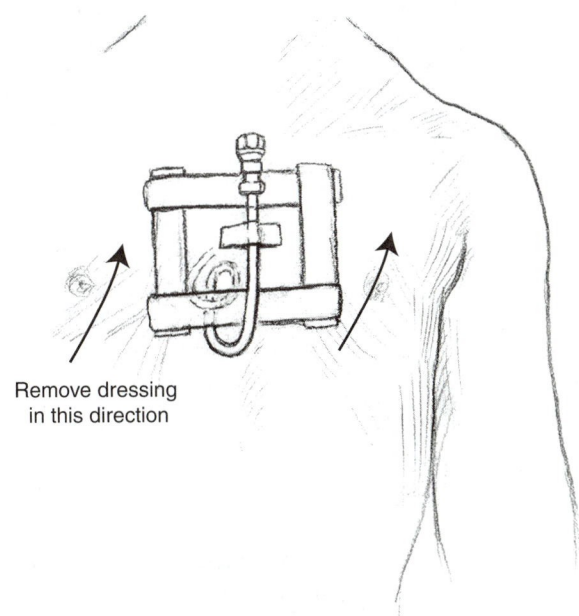

Remove dressing in this direction

Figure 15-9 | Technique for removal of IV dressing

to prevent complications. The less covered the site is with tape and gauze, the easier it is for the nurse to monitor the site. The nurse must examine the risks and the benefits of safely protecting the IV system as well as the patient against the possibility of dislodging the IV.

The following paragraphs discuss the complications of IV therapy as they relate to children. (See Chapter 5 for a detailed discussion of the risks and complications of infusion therapy.)

Infiltration is the leakage of IV fluid into the surrounding tissue. It is difficult to detect in the infant and small child because they have a large amount of subcutaneous fat. The pediatric patient is at greater risk for potential complications related to IV therapy and should be monitored, at least, every 2 hours, and more frequently, depending on the patient's age and size, or type of therapy. When an infiltration is present, the infusion slows or stops, and the child usually complains of tenderness or pain at the site. The infant or younger child, however, may not be as specific in identifying their pain, therefore the only visible sign of discomfort may be generalized crying and irritability. The nurse must remove all the tape used to secure the site and visually evaluate and touch the skin in order to assess for redness, drainage, hardness, or inflammation. The area is compared with the opposite extremity for diameter, color, temperature, and softness of the child's skin. If any of these complications are present, the cannula is to be removed and the patient is evaluated for insertion of a new cannula in a different location. The site of the infiltration should be treated according to agency policy and physician preference.

Overhydration is another complication of IV therapy. IV complications in the pediatric patient are often attributed to dosing or fluid administration. The volume of the solution should be based on the age, height and weight of the patient, and the container should hold no more than 500 ml of fluid. Consideration is given to the use of smaller volume containers in infants and premature infants owing to the ever-present complications of fluid volume overload. Consideration should also be given to the use of pediatric-specific equipment for the delivery of infusion therapy.

Signs of overhydration include bounding pulses, increased urine output, tachycardia, tachypnea, puffy eyes, bulging fontanels, and rales on auscultation of the lungs. Prevention of overhydration is possible through close monitoring of the IV line, using volume control administration sets and EIDs, and assuring that both the delivery container and the volume to be infused (VTBI) has no more than a 2-hour supply of fluid. The nurse must also be careful in setting the rate on infusion machines, as many machines deliver in increments of ones, tens, and hundreds (10.0 ml can easily be confused as 100 ml if the nurse is not careful to look for the decimal point).

NURSING TIP

Assessing and Documenting Peripheral IV Sites in Children

1. Complete assessment and documentation of IV site should be performed at *least* every 2 hours.
2. Deviation from baseline vital signs can indicate circulatory overload or dehydration. Dehydration is manifested by tachycardia and hypotension. Circulatory overload can be manifested by tachypnea and hypertension.
3. All senses, especially visual and tactile, must be used when assessing an IV site. Check for drainage, redness, hardness, inflammation, and overall affect of the child. A child with fluid overload may have periorbital or sacral edema.
4. Special attention to circulation, particularly to the distal limb, must be taken. Assess and document capillary refill, mobility, sensation, color and temperature to the extremity where the IV cannula is located. Compare this extremity with the others.
5. Check patency of an IV site by flushing only with normal saline solutions. Extravasation of any other medication (i.e., inotropes, antibiotics, anticonvulsants, electrolytes, etc.) can cause severe loss and/or function of all or part of the extremity. Furthermore, a rapid bolus of a certain medication could negatively affect the patient's hemodynamic and/or neurologic status.
6. Listen carefully for alarms from the electronic infusion device. Investigate all alarms methodically and thoroughly.

MEDICATION ADMINISTRATION

Administering medications via the intravenous route is a common therapy used in pediatric nursing. Most drugs require a specific minimum dilution and a prescribed flow rate. Issues to keep in mind when administering IV medications in pediatric patients are: (1) drug to be administered, (2) volume of drug, (3) minimum dilution, (4) compatible infusates, (5) duration of administration, (6) volume capacity of the IV tubing, (7) condition of the patient's veins, (8) the flow rate that the vein can tolerate, (9) other medications that the patient is receiving, (10) time, and (11) potential side effects.

There are several methods the nurse can use to administer medications via the intravenous route. The procedures for

Administering Total Fluid Volume

Michael is to receive 30 mg gentamicin over a 30-minute period. The medication is diluted in a 10 mg/ml concentration (3 ml of medication). The medication is to be given via a Buretrol®, and the priming volume of this tubing is 10 ml. What is the total fluid volume to be administered?

A total of 13 ml needs to be administered over 30 minutes. If the medication is being delivered via a machine that infuses ml/hr, the flow rate will have to be set at 26 ml/hr so the medication infuses over 30 minutes. Once the medication has infused, 10 ml is added to the Buretrol and allowed to go in at the same rate to flush all the medication through the tubing to the patient.

IV push and minibag (or "piggyback") methods are the same for the child as for the adult. When a drug is to be administered over a specified amount of time, all tubing volumes must be taken into consideration.

Retrograde Technique

Medications can also be administered via the retrograde technique (Figure 15-10), a method of infusing small amounts of medication (less than 1 ml) directly into the patient's IV tubing. The tubing is clamped below the site of administration, and the medication is injected via a Y-port in the direction away from the child. The medication is diluted with the fluid in the tubing. The rate may still need to be adjusted, but a smaller volume of fluid is required than with the Buretrol® technique. The retrograde technique is performed as follows:

1. Pause the infusion of IV fluids.
2. Clamp the patient's IV tubing as close to the actual infusion site as possible.
3. Inject the small volume of medication with a syringe away from the patient and up the tubing (retrograde— away from the patient). Ensure that the tubing is not kinked or clamped anywhere *above* the injection site; otherwise, the tubing can rupture or resistance will be met as the medication is injected.
4. Unclamp the tubing.
5. Restart the infusion at the appropriate rate.

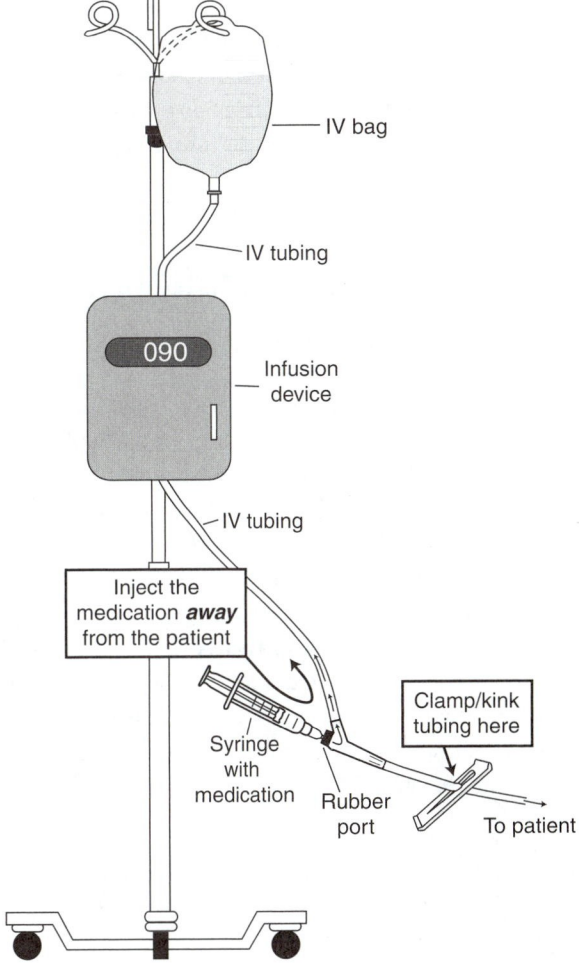

Figure 15-10 | Retrograde technique for medication administration

Direct Technique

With the direct technique, the correct volume of previously diluted medication is injected directly into the tubing through a Y connection or a stopcock in the direction of the child. Syringe pumps are available that administer the medication over a set time or at a rate of ml/hr, mcg/kg/min, or units/hr. This is the most convenient way of administering IV medications, as the nurse has greater control and the amount of fluid required for flushing is less, thus decreasing the risk of overhydration. Another advantage of syringe pumps is that resulting therapeutic serum drug levels are more successfully maintained than with other medication administration techniques.

Use of Volume Control Sets

With the technology advancing rapidly in the area of intravenous infusion devices, volume control sets are becoming obsolete. The trend is for electronic infusion devices to have very sensitive alarms and settings, such that the nurse can program the amount of fluid to be infused down to a tenth of a milliliter. Many children's hospitals are phasing out the use of volume control sets as electronic infusion devices become more sophisticated.

BLOOD AND BLOOD PRODUCT ADMINISTRATION

Principles of administration of blood and blood products are quite similar in the pediatric patient as in the adult patient (see Chapter 14). Generally, any gauge catheter can be used for delivery of blood products in pediatric patients. However, dosing of these products must be carefully calculated so as not to cause circulatory overload (see Table 15-11). When initiating a transfusion, baseline vital signs are obtained, and then three times at 5 minute intervals every 30 minutes, and again at the end of the transfusion. The reason for this is that most transfusion reactions occur within the first 30 minutes of the transfusion. Each institution provides strict protocols guiding the pediatric nurse.

INTRAVENOUS THERAPY IN HOME CARE

Today, many children receive IV therapy in the comfort of their own home. Infusion therapy runs the gamut from antibiotics to total parenteral nutrition to chemotherapy. Nurses work closely with patients and their parents or significant others in ensuring the therapy is carried out in a safe and effective manner. The goal of home care is to allow the therapy to be carried out in a familiar, low-stress environment and to decrease exposure to pathogens.

Before a patient can receive IV home therapy the household environment must be assessed to be sure the therapy can be safely carried out. The parents must be educated about the use and care of IV therapy and accept involvement in and responsibility for the treatment regimen. The nurse assists the family in the decision-making process in order to maintain as normal a home environment as possible.

Even though the goal of home care is to allow for therapy to be carried out in a low-stress environment, the appropriateness of matching home care therapy and the equipment involved to the pediatric patient and his family is critical. Consequently, not all pediatric patients and their families are candidates to receive home care therapy, due to the nature of its unique needs, such as skilled nursing assessment, hands-on procedures, and highly precise equipment needed to carry

out therapeutic care. Teamwork and providing highly skilled nurses for the home environment can assure quality nursing care is provided to the pediatric patient.

CHILDREN WITH CANCER

Cancer is the leading cause of death from disease in children. Although some theories hypothesize the causes of cancer, the actual causes remain unknown. Cancer occurs most frequently in the rapidly growing tissues of children, such as the bone marrow. The following paragraphs address chemotherapy as a mode of therapy for childhood cancer and include an overview of chemotherapy administration.

Chemotherapy

Chemotherapy is the use of chemical agents to destroy malignant or cancerous cells. It is often used in conjunction with other modes of therapy, such as radiotherapy and surgery, for remission, cure, control, or palliation of cancer. It is usually given at intervals for an extended period of time to minimize the damage to normal cells. A large number of chemotherapeutic agents are used for the treatment of cancer. Almost all of them work by affecting the synthesis of DNA. Often, several agents are given in combination to maximize the effects of the therapy.

Chemotherapy has advantages and disadvantages. Malignant cells have rapid growth patterns and weak cellular structures, making them sensitive to the effects of chemotherapy. However, normal cells are equally affected by chemotherapy: side effects are uncomfortable and can be detrimental for the child receiving treatment.

Administration of chemotherapy is not without risk because many of the chemotherapeutic agents are highly toxic. In order for them to be safely administered, the nurse must be familiar with their expected action, major side effects, recommended dosages, signs of toxicity, and other nursing concerns. Although screening techniques have decreased the risk for error, there is still a chance for incorrect administration of chemotherapy. Because of the many chemotherapeutic regimens that are investigational, few therapies are standardized, thus making it more significant that the nurse use extreme caution and make every effort to avoid improper administration of chemotherapy.

Although nurses are not responsible for prescribing the chemotherapeutic agents to be administered, they are responsible for administering them in a safe manner. Children must be carefully monitored during the administration of chemotherapy. Safe administration requires a broad base of knowledge on the part of nurses that includes referencing specific drug handbooks, pediatric literature, and pharmacists for in-depth information regarding chemotherapeutics.

Table 15-11 | Dosing of Blood Products

BLOOD PRODUCT	INDICATION	DOSE	RATE OF ADMINISTRATION
Whole blood	Acute hypovolemia from hemorrhage or exchange transfusion	10-20 ml/kg (consider diuretics) (10 ml/kg should raise the hematocrit by 10 points)	As fast as tolerated
PRBCs	Acute or chronic anemia	10 ml/kg	2–4 hours, not greater than 6 hours
Platelets	Thrombocytopenia	1 unit/5 kg, max 10 units	As fast as tolerated, generally 1 ml/kg/min
Fresh frozen plasma	DIC or acute hemorrhage	15–30 ml/kg (consider diuretics if concerned with potential fluid overload)	As fast as tolerated, generally 1 ml/kg/min
	Clotting deficiency	10–15 ml/kg (consider diuretics if concerned with potential fluid overload)	As fast as tolerated, generally 1 ml/kg/min
Cryoprecipitate	DIC or other clotting deficiency	1 unit/5 kg (titrate to achieve improvement in fibrinogen level)	As fast as tolerated, generally 1 ml/kg/min
Albumin 5%	Hypovolemia	10–20 ml/kg (consider diuretics if concerned with potential fluid overload)	As fast as tolerated
Albumin 25%	Hypovolemia or hypoalbuminemia in fluid-restricted patients	2–4 ml/kg (consider diuretics if concerned with potential fluid overload)	20–60 minutes

Classifications of Chemotherapy

Chemotherapeutic agents are classified according to the source of the drug, its cytotoxic action within the body, or cell-cycle specificity. Table 15-12 illustrates the classification of various chemotherapeutic agents and their use.

Precautions in Administering and Handling Chemotherapeutic Agents

Before any child receives chemotherapy, several factors must be considered. Administration of chemotherapy is a team effort. Many institutions require that only nurses who have undergone formal training and who are experienced with

Table 15-12 | Classifications of Chemotherapy and Their Use

CLASSIFICATION	EXAMPLES	USE
Alkylating Agents: Interfere with protein synthesis, resulting in cell death	Cyclophosphamide Procarbazine	Chronic leukemias Hodgkin's disease Non-Hodgkin's lymphoma
Antimetabolites: Interfere with protein, RNA and/or DNA synthesis	Methotrexate 6-mercaptopurine 5-fluorouracil	Chronic leukemias
Antitumor Antibiotics: Inhibit replication of DNA and/or transcription of RNA	Adriamycin Daunorubicin Bleomycin Idarubicin	Leukemias Lymphomas Hodgkin's disease Neuroblastomas Sarcomas
Plant Alkaloids: Inhibit mitosis	Vincristine Vinblastine Etoposide	ALL Hodgkin's disease Lymphoma Neuroblastoma Wilms' tumor
Steroid Hormones: Have antineoplastic properties but precise mechanism remains unknown	Adrenocorticosteroids Estrogens	Leukemias Lymphomas Hodgkin's disease
Miscellaneous: Prevents synthesis of protein	L-asparaginase, Erwinia, Oncaspar (can all cause severe anaphylaxis)	Leukemia

administration of chemotherapy should administer these drugs. Guidelines are available from the Association of Pediatric Oncology Nurses for the administration of chemotherapy in children. Nurses must provide each other with a check-off system that allows them to frequently document their competency in administering chemotherapeutic agents. Responsibility for ensuring the safe administration of these medications rests with the family, the physicians, the nurses, the pharmacists, and other personnel.

Each team member must be familiar with the patient's treatment schedule and the results of the pretreatment evaluation, which include tests such as complete blood count (CBC), chemistry panel, renal and liver function, echocardiograms, electrocardiograms, x-rays, and biopsy results. Furthermore, physiologic and psychological preparation must be complete prior to the administration of chemotherapy.

Assessment

The patient must be thoroughly assessed prior to the administration of chemotherapy. A history relevant to the planned chemotherapy is obtained, which reflects allergies, cardiac disease, and previous radiation therapy. The child's previous experience with chemotherapy, including types of drugs administered and the physical and emotional responses and

NURSING TIP

Administration of Chemotherapy

Nurses involved in caring for hematology/oncology patients should review their state's nurse practice act for the special training required to administer chemotherapy.

interventions that alleviated any side effects, is included. The parents', child's, and siblings' knowledge base regarding the malignancy and chemotherapy administration is also explored. Current lab values and diagnostic exams are reviewed. An informed consent is obtained when appropriate, as in the case of administration of investigational drugs or regimens. An accurate height and weight must be obtained, and the child's body surface area is calculated. A thorough head-to-toe exam is also documented and discussed with the members of the team.

Interventions

Once a definitive diagnosis is made, the child is then psychologically prepared for chemotherapy administration. A Child Life Specialist can be consulted for the psychological preparation of the treatment schedule. Nursing staff can assist in

NURSING TIP

The Five Rights of Chemotherapy Administration

1. *Right Patient.* Verify patient identification by checking the patient's ID armband and asking the patient's name. Never assume that the child in Nicole's bed is actually Nicole! If the identification band is missing, correctly identify the patient by other means (e.g., asking the child's parent/s) and replace the missing identification band immediately.

2. *Right Drug.* Follow the RL^3 (READ THE LABEL 3 TIMES!!) program. *Always check the label on the bag or container 3 times:*
   a. When you remove the medication from the bag or patient's drawer
   b. While preparing the medication
   c. Immediately before administering it

   Note: It is also a good idea to check the label when you discard the container or the bag to ensure the right medication was in fact given.

   Always be suspicious of confusing or poor labeling. If the label is not clear, DO NOT give the medication. Always check the color and consistency of the drug and be aware of signs of deterioration. Check the drug's expiration date on the container. If the patient or the family questions your actions or says, "That medication looks funny," RECHECK THE DRUG!!

3. *Right Dose.* Always be aware of how much medication is an appropriate dose for each patient. If you are in doubt, *always* check a reference *before* you give the medication. *Always* check chemotherapy doses with another registered nurse. When you are ready to administer the drug, recalculate the dose, and compare the information on the bag or syringe and the label with the written order.

   Be aware of the reasons why dosage errors occur:
   a. Improper calculation of a dosage—we are all humans and humans make mistakes. Take your time when calculating drug dosages! Think about what you are doing during drug calculations!

   b. Phantom decimals—decimal points in the original orders may not be seen if they are written too lightly or written over a line. *Always* clarify poorly written orders and watch closely for decimal points.
   c. Hazardous abbreviation—follow the list of approved abbreviations in each facility.
   d. Mixing incompatible drugs—many drugs are incompatible with one another. As a rule of thumb, liquid oral medications should never be mixed together. Injectable medication must be diluted with an appropriate diluent. Always check your resources before giving a medication that was diluted or before mixing any medication.

4. *Right Route.* Some drugs are never given by certain routes of administration. For example, drugs such as Elspar, Erwinia, and Oncaspar are given only via the IM or SQ routes. Always question any order that does not seem appropriate; e.g., "10 units regular insulin po now" or "Elspar 10 mg IV now."

5. *Right Time.* Omission of drug doses is believed to be one of the most common of all medication errors. These errors are usually discovered when the next dose is due. Reasons for omissions include:
   • Drug administration schedules are disorganized
   • Drug is not available on the unit

   Using forms that all personnel are familiar with when administering chemotherapy can assist in ensuring that schedules are strictly followed. In addition, communicating closely with the pharmacy can help ensure that medications are administered as scheduled.

   Chemotherapy must be given through a free-flowing line. The nurse must frequently check the IV, whether it is a central or peripheral line, to ascertain patency prior to, during, and after administration.

teaching the patient and his family about the possible side effects of chemotherapy. A plan for hydration, diuresis, and electrolyte supplementation, also part of the treatment regimen, is in place prior to chemotherapy administration.

Calculation of Dosages

Once the patient has been prepared physically and psychologically, chemotherapy can begin. Most chemotherapy dosage calculations are based on the patient's body surface area. The nurse must check and double-check to ensure the Five Rights of medication administration (see the accompanying box) are followed during chemotherapy administration.

The nurse must be fully aware of the side effects and adverse reactions that can occur with the drugs the child is about to receive. For drugs that are irritating to the veins, appropriate interventions must be taken. When vesicants

NURSING TIP

Effective Chemotherapy Administration

1. Use maximum care and strict aseptic technique in handling chemotherapeutic agents.
2. Chemotherapy must be prepared in a properly ventilated room by only those persons who have formal orientation to and training for the preparation of chemotherapy.
3. Eye shields, gowns, and disposable gloves must be used when handling any chemotherapeutic agent.
4. All equipment and supplies that have come in contact with chemotherapeutic agents must be properly discarded, following MSDS guidelines.

5. When priming IV tubing to be used for chemotherapy administration, never prime excess fluid into a sink. Rather, use the backflush method, using maintenance solution (see Chapter 9, Secondary Medication Administration). This will prevent accidental spillage of chemotherapeutic agents.
6. When administering chemotherapy by the IV push method, place gauze under the Y or injection port of IV tubing. After pushing the chemotherapeutic agent, draw back 1 to 2 ml of maintenance solution as you are pulling the needle out. Discard needle and syringe in containers approved for these items. Pull glove over gauze and discard appropriately.

(those that can cause necrosis or sloughing of tissue if the drug infiltrates out of the vein) are used, the nurse must continually assess for extravasation and follow the established institutional treatment protocols should it occur.

Evaluation

The effectiveness of nursing interventions during chemotherapy administration must be evaluated. Continuous reassessment of the patient will determine patient outcomes. The patient must return frequently to the clinic or physician's office for re-evaluation of interventions and to check his progress.

Key Concepts

* The nurse providing care for the pediatric patient receiving intravenous therapy must be knowledgeable in physiologic, cognitive, and psychosocial needs of the pediatric patient.

* Children are not small adults. They have their own physical, physiologic, and emotional mechanisms that greatly affect their response to illness or injury.

* Dehydration is a common cause of fluid and electrolyte imbalance in children and is due to their special physical and physiological needs.

* Dehydration is classified by severity: mild, moderate, and severe; and types: isotonic, hypotonic, and hypertonic.

* The treatment of dehydration involves steps to provide carefully for fluid and electrolyte homeostasis.

* Acute gastroenteritis (AGE) is caused by a hostile organism in the gastrointestinal tract. The illness can take one of three pathophysiologic pathways, which typically lead to dehydration.

* Assessment of a child's hydration status involves a systematic head-to-toe approach.

* The nursing process allows for an organized approach for implementing safe and effective nursing care to the child requiring fluid and electrolyte therapy.

* Vital signs, weight, and clinical presentation must be evaluated carefully to obtain accurate physiologic status of a child's hydration.

* Therapeutic play allows children to release and express their anxieties and fears related to parenteral fluid therapy.

✴ Parenteral fluid therapy in pediatric patients can be achieved by way of the peripheral, intraosseous, and central routes.

✴ Complications of intravenous therapy include infiltration, infection, thrombophlebitis, air embolus, and overhydration.

✴ Regardless of the route, nursing care of patients with parenteral fluid therapy requires organizational skills, a strong knowledge base, a caring attitude, and strong teamwork.

✴ Chemotherapy administration must be taken very seriously. When a child is receiving chemotherapy, an interdisciplinary approach must be taken to improve communication and avoid unnecessary complications.

✴ Nurses who administer chemotherapy must be well versed in its action, uses, dosages, and potential side effects.

✴ Nurses who administer chemotherapy as well as any other medication must *actively* think about the Five Rights and the RL[3] of medication administration.

Review Questions and Activities

1. Calculate Alex's fluid maintenance needs using both the formula and BSA, with 16 kg the child's weight and 104 cm for his height.

   (a) The weight is broken down by 10's: 10 kg

   6 kg

   (b) For the first 10 kg give 100 ml/kg/day.

   $10 \text{ kg} \times 100 \text{ ml} = 1000 \text{ ml}$

   For the second 10 kg give 50 ml/kg/day.

   $6 \text{ kg} \times 50 \text{ ml} = 300 \text{ ml}$

   (c) Add the products in step (b) to obtain total fluid for 24 hours.

   $1,000 \text{ ml} + 300 \text{ ml} = 1,300 \text{ ml}/24 \text{ hr} = 54 \text{ cc/hr}$

2. Calculate Alex's BSA.

   (a) Using the BSA nomogram (Figure 15-2), Alex's BSA is 0.68 m2.

   (b) $1,500 \text{ ml} \times 0.68 = 1,020 \text{ ml}/24 \text{ hr} = 43 \text{ cc/hr}$

3. *Case Study*

Assessment

Tommy, a 10-kg child, is brought in to the ED with a history of vomiting and diarrhea for 2 days. Mom reports that Tommy has not wet his diapers very much today. He is 80 cm long, his vital signs are: temperature 103.8°F, heart rate 190 beats per minute, respiratory rate 45 per minute, blood pressure 60/30. The child is limp and does not respond when his mother is asked to step out of the room for an interview. Upon assessment, Tommy's fontanels are sunken, the periorbital area is sunken, mucous membranes are parched, there is evidence of skin tenting, capillary refill is 6 seconds, pulses in the upper extremities are weak and thready, and the pulses in the lower extremities are hard to find. Serum sodium concentration is 135 mEq/L, but all other electrolytes are within normal limits.

The following nursing care plan focuses only on the calculation of fluid replacement and maintenance for this child. All of the interventions are based on interdisciplinary team decision-making processes (medical and nursing), with independent, dependent, and collaborative nursing actions.

Nursing Diagnoses

1. Ineffective Tissue Perfusion Related to Gastrointestinal Fluid Losses

2. Deficient Fluid Volume Related to Vomiting and Diarrhea

Planning

1. Improve tissue perfusion, as evidenced by (AEB):

   Stabilized vital signs

   Palpable peripheral pulses

   Adequate urine output

   Normal capillary refill

2. Maintain adequate fluid volume AEB:

   Moist mucous membranes

   Balanced intake and output

   Normal skin turgor

   Vital signs within normal limits

   Urine of normal amount and concentration

Intervention

A bolus of 200 ml (20 ml/kg) of LR or NS must be administered and repeated until systemic perfusion has returned.

Rationale

Because the patient is in a state of shock (refer back to Table 15-2), systemic perfusion must be returned.

Evaluation

Upon completion of the bolus, a reassessment reveals that Tommy now recognizes his mother and cries out to her. The nurse assesses that the child now has a temperature of 103.5°F, heart rate of 175, respiratory rate of 35, blood pressure of 90/60, a capillary refill of 3 seconds, and pulses are palpable to all four extremities. The nurse also notices that Tommy's diaper is wet with urine. This is evidence that the child is now perfusing and out of a shock state. A diagnosis of acute gastroenteritis (AGE), unknown cause, is made by the physician. Further management can now continue.

Tommy is in a state of isotonic dehydration of 15%. His fluid deficit, therefore, is calculated to be 1,500 ml (15% of his weight or 150 ml/kg = 150 ml × 10 kg = 1,500). Half of this 1,500 ml must be replaced within the first 8 hours, the other half within the next 16 hours using either NS or LR.

Intervention

His fluid deficit must be replaced over the next 24 hours: half within the first 8 hours, the other half within the next 16 hours. Calculate $^1/_2$ of 1,500 ml equals 750 ml.

750 ml replaced over first 8 hours

750 ÷ 8 = 93.8 ml/hr for 8 hours

750 ml replaced over next 16 hours

750 ÷ 16 = 46.9 for 16 hours

Note: These numbers must be taken into consideration and *added* to the fluid maintenance.

Rationale

Now that Tommy is out of a shock state (based on the improvement of his clinical condition), the fluid he lost initially through vomiting and diarrhea must be replaced. Replacement should be over the next 24 hours to avoid fluid overload.

Evaluation

Tommy must be closely monitored for signs of dehydration and signs of overhydration. The balance must be exact to avoid further complications in Tommy's health status.

Intervention

Tommy's fluid needs must now be maintained through the parenteral route. He will be placed NPO to allow his gastrointestinal function to return to normal.

Tommy's fluid maintenance will be calculated using the formula based on his weight.

(a) Break down the patient's weight in kilograms by tens. Because Tommy weighs 10 kg, the calculation will be:

(b) 100 ml × 10 kg = 1,000 ml/day

(c) 1,000 ÷ 24 hr = 41.6 ml/hr

The nurse must now add the deficit *plus* the maintenance and run the IV at that calculated rate:

93.8 ml/hr (fluid deficit calculated previously)

+ 41.6 ml/hr (the child's fluid maintenance needs)

= 135.4 ml/hr

The IV must run at this rate for the first 8 hours, counting from the time that the patient was no longer in shock. For example, the child came in to the ED at 0700, he was assessed, an IV was started, and the bolus was given at 0800. If at 0800, 24 hours later, it was determined that he was no longer in a shock state, then the IV would run from 0800 to 1600 at 135 ml/hr.

After the first 8 hours, the physician, nurse practitioner, and/or nurse must then calculate what the IV rate will be based on the previous calculations:

46.9 ml/hr (fluid deficit calculated previously)

+ 41.6 ml/hr) (the child's fluid maintenance needs)

= 88.5 ml/hr.

Using the preceding times, the IV would run at 89 ml/hr from 1600 to 0800 the next day.

Evaluation

Tommy must be closely monitored for signs of dehydration and signs of overhydration. The balance must be exact so as to avoid further complications in Tommy's health status.

Note: To fully address the needs of this child and his mother, the following nursing diagnoses (with appropriate planning strategies, interventions, and evaluations) would also be included:

- Imbalanced Body Temperature (fever) related to age (with planning and interventions used to reduce fever and maintain normal body temperature).
- Disorganized Infant Behavior (Lack of Affect/Response) related to physiologic factors associated with illness/disease process (with planning and interventions used to improve age-appropriate demeanor AEB: normal separation anxiety response and relaxed demeanor when mother is present).
- Deficient Fluid Volume (Vomiting and Diarrhea) related to inflammation and irritation of the gastrointestinal tract (with planning and interventions used to alleviate the problems while keeping the child comfortable).
- Imbalanced Nutrition less than body requirements (Potential Deficit) related to vomiting and diarrhea (with planning and interventions used to reestablish nutritional balance and provide to child's oral needs while NPO).

Write a teaching plan for a child such as Tommy that addresses the following:

a. Hand hygiene (and why it is important)

b. Food preparation (including the importance of cooking foods well such as meat/poultry products, and the proper handling and storage of eggs and other dairy products

c. The child's IV therapy needs while hospitalized

d. The child's NPO status

e. The child's (and parents') anxiety

f. The importance of laboratory testing and the appropriate measures needed regarding specimen collection

g. Safety measures (such as side rails being raised on the child's bed)

4. List at least two pathologic mechanisms by which bacteria cause diarrhea.

(a) Multiplication of bacteria after invasion of the GI epithelium, which leads to cell destruction and inflammation of the GI tract

(b) Bacterial production of an enterotoxin that causes local tissue damage and destruction of intestinal cells

5. Identify at least four bacteria that commonly cause diarrhea in infants and children.

(a) *E. coli*

(b) *Shigella*

(c) *Salmonella*

(d) *Vibrio cholerae*

6. How do you anticipate his AGE will be managed?

(a) NPO and advance to a lactose-free diet (to restore bowel to normal function)

(b) IV fluid therapy

(c) Possible use of antibiotics

(d) Monitor electrolytes (to ensure fluid and electrolyte balance is restored)

(e) Strict intake and output: monitor urine and stool output

(f) Anticipate metabolic acidosis and look for early signs

(g) Frequent head-to-toe assessment; trends are monitored, abnormal findings reported immediately

7. What should the nurse include in the patient education plan?

(a) Importance of good handwashing

(b) Cooking foods well, especially beef and poultry products, including eggs and other dairy products

(c) IV therapy while in the hospital

(d) NPO status

(e) Lab testing

(f) Keeping side rail up

(g) Psychosocial needs of the patient and family

Answer the following for each of these questions:

a. What is the patient's body surface area?

b. What is the fluid maintenance need for a 24-hour period (1,500 ml/m2/24 hr)?

c. What would the hourly IV fluid rate be if giving full maintenance (1,500 ml/ m2/24hr)?

8. Newborn weighs 3.5 kg, height = 60 cm
a. 0.24 m² b. 362 cc/24 hr c. 15 cc/hr

9. Toddler weighs 12 kg, height = 80 cm
a. 0.52 m² b. 775 cc/24 hr c. 32 cc/hr

10. School-age child weighs 25 kg, height = 100 cm
a. 0.83 m² b. 1,250 cc/24 hr c. 52 cc/hr

11. Teenager weighs 70 kg, height = 150 cm
a. 1.71 m² b. 2,561 cc/24 hr c. 107 cc/hr

Chapter 16

Intravenous Therapy for the Elderly Patient: Special Considerations

Cerena Henderson Suarez, RN, MSN, CS

COMPETENCIES

Upon completion of this chapter, the reader should be able to:

- Describe population trends that make the study of the elderly a vital component of nursing education.

- Define the terms geriatric, gerontologic, and gerontic.

- Describe physiologic changes associated with aging.

- Identify disorders commonly found in the hospitalized elderly.

- List indications for intravenous therapy for the elderly.

- Compare and contrast venous access sites in the elderly.

- Compare and contrast venous access devices in the elderly.

- Describe procedures for insertion of peripheral intravenous catheters in the elderly.

- Describe precautions for intravenous administration of fluids, blood, medications, and nutrition to the elderly.

- Discuss problems associated with medicating the elderly.

- Describe a clinical pathway and the expected outcomes for an elderly patient receiving intravenous therapy.

KEY TERMS

activities of daily living (ADLs)
adverse drug reaction
clinical pathway
competency
drug interaction
elder abuse

elder neglect
elderly
frail elderly
geriatrics
gerontic nursing
gerontologic nursing

gerontology
instrumental activities of daily living
medication review
polypharmacy
risk-benefit analysis

The United States is on the threshold of a longevity transformation. The older population—persons 65 years or older—was figured to be 35 million in 2000. (U.S. Bureau of the Census, 2000). This group represented 12.4% of the U.S. population, or about one in every eight Americans. People over 85 comprise the fastest growing group of the population. By 2030, there will likely be 8.5 million people over the age of 85 (ANA, 2001).

The growing number and proportion of older adults are carrying the weight of long-term illness, disability, diminished quality of life, and greatly increased health care costs. The need to address the unique needs of the elderly population was first recognized by nursing as early as the 1920s. Clearly now, more than ever before, there is a need for nurses to address the unique characteristics of such a large segment of the population.

GERONTOLOGY

Geriatrics is defined as the branch of medicine concerned with medical problems and care of old people. **Gerontology** is the scientific study of the process and problems of aging. **Gerontologic nursing** is the application of scientific, logical practice to the nursing care of the elderly. **Gerontic nursing** is the care of the elderly.

Elderly is generally understood to mean people 65 years of age and older. There is nothing scientific about that number, however, and the following labels are often used for groups of elderly:

- 55–64   young old
- 65–74   elderly
- 75–84   middle old
- 85–100   old, old
- over 100   centenarians

Another term used to describe the elderly is frail. **Frail elderly** refers to those who are over 85 or who are at high risk for health problems.

Advanced education to prepare nurse specialists and nurse practitioners to meet the health care needs of the elderly in the many settings in which they are encountered is gaining momentum. Care of the elderly is of the highest quality when those caring for them have specialized training in geriatrics or gerontologic nursing. The American Nurses Association's *Standards and Scope of Gerontological Nursing Practice* (2001) is the basis of gerontologic nursing practice in all settings. In light of the anticipated growth in the elderly population and the impact health care reform is likely to have in the future, advanced-practice nurses specializing in gerontology are, and will be, in great demand.

The peculiar thing about aging is that it seems to be something happening to everyone else. Perception of age is individual and has little to do with years and everything to do with functional capacity. The reader should understand that aging is not something that happens to old people, but begins as soon as an individual is born.

PHYSIOLOGIC CHANGES OF AGING

Many commonly accepted disorders of the elderly are not part of the aging process at all and go untreated owing to misconceptions about what normal old age is. Nurses must be able to recognize normal physiologic changes in order to facilitate identification of abnormal changes that limit the functional capacities of the elderly patient.

Cardiac System

The heart muscle of an elderly person shows signs of atrophy and decreased contractility. An elderly person has a decreased ability to adapt to stress. The heart rate does not increase in response to stress as quickly as the younger heart. After the stress is relieved, the heart rate is slow to return to normal. There is less cardiac reserve, there are fewer pacemaker cells, and the valves of the heart stiffen.

These changes require older persons to make adjustments in activities of daily living. When caring for geriatric patients, plan activities to conserve energy and allow for rest periods. Avoid stressors as much as possible. Allow adequate time for the individual to recover from stressors when they occur. When initiating intravenous therapy, allow time between attempts and afterward for the elder to adapt and for vital signs to return to normal. Monitor activity tolerance, as well as heart rate, rhythm, and blood pressure.

Vascular System

There is a decrease in tone and elasticity of the aorta and the great vessels with aging. Less vascular elasticity promotes venous pooling in lower extremities, which may lead to edema, orthostatic hypotension, varicose veins, venous stasis, and thrombosis. Venous valves are less competent, which further contributes to these problems. Superficial veins often

used for peripheral intravenous therapy are small and fragile. Injury to a vessel is more likely to cause phlebitis. When caring for elders receiving intravenous therapy, vein selection and avoiding unnecessary trauma to the vascular system is critical.

Loss of vascular elasticity and decreased response to stress contributes to hypertension. Hypertension is seen as injury to various organs, especially the kidneys, brain, and eyes.

Teach elderly patients to make allowances for changes to the vascular system. Garters, tight clothing, and crossing the legs should be avoided. Have patients alternate sitting and standing, with intervals of walking to decrease venous pooling in the legs. Orthostatic hypotension may be avoided by teaching the elderly person to change positions slowly. Signs of thrombophlebitis should be reported to the individual's primary health care provider.

Pulmonary System

Aging causes decreased mobility of the chest wall, increased anterior-posterior diameter, decreased vital capacity, increased residual volume, and a decreased cough response. These changes make the elderly individual vulnerable to respiratory infections and pneumonia.

Encourage influenza immunizations for elderly patients. Teach the elderly to avoid respiratory irritants such as smoking, second-hand smoke, and environmental pollutants. Avoiding people with known respiratory infections and crowds during the flu season should be stressed. If hospitalized, the elderly become extremely vulnerable to respiratory infection. Deep breathing exercises and coughing should be part of the nursing care plan. Avoid immobilizing an elderly person at all costs since it will further compromise respiratory function. Select veins for intravenous therapy which allow for maximum mobility and encourage movement. Monitor the elder closely for respiratory distress, which may signal fluid overload.

Renal System

Aging causes a decrease in the number of nephrons and in the weight of the kidneys. Renal blood flow diminishes and glomerular filtration rate decreases. The kidneys are unable to adapt to extreme situations such as fluid overload and dehydration.

Instruct elderly patients at risk for fluid imbalance to monitor their weights daily and to respond to sudden changes quickly. Decreased renal function means that drugs that are excreted through the kidneys have extended half-lives, and smaller doses are usually required. Monitor therapeutic drug levels to prevent drug toxicity. During infusion therapy, it is critical to monitor intake and output closely. Be

---

CRITICAL THINKING

How Do You Conquer Immobility in the Elderly?

When hospitalized, maintaining mobility in an elderly patient may be difficult due to the illness or for a number of other reasons. Patients may be tired, weak, depressed, or afraid of falling. They may expect that in the hospital they can rest and not have to exert themselves. Often this perception may be perpetuated by the patient's family. How do you explain to a fearful patient and family that mobility is critical to prevent complications and maintain function? What referrals would be appropriate to facilitate the patient's cooperation?

Explain to the patient and family that mobility is needed to prevent bedsores, pneumonia, weakness, stiffness, blood clots and many other problems. Remind them of the adage, *use it or lose it*. Explain that a prolonged period of immobility may make the previous level of activity impossible. Referrals to a physical therapist, an occupational therapist, and a counselor would be appropriate to ensure activity progresses at a safe pace and that the patient's fears or depression are recognized and addressed.

sure to include amounts infused in piggyback medication in the calculations. Monitor frequently for signs of excess fluid volume, such as weight gain, increased respiratory rate, or crackles heard on auscultation of the lungs.

Musculoskeletal System

Elderly people experience a decrease in strength owing to a decrease in the number of and the mass of muscle fibers. There is compression of the discs in the spine, with loss in height, and kyphosis. Bone becomes porous and brittle from the loss of calcium. Some bone loss is attributable to hormonal changes, since estrogen protects the bone from demineralization; some loss is due to decreased calcium intake and lack of weight-bearing exercise.

Arthritis and degenerative joint disease are more common in the older population. Mobility may be painful or limited. Exercise programs individualized to the needs of the person will help preserve muscle strength and bone density, as well as maintain range of motion and flexibility. Safety precautions to prevent falls should be implemented. Immobility is the enemy of the aged and must be avoided. When caring for elderly patients receiving intravenous therapy, use equipment which is the least restrictive and which will allow for easy, safe patient mobility.

Integumentary System

There is generalized thinning of the skin, loss of subcutaneous fat, and a decrease in sweat glands with aging. Skin is dry and fragile. Immobility, again, puts this population at risk. Pressure over bony prominences leads to skin breakdown. Aggressive measures to maintain skin integrity should be taken anytime an elder is immobilized, even for short periods. A risk assessment tool, such as the Braden Scale or the Norten Scale, identifies patients at risk for skin breakdown and allows nurses to institute preventive measures upon admission to the hospital or long-term care facility. Routine procedures, such as daily bathing, applying tape to the skin, pulling patients up in bed, and having patients slide themselves from bed to stretcher put the elder at risk for skin breakdown. During intravenous therapy, pay attention to securing lines with paper tape and follow rigid infection control guidelines, as detailed in the Infusion Nursing Standards and Practice.

Immune System

The immune system becomes less effective as an individual ages. Cell-mediated immunity decreases, and there are changes in the T lymphocytes. The geriatric population is at risk for infection; reactivation of latent infections, such as varicella zoster; and for the development of malignancies. Because of the effects of aging on other systems and changes in the inflammatory response, infections may present atypically. A change in mental status is often the first sign of infection in an elderly person, instead of fever.

Teach elderly clients to get an annual influenza vaccine and a pneumococcal vaccine to prevent infection. Skin care, hygiene, and good nutrition are also necessary to help elderly patients avoid infections.

For the hospitalized elderly, strict adherence to infection control standards and close monitoring are required. Weigh the risks and benefits of each invasive procedure prior to initiation.

Cognition

Normal changes in cognition are subtle and are not likely to impair the ability of the individual to function independently. There is an increase in reaction time, learning takes longer, and problem solving is less effective. Recall of recent events may be affected. These changes have implications for patient teaching. Teaching should be done slowly, in short sessions. Base teaching on prior experience of the patient. Be concise and do not give extraneous information, which is nice to know, but not needed to perform the skill. Give positive feedback periodically during the session and review learning at frequent intervals.

Sense Organs

Sensory changes may be mistaken for cognitive changes. An elderly person who does not hear well may be mistaken for confused or senile. In fact, hearing normally diminishes with age. Appropriate referrals for diagnosis of the hearing problem and prescription of a hearing aid should be made. When caring for elderly people who are hard of hearing, speak slowly and distinctly and use gestures. Make sure the elder can see the face of the speaker. Minimize extraneous sounds by turning off the television and shutting the door. If the patient has a hearing aid, make sure she has it on.

Other senses are also affected by the aging process. Visual acuity decreases, as does accommodation. Cataracts are common in the aged. Eyes are more sensitive to glare. When caring for elderly patients, minimize glare while keeping the room well lighted. Glasses should be used and kept clean. Regular examinations will ensure eyes are healthy and that glasses are the correct prescription.

There is a decreased sensitivity to touch with advancing age. Teach elderly patients to use care when applying hot or cold or when getting into a tub of water. Foot care requires attention as well, since blisters or other foot injuries may go unnoticed by the elder. Trimming toenails is a task best left to a professional.

Taste is also affected by the aging process. Elderly people experience increased sensitivity to bitterness and a decreased sensitivity to sweetness and salt. The sense of smell diminishes. Foods often taste bland unless they are very sweet or very salty. The lack of taste is the reason some elders give for losing interest in eating. This is especially problematic if diet restrictions are being imposed upon the elderly patient, such as a low-salt diet.

Another issue related to taste is dental health. Regular dental exams are important to ensure teeth and gums are healthy or that dentures fit properly.

Psychodynamics

The elderly individual faces many losses: loved ones, friends, job, earnings, functional abilities, and sometimes health. Psychological well-being rests upon the ability to cope with these losses and the ability to find meaning in life. When hospitalized, an elderly patient may experience all of these losses as well as fear, hopelessness, and powerlessness. Psychological factors of aging, such as short-term memory loss, depression, and mental deterioration, make it extremely important for the nurse to have a knowledgeable understanding of the aging process.

Depression is common in this age group, though often not diagnosed. Changes associated with depression may be attributed to the aging process alone. When caring for an older individual, communicate worth and respect. Call the person by name, respect decisions and choices made, and encourage independence. When hospitalized, the tendency for the nursing staff to take control of all activities for the elderly patient should be avoided.

Differentiating normal changes of aging from serious signs of disease will ensure that the elderly patient will receive prompt intervention and treatment from the nurse who cares for him. See Table 16-1 for a summary of key points related to IV therapy.

INTRAVENOUS THERAPY

Indications

Indications for intravenous therapy in the elderly include fluid replacement, medication administration, parenteral nutrition, blood therapy, and vascular support. Changes related to fluid balance, blood vessels, the immune system, mental status, sensory systems, and the skin affect the older adult's response to infusion therapy.

Fluid Replacement

Fluid replacement is indicated for acute or chronic depletion. Acute dehydration may be the result of vomiting, diarrhea, or bleeding. Infections with fever require more fluid than usual and may result in a depleted state. Iatrogenic causes include infusion of hypertonic solutions or tube feedings. Hyperglycemia may also cause dehydration. Individuals with acute dehydration may be hypotensive and even in shock. Perfusion of vital organs is diminished. The kidneys are especially vulnerable, and acute renal failure may result.

Chronic dehydration is usually associated with inadequate intake or long-term diuretic use. Some elderly people have difficulty getting fluids and drinking fluids due to arthritis or other mobility problems. People receiving tube feedings are at risk for dehydration if sufficient water is not given through the tube as well. Individuals taking diuretics for long periods may develop dehydration when their patterns of fluid intake change, the medication is not taken as prescribed, or the condition requiring the use of diuretics is not monitored frequently.

Medication Administration

IV medication administration is indicated for patients who are unable to tolerate medications orally or who need more effective drug distribution. Intravenous antibiotics are indicated for the treatment of pneumonia, septicemia, or other serious infections. Medications for acute management of cardiac dysrhythmias or shock related to acute myocardial infarction are effective only when given intravenously.

Parenteral Nutrition

Parenteral nutrition should be considered without delay when oral intake is not possible and the enteral route is not available. Indications for parenteral nutrition in the elderly include major surgery requiring several days without oral intake, multiple trauma, and other conditions that make oral intake impossible for a prolonged period of time. Careful attention to nursing protocols that protect patients from complications associated with parenteral nutrition is vital. The physical changes associated with aging make the elderly patient particularly vulnerable to complications of parenteral nutrition (see Chapter 13).

Blood Therapy

The administration of blood or blood products is indicated to correct acute deficiencies associated with trauma, gastrointestinal bleeding, or surgery. Protocols may need to be modified to take into account the total additional volume the patient will receive. If needed, units of blood may be given slowly over a four-hour period. Monitor for signs of fluid overload such as rales, shortness of breath, jugular vein distention, and mental status change. Observe closely for transfusion reactions, which may have an atypical presentation in the elderly patient (see Chapter 14).

Table 16-1 | Physiologic changes associated with aging

SYSTEM	CHANGES	NURSING CARE
Cardiac	• Atrophy of cardiac muscle • Decreased contractility • Decreased ability to adapt to stress • Diminished cardiac reserve • Fewer pacemaker cells • Stiffer valves	• Plan activities to allow for rest periods • Avoid stressors • Allow time to recover from stressors • Monitor heart rate, rhythm, BP • Monitor activity tolerance • Allow time after IV starts for adaptation to occur
Vascular	• Decreased tone • Decreased elasticity of vessels • Less competent • Fragile superficial veins	• Alternate sitting and standing with walking • Avoid garters, tight clothing, crossing legs • Change position slowly • Monitor for orthostatic hypotension • Avoid unnecessary trauma to vessels • Monitor for phlebitis and deep-vein thrombosis
Pulmonary	• Decreased mobility of chest • Increased A–P diameter • Decreased vital capacity • Increased residual volume • Diminished cough reflex	• Monitor for respiratory infection • Immunize for influenza and pneumococcus • Teach to avoid respiratory irritants, crowds • Avoid immobility • Teach coughing and deep breathing
Renal	• Fewer nephrons • Diminished blood flow • Decreased glomerular filtration rate • Inability to adapt to extremes	• Monitor fluid balance • Monitor therapeutic drug levels • Teach to drink 2–3 liters each day • Monitor for fluid overload
Musculoskeletal	• Decreased strength • Compression of discs • Osteoporosis • Arthritis • Degenerative joint disease	• Refer for appropriate exercise program • Avoid immobility • Monitor gait, balance, strength • Teach safety precautions to prevent falls • Select IV sites that allow maximum mobility
Integumentary	• Thinning skin • Loss of subcutaneous fat • Decreased sweat gland activity	• Assess for skin breakdown risk • Avoid immobility • Avoid daily bathing • Implement measures to prevent skin breakdown • Use paper tape • Monitor IV sites frequently for complications
Immune	• Decreased cell-mediated immunity • Changes in T lymphocytes • At risk for infection, reactivation of latent infections, malignancies	• Protect from infection • Teach lifestyles that protect from infection • Analyze risk-benefit ratio prior to invasive procedures
Cognitive	• Increased reaction time • Slowed learning • Recent recall impaired • Less effective problem solving	• Teach slowly in short sessions • Base teaching on prior experience • Be concise with instructions • Give feedback • Review learning
Sensory	• Diminished hearing • Decreased visual acuity • Increased sensitivity to glare • Decreased sensitivity to touch • Increased sensitivity to bitterness • Decreased sensitivity to salt and sweetness	• Safety precautions • Referrals for appropriate evaluation of hearing and visual problems • Include patient in planning dietary modifications
Psychological	• Experience many losses • Depression common	• Communicate worth and respect • Respect choices and decisions • Encourage independence

Vascular Support

In the event of vascular collapse, intravenous therapy is needed to administer fluids to expand circulating volume and give medications to support vital organ function. Monitoring cardiac status through a flow-directed catheter such as a Swan-Ganz catheter may be indicated. Very accurate information about fluid status and cardiac output can be obtained with a Swan-Ganz catheter, making decisions regarding fluid balance easier (i.e., low pressure readings indicate a need for additional fluid).

Intravenous Access

Peripheral venous access is associated with fewer risks, is easily placed, and is easily maintained. The choice of sites for elderly patients is the same as younger adults. Choose distal sites first, especially if long-term therapy is anticipated. Avoid placing intravenous catheters over or near joints as flow rates will be erratic, or the extremity will have to be immobilized. Immobilization of any joint can be painful and has the potential to cause long-term loss of function of that joint.

The following diagnoses in elderly patients suggest that long-term therapy will be needed:

- Major surgery
- Dehydration
- Pneumonia
- Septicemia
- Acute myocardial infarction
- Trauma
- Gastrointestinal hemorrhage
- Cancer chemotherapy
- Stroke

Sepsis requires several days or weeks of intravenous antibiotics. Pneumonia, dehydration, and any surgical procedure will require long-term intravenous therapy. Consideration should be given to a device that can remain in place for several days or weeks.

Central lines can remain in place for extended periods of time, thus avoiding the trauma and potential for complications associated with repeated peripheral cannulation. The options available for the type of central line are essentially the same as those for a younger person. These include closed- and open-end catheters, accessed via the subclavian and internal or external jugular veins, and placed in the superior vena cava (SVC); peripherally inserted central catheters (PICCs); and subcutaneously implanted ports.

The risks and complications associated with central lines can occur in any age group, but may be more prevalent and serious in the elderly. The older person who already has a

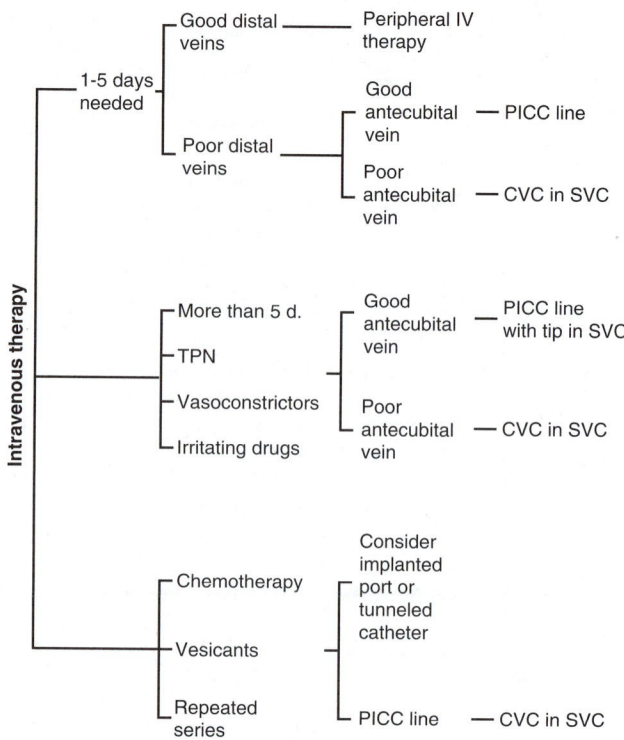

Figure 16-1 | Decision tree: Choosing the site and appropriate intravenous device

significant decline in respiratory reserve is at greater risk for complications of fluid overload, pneumothorax, infection, and sepsis (see Chapter 12).

The PICC line, with the tip in the SVC, has become a popular option for central access in the elderly. The catheter material is soft and flexible, and patients are encouraged to use the extremity fully. With its successful use in home care and outpatient settings, especially with children and with cancer patients, the PICC line is a viable option. Patients who are likely to require five or more days of IV therapy or who have poor peripheral access should be considered PICC line candidates. Many of the hospitalized elderly meet these criteria.

Surgically implanted ports or tunneled catheters should be considered for elderly patients with chronic disorders that are likely to require repeated periods of intravenous therapy or for those with cancer who will require chemotherapy. The risk of infection is lessened when compared with a percutaneously inserted CVC, and a reliable venous access is assured. See Figure 16-1 for a decision tree related to appropriate intravenous access.

Intravenous Devices

In the critical care areas within acute care settings, the tendency is to use the largest-gauge intravenous device that can be placed. In the elderly, this is rarely a good rule. (This is not a good practice in any age group; as a rule, the smallest cannula needed to deliver the prescribed infusate should be used.) If the individual needs blood therapy, is in shock, or may need major surgery, then an 18 ga. cannula or larger is needed. For fluid therapy, administration of medications, or correction of electrolyte imbalances, a small-bore device is more acceptable (20 or 22 ga.). The smaller, fragile veins are easily inflamed, and a small-bore catheter causes less injury. A 24-ga. (¾-inch) catheter is most appropriate and can deliver up to 250 ml of fluid per hour.

With the complexity of problems experienced by elderly patients in acute care, multilumen CVC catheters are popular. These allow two or more incompatible solutions to be infused simultaneously without the inconvenience and risk of having different sites. Central lines are available with double, triple, or quadruple lumens. PICC lines are available with double lumens, and even peripheral catheters can be inserted that have a double lumen.

N U R S I N G   A L E R T

Choosing the Number of Lumens

Consider the number of lumens needed to provide care for the patient and choose the least number possible. The more lumens, the more portals of entry for infection.

PROCEDURES FOR THE ELDERLY

The procedures for placing a peripheral line require a few modifications for an elderly patient. Since peripheral veins are fragile, the use of a tourniquet may cause pressure to build up and the vein to rupture when venipuncture is attempted. If, as is sometimes the case, the patient's distal veins are distended without a tourniquet, then the venipuncture should be done without one. If the veins are not distended, then a light tourniquet (as opposed to one that totally obstructs venous flow) may be used. Care should be taken to perform the venipuncture as soon as possible after applying the tourniquet to decrease the possibility that excessive pressure will cause the vein to rupture when the needle punctures it. Cannulating a fragile vein with the bevel of the needle down, rather than up, may be advisable to prevent penetration of the opposite vein wall.

Other helpful techniques include strategies to promote venous filling, such as warm towels placed over the site, placing the arm in a dependent position, relaxation exercises,

---

N U R S I N G   T I P

Use of a Tourniquet

If distal veins are distended without a tourniquet, consider inserting the intravenous catheter without the use of a tourniquet.

---

and distraction. Attention should be paid to pain management. A patient who is in pain will be more anxious, and the vessels will constrict more readily. If the patient is anticipating the pain of the venipuncture, veins may constrict. This supports the use of anesthetic injections or creams for venipuncture. Distraction and relaxation may be effective pain management strategies for some patients.

Securing the intravenous catheter is complicated by the elderly patient's skin characteristics. Cover the site with an appropriate dressing in accordance with the institution's policies. Use tape to stabilize the device and to prevent tension on the catheter by the infusion tubing. Paper tape is usually best tolerated by older people. A skin barrier, such as Skin Prep, may be used to protect the skin from the effects of the tape.

COMPLICATIONS OF INTRAVENOUS THERAPY

Fluid Overload

Fluid overload is a serious complication of intravenous therapy in the elderly. As discussed earlier, extremes of fluid imbalance are not well tolerated by older people. All infusions should be on an electronic infusion device (EID) or pump. Use of an EID, however, does not mean the patient is safe from fluid overload. Many things can happen to cause

---

N U R S I N G   T I P

Assessing the Elderly Patient for Fluid Overload

Assess an elderly patient at least hourly for signs of fluid overload. Include intake and output, breath sounds, jugular vein distention, mental status, and respiratory status.

even a well-controlled rate to overload the patient. For instance, the patient may be getting several intravenous medications piggyback in 50- to 250-ml volumes in addition to the primary infusion. Some infusion systems allow piggybacks to be given without interrupting the primary infusion or they allow a faster rate to be set for the piggyback to enable the nurse to administer the medications over a period of time. In other instances, patients improve, and they begin taking in normal amounts of oral fluids without a subsequent decrease in the intravenous fluid rates. Third, the patient's condition may deteriorate, and the heart, kidneys, or both begin to fail, causing fluid overload.

Phlebitis

Phlebitis is the inflammation that occurs when a vein is damaged. It is caused by mechanical irritation from the cannula, chemical irritation from the infusion, or microscopic contaminants. Intravenous sites should be observed frequently for signs of phlebitis, and patients should be taught to notify the nurse of pain, swelling, or feelings of warmth or tightness at the site. Discontinue intravenous catheters at the first sign of phlebitis. Progression to thrombophlebitis, which is more severe and more painful, may result. After removal of the catheter, phlebitis can be treated according to agency policy and physician preference. If severe, the administration of antibiotics may be needed.

Infiltration

Infiltration occurs when the catheter pulls out of the vein or punctures the vein wall. The discomfort felt by the patient depends upon the solution that infiltrates. Isotonic fluids may not cause any discomfort, only swelling around the site. Fluids containing potassium or other irritating medications may cause pain at the site.

Hematoma

Hematomas and ecchymoses are seen often on the hospitalized elderly. Fragile veins are easily injured and may bleed into the surrounding tissue. Careful use of tourniquets will help prevent complications. Application of pressure after venipuncture for one to two minutes is required. Patients receiving aspirin or anticoagulant therapy will require pressure be held for longer periods. Do not apply a tourniquet above the injured site until hemostasis occurs.

Infection

Infection, either local or systemic, is another potential complication of intravenous therapy in the elderly. The alterations in the immune system caused by aging place this population at particular risk for intravenous-related infections. Infection rates with peripheral catheters can be kept very low with strict adherence to infection control standards and the INS standards, which include changing peripheral sites at least every 72 hours.

In practice, peripheral IV sites rarely last 72 hours in the hospitalized elderly. When they do, nurses and patients are reluctant to remove a functioning line. If left in place, the infection rate climbs drastically. The nurse must determine if the risk is warranted in light of the lack of other suitable intravenous sites. Careful attention should continue, maintaining strict standards of care and documentation. It is advisable to discuss the placement of a midline catheter, especially if intravenous therapy will be needed for additional days instead of hours.

Catheter-related sepsis is also a risk in the elderly population. This risk is higher with subclavian entry central lines than with peripheral lines. Strict adherence to asepsis during insertion has been related to a lower incidence of catheter-related sepsis. Careful site care according to the CDC, INS, and institutional standards will also help prevent sepsis. Manipulating lines to change tubing or administer medication requires careful attention to asepsis to prevent introduction of microorganisms into the system.

MEDICATIONS

Physiologic changes associated with aging affect the way the body deals with medications. Older people have less total body water, more total body fat, diminished renal and liver blood flow, and decreased glomerular filtration rate compared with younger adults. These changes affect drug absorption, binding, distribution, and half-life. Elderly patients require smaller doses or longer periods between doses for most drugs.

Case Study

IV INFILTRATION IN THE ELDERLY

Case Presentation

A 70-year-old woman in the intensive care unit had been discharged to the regular nursing unit. Because of a lack of available beds, the patient was spending another night in the ICU as an overflow patient. The woman had an IV infusing at 100 ml/hr and remained on a cardiac monitor. Since the patient was an overflow patient, and she had had little sleep over the previous days in the ICU, the nurse did not disturb her between midnight and 6 A.M. When he woke the patient, the patient complained of severe pain in the arm with the IV. The IV had infiltrated during the night, and because the skin turgor was so loose, a large volume of IV fluid had infused into the tissue, leaving the patient's arm at least twice the normal size, with blisters noted on the posterior aspect of the arm.

Nursing Diagnosis #1

Impaired Skin Integrity Related to IV Infiltration as Evidenced by Blisters on Arm

Expected Outcome

1. Patient's skin will heal without signs of infection or further alteration in skin integrity.

Interventions

1. Apply dressings that promote moist wound healing and protect skin from further injury.
2. Handle skin with care.
3. Do not apply tape to affected arm.
4. Do not use arm for blood pressure or other procedures.

Nursing Diagnosis #2

Acute Pain Related to IV Infiltration as Evidenced by Patient Complaining of Discomfort and Tightness

Expected Outcome

1. Patient will verbalize relief of discomfort.

Interventions

1. Elevate extremity on pillows.
2. Apply moist heat to extremity for 20 minutes three times daily.

Evaluation

Skin is warm, dry, and normal in appearance. Patient is asleep.

Problems with medications arise with elderly patients because they are often receiving more than one drug for more than one condition prescribed by more than one physician. **Polypharmacy** is the use of similar or identical medications for the same person for no apparent reason, or as a treatment for side effects of another drug. **Drug interactions** are more likely when polypharmacy is practiced, and **adverse drug reactions** become real possibilities. Adverse drug reactions are estimated to cause as much as 30% of the hospital admissions for the elderly. A change in mental status, usually seen as acute confusion, is a common presentation for adverse drug reactions in the elderly. Identification of the specific cause may be difficult owing to the number of prescribed medications, over-the-counter medications, and the use of alcohol, caffeine, and tobacco. The nurse must have knowledge of potential drug interactions when caring for the geriatric patient taking multiple medications.

Risk-benefit analysis should accompany each drug prescribed. Review the elderly patient's medications at regular intervals and upon admission to the hospital. Ask the patient how each drug is taken. Assess, also, the patient's understanding of what each medication is for, how and when it should be taken, what the expected effects are, and what side effects should be reported.

A **medication review** matches each medication to a specific condition that the patient is known to have. Drugs with the same effect should be identified. Medications without a clear indication for the patient should be identified. Flag drugs that seem to be taken to treat a side effect of another drug. Review the list for potential drug interactions

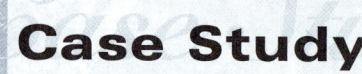

Case Study

COMPOUNDING MEDICATION PROBLEMS IN THE ELDERLY

Case Presentation

A 68-year-old woman in an acute care hospital was experiencing severe pain. She was treated with intravenous morphine sulfate. During her treatment, she complained of nausea, a common side effect of morphine. She was treated with intravenous metoclopramide. She later complained of itching, another common side effect of narcotics, and received small doses of intravenous diphenhydramine. Urinary retention was also a problem, and she was treated with Urecholine and intermittent urinary catheterization. After several hours, the patient became progressively more confused, agitated, and unable to communicate with family members.

Nursing Diagnosis

Risk for Injury Related to Acute Confusion as Evidenced by Disorientiation and Agitation

Expected Outcomes

1. Patient will not experience injury during acute confusion.
2. Patient will be oriented with her baseline cognitive function.

Interventions

1. Enlist family members to stay with the patient and frequently reorient her.
2. Consult with the physician and pharmacist about the drug regimen and potential adverse drug reactions.
3. Eliminate all unnecessary medications and procedures.
4. Consult with the dietitian to ensure nutritional needs are met.
5. Ensure fluid balance is maintained by offering fluids frequently.
6. Assist the patient to the bathroom every two to four hours.

Evaluation

The goal was met. The patient is alert and responding to family members. Balanced I&O.

and consult a pharmacist for assistance with the drug review as needed.

Compliance with a prescribed regimen is often cited by health care professionals as problematic with this age group. Physiologic changes of aging may affect compliance. Ensure that labels are printed large enough for the patient to read. Make sure the individual can remove the safety cap or have medications dispensed without safety caps if there are no small children in the patient's home. Remembering to take medications can be facilitated by scheduling them around other activities such as meals and bedtime. Placing a day's regimen in a box labeled for each time of day will help the elder to identify if all doses have been taken. Other issues to consider when compliance is questioned are whether the individual can afford the medications, whether she can get to the pharmacy to buy them, whether she believes that the medication will help, and whether she understands what she is supposed to do.

Taking the preceding information into account, the following general principles should be practiced when medicating the elderly:

- Determine whether the expected benefit outweighs the risks
- Keep the regimen simple
- Review all medications before adding another
- Use small doses
- Monitor effects
- Teach, teach, and teach again
- Include family members or caregivers
- Refer to appropriate resources to maximize the possibility for compliance

COMMON NURSING CONCERNS

Caring for the elderly patient receiving intravenous therapy requires astute assessment skills and ongoing monitoring. Care plans are often complicated by other nursing concerns.

Confusion

Confusion in the elderly may be caused by many things including infection, medications, trauma, stress, dehydration, electrolyte imbalances, hypoxia, hypothermia, surgery, or fever. As many as 80% of hospitalized elderly patients experience confusion (Evans, Kenny, & Rizutto, 1993). Often, acute confusion is not detected or is treated as a normal condition of aging. Many of the causes of confusion in the elderly are correctable if treatment is initiated before permanent damage has occurred. Untreated, confusion may result in falls, dehydration, malnutrition, and surgical complications. Care is directed toward identifying the cause of the confusion and correcting it.

Safety is the nurse's number one priority when caring for a confused patient. Policies in some institutions require the use of restraints for a confused patient. Serious consideration should be given to the effects of restraints on the geriatric patient. Restraints force immobility, may cause skin breakdown, and may result in decline of functional status. A patient who is restrained is frequently more agitated and paranoid, and the restraints may cause physical injury to a person in this state. Incontinence is a common consequence of the use of restraints. The biggest argument against the use of restraints is the emotional stress it causes an individual who is already having a difficult time adapting to stress. Chemical restraints or sedation place the individual at risk for further complications such as adverse drug reactions, respiratory depression, aspiration, falls, and the likelihood that the true cause of the confusion will not be corrected.

That confused patients may disturb intravenous lines or surgical drains are other reasons for the use of restraints in acute care. Staffing patterns and increasing patient acuity make restraints seem like the only solution for some nurses. Alternatives need to be identified, however. When the use of restraints is necessary, the written policy of the agency must be followed, supported by a medical order. The patient must be assessed frequently and the assessments must be documented. Nurses in acute care who have found an elderly patient on the floor after a fall have experienced litigation related to the event.

Encouraging family members to stay with the patient may eliminate the need for restraints and serve to comfort the patient during a stressful time. If family members cannot stay with the patient, the institution might benefit from incurring the cost of a sitter compared to paying for the cost of a fall or the complications of restraints. After the confusion clears, the patient usually remembers the event and needs time to talk about the feelings and fears she experienced.

Functional Abilities

Many gerontic nurses have witnessed a patient's loss of functional ability, which hospitalization can cause. The phenomenon of *use it or lose it* is very applicable to the geriatric population. When an elder is hospitalized, it is often quicker and easier for the staff to do things for the patient than to stand by and wait for the elder to do it for herself. Immobility often lasts longer than necessary, and the elderly patient loses what functional capacity she had.

Initial nursing assessment must focus on functional abilities. **Basic activities of daily living** (ADL) include bathing, dressing, toileting, and eating. **Instrumental activities of daily living** include the ability to prepare a meal, shop, pay bills, and drive. The nurse should question the patient about her ability in both areas of ADLs. Physical therapy and occupational therapy consultations should be considered to assess problem areas such as balance and gait.

The care plan must be individualized and include interventions designed to maintain or improve the patient's level of function. These interventions may include planned exercise, self-care, progressive ambulation, and socialization. An assessment of the home environment may be indicated to plan for discharge. Any referrals that will help the elderly patient remain independent, such as Meals on Wheels, homemaker services, personal alarms, or home health services, should be made.

Elder Abuse or Neglect

Abuse is defined as "deliberate and willful act of a caregiver in inflicting injury." **Neglect** is "failure to provide the necessities of life such as food, clothing, shelter, hygiene, and medical care" (Loftis & Glover, 1993). Statistics indicate that the elderly person who is at risk for abuse or neglect is female, over 75, with a mental or physical impairment, and living with a relative.

The nurse should suspect abuse when an elderly person is seen with injuries that do not match the information given. The patient may be suspicious, withdrawn, or frightened. Injuries include bruises and skin lesions, especially over soft tissue or over the wrists and ankles from restraints. There may be fractures, burns, drug toxicities, or overdose. The victim of neglect may present with very poor hygiene, pressure ulcers, dehydration, malnutrition, or evidence that medications have been withheld. Neglect may be intentional or the result of an overwhelmed or ignorant caregiver.

Suspected abuse or neglect must be reported to a state agency of Adult Protective Services. It is the job of the agency to investigate all of the circumstances and to make a determination about guardianship. A social worker should be consulted to explore with the family the options of alternative living arrangements, respite, or community support. If neglect is due to a knowledge deficit, then intensive education about the needs of the patient and about available community services is needed.

Advance Directives

For many elderly, end-of-life decisions become urgent. The incidence of terminal conditions rises in the geriatric age group. Issues determining living wills, do-not-resuscitate orders, informed consent and competency are daily occurrences in geriatric nursing. The Patient Self-Determination Act of 1989 requires that upon admission to a hospital or long-term care facility, individuals are asked if they have executed a document called an Advance Directive to the Physician, or they are given the opportunity to find out about advance directives. A Directive to the Physician delineates in advance a person's wishes about medical care should a terminal condition be diagnosed and the patient is unable to express his wishes.

In a hospital or long-term care facility, the Directive to the Physician must be executed by a physician's order. Individual institutions' policies should be followed.

Competency is a legal determination of an individual's capacity to make informed decisions. A determination of incompetence is usually required for a guardianship to be implemented. For health care workers, if a guardian has been appointed, the guardian gives consent for procedures that are done to his ward.

Another document the nurse must be familiar with is the durable power of attorney for health care decisions. A person previously named by the patient can make decisions for the patient if he is unable to express himself.

COMMON DISORDERS OF THE ELDERLY

Dehydration

Dehydration may be the reason for hospitalization, or it may develop during treatment. Fluid depletion is caused by a number of things, either acute or chronic, such as the following:

- Sudden losses due to vomiting, diarrhea
- Infections with fever
- Hyperglycemia
- Restricting intake to treat incontinence
- Long-term diuretic therapy
- Inadequate intake in hot weather
- Gastrointestinal bleeding
- Inadequate intake due to immobility or confusion
- Hypertonic infusions
- Tube feedings

Dehydration in the elderly is not easily recognized. Skin turgor is not a reliable indicator, and eyes normally appear sunken. Decreased urinary output, hypotension, orthostatic hypotension, and a change in mental status are the most reliable clinical signs. Thirst may be present in an alert patient. Weight loss will be present. Laboratory values will show an elevated hematocrit, an elevated sodium level, and an elevated urine specific gravity.

Intravenous replacement is indicated for acute dehydration and for chronic depletion. The fluid of choice depends upon the loss. Fluid loss from vomiting is generally replaced with normal saline. Losses from diarrhea should be replaced with Ringer's lactate. Urinary output of 50 ml/hr should be the goal for acute situations, whereas 25 to 50 ml/hr is adequate for those with a chronic problem. Pay close attention to electrolyte balance as hydration occurs since potassium will usually need to be added to replacement fluids.

Discharge planning includes appropriate patient teaching regarding preventing future occurrences of dehydration. Teach patients to drink 2 to 3 L of fluid each day unless there are cardiac or renal contraindications. Help patients plan when and how to obtain fluids. Caregivers of patients should be taught to ensure that the elderly patient receives adequate fluids and water each day. Teach individuals who are diabetic or taking diuretics to weigh themselves daily and respond to sudden weight loss by increasing fluid intake. Patients who may be limiting their fluid intake to avoid incontinence should be referred to a care provider who can evaluate the problem in accordance with the Agency for Health Care Policy and Research Guidelines on Urinary Incontinence in

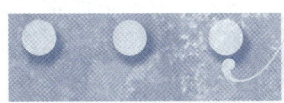

Nursing Care Plan

ELDERLY PATIENT WITH DEHYDRATION

Nursing Diagnosis #1

Deficient Fluid Volume Related to Acute Losses as Evidenced by Confusion, Oliguria, Elevated Hematocrit, Weight Loss, Thirst

Expected Outcomes

1. Urine output will be at least 25–50 ml/hr.
2. Hematocrit will be within normal limits.
3. Intake will be 500 ml more than output.

Interventions

1. Record patient's intake and output.
2. Administer intravenous fluids as prescribed with electronic controller or pump.
3. Assess patient each hour for jugular vein distention, mental status, breath sounds, respiratory status, intravenous complications.
4. Offer patient oral fluids every hour.

Nursing Diagnosis #2

Risk for Impaired Skin Integrity Related to Changes of Aging, Pressure Ulcer Risks

Expected Outcome

1. Skin will remain intact.

Interventions

1. Assess patient on admission for risk factors.
2. Turn and reposition patient every two hours.
3. Keep patient's skin clean and moisturized.
4. Use paper tape on patient's skin.
5. Bathe patient every other day with clear water only.
6. Assess patient's skin condition every four hours, particularly over bony prominences or under restraints.

Nursing Diagnosis #3

Risk for Injury Related to Confusion

Expected Outcome

1. Patient will not sustain injury during hospitalization.

Interventions

1. Assess patient for fall risk potential on admission and every shift.
2. Have a family member or sitter stay with the patient at all times.
3. Reorient the patient with each contact.
4. Ensure the patient has sensory aids as needed.
5. Notify the physician regarding the patient's confusion and discuss diagnostic strategies.
6. Consult with the pharmacist and physician for medication review.

Nursing Diagnosis #4

Disturbed Thought Processes Related to Confusion

Expected Outcomes

1. The patient will be able to converse appropriately.
2. The patient will be able to identify time, place, and person.

Interventions

1. Attempt to reorient the patient with each contact.
2. Encourage activity as tolerated.
3. Avoid restraints.
4. Allow the patient to verbalize feelings and acknowledge those feelings.

Nursing Diagnosis #5

Deficient Knowledge Related to Self Care and Medications

Expected Outcomes

1. Patient will be able to identify what medications are for, when and how to take medications, and side effects to report.

(continues)

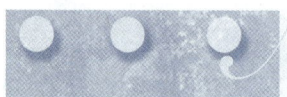

Nursing Care Plan

ELDERLY PATIENT WITH DEHYDRATION (continued)

2. Patient will be able to identify times when fluid intake must be increased.

Interventions

1. Teach the patient about medications.
2. Teach the patient to drink 2 to 3 L of fluid each day.
3. Teach the patient to increase fluid intake in hot weather, when fever is present, or as soon as possible after sudden losses.

Nursing Diagnosis #6

Impaired Home Maintenance Management Related to Declining Functional Capacity as Evidenced by Admission for Dehydration

Expected Outcome

1. Patient will have sufficient support to maintain current living arrangements.

Interventions

1. Consult social services, discharge planner, or case manager on admission.
2. Refer to home health agency.
3. Refer to appropriate community support services (Meals on Wheels, Adult Day Care, etc.).
4. Assess home environment prior to discharge for safety and accessibility to patient.

Nursing Diagnosis #7

Hopelessness Related to Declining Health as Evidenced by Expressions of Worthlessness and Apathy

Expected Outcome

1. Patient will express feelings of worth and hope.

Interventions

1. Assist the patient to plan activities meaningful to him, such as volunteering, worship.
2. Assist the patient to verbalize fears and concerns.
3. Assist the patient to examine contributions he has made in his lifetime.

Adults (1992). Other referrals to home health agencies or community agencies for support and monitoring are appropriate to prevent recurrences.

Pneumonia

Physiologic changes of aging put elderly patients at risk for pneumonia. Hospitalization increases this risk. Pneumonia is a leading cause of death in the elderly population. Hospitalized elderly with pneumonia will require several days of intravenous therapy to correct or maintain fluid balance, correct or maintain electrolyte balance, and for the administration of intravenous antibiotics. Hydration is especially important since it will facilitate thinning of respiratory secretions. Oxygen therapy will usually be required and aerosolized saline therapy will facilitate removal of respiratory secretions. After two or three days, patients will begin to feel better, and the progressive return to previous activities should begin. Prior to discharge, teach patients

how to avoid future infections, about immunizations for pneumococcus and influenza, and to recognize signs of pneumonia to report to their health care provider.

Congestive Heart Failure

Many factors predispose elderly patients to congestive heart failure. Physiologic changes of the heart and vasculature, coronary artery disease, and polypharmacy may all contribute. When hospitalized, the patient will require intravenous therapy for the administration of diuretics and anti-arrhythmics, and for emergency access. Oxygen therapy is required and activity limited to decrease cardiac and respiratory demands. As soon as the patient is stabilized, progressive activity should be instituted with careful monitoring of heart rate, rhythm, and blood pressure. Patient teaching includes medications, daily weights, diet alterations, and energy conservation measures. Cardiac rehabilitation referral is indicated.

Septicemia

Geriatric patients who are at risk for infection are also at risk for the development of septicemia. Chronic problems such as urinary retention, skin breakdown, indwelling catheters, and immobility are risk factors. Any infection in the elderly can progress quickly to septicemia. Presentation may be atypical. Confusion is frequently the first sign, not fever. When hospitalized, intravenous therapy is indicated to hydrate and administer antibiotics. The patient should be observed closely for signs of septic shock, in which case intravenous access will be needed to administer volume and vasoconstrictors to support vital organs. Discharge planning is directed toward teaching the individual or caregiver to prevent infection and to recognize what may be atypical signs of infection.

Stroke

A cerebrovascular accident or stroke is a term used to describe an event that has disrupted the blood flow to part of the brain. The event may be a thrombus occluding a vessel or a ruptured vessel with a resultant cerebral hemorrhage. Depending on the cause and the patient's condition, intravenous therapy is needed to administer medication to prevent further thrombus formation, stop bleeding, decrease cerebral edema, and administer fluids and electrolytes. As the patient stabilizes, rehabilitation begins. Physical therapy, occupational therapy, and speech therapy evaluations should begin as soon as the patient's vital functions have stabilized. Discharge planning includes physical aids to promote independence, patient and family education about medications and lifestyle changes and referral to support groups and community services.

Trauma

Falls are the most common trauma experienced by the geriatric population. Motor vehicle accidents and other trauma are not uncommon, however. For the elderly, intravenous therapy is required for hydration, electrolyte balance, monitoring of fluid status, blood therapy, and administration of prophylactic antibiotics.

As soon as fractures are stabilized, physical therapy and occupational therapy evaluation and treatment should begin. The elderly patient should be evaluated to determine the cause of the fall. Consideration should be given to balance, gait, medication, use of alcohol, and safety hazards in the home prior to discharge.

CASE MANAGEMENT

Case management is the method of nursing care delivery that seeks to maximize patient outcomes while ensuring cost-effective utilization of health care resources. It is a system used by insurance agencies, businesses, health maintenance organizations, and health care facilities to control cost and utilization. The elderly population as a group benefits greatly from case management, especially in models that use nurses as case managers to serve as patient advocates and facilitators.

One of the tools often used by hospitals to facilitate case management is a **clinical pathway**. The clinical pathway is a case management tool that describes a sequence of events leading to desired outcomes for patients with similar problems and treatment plans (Goodwin, 1992). The concept is based on the program planning format of the critical pathway, often used in business and industry (Moulton, Wray-Langevine, & Boyer, 1997). The pathway defines activities that should be done on each day of a hospital stay for a particular diagnosis. The purpose is to define the average length of stay and to identify early those patients who deviate from the pathway so that corrective action can be taken. It provides a framework that ensures the delivery of appropriate but cost-effective care within a specified time period.

The concept can be applied with success to the elderly population if one understands that many have coexisting conditions and will require additional activities to enable a timely discharge. For instance, an elderly patient who cannot ambulate on the day she is expected may need a physical therapy consultation and home health referral to allow her to go home within the designated time frame (Table 16-2).

CRITICAL THINKING

Facilitating Discharge for the Elderly Patient

The elderly patient you are caring for, using the septicemia clinical pathway, is unable to tolerate liquids on the second day. What nursing interventions might you implement to facilitate discharge within the expected time frame? The situation calls for reassessment of gastrointestinal function and consultation with the physician, since intravenous fluids will need to be continued. A dietitian should be consulted to assess the patient's nutritional status and ensure nutritional needs are met until the patient can resume oral feedings. Assessment of the patient's psychological status should also be completed, since depression may be a contributing factor. When assessment is complete, a plan can be developed to address the identified problems and facilitate timely discharge.

Table 16-2 | Example of a clinical pathway for septicemia

	ADMISSION OR DAY 1	DAY 2	DAY 3	DAY 4	DAY 5	DAY 6	DAY 7
Tests	In ER or within 1 hour: CBC, chemistries, ABGs, urinalysis Culture and sensitivity: Sputum, urine, blood × 3, 15 min apart, any wound Chest X-ray ECG Other studies as indicated by presentation	Therapeutic drug levels after third dose of amnioglycosides Blood culture prn temp >101 Cell preliminary culture reports	BUN, creatinine if on amnioglycosies Review serial culture reports		BUN and creatinine if on on aminoglycosides	CBC	
Treatments	Oxygen by nasal cannula or mask IV fluids for hydration and electrolytes		Change IV to hep lock DC oxygen		Consider DC hep lock	DC IV access	Discharge
Consults	Infectious disease specialist if etiology or therapy not clear from presentation		Infectious disease if no improvement				
Meds	IV antibiotics Antipyretics Continue home meds	Adjust antibiotics based on 24 hr culture reports	Adjust antibiotics based on 48 hr culture reports		Consider start P.O. antibiotics	P.O. antifbiotics Adjust home meds	
Nursing Assessment	Nursing admission assessment to include skin risk, fall risk, and functional assessment VS q 4 hr Monitor closely for signs of septic shock, dehydration, fluid overload, confusion, hypothermia, and hypotension I & O				DC I & O		
Nursing Care	Bed rest with active or passive ROM Complete care IV protocol Fall prevention Skin breakdown prevention Oxygen therapy protocol Encourage oral fluids Diet as tolerated Consider dietician referral	Up in chair Assist with bath and hygiene Advance diet as tolerated and monitor intake	Ambulate tid with assistance Encourage self-care DC oxygen protocol	Progress activity as tolerated	DC IV protocol when access removed		
Teaching	Hospital routines Procedures Septicemia causes and treatment	Continue previous teaching and review Assess knowledge aabout medications, other existing conditions, self-care	Medications Diet	Review previous teaching Preventing infection and septiicemia	Review	Review meds Assess learning outcomes	Review Follow up instructions
Discharge Planning	Consult SS, DCP, or case manager	Assess home situation Begin planning with patient and family for discharge			Finalize home care plans		Notify support agencies of discharge

Key Concepts

✴ Aging begins as soon as an individual is born.

✴ Misconceptions of what is normal aging cause many disorders to go untreated.

✴ Immobility in the elderly should be avoided at all costs.

✴ Fluid overload is a serious complication of intravenous therapy in the elderly.

✴ Elderly patients usually require smaller doses or longer periods between doses of medications.

✴ Care of the confused elderly patient is directed toward identifying the cause of the confusion, treating the cause, and keeping the individual safe.

✴ If possible, promote venous filling without a tourniquet when performing venipunctures on elderly patients.

✴ The skin of elderly patients requires special care to protect it from pressure, shear, moisture, and tape.

✴ Protect elderly patients from complications of intravenous therapy by using electronic pumps or controllers, selecting appropriate intravenous devices and sites, and careful monitoring.

Review Questions and Activities

1. List two changes associated with aging for each of the following:

   Cardiac system

   Vascular system

   Pulmonary system

   Renal system

   Musculoskeletal system

   Integumentary system

   Immune system

   Cognitive ability

   Sensory capacity

   Psychological status

2. What are the indications for intravenous therapy in the elderly?

3. What are the advantages and disadvantages of a peripherally inserted central line in the elderly?

4. Why is fluid volume overload a concern when administering intravenous therapy to an elderly person?

5. What is polypharmacy?

6. List six principles to practice when medicating the elderly.

7. List four nursing interventions that may protect a confused elderly patient in a hospital.

8. How is venipuncture to initiate intravenous therapy different for an elderly individual?

9. List four potential complications for elderly patients receiving intravenous therapy.

10. What are three nursing diagnoses common to elderly patients receiving intravenous therapy?

Appendix A

Abbreviations

AAP	American Academy of Pediatrics	CRI	catheter-related infection
ADH	antidiuretic hormone	CVC	central venous catheter
ADL	activities of daily living	CVP	central venous pressure
ADP	adenosine diphosphate	CXR	chest x-ray
AFB	acid-fast bacillus	dc'd	discontinued
AGE	acute gastroenteritis	DCP	discharge planning
AHA	American Hospital Association	DEHP	Di (2-ethylhexyl) phthlate
AHF	antihemophilic factor	DHEW	Department of Health, Education, and Welfare
AIDS	acquired immune deficiency syndrome		
ANA	American Nurses Association	DHHS	Department of Health and Human Services
ANH	acute normovolemic hemodilution	DIC	disseminated intravascular coagulation
ANS	autonomic nervous system	DSD	dry sterile dressing
APIC	Association for Practitioners in Infection Control and Epidemiology, Inc.	DVT	deep-vein thrombosis
		ECF	extracellular fluid
ARDS	adult respiratory distress syndrome	ED	emergency department
ATP	adenosine triphosphate	EID	electronic infusion device
BRAT	bananas, rice, applesauce, toast diet	EKG	electrocardiogram
BRM	biologic response modifier	EPA	Environmental Protection Agency
BSA	body surface area	°F	degree Fahrenheit
BSI	bloodstream infection	FDA	Food and Drug Administration
BSI	body substance isolation	FFP	fresh frozen plasma
°C	degree Celsius	GFR	glomerular filtration rate
CBC	complete blood count	GPICRI	Guidelines for the Prevention of Intravascular Catheter-Related Infections
CCS	cell cycle specific		
CCNS	cell cycle nonspecific	HBsAG	hepatitis B surface antigen
CDC	Centers for Disease Control and Prevention	HBV	hepatitis B virus
CHF	congestive heart failure	HCV	hepatitis C virus
CHG	chlorhexidine gluconate	HCW	health care worker
CMS	circulation, mobility, sensation	HDV	hepatitis D virus
CMV	cytomegalovirus	HES	hetastarch
CNS	central nervous system	HEV	hepatitis E virus
COPD	chronic obstructive pulmonary disease	HICPAC	Hospital Infection Control Practices Advisory Committee
CPM	continuous passive motion		
CRBSI	catheter-related bloodstream infection	HIV	human immunodeficiency virus

HLA	human leukocytic antigen	Osm	osmole
HPT	home parenteral therapy	OTC	over-the-counter (medications)
I & O	intake and output	PABD	preoperative autologous blood donation
ICF	intracellular fluid	PCA	patient controlled analgesia
ICRI	intravascular catheter-related infections	PEP	postexposure prophylaxis
IDSA	Infectious Disease Society of America	P–E–S	problem–etiology–signs/symptoms
IICP	increased intracranial pressure	PHS	Public Health Service
IIP	increased intracranial pressure	PICC	peripherally inserted central catheter
INS	Infusion Nurses Society	PIP	post-insertion phlebitis
IOM	Institute of Medicine	PPF	plasma protein fraction
ISF	interstitial fluid	PPN	peripheral parenteral nutrition
ISG	immune serum globulin	ppm	parts per million
ITP	idiopathic thrombocytopenia purpura	psi	pounds per square inch
IVAD	intravascular access device	PTC	plasma thromboplastin component
IV	intravenous	PT	prothrombin time
IVF	intravascular fluid	PTH	parathyroid hormone
IVPB	intravenous piggyback	PTT	partial thromboplastin time
JCAHO	Joint Commission on Accreditation of Healthcare Organizations	PVC	polyvinyl chloride
JVD	jugular vein distention	RDA	recommended daily allowance
KVO	keep vein open	RBC	red blood cell (erythrocyte)
LCD	liquid crystal display	RL	Ringer's lactate
LED	light-emitting diode	RN	registered nurse
LOC	level of consciousness	ROM	range of motion
LOC	loss of consciousness	SCD	sequential compression device
LR	lactated Ringer's	SCIR	Society of Cardiovascular and Interventional Radiology
LPN	licensed practical nurse	SE	silicone elastomer
LVN	licensed vocational nurse	SIADH	syndrome of inadequate antidiuretic hormone (secretion)
MAC	monitored anesthesia care		
MAR	medication administration record	SIRS	systemic inflammatory response syndrome
MHC	major histocompatibility complex (antigen)	SS	social services
MMWR	*Morbidity and Mortality Weekly Report*	SVC	superior vena cava
MODS	multiple organ dysfunction syndrome	SW	sterile water
mOsm	milliosmol	T & C	type and crossmatch
MRSA	methicillin-resistant *Staphylococcus aureus*	TFD	transparent film dressing
NAHC	National Association for Home Care	TKO	to keep open
NANDA	North American Nursing Diagnosis Association	TMD	transparent membrane dressing
		TNA	total nutrient admixture
NBREP	National Blood Resource Education Program	TNC	through-the-needle catheter
		TNF	tumor necrosis factor
NCHSS	National Center on Health Status Surveillance	TPN	total parenteral nutrition
		TSF	transcellular fluid
NCID	National Center for Infectious Diseases	TSM	transparent semipermeable membrane (dressing)
NIC	Nosocomial Infection Control		
NIH	National Institutes of Health	TSS	toxic shock syndrome
NKA	no known allergies	USCB	United States Census Bureau
NNISS	National Nosocomial Infection Surveillance System	USPHS	United States Public Health Service
		VAD	vascular access device
NPO	nothing by mouth	VAP	vascular access port
NS	normal saline	VRE	vancomycin-resistant enterococci
ONC	over-the-needle catheter	VWD	von Willebrand disease
OSHA	Occupational Safety and Health Administration	WBC	white blood cell (leukocyte)
		XRO	x-ray opaque

Combining Forms, Suffixes, or Prefixes

a-; an-	without; no; not		infra-	below; inferior to; beneath
ad-; af-	to; toward		inter-	between
-algia	pain		intra-	into; within
ante-	before		-itis	inflammation
anter/o	before; in front of			
anti-	against		necr/o	death
arteri/o	artery			
			-ostomy	artificial opening
bi-	two; double; twice			
bi/o	life; living		peri-	surrounding
			phleb/o	vein
cardi/o	heart		poster/o	behind; in back of
cephal/o	head		psych/o	mind
-cerebr/o	brain		pulm/o	lung
-cide, -cida	destruction or killing			
crani/o	brain		ren/o	kidney
de-	down; lack of; less; removal of		semi-	half
derm/o	skin		seps/o	infection
di-	twice; double; two		sub-	under; below
			supra-	above; upper
ef-; ex-	out; away from			
			-tomy	process of cutting; incision
gastr/o	stomach		trans-	across
			tri-	three; triple
hepat/o	liver			
hist/o	tissue		uni-	one; single; once
hydr/o	water			
hyper-	above; excessive		vas/o	vessel
hypo-	below; deficient; under		ven/o	vein

Symbols

$<$	is less than	Ca^{++}	calcium
$>$	is greater than	cc	cubic centimeter
$\leq$	is less than or equal to	Cl^-	chloride
$\geq$	is greater than or equal to	CO^2	carbon dioxide
$\not<$	is not less than	dl	deciliter
$\not>$	is not greater than	D_5W	5% dextrose in water
$\prec$	precedes	H^+	hydrogen
$\succ$	succeeds	H_2O	water
$\equiv$	is identical with; equivalent (also ==)	HCO_3	bicarbonate
$\not\equiv$	is not identical with; is not equivalent to	Hg	mercury
$\pm$	plus or minus	K^+	potassium
#	number; pounds; weight	L	liter
$\uparrow$	increase	$\square$, ♂	male
$\downarrow$	decrease	○, ♀	female
$\nearrow$	increasing	mEq	milliequivalent
$\searrow$	decreasing	Mg^{++}	magnesium
$\rightarrow$	causes; direction of flow; followed by; radiating to; toward; to the right	ml	milliliter
		mm	millimeter
$\leftarrow$	caused by; direction of flow; derived from; reaction produced by; to the left	mm Hg	millimeters of mercury
		mmOl	millimole
$=$	equals	mOsm	milliosmol
$\approx$	approximately equal	Na^+	sodium
$\neq$	not equal to	O_2	oxygen
$\sim$	about; is similar to	OH^-	hydroxyl
/	per, or	$PaCO_2$	partial pressure of carbon dioxide
$\therefore$	therefore	pH	potential of hydrogen
:	the ratio of; is to	$\rightleftharpoons$	reversible reaction
::	proportion, equality between ratios	$t\frac{1}{2}$	drug half-life

Antineoplastic and Chemotherapeutic Agents

Antineoplastic therapy is a treatment modality used to prevent the development, growth, or proliferation of malignant cells. Chemotherapy is a form of antineoplastic drug therapy used to treat malignant disease processes. It involves the administration of chemical agents that exert a cytotoxic effect on neoplastic cells. Its goal is the destruction of all malignant cells.

In the process of targeting the disease-causing cells, these agents also interfere with normal cells. Because neoplastic cells are more active and multiply at a faster rate than normal cells, they are more prone to the effects of the agents. Normal tissue cells that are naturally vigorous, such as bone marrow, the mucosal epithelium of the gastrointestinal tract, the hair follicles, and the reproductive cells, are particularly sensitive to the effects of antineoplastic agents. Bone marrow depression, or *myelosuppression*, is carefully watched to determine the point at which the blood count reaches its lowest point, clinically referred to as the *nadir*, in order to manage toxic side effects. Many organ system toxicities are also associated with chemotherapy, some of which may be reversible or irreversible and permanent.

Antineoplastic agents should be handled only by trained individuals who are knowledgeable regarding all aspects of the drugs. This includes, but is not limited to, the storage, preparation, use, patient care protocols, extravasation guidelines, management of spills, and mechanisms of disposal for anything that comes in contact with the agents. Many of these products possess carcinogenic, mutagenic, and teratogenic properties. Exposure may occur via absorption into the skin and mucous membranes or through inhalation and ingestion.

Only RNs who are authorized by their employers may administer chemotherapy. Most antineoplastics are given intravenously, so the nurse must have expert clinical skills regarding venipuncture and infusion therapy. The dosage and sequencing of chemotherapy are critical to the outcome. Many agents have irritant or vesicant properties so measures to prevent the extravasation of such drugs must always be a prime consideration. Should inadvertent leakage occur, protocols must be followed to swiftly handle the problem so as to prevent tissue damage.

Antineoplastics fall into several broad categories, including alkylating agents, antimetabolites, antitumor antibiotics, biologic (natural) products, hormonal and antihormonal agents, nitrosureas, plant alkaloids, radioactive isotopes, and miscellaneous agents. Nearly all chemotherapeutic agents kill neoplasms through their effect on the function or synthesis of DNA. They vary as to their mechanism within cell cycles. Cell cycle specific (CCS) agents work only during certain phases of the cycle, while cell cycle nonspecific (CCNS) drugs exert their effect on dividing or resting cells in all phases of the cell cycle. Many agents are used in combination so their cell cycle attributes and toxicities are united to produce maximum tumor destruction with minimal toxicity to the body as a whole.

For the latest information regarding specific drugs, refer to a drug reference book such as *PDR® Nurse's Drug Handbook*™ or access Delmar's Web site at www.NursesPDR.com.

Alkylating Agents

Alkylating agents are cell cycle nonspecific. They directly attack DNA, breaking the DNA strands. A list of alkylating agents follows.

aziridinylbenzoquinone (AZQ)
busulfan (BUS)
carboplatin

chlorambucil (CHL)
cisplatin
cyclophosphamide (CYC)
dacarbazine (DTIC)
estramustine phosphate sodium
ifosfamide (used with antidote Mensa)
mechlorethamine hydrochloride
melphalan
nitrogen mustard
temozolomide
thiotepa
uracil mustard

Antimetabolites

Antimetabolites are cell cycle specific. They impede cellular development by interfering with DNA synthesis and other metabolic processes. Once they enter a cell, they stop normal development and reproduction. A list of antimetabolites follows.

capecitabine
cladribine
cytarabine
floxuridine (FUDR)
fludarabine phosphate
fluorouracil (FU)
5-Fluorouracil (5-FU)
gemcitabine hydrochloride
hydroxyurea
6-Mercaptopurine (6-MP)
methotrexate, Methrotrexate sodium
pentostatin
6-Thioguanine

Antitumor Antibiotics

Antitumor antibiotics are used to treat a wide variety of malignancies. Most of them are cell cycle nonspecific. They usually act by binding with DNA and hindering RNA synthesis. A list of antitumor antibiotics follows.

bleomycin sulfate (BLM)
dactinomycin
daunorubicin
doxorubicin hydrochloride (ADR)
epirubicin
hydroxyurea (HYD)
idarubicin
mithramycin
mitomycin (MTC)
mitoxantrone hydrochloride
pentostatin
plicamycin
valrubicin

Hormonal Agents

anastrozole
diethylstilbestrol
estramustine (hormone + alkylating agent)
ethinyl estradiol
fluoxymesterone
flutamide
goserelin acetate
irinotecan hydrochloride
leuprolide acetate
medroxyprogesterone acetate
nilutamide (hormone + alkylating agent)
prednisone
testolactone
testosterone
topotecan hydrochloride

Antihormonal Agents

aminoglutethimide
anastrozole
bicalutamide
exesestane
flutamide
goserelin acetate
letrozole
mitotane
nilutamide
tamoxifen (also considered a Biologic Response Modifier)
toremifene

Nitrosureas

Nitrosureas act in a similar manner to alkylating agents. They inhibit enzymatic changes that are needed for DNA repair. Since they cross the blood-brain barrier, they are used to treat brain tumors, lymphomas, multiple myeloma, and malignant melanomas. Nitrosureas include the following drugs:

carmustine
lomustine—CCNU
streptozocin

Plant Alkaloids

Plant alkaloids are cell cycle specific substances that block cell division by inhibiting spindle formation during mitosis. They include the following:

docetaxel
etoposide (VP-16-213)
irinotecan hydrochloride

paclitaxel
teniposide
topotecan hydrochloride
vinblastine sulfate (VLB)
vincristine sulfate (VCR)
vindesine
vinorelbine tartrate

Radioactive Isotopes

strontium-89 chloride

Miscellaneous Agents

altretamine
amifostine
amsacrine (M-AMSA)
asparaginase
cladribine
docetaxel
gemcitabine hydrochloride
hydroxyurea
l-asparaginase
idarubicin hydrochloride
ievamisole hydrochloride (adjunct to 5-FU)
imatinib
Mitotane
octreotide acetate
paclitaxel
pegaspargase
porfimer sodium
procarbazine hydrochloride
Rituximab
Trastuzumab

Biologic Response Modifiers (BRMs)

Biologic response modifiers (BRMs) alter the affiliation between the host and the tumor by strengthening the host's biologic response to tumor cells. They either (1) augment, modulate, or restore the host's normal immunological mechanisms; (2) have direct antitumor effects; or (3) have other biologic capabilities (e.g., hinder a tumor cell's ability to metastasize or survive after metastasis, foster cell differentiation, or interfere with neoplastic transformation in cells). Most BRMs, with the exception of some interferons, are under clinical investigation in patients with advanced neo-

plastic disease or disease that is unresponsive to conventional therapy.

Interleukin-2 (IL-2)

Interleukins are cytokines that are numerically listed according to the number of amino acid sequences in them. Interleukin 1 through 7 have been discovered. IL-2 has been the focus of a great deal of clinical trial and exposure. Interleukin-2, originally named T-cell growth factor, is an essential component for the growth of T cells and augmentation of their functions, making it a strong modulator of immune responses. IL-2 is produced by lymphocytes.

Aldesleukin (Interleukin-2)

Colony Stimulating Factors (CSFs)

Colony stimulating factors (CSFs) are glycoprotein hormones or growth factors that act as intermediaries in the activation, maturation, propagation, and regulation of hematopoietic cells.

Interferons

Interferons (IFNs) are small proteins that inhibit viral replication and promote cellular (T-cell) immune responses. These include the following:

Interferon alfa-2a recombinant
Interferon alfa-2b recombinant
Interferon alfa-n3

Monoclonal Antibodies (MoAbs)

MoAbs are specifically developed antibodies that are directed against antigens located on the surface of tumor cells. Samples of the patient's tumor cells are retrieved and processed to expose specific antibodies to the tumor-affiliated antigens.

Tumor Necrosis Factor (TNF)

Tumor necrosis factor is a substance naturally secreted by macrophages. Macrophages release TNF when activated by endotoxins. The TNF binds to receptors on cell membranes and initiates cellular activity.

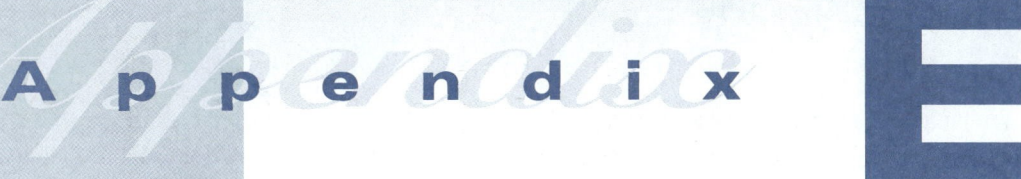

Study Questions
for Further Review

CHAPTER 1: INTRODUCTION TO INTRAVENOUS INFUSION THERAPY

THE NURSING PROCESS
Matching

_____ 1. Nursing process

_____ 2. Assessment

_____ 3. Analysis

_____ 4. Nursing diagnosis

_____ 5. Planning

_____ 6. Intervention

_____ 7. Evaluation

_____ 8. Subjective data

_____ 9. Objective data

_____ 10. Communication

a. statement of an actual or potential health impairment that the nurse can legally identify and treat

b. carrying out the written plan of care

c. process of gathering information about the patient from the nursing interview, history, physical examination, and investigation of objective and subjective data

d. information detected by means of sensory input

e. determination of goal achievement

f. dynamic interchange of self-expression, emotions, beliefs, information, and knowledge between individuals

g. organized, systematized, five-step approach to managing nursing care, composed of assessment, analysis (nursing diagnosis), planning, intervention, and evaluation

h. identification of the patient's strengths, weaknesses, and problems so a plan of care can be established

i. information obtained from verbalizations with the patient, family, or significant others that includes beliefs, feelings, and opinions

j. formalization of a goal-directed nursing care plan consisting of all the measurable actions that will move the patient toward the desired goal(s)

GENERAL CONCEPTS REGARDING IV THERAPY

Multiple Choice

1. Venipuncture and intravenous therapy are indicated for
    a. blood sampling for diagnostic tests, donor phlebotomy for transfusion, and fluid volume maintenance.
    b. fluid volume replacement, medication administration, and blood-blood product administration.
    c. nutritional supplementation and to keep a vein open for an emergency situation, should it arise.
    d. all of the above.
    e. a and b only.
    f. b and c only.

True/False

_____ 2. The nurse is expected to understand only the indications and interventions regarding IV therapy; the physician is responsible for determining possible side effects and adverse reactions.

_____ 3. Accountability is the act of being professionally responsible and answerable for one's actions, inactions, decisions, and judgments.

_____ 4. Accountability, as it relates to IV therapy, includes knowing what is ordered, why it is indicated, its intended impact on the patient, and any possible side effects or adverse reactions, as well as the physical and psychological preparation of the patient and all reporting and documentation regarding the therapy.

_____ 5. The RN and the LVN (LPN) both hold the first line of responsibility for IV therapy and are expected to know and understand all the necessary principles and procedures regarding its management, as well as delegation of tasks to unlicensed individuals.

Fill in the Blank

List three advantages of IV therapy

6. _____

7. _____

8. _____

List three disadvantages of IV therapy

9. _____

10. _____

11. _____

CHAPTER 2: FLUID & ELECTROLYTE FUNDAMENTALS RELATED TO INTRAVENOUS INFUSION THERAPY

FUNDAMENTAL CONCEPTS OF FLUID AND ELECTROLYTE BALANCE

Multiple Choice

1. The primary chemical component within the human organism that accounts for 50% to 70% of the adult body weight is
    a. protein.
    b. fat.
    c. water.
    d. muscle.

2. The principal constituent of all body fluids is
   a. water.
   b. blood.
   c. lymph.
   d. tissue fluid.
3. Water balance is regulated through
   a. kidney function.
   b. cardiovascular circulation.
   c. ADH action on the kidneys and renal regulation of sodium.
   d. alpha and beta receptors in the cardiovascular system.
4. The percentage of body water in the average adult is
   a. 35% to 50%.
   b. 50% to 70%.
   c. 70% to 85%.
   d. 75% to 90%.
5. The percentage of body water in an infant (1 to 12 months) is
   a. 40% to 50%.
   b. 50% to 60%.
   c. 60% to 65%.
   d. 75% to 80%.
6. Extracellular fluid (ECF) comprises approximately
   a. one-third of total body fluid and 20% of total body weight.
   b. one-half of total body fluid and 50% of total body weight.
   c. two-thirds of total body fluid and 60% of total body weight.
   d. three-quarters of total body fluid and 75% of total body weight.
7. The ECF functions to
   a. maintain cell membrane permeability and membrane potential.
   b. serve as a vehicle for movement of substances to and from body areas.
   c. both a and b.
8. The intravascular fluid (IVF) or plasma
   a. is the liquid portion of blood and lymph.
   b. contains serum (the water portion of the blood left after coagulation), protein, and chemical products.
   c. serves as a vehicle for the transport and exchange of nutrients.
   d. all of the above.
   e. a and b only.
   f. a and c only.
   g. b and c only.
9. The interstitial fluid (ISF)
   a. is the fluid that exists in the small spaces and gaps between body structures, cells, and tissues.
   b. is the same as lymph.
   c. contains proteins, salts, organic substances, and water.
   d. all of the above.
   e. a and b only.
   f. a and c only.
   g. b and c only.
10. The mechanism that maintains a balanced concentration of ions and is vital to cellular respiration and metabolism is the
    a. cell membrane.
    b. sodium pump.
    c. sodium-potassium pump.
    d. cell cycle.

11. The highly specialized molecules that coordinate and control cellular chemical reactions are known as
   a. ions.
   b. electrons.
   c. enzymes.
   d. catalytic charges.

Matching

Match the item with the correct serum value range.

_____ 12. Sodium (Na^+)
_____ 13. Potassium (K^+)
_____ 14. Calcium (Ca^{++})
_____ 15. Magnesium (Mg^{++})
_____ 16. Chloride (Cl-)
_____ 17. Phosphate (PO_4)
_____ 18. Hydrogen ion concentration or potential of hydrogen (pH)
_____ 19. Partial pressure of oxygen (PaO_2)
_____ 20. Carbon dioxide (CO_2)
_____ 21. Partial pressure of carbon dioxide ($PaCO^2$)
_____ 22. Bicarbonate (HCO_3)
_____ 23. Carbonic acid (H_2CO_3)
_____ 24. Bicarbonate (HCO_3) carbonic acid (H_2CO_3) ratio
_____ 25. BUN
_____ 26. Creatinine
_____ 27. BUN—creatinine ratio (approximate)
_____ 28. Glucose
_____ 29. Serum osmolality
_____ 30. Hematocrit percentage (Hct)
_____ 31. Anion gap

a. 20:1
b. 7.35–7.45
c. 24–30 mEq/L
d. 10:1
e. 30 ± 2 mEq/L
f. 24 mEq/L
g. 35–45 mm Hg
h. 150–165 mEq/L
i. 135–145 mEq/L
j. 280–300 mOsm/kg
k. 1.2 mEq/L
l. 36%–52%
m. 3.5–5.0 mEq/L
n. 8.5–10.5 mg/dl
o. 65–110 mg/dl
p. 30:1
q. 305–320 mOsm/kg
r. 2.5–4.5 mg/dl
s. 8–25 mg/dl
t. 8.25–8.35
u. 12 ± 2 mEq/L
v. 1.3–2.1 mEq/L
w. 0.6–1.5 mg/dl
x. 80–100 mm Hg
y. 265–280 mOsm/kg
z. 97–110 mEq/L

Matching

Match the term with the definition.

a. active transport
b. diffusion
c. osmosis
d. osmotic pressure
e. colloid
f. osmolality
g. osmolarity
h. solvent
i. solute
j. solution
k. permeability
l. hydrostatic pressure
m. hydraulic pressure
n. colloid osmotic (oncotic) pressure

_____ 32. the random movement of molecules in all directions across a selectively permeable membrane with the molecules moving faster from an area of higher concentration to an area of lower concentration
_____ 33. the capability of a substance, molecule, or ion to diffuse through a membrane

_____ 34. the passage of a solvent through a partition from a solution of lesser solute concentration to one of greater solute concentration

_____ 35. a liquid with a substance in solution

_____ 36. a substance dissolved in a solution or in body fluids (electrolytes and nonelectrolytes)

_____ 37. the pressure or force that develops when two solutions of different strengths or concentrations are separated by a selectively permeable membrane, or the force that draws water (fluid) across a selectively permeable membrane

_____ 38. a nondiffusible substance; a solute suspended in solution

_____ 39. the osmotic pressure of a colloid (protein), or suspended molecule that does not dissolve, in body fluid

_____ 40. pressure created by the physical force of water as it pushes against vessel walls or membranes

_____ 41. the combination of hydrostatic pressure (force of gravity acting on the fluid) and the pressure created by the pumping action of the heart that influences the movement of fluid across the capillary membrane

_____ 42. the number of particles contained in body fluids or the concentration, measured in a kilogram of water (mOsm/kg)

_____ 43. the term used to describe the concentration of solutions, reflecting the number of particles in a liter of solution (mOsm/L)

_____ 44. the movement of solutes across the cell membrane—usually against a concentration gradient, pressure gradient, or electrochemical gradient—that requires cellular energy sources for the transport of the substances

_____ 45. solutes dissolved in a solvent

Fill in the Blanks

46. _____ is the major cation and mineral in the ECF responsible for maintaining blood volume and ISF volume, regulating water shifts between compartments, and influencing the excretion of water. It helps regulate acid-base balance and is an important factor in nerve conduction.

47. _____ is the major cation and electrolyte in the ECF responsible for neuromuscular excitability and acts to regulate acid-base balance.

48. _____ is the major ECF anion responsible for fluid balance and maintaining the osmotic pressure of the blood.

49. _____ is an active transport system, vital to physiologic functioning, that results in most of the body's potassium remaining in the ICF and most of the sodium remaining in the ECF. It is vital for the transmission of electrical impulses, to the secretory functioning of glands, and to prevent all cells from swelling and bursting.

50. _____, a mineralocorticoid secreted by the adrenal glands, increases both sodium and chloride levels (and thus water), thereby playing a major role in regulating the osmotic pressure of the blood, total blood volume, and arterial pressure.

51. In the first two to four postoperative days, patients have higher-than-normal levels of _____ —as much as 5 to 50 times their preoperative values.

Multiple Choice

52. With the facilitated diffusion of glucose,
    a. there is a net movement from the region of low to the region of high concentration.
    b. carrier proteins in the cell membrane are required.
    c. energy obtained from ATP is required.

53. RBCs crenate in
    a. an isotonic solution.
    b. a hypotonic solution.
    c. a hypertonic solution.

54. An increase in blood osmolality
    a. can occur as a result of dehydration.
    b. causes a decrease in blood osmotic pressure.
    c. is accompanied by a decrease in ADH secretion.
    d. all of the above.

CLINICAL MANIFESTATIONS OF FLUID AND ELECTROLYTE IMBALANCES

Potassium Imbalances

True/False

_____ 1. Cardiac arrest may occur if the serum potassium level is less than 2.5 mEq/L or greater than 7.0 mEq/L.

_____ 2. Potassium enters the cells during periods of starvation, trauma, and wasting disease.

_____ 3. During periods of physical or emotional stress, an excessive amount of potassium is lost through the kidneys.

_____ 4. Steroids, especially aldosterone and cortisone, influence the kidneys to excrete potassium and retain sodium.

_____ 5. Potassium is well conserved by the body.

_____ 6. Extra potassium is needed to repair cells and tissues that have been injured, damaged, or traumatized as a result of crushing injuries, burns, or surgery.

_____ 7. Metabolic acidosis promotes the movement of potassium into the cells.

_____ 8. Diuretic use is the major cause of hypokalemia, with gastrointestinal losses accounting for the second major cause of a deficit.

_____ 9. Potassium in IV fluids administered at a rate greater than 20 mEq/L/hr for 24 to 72 hours can result in hyperkalemia.

_____ 10. Tight application of a tourniquet can cause a temporary increase in the serum potassium level.

_____ 11. Drawing blood with a small needle can cause a pseudohyperkalemia.

_____ 12. In acidosis, the hydrogen ion moves into the cells and the potassium moves out, increasing the serum potassium level.

_____ 13. In hyperglycemia, the cells cannot utilize glucose, catabolism occurs, potassium leaves the cells, and polyuria occurs.

_____ 14. Administering glucose and insulin to a diabetic patient may lead to the rapid transfer of potassium from the ECF to the cell, with potassium rapidly decreasing.

Matching

Match the clinical manifestation with the potassium imbalance (a. hypokalemia or b. hyperkalemia).

_____ 15. Anorexia, vomiting

_____ 16. Abdominal cramps

_____ 17. Decreased peristalsis or silent ileus

_____ 18. EKG with flat or inverted T wave; depressed ST segment

_____ 19. EKG with peaked, narrow T wave, shortened QT interval, prolonged PR interval followed by disappearance of P wave; prolonged QRS level

_____ 20. Oliguria or anuria

_____ 21. Polyuria

_____ 22. Malaise, muscular weakness, diminished deep tendon reflexes, respiratory paralysis

_____ 23. Drowsiness, confusion, mental depression

_____ 24. Muscle cramps, numbness or tingling sensation

_____ 25. Serum: K <3.5 mEq/L, osmolality <280 mOsm/L

_____ 26. Serum: K >5.5 mEq/L, osmolality >295 mOsm/L

_____ 27. Membrane potential decreases

Sodium Imbalances

True/False

_____ 1. The kidneys maintain homeostasis through excretion and absorption of water and sodium from renal tubules in response to an excess or deficiency of serum sodium.

_____ 2. The pathophysiologic effects of hyponatremia are evidenced in the membranes of the CNS, neuromuscular tissues, and the smooth muscles of the gastrointestinal tract.

_____ 3. The cells of the CNS are more sensitive than other cells to a decreased sodium level.

_____ 4. The cardiac muscle is highly affected by changes in the serum sodium level.

_____ 5. Hyponatremia can occur when the kidneys are unable to excrete enough urine, thus increasing the amount of body water and diluting the serum sodium.

_____ 6. The administration of large volumes of IV D₅W, as well as excessive drinking of electrolyte-free water, can cause or aggravate hyponatremia.

_____ 7. Vomiting and diarrhea decrease serum sodium levels.

_____ 8. Wound drainage and postoperative bleeding can cause sodium retention.

_____ 9. Excessive or continuous ADH secretion, associated with the syndrome of inadequate antidiuretic hormone secretion (SIADH), causes water to be reabsorbed from the kidney, thus diluting the ECF and causing a sodium deficit.

_____ 10. Addison's disease occurs when there is an insufficient level of ADH and a sodium loss.

_____ 11. Patients recovering from burn injuries experience numerous fluid shifts as the body attempts to compensate for trauma to its tissues, promoting increased water and sodium loss due to oozing at the burn surface, or because sodium replaces potassium in the damaged cells.

_____ 12. Repeated tap water enemas can result in a sodium gain.

Matching

Match the clinical manifestation with the sodium imbalance (a. hypernatremia or b. hyponatremia).

_____ 13. Altered cellular function, CHF, hypertension

_____ 14. Increased ADH production, oral or IV cortisone

_____ 15. Diuretic use, continuous D5W infusions, neuromuscular weakness

_____ 16. Fatigue, headache, apprehension, confusion, convulsions

_____ 17. Agitation, restlessness, stupor

_____ 18. Dry, edematous, red tongue, fever, coma, intracranial hemorrhage

_____ 19. Decreased renal glomerular filtration

_____ 20. Serum Na: >146 mEq/L, urine Na: <40 mEq/L, serum osmolality: >295 mOsm/kg, urine specific gravity: >1.125

Calcium Imbalances

True/False

_____ 1. Vitamin C is the element needed for calcium absorption from the gastrointestinal tract.

_____ 2. The thyroid gland, which secretes parathyroid hormone, is responsible for the homeostatic regulation of the calcium ion in body fluids.

_____ 3. Calcitonin from the thyroid gland increases calcium return to the bone, thus decreasing the serum calcium level.

_____ 4. The parathyroid hormone (PTH) can increase the serum calcium level by promoting calcium release from the bone as needed.

_____ 5. Calcium is needed for normal nerve and muscle activity, causing the transmission of nerve impulses and the contraction of skeletal muscles, as well as the contraction of heart muscle.

Matching

Match the clinical manifestation with the calcium imbalance (a. hypocalcemia or b. hypercalcemia)

_____ 6. Bleeding, decreased blood coagulation, reduction of prothrombin

_____ 7. Weak cardiac contractions

_____ 8. EKG: decreased or diminished ST segment or shortened QT interval, signs of heart block

_____ 9. Anxiety, irritability, tetany, circumoral tingling, numbness and tingling of the fingers

_____ 10. Carpopedal spasm, laryngeal spasm, convulsions

_____ 11. Abdominal cramping, muscle cramps

_____ 12. Positive Chvostek's sign and positive Trousseau's sign

_____ 13. Apathy, depression, flabby muscles
_____ 14. Bone tumors, prolonged immobilization, increased PTH secretion
_____ 15. Flank pain, calcium renal lithiasis (stone formation)

Magnesium Imbalances

True/False

_____ 1. Magnesium is the second most plentiful ICF cation and has functions similar to potassium.
_____ 2. Hypomagnesemia is probably the most undiagnosed electrolyte deficiency, with the patient being asymptomatic until the magnesium level nears 1.0 mEq/L.
_____ 3. Magnesium has a higher concentration in the CSF than in the blood plasma, and is a mediator of neural transmission.
_____ 4. Magnesium relaxes the myocardium.
_____ 5. Magnesium is important for enzyme activity and acts as a coenzyme in the metabolism of carbohydrates and protein.

Matching

Match the clinical manifestation with the imbalance (a. hypomagnesemia or b. hypermagnesemia).

_____ 6. CNS depression, drowsiness, lethargy
_____ 7. Loss of deep tendon reflexes, paralysis
_____ 8. Hyperirritability, tremors, facial twitching, spasticity, increased tendon reflexes
_____ 9. Hypertension, cardiac dysrhythmias (PVCs, V-tachycardia, V-fibrillation)
_____ 10. Hypotension (severe or prolonged), complete heart block
_____ 11. Flushing, respiratory depression
_____ 12. Long-term administration of IV saline administration
_____ 13. Antibiotic, corticosteroid, digitalis, diuretic, and laxative use

Phosphorus Imbalances

True/False

_____ 1. Phosphorus balance is influenced by the parathyroid hormone (PTH), which stimulates calcitrol (a vitamin D derivative) to increase phosphorus absorption from the gastrointestinal tract.
_____ 2. Along with the cations potassium and sodium, phosphorus functions to maintain neuromuscular activity.
_____ 3. Phosphorus is important for the utilization of vitamin A and vitamin C.
_____ 4. Phosphorus deficits can occur from IV hyperalimentation (TPN) infusions.
_____ 5. Phosphorus excesses can occur with the oral intake of aluminum, calcium, and magnesium antacids.

Matching

Match the clinical manifestation with the phosphorus imbalance (a. hypophosphatemia or b. hyperphosphatemia).

_____ 6. Anorexia, dysphagia
_____ 7. Abdominal cramps, diarrhea, nausea
_____ 8. Tachycardia
_____ 9. Hyperventilation, weak pulse, myocardial dysfunction
_____ 10. Flaccid paralysis, hyperreflexia, muscular weakness, tetany
_____ 11. Bone pain, hyporeflexia, paresthesia, tremors, seizures
_____ 12. Bleeding due to possible platelet dysfunction, possible infection, tissue hypoxia

Chloride Imbalances

True/False

_____ 1. When RBCs are oxygenated, chloride travels from the RBCs to the plasma and the bicarbonate leaves the plasma and moves to the RBCs.

_____ 2. Chloride is important for serum osmolality, water balance, acid-base balance, and gastric juice acidity.

_____ 3. A chloride deficit can occur with prolonged use of IV D5W because dextrose in water dilutes the serum levels of chloride, sodium, and potassium

_____ 4. Hypochloremia usually indicates acidosis due to increased levels of bicarbonate.

_____ 5. A potassium deficit cannot be fully corrected until a chloride deficit is corrected.

_____ 6. Hypochloremia can be prevented by administering D5W in normal saline or half-normal saline.

Matching

Match the clinical manifestation with the chloride imbalance (a. hypochloremia or b. hyperchloremia).

_____ 7. Lethargy, weakness, loss of consciousness

_____ 8. Hyperexcitability of the nerves and muscles, with tremors and twitching

_____ 9. Slow, shallow respirations

_____ 10. Deep, rapid, vigorous respirations

_____ 11. Alkalosis due to persistent vomiting and gastric suctioning

CONCEPTS OF ACID-BASE BALANCE

Fill in the Blank

Fill in the blanks using the following terms. Some answers will be used more than once.

- HCO_3 of the arterial blood gas (ABG)
- Serum CO_2
- Bicarbonate-carbonic acid buffer system
- Phosphate buffer system
- Protein buffer system
- Chloride shift
- Hemoglobin-oxyhemoglobin buffer system
- pH
- $PaCO_2$
- Buffer system
- Renal regulatory mechanism for pH control
- Base excess (BE) of the ABG
- Ion exchange regulatory mechanism
- Respiratory regulatory mechanism

1. The system that protects body fluids against changes in pH by soaking up surplus H+ and releasing them as needed is called a _____.

2. The _____ is the most important buffer system in the body, maintaining acid-base balance 55% of the time, where acids combine with bicarbonates in blood to form neutral salts (bicarbonate salt) and carbonic acid (weak acid).

3. The _____ maintains acid-base balance by combining excess H^+ with sodium salts to form NaH_2PO_4, making the ECF more alkaline by excreting excess acid in the urine.

4. The _____ maintains the same pH level in venous blood as in arterial blood.

5. The _____ is the mechanism whereby proteins exist in the form of acids (H protein) or alkaline salts (B protein), carrying an acidic and a basic charge, and has the ability to bind or release excess H^+.

6. _____ is the process that occurs when CO_2 enters the RBC and HCO_3 diffuses out of the cell and the Cl ion enters the cell.

7. The regulatory mechanism, in which there is a redistribution of anions in response to elevated serum concentrations of carbon dioxide (where CO_2 enters the RBCs, combining with water [H_2O] to form H_2CO_3), is _____.

8. The system that takes one to three minutes for readjustment of H^+ concentration, by controlling the rate and depth of respiration, and is sensitive to changes in blood pH or CO_2 concentration is the _____.

9. The system whereby the kidneys regulate pH through the acidification of phosphate buffer salts, the reabsorption of bicarbonate, and the secretion of ammonia, is known as the _____.

10. To determine if acidosis or alkalosis is present, the nurse should first assess the level of _____.
11. Next, the nurse should check the _____ to determine if the acid-base imbalance is respiratory acidosis or alkalosis.

The third step toward determining the type of acid-base imbalance is to check one or all (if available) of the following:

12. _____.
13. _____.
14. _____.

Respiratory acidosis and alkalosis are determined by two tests, the

15. _____ and the
16. _____.

Metabolic acidosis and alkalosis are determined by the following four tests, the

17. _____,
18. _____,
19. _____, and the
20. _____.

CLINICAL MANIFESTATIONS AND TREATMENT OF ACID-BASE IMBALANCES

Multiple Choice

1. Metabolic acidosis may be manifested by
   a. CNS stimulation, hyperactive reflexes, and shallow, breathing.
   b. CNS depression, confusion, stupor, and Kussmaul's respirations.
   c. irritability, seizures, and pH >7.45.
2. Treatment modalities for metabolic acidosis include
   a. IV fluid alkalinization with an infusate, such as $NaHCO_3$.
   b. water restoration.
   c. electrolyte restoration.
   d. all of the above.
3. When caring for a patient with metabolic acidosis, the nurse's responsibilities include
   a. treatment of diabetic ketoacidosis, infection, and cardiac dysrhythmias.
   b. providing for frequent periods of activity, encouraging frequent deep breathing, and monitoring vital signs.
   c. administering adequate fluid replacement; maintaining accurate vital signs and I & O; monitoring laboratory results regarding electrolytes, ABGs, and glucose; and providing comfort.
   d. all of the above.
4. Metabolic alkalosis may be manifested by
   a. CNS excitability, confusion, hyperactive reflexes, and hypoventilation.
   b. sluggish reflexes, lethargy, apathy, and pH <7.30.
   c. CNS depression, hyperventilation, and restlessness.
   d. all of the above.
5. Treatment modalities for metabolic alkalosis include
   a. removal of the cause.
   b. IV fluid administration with NaCl.
   c. replacement of potassium deficit.
   d. all of the above.
6. When caring for a patient with metabolic alkalosis, nursing responsibilities include
   a. taking proper seizure precautions, accurate monitoring of vital signs, maintaining accurate I & O, assessing potassium and hydrogen ion losses, and administering IV fluids as ordered by the physician.

b. frequently ambulating the patient, monitoring I & O, administering 3% IV NaCl, and assessing Hbg and Hct levels.

c. administering CNS depressants, oral antacids, and IV bicarbonate preparations, and monitoring of accurate intake and output.

d. all of the above.

7. The cause of respiratory acidosis is often related to

a. pain and anxiety with hyperventilation and overbreathing.

b. Salicylate poisoning or hyperthyroidism.

c. CNS depressants, hypoventilation, pneumonia or chronic obstructive pulmonary diseases (COPD), and chest injuries.

d. all of the above.

8. The signs and symptoms of respiratory acidosis include

a. decreased $PaCO_2$ and PaO_2.

b. decreased ventilation, changes in sensorium, and somnolence.

c. diaphoresis, restlessness, tachycardia, and dysrhythmias.

d. all of the above.

9. When caring for a patient with respiratory acidosis, nursing responsibilities include

a. administering sedatives to lower the patient's anxiety level, keeping the patient in a flat, supine position, limiting oral fluid intake, and frequently monitoring vital signs.

b. accurately monitoring vital signs and I & O; prn use of oxygen and suctioning; encouraging oral hydration, encouraging and frequently assisting the patient to turn, cough, and breathe deeply; and positioning the patient in semi-Fowler's position.

c. monitoring for respiratory distress and tachycardia.

d. none of the above.

10. The etiology of respiratory alkalosis is usually

a. hypoventilation.

b. hyperventilation.

c. exposure to cold.

d. stress.

11. The usual treatment of respiratory alkalosis includes

a. administering CNS stimulants, oxygen therapy, and deep breathing treatments.

b. IV administration of Ringer's lactate, bronchodilators, and oxygen.

c. sedation, psychological reassurance, and administering O_2.

d. sedation, reassurance, CO_2 treatments, voluntary breath-holding, or use of a rebreathing mask.

12. When caring for a patient with respiratory alkalosis, nursing responsibilities include

a. providing emotional support and education regarding breathing patterns.

b. administering CNS stimulants and oxygen.

c. instructing the patient to "calm down and breathe deeply, as this is just a stress response."

d. all of the above.

True/False

_____ 13. To correct metabolic acidosis the IV fluid of choice is $NaHCO_3$.

_____ 14. The IV fluid replacement regimen for metabolic alkalosis includes potassium, chloride, and an acidifying infusate such as ammonium chloride.

_____ 15. The administration of IV fluids must be monitored carefully to prevent the development of pulmonary edema in patients with respiratory acidosis, due to COPD, pneumonia, or pulmonary edema.

_____ 16. The treatment of respiratory alkalosis is always an emergency situation.

CHAPTER 3: LEGAL IMPLICATIONS OF INTRAVENOUS INFUSION THERAPY

LEGAL CONSIDERATIONS

True/False

_____ 1. The standard of care determines the nurse's liability for negligent acts.

_____ 2. The careless administration of an IV drug is considered a breach of duty.

_____ 3. Negligence is any professional misconduct; unreasonable lack of skill or fidelity in professional or judiciary duties; or evil, illegal, or immoral conduct that results in unnecessary suffering or death to a patient and proceeds from ignorance, carelessness, lack of professional skill, disregard of established rules and principles, neglect, or a malicious or criminal intent.

_____ 4. Malpractice is the term that denotes carelessness or conduct lacking in due care and a deviation from the standard of care that a reasonable person would use.

_____ 5. A nurse may be in violation of criminal law if she violates a state's nurse practice act or violates safe nursing practices.

Fill in the Blank

6. The nurse threatens to start an IV on a patient who refuses to take oral medication. This is an example of _____.

7. The nurse forces a patient to take a medication, against his will. This is an example of _____.

8. The nurse tells a patient he may not have visitors if he does not take the medications the nurse is supposed to administer to him. When he refuses to take the meds, the nurse does not allow him to see his family when they come to visit. This is an example of _____.

9. The nurse administers an IV sedative to a patient who is agitated and confused postoperatively. When the patient becomes more agitated, the nurse leaves the room to call the physician. The patient has a seizure and suffers a concussion. This is an example of _____.

10. The RN is very busy and needs to administer blood to two patients and start several IVs on new admissions. A newly hired LPN offers to start some of the IVs saying, "I did it all the time where I worked before. I even started blood when the RNs were too busy." The RN delegates the starting of one of the STAT transfusions. The LPN does not stay with the patient after starting the blood and the patient has a severe hemolytic reaction. This is an example of liability under the notion of _____.

CHAPTER 4: INFECTION CONTROL AND SAFETY MEASURES RELATED TO INTRAVENOUS INFUSION THERAPY

INFECTION CONTROL PRINCIPLES

Multiple Choice

1. The epidemiologic triangle consists of the
   a. organism, inflammation, and infection.
   b. host, signs, and symptoms.
   c. agent, host, and environment.
   d. disease, organism, and outcome.

2. Death caused by sepsis is most often attributed to
   a. *E. coli, Pseudomonas*, and *Klebsiella* species.
   b. *Pseudomonas, Staphylococcus aureus*, and *epidermidis*.
   c. *Candida* strains and *Streptococci* species.
   d. all of the above.

3. A common microbe, present on the skin, that poses the greatest threat to the patient receiving IV therapy belongs to the genus of
   a. coagulase-negative streptococci.
   b. coagulase-negative staphylococci.
   c. *Bacillus.*
   d. all of the above.

4. Blood serves as the reservoir for the pathogens
   a. HAV and HBV.
   b. HBV and HCV.
   c. HBV and HIV.
   d. all of the above.

5. A nosocomial infection is one that is
   a. person-to-person acquired.
   b. health care setting acquired.
   c. community acquired.
   d. fomite acquired.

6. The organism that accounts for the majority of IV cannula-related nosocomial infections is
   a. *Escherichia coli.*
   b. *Pseudomonas aeruginosa.*
   c. *Enterococcus* species.
   d. *Staphylococcus epidermidis.*

7. The single most important means of preventing the spread of nosocomial infections is
   a. wearing gloves.
   b. not wearing artificial fingernails.
   c. proper hand hygiene.
   d. following germicidal precautions.

8. Standard Blood and Body Fluid Precautions is the CDC guideline that says the blood and body fluids that are to be considered potentially harmful come from
   a. persons known to have HIV.
   b. persons known to have HBV.
   c. persons with suspected HIV or AIDS.
   d. all persons.

9. The CDC-recommended precannulation antiseptic agent is
   a. 2% aqueous chlorhexidine gluconate (CHG)
   b. 70% isopropyl alcohol.
   c. 10% povidone-iodine or 2% tincture of iodine or iodophors.
   d. all of the above.

10. According to the CDC, dressings used to cover IV sites should be changed
    a. every 24 hours.
    b. every 48 hours.
    c. every 72 hours.
    d. when they become damp, loose, soiled, or when the IV is changed.

11. According to the CDC, the IV cannula device for peripheral IVs should be changed
    a. at 24- to 48-hour intervals.
    b. at 48- to 72-hour intervals.
    c. at 72- to 96-hour intervals.
    d. prn.

12. The best way to prevent needlestick exposure is
    a. through the use of needleless systems in all agencies.
    b. through the use of care and precaution in handling needles and disposing of needles in approved sharps containers.
    c. by not recapping used needles.
    d. all of the above.

CHAPTER 5: RISKS, COMPLICATIONS, AND ADVERSE REACTIONS ASSOCIATED WITH INTRAVENOUS INFUSION THERAPY

COMPLICATIONS OF IV THERAPY

Matching

Match the description of the problem with one of the listed complications.

a. cellulitis   f. thrombophlebitis
b. hematoma   g. venous spasm
c. infiltration   h. pain
d. occlusion   i. vessel collapse
e. phlebitis

_____ 1. Patient's subjective description (ache, burn, hurt, stinging, etc.) of discomfort

_____ 2. Swelling or edema; skin feels taut or rigid with blanching; cool skin temperature around IV site; damp dressing; slowed infusion rate

_____ 3. Slowed rate or stopped infusion; infusion site pain with normal appearance; blood backs up into IV tubing

_____ 4. Erythema at IV insertion site and along the vein, with warmth, pain, or burning; vein edema; indurated and cord-like vein; temperature 1° or more above baseline

_____ 5. Slowed/stopped infusion; aching/burning at IV site; erythema and warmth at site; cording of infusion vein; fever; swelling of extremity; mottling/cyanosis of extremity; diminished pulse; pallor

_____ 6. Ecchymosis over and around insertion area with area raised and hardening at insertion site; inability to advance cannula into the vein on insertion; inability to flush IV line

_____ 7. Slowed/stopped infusion; severe pain from the IV insertion site that radiates up the extremity; blanching over IV site; redness around IV site; patient complains of feeling like an *electric shock* is radiating up the extremity

_____ 8. Inability to see or palpate the vein; loss of vessel elasticity; vessel feels flat or flaccid; slowed/stopped infusion

_____ 9. Tenderness, pain, warmth, edema, induration, and red streaking on skin, *peau d'orange* skin; vesicles; abscesses formation with pus, ulceration; fever, chills, malaise

Multiple Choice

10. In order to prevent excess pressure that can damage the intima of the vein, the syringe barrel used to irrigate a peripheral IV line should be
    a. 1 ml in size or smaller.
    b. 3 ml in size or smaller.
    c. 3 ml in size or larger.
    d. none of the above.

11. If a patient has a lot of body hair growing around the intended cannulation site, it should
    a. not be removed in order to prevent infection.
    b. shaved off smoothly with a safety razor using an antibacterial soap.
    c. clipped close to the skin with a scissor.
    d. any of the above.

12. When a patient who has an IV presents with fever, chills, malaise, tachycardia, tachypnea, hypotension, and altered mental status, the nurse should suspect
    a. infection.
    b. sepsis.
    c. DIC.
    d. inflammatory response syndrome.

13. If the nurse suspects a hypersensitivity reaction in a patient receiving IV medications, she should
    a. stop the infusate, discontinue the IV, and notify the physician.
    b. stop the infusion, keep the vein open with normal saline, notify the physician, stay with the patient, and monitor his vital signs.
    c. stop the infusion and discontinue the IV, start a new IV with 5% dextrose in normal saline, and give IV Benadryl.
    d. slow the infusion, administer adrenaline, take vital signs, and notify the physician.

14. An air embolism can be caused by
    a. a severed IV line.
    b. IV tubing that is not primed with fluid.
    c. vented IV containers that run dry.
    d. all of the above.

15. The signs and symptoms of an air embolism are
    a. dyspnea, tachypnea, cough, and diaphoresis.
    b. cardiac dysrhythmia, hypotension, anxiety, and substernal pressure.
    c. localized decreased breath sounds, chest pain with inhalation and exhalation, pleural friction rub, and a cog wheel murmur.
    d. all of the above.

CHAPTER 6: INTRAVENOUS INFUSION PREPARATIONS

IV INFUSION PREPARATIONS

Multiple Choice

1. A true solution that is usually an isotonic, hypotonic, or hypertonic electrolyte solution is a
    a. crystalloid solution.
    b. colloid solution.
    c. hydrating solution.

2. An IV solution used to raise osmotic pressure and expand volume is a
    a. crystalloid solution.
    b. colloid solution.
    c. hydrating solution.

3. An IV solution, usually an infusate containing glucose, given to supplement calorie intake, supply nutrients, provide free water for maintenance or rehydration, or promote effective renal output is a
    a. crystalloid solution.
    b. colloid solution.
    c. hydrating solution.

4. An IV fluid that, once infused, remains within the intravascular space and is used to treat hypotension resulting from hypovolemia is an example of a(n)
    a. isotonic infusate.
    b. hypotonic infusate.
    c. hypertonic infusate.

5. An IV fluid that lowers serum osmolality by causing fluid to shift out of the blood and into the cells and ISF spaces, used to hydrate the ICF and ISF compartments and lower sodium levels is a(n)
    a. isotonic infusate.
    b. hypotonic infusate.
    c. hypertonic infusate.
6. An IV fluid that acts to expand the intravascular compartment by causing a pull of fluids from the ICF and ISF compartments into the blood vessels is a(n)
    a. isotonic infusate.
    b. hypotonic infusate.
    c. hypertonic infusate.

Matching

Match the infusate preparations in questions 7–25 with the appropriate osmolarity.

  a. isotonic infusate
  b. hypotonic infusate
  c. hypertonic infusate

_____ 7. 5% dextrose in water (in container)
_____ 8. 5% dextrose in water (infused)
_____ 9. 2.5% dextrose in water
_____ 10. 5% dextrose in 0.2% sodium chloride
_____ 11. 5% dextrose in 0.9% sodium chloride
_____ 12. 10% dextrose in water
_____ 13. 0.9% sodium chloride
_____ 14. 10% dextrose in 0.9% sodium chloride
_____ 15. 0.45% sodium chloride (half-normal saline)
_____ 16. Isolyte E®
_____ 17. 10% mannitol
_____ 18. Ringer's solution
_____ 19. 3% sodium chloride
_____ 20. 5% mannitol in 0.45% sodium chloride
_____ 21. Aminosyn® or FreAmine®
_____ 22. 5% sodium bicarbonate
_____ 23. Hetastarch 6% in 0.9% sodium chloride
_____ 24. 5% dextrose in Ringer's lactate
_____ 25. Sterile water for injection

CHAPTER 7: PATIENT PREPARATION AND SITE SELECTION FOR PERIPHERAL INTRAVENOUS INFUSION THERAPY

PATIENT PREPARATION, DELIVERY AND CARE

Multiple Choice

1. When administering IV therapy the nurse must follow the
    a. standards set forth by the state nurse practice act.
    b. CDC guidelines and OSHA standards.
    c. INS standards and agency policies and procedures.
    d. all of the above.

2. In order for a nurse to start an IV, there must be
   a. a medical order that is appropriate for the patient.
   b. a medical order that includes the date, name of the infusate, the frequency, and the delivery rate.
   c. a physician's order that is appropriate for the patient, written on the medical record (chart), that includes the date, name of the infusate, the dose, the delivery rate, and the physician's signature.
   d. approval by the employer.

3. If a patient isn't both psychologically and physically prepared for an IV, venous selection may be difficult because
   a. the patient may not cooperate.
   b. a sympathetic response may be elicited.
   c. peripheral vasoconstriction may occur.
   d. all of the above.

4. When starting an IV, a vascular access device must not be introduced into a vessel in
   a. the nondominant hand or arm.
   b. the arm on the side of a mastectomy without lymph node dissection.
   c. the arm where there is lymphedema and inadequate venous return or vessel damage.
   d. the arm used for previous IVs.

5. The correct position for a patient to be in prior to starting a peripheral IV is
   a. supine.
   b. whatever is comfortable for him.
   c. Fowler's or semi-Fowler's.
   d. —it doesn't matter as long as the IV gets placed.

6. Veins that are ideal for short-term use with a small-gauge cannula are the
   a. basilic and median basilic.
   b. cephalic and accessory cephalic.
   c. digital and metacarpal.
   d. antecubital.

7. The first vein of choice for early access and good visibility would be the
   a. antecubital.
   b. basilic.
   c. cephalic.
   d. metacarpal.

8. When a mildly hypertonic or irritating infusate must be administered, the peripheral vein(s) of choice would be the
   a. basilic and cephalic.
   b. metacarpal and radial.
   c. the digital and metacarpal.
   d. any of the above.

9. The ideal vein for phlebotomy is the
   a. basilic.
   b. cephalic.
   c. antecubital.
   d. radial.

10. When initiating IV therapy the nurse should select
    a. proximal veins of the upper extremities first, with subsequent venipunctures distal to the previous sites.
    b. distal veins of the upper extremities first, with subsequent venipunctures proximal to the previous sites.
    c. distal veins of the lower extremities with subsequent venipunctures in the upper extremities.
    d. none of the above.

11. Dilating a vein in preparation for venipuncture may be accomplished by all of the following except
    a. to have the patient open and close his fist several times.
    b. to instruct the patient to elevate his hand above the level of his heart.
    c. to apply warm compresses to the site for 10 minutes.
    d. to apply a tourniquet for a short period of time while rubbing the area with an alcohol sponge.

12. The most important thing to remember when using a tourniquet is to apply it so that it
    a. suppresses only arterial blood flow.
    b. suppresses only venous blood flow.
    c. suppresses arterial and venous blood flow.
    d. is tight enough to engorge the veins.

13. Because enhanced bleeding may occur in patients undergoing anticoagulant therapy, the nurse who initiates IV therapy should
    a. avoid the use of a tourniquet or apply it loosely.
    b. avoid excess pressure when cleansing the skin.
    c. use adhesive remover when removing adhesive dressings.
    d. all of the above.

14. When performing skin antisepsis the sequence of antimicrobial use should be
    a. 70% alcohol, then tincture of iodine, iodophor complex, or approved chlorhexidine preparation.
    b. tincture of iodine or iodophor complex, then 70% alcohol.
    c. either of the above in either order.

15. When entering the skin and cannulating a vein, the usual needle position is
    a. bevel up.
    b. bevel down.
    c. either bevel up or bevel down.

16. When applying an IV site dressing, the dressing should be placed so that it
    a. covers only the area surrounding the IV entry site.
    b. covers the area surrounding the IV entry site up to the top margin of the cannula hub.
    c. covers the IV entry site, the catheter hub, and the connection between the IV device and the administration set tubing.

17. When a patient is receiving IV therapy, both the patient and the IV site should be monitored
    a. every hour or more frequently if his condition warrants it.
    b. every shift, or every 8 to 12 hours.
    c. every 24 hours.

18. When the nurse must add medication(s) to an infusate container, the protocol is to
    a. check for compatibility.
    b. check to be sure that the addition of medication would render a safe concentration, depending on the amount of infusate left in the hanging container.
    c. determine how long the added medication will be stable in the container.
    d. all of the above.

19. When adding a medication to a hanging IV container, the nurse must
    a. add the medication to the hanging container through the additive port in the bag.
    b. clamp the administration set tubing, add the medication through the additive port in the hanging bag, then unclamp the tubing.
    c. clamp the administration set tubing, add the medication through the additive port in the hanging bag, remove the bag from the IV pole and rotate it several times, hang the bag back on the IV pole, then unclamp the tubing and regulate the rate.

20. When an intermittent infusion plug (heparin lock) is inserted into an IV device, but the cannula is not being used, the catheter should be flushed with saline
    a. every 8 hours.
    b. every 24 hours.
    c. every 36 hours.

21. When medications are administered into an intermittent infusion device, the protocol is to
    a. instill 2 cc of NS, administer the medication, and instill another 2 cc of NS.

b. administer the medication and follow with 2 cc of NS.

c. assess the site, aspirate to verify patency, administer the medication, and instill 2 cc of NS.

d. assess the site, aspirate to verify cannula patency, instill 2 cc of NS, administer the medication, and instill 2 cc of NS.

True/False

_____ 22. Veins should be palpated prior to initiating venipuncture in order to determine the condition of the veins and differentiate them from arteries.

_____ 23. When starting an IV, the nurse should use the largest cannula that will deliver the prescribed infusate.

_____ 24. The cannula size for an infusion should be as large as will fit into the vein.

_____ 25. In order to preserve the veins, IV sites should be rotated, using both the arm veins and the vessels of the lower extremities, in adults and children who are able to walk.

_____ 26. If a patient doesn't know whether or not he is allergic to iodine, the nurse should ask if he has any allergies to shellfish.

_____ 27. To ensure that a tourniquet is properly placed, the nurse must be able to palpate a pulse distal to the tourniquet.

_____ 28. For a vein to be viable, it must be able to be blanched when downward pressure is applied over or on each side of it.

_____ 29. To determine that an IV medication is administered directly into the vein, inject the medication slowly and observe for unusual reactions surrounding the IV site.

_____ 30. To properly identify a patient the nurse should call him by name.

_____ 31. Proper anchoring of the vein is usually the key to successful cannulation.

_____ 32. For elderly patients or those with fragile or thin-walled veins, successful venous cannulation is often accomplished by entering the vein with the bevel of the needle down.

_____ 33. Cannulation may be attempted only one more time with the same needle following an unsuccessful venipuncture.

_____ 34. Following unsuccessful venous access, the same nurse should attempt to cannulate the vein three or four more times before asking someone else to try.

_____ 35. Whenever an IV is started, the IV device should be secured with the patient's arm secured to an armboard.

_____ 36. Failure to check for compatibility with the infusate that is being delivered, when administering IV push medications through a port in the IV tubing, could result in a precipitate that obstructs the line or causes damage to the vein and embolization in the patient.

_____ 37. During removal of the cannula, when discontinuing an IV, the exit site should be covered with an alcohol swab and held in place after removal of the cannula until bleeding stops.

CHAPTER 8: EQUIPMENT AND SUPPLIES EMPLOYED IN THE PREPARATION AND ADMINISTRATION OF INTRAVENOUS INFUSION THERAPY

IV THERAPY EQUIPMENT AND SUPPLIES

True/False

_____ 1. When using a plastic IV container, the nurse should label it by writing directly on the bag using a ballpoint pen or an indelible marker.

_____ 2. The drop factor is the number of drops per minute that an IV tubing delivers.

_____ 3. In order to calculate the rate of an infusion, the nurse must know the volume to be infused, the time needed for it to be infused, the drop factor, and the mathematical formula needed to calculate the rate.

_____ 4. Y-type infusate administration sets are not vented and must be used only with collapsible infusion containers.

_____ 5. Unless absolutely necessary, the CDC does not recommend the routine use of extension sets or extra tubings with IV administration sets.

_____ 6. The priming volume of an IV device is the amount of infusate needed to replace air in the mechanism.

_____ 7. The ONC is a steel needle that encases a flexible cannula and is the most commonly used peripheral IV device.

_____ 8. According to the CDC, the dressing used to cover an IV insertion site should be only a transparent membrane dressing.

_____ 9. An EID with a controller mode functions as an electronic eye that "watches" the drops flow, according to a preset rate through a drop sensor system.

_____ 10. An EID that functions as a pump provides a driving force to overcome resistance to pressure in order to propel the infusate.

_____ 11. With a PCA, a patient is able to self-administer as much medication as needed for pain control.

_____ 12. An IV pole should be positioned so that the IV infusate container hangs 48 to 60 inches above the IV site.

_____ 13. When the nurse starts an IV, labels must be affixed to the IV site, the IV tubing, and the IV container to alert all nurses to changing times.

_____ 14. To prevent disconnection and the possibility of air embolism or contamination, Luer-Lok® connectors and adapters should be used.

CHAPTER 9: DELIVERY, CARE, MAINTENANCE, AND DISCONTINUATION OF INTRAVENOUS INFUSION THERAPY

Multiple Choice

1. When applying a tourniquet, the nurse should apply it so that
   a. arterial circulation is suppressed proximal to the tourniquet.
   b. venous circulation is suppressed proximal to the tourniquet.
   c. arterial circulation is suppressed distal to the tourniquet.
   d. venous circulation is suppressed distal to the tourniquet.

2. For a vein to be viable for venipuncture it should
   a. be able to be distended.
   b. be able to be blanched.
   c. be only mildly sclerosed.
   d. be free of valves.

3. When it is necessary to remove body hair from the intended site of venipuncture and venous cannulation, the nurse's best choice is to
   a. gently clip the hair with a scissor.
   b. shave the area using a sterile safety razor.
   c. shave the area using a safety razor or electric razor.
   d. apply a surgical-grade depilatory.

4. When attempting venipuncture, the nurse may puncture the skin with the same cannula
   a. only once.
   b. no more than two times.
   c. a maximum of three times.
   d. as many times as necessary as long as the cannula is intact and is wiped clean with an approved sterile antiseptic between sticks.

5. When adding a medication to an infusate that is running, the nursing interventions should include
   a. swabbing the injection port with antiseptic solution, injecting the medication, and labeling the container.
   b. clamping the IV tubing, injecting the medication into the injection port, and unclamping the tubing.
   c. clamping the IV tubing, injecting the medication into the port, agitating the hanging IV container vigorously, then opening the tubing, and labeling it.
   d. clamping the IV tubing, cleansing the injection port with an antiseptic, injecting the medication into the injection port, removing the hanging IV container—gently rotating it back and forth to mix the contents, rehanging the IV container, opening the tubing clamp, regulating the IV, and affixing a medication-added label to the IV container.

CHAPTER 10: MATHEMATICAL CALCULATIONS FOR THE ADMINISTATION, REGULATION, AND MAINTENANCE OF INTRAVENOUS INFUSION THERAPY

MATHEMATICAL CALCULATIONS

Fill in the Blank

1. Order: 1,500 ml NS to run for 24 hours.
   Drop Factor: 10.
   Give _____ gtt/min.

2. Order: 100 ml NS antibiotic solution to infuse over 30 minutes.
   Drop Factor: 15.
   Give _____ gtt/min.

3. Order: 1,000 ml NS to infuse over 8 hours.
   Drop Factor: 10.
   Give 21 gtt/min
   After 4 hours, when there should be 500 ml left, there is 600 ml remaining.
   Recalculate, so that the remaining 600 ml infuses in 4 hours.
   Give _____ gtt/min.

4. Order: Antibiotic: 0.5 g in 100 ml D_5W IVPB to infuse over 30 min.
   Drop Factor: 10.
   Give _____ gtt/min.

5. Order: Kefzol 250 mg q 8hr in 50 ml D_5W to infuse per Buretrol over 60 minutes followed by a 15 ml NS flush.
   Supply: Kefzol is reconstituted to 125 mg/ml
   a. Calculate the total volume for one dose of the intermittent IV medication and the IV flush.
   b. What is the daily amount of the intermittent IV medication and the IV flush?
   c. Calculate the flow rate of the IV medication and the flush.
   d. Calculate the volume of the medication to be administered.
   e. Calculate the volume of NS to add to the Buretrol chamber for a dilution volume of 50 ml.

6. Order: Heparin IV to infuse at 1,000 U/hr.
   Available: 500 ml bag of D_5W with 25,000 U heparin.
   Drop Factor: 15.
   a. Give _____ ml/hr.
   b. Give _____ gtt/min.

7. Order: 1,000 ml NS to infuse at 60 ml/hr to begin at 0600 hours.
   When will the IV be finished?

8. Order: Lidocaine 2 g IV in 500 ml D_5W at 2 mg/min per infusion pump.
   Drop Factor: 10.
   a. Calculate the ml/min.
   b. Calculate the ml/hr.
   c. Calculate the drops per minute.

9. Order: 2,000 ml NS IV to infuse over 24 hours with 80 mg gentamicin in 80 ml IVPB NS to infuse over 30 minutes. Maintain fluid limitation at 200 ml/day.
   Drop Factor: 15.
   a. Calculate the daily volume for the IVPB infusion.
   b. Calculate the flow rate for the IVPB.
   c. Calculate the daily volume for the regular IV.
   d. Calculate the flow rate for the regular IV.
   e. How would this IV be regulated over 24 hours?

10. The nurse is working the day shift from 0700 to 1530 hours. One patient assigned to him, who is receiving an IV infusion with a Buretrol volume control set, has the following orders:
    1. D_5W IV to infuse @ 50 ml/hr for continuous infusion.

2. Pipracil 1 g IV q6hr.

The pharmacy supplies the Pipracil in a prefilled syringe labeled 1 g/5 ml with instructions to "add Pipracil to Buretrol and infuse over 30 minutes."

a. What is the drop factor of the Buretrol?

b. What amount of Pipracil will the nurse add to the Buretrol?

c. How much D_5W IV fluid will the nurse add to the Buretrol with the Pipracil?

d. To maintain the flow rate of the IV at 50 ml/hr, the nurse will time the Pipracil to infuse at what rate (in gtt/min)?

e. If the patient received the last dose of Pipracil at 0600 hours, how many doses will the nurse give during his shift?

CHAPTER 11: PHARMACOLOGIC PRINCIPLES RELATED TO THE PREPARATION AND ADMINISTRATION OF INTRAVENOUS MEDICATIONS

PHARMACOLOGY

Multiple Choice

1. Which of the following is not the primary responsibility of the nurse regarding medication administration?
   a. Recognize the desired/undesired drug effects.
   b. Alter dosages to achieve desired responses.
   c. Determine the correct dosage and route of administration.
   d. Provide patient teaching regarding side effects of the drug.

2. The pharmacokinetics aspect of drug administration describes
   a. the process involved in absorbing, distributing, metabolizing, and eliminating a drug from the body.
   b. the study of accelerated drug metabolism and elimination in those with liver disfunction.
   c. the process of converting a solid form of drug into a solution for enhanced absorption.
   d. determining the optimal drug dose to achieve the desired therapeutic effects.

3. Which statement regarding drug absorption is incorrect?
   a. Specialized transport proteins exist to actively "pump" some drugs through cell membranes.
   b. Energy in the form of ATP is required during all absorption processes.
   c. Drug molecules move across membranes from areas of low to high concentrations during active transport.
   d. Passive diffusion allows drugs to move from areas of high to low concentrations.

4. The major method of cellular drug absorption for most medications administered is through
   a. active transport.
   b. passive diffusion.
   c. special carrier proteins.
   d. membrane pores.

5. If an IV medication is administered at scheduled intervals over a period of time, the peak plasma concentration occurs
   a. immediately following administration of a dose.
   b. within 30 to 60 minutes following administration of the drug.
   c. at the point between administration of one dose and the administration of the next, or halfway between doses.
   d. just before the next dose is given.

6. The trough plasma concentration of an IV medication, given at regularly scheduled intervals, occurs
   a. one hour after administration of a dose.
   b. at the halfway point between doses.
   c. just before the next dose is administered.
   d. 24 hours after the final dose is given.

7. The half-life refers to the time
   a. it takes for a medication to break down after it is reconstituted.
   b. interval between doses of a medication.
   c. it takes for the body to ingest and absorb one-half of the original concentration of an administered drug.
   d. it takes for the body to metabolize and eliminate one-half of the original concentration of an administered drug.

8. When a physician writes an ambiguous medication order, the nurse should
   a. clarify the order with any physician who happens to be on the unit.
   b. ask the head nurse or supervisor if the order is correct.
   c. get a second opinion from the pharmacist.
   d. call the physician who wrote the order.

9. All state nurse practice acts provide for revocation of a license or probation if a nurse
   a. practices while under the influence of alcohol.
   b. loses a malpractice suit.
   c. is accused of negligent practice.
   d. gives the wrong medication to a patient.

10. A patient with NKA is receiving the first dose of an IV antibiotic. The nurse notices a fine red rash on his neck and he complains of rhinitis. The first thing the nurse should do is
    a. call the patient's physician.
    b. discontinue the medication.
    c. continue the drug at a slower rate and observe the patient.
    d. administer diphenhydramine.

11. In case an IV infusion of norepinephrine (Levophed) extravasates, the nurse should be prepared to administer
    a. propranolol (Inderal).
    b. phentolamine (Regitine).
    c. phenylephrine (Neo-Synephrine).
    d. physostigmine (Antilirium).

12. The best drug for managing tissue necrosis due to extravasation of dopamine (Intropin) infusion is
    a. phenylephrine (Neo-Synephrine).
    b. phentolamine (Regitine).
    c. atropine.
    d. methoxamine (Vasoxyl).

13. The nurse should be aware of which effect of procaine (Novocain) and other local anesthetics?
    a. It blocks potassium transport into nerves.
    b. It causes CNS depression.
    c. It prevents nerve cell depolarization.
    d. It stimulates the conduction of nerve action potentials.

14. Within one to two minutes after receiving a local anesthetic, the patient experiences *tightness* in the chest, progressing to severe bronchoconstriction and hypotension. Which is least likely to alleviate these symptoms and signs?
    a. Diphenhydramine.
    b. Oxygen.
    c. Epinephrine.
    d. IV fluids.

15. Overdoses of a local anesthetic such as lidocaine (Xylocaine) are likely to cause all of the following except
    a. hypertension.
    b. convulsions.
    c. respiratory depression.
    d. cardiac depression.

16. The peripheral vasodilating effects of some anesthetic agents, such as halothane, would require which of the following changes in managing pain in the immediate postoperative period?
    a. A higher dose will be needed to relieve pain.
    b. IV analgesia will have to be used as IM injections for analgesia will not be effective.

c. IV medications will be too potent.

d. The patient will have little or no pain until the drug wears off.

17. The nurse anesthetist chooses midazolam (Versed) over diazepam (Valium) as a preanesthetic induction agent because midazolam

 a. can be given IM.

 b. is less irritating to the veins than diazepam with IV injection.

 c. diazepam cannot be given IV.

 d. does not cause respiratory depression.

18. Before administering IV morphine sulfate, the most important nursing assessment would be to

 a. check urinary output.

 b. take apical and radial pulses.

 c. check skin color and turgor.

 d. assess respirations.

19. Should any opioid side effect occur, the antagonist of choice is IV

 a. atropine sulfate.

 b. methadone (Dolophine).

 c. naloxone (Narcan).

 d. disulfiram (Antabuse).

20. When giving IV digoxin (Lanoxin), nursing actions include all of the following except

 a. taking an apical pulse for one full minute prior to administration.

 b. not giving the drug if the heart rate is below 45 beats per minute.

 c. administering the drug over a period of five minutes or longer.

 d. giving the drug only when the patient is being monitored electrocardiographically.

21. When administering IV phenytoin (Dilantin) the nurse must remember all of the following except

 a. it can be diluted only with a special manufacturer-supplied diluent or preservative-free 0.9% NaCl.

 b. it must be injected slowly (not to exceed 50 mg/min) and directly into a large vein through a large-gauge cannula.

 c. it must not be added to an already running infusion.

 d. it cannot be given IV.

22. When administering IV amphotericin B, the nurse must

 a. know that rapid infusion may result in hypotension, hypokalemia, dysrhythmias, and shock.

 b. remember that strict aseptic technique must be used in preparation and administration because there is no bacteriostatic agent in the medication.

 c. determine that a 1-mg test dose is administered to assess the patient's tolerance to the drug before a scheduled regimen of therapy is started.

 d. all of the above.

23. The IV administration of diazepam (Valium) is the drug of choice for treating

 a. severe dyskinesia.

 b. severe recurrent seizures and status epilepticus.

 c. postoperative psychosis.

 d. all of the above.

24. When administering diazepam, the nurse must

 a. administer it slowly (not to exceed 5 mg/min), directly into large veins, using a glass syringe.

 b. carefully monitor vital signs and have emergency equipment available in the event of bradycardia, respiratory depression or arrest, and cardiac arrest.

 c. never mix it with other drugs or infusates as it is very unstable and a precipitate may form in the vein during infusion.

 d. all of the above.

25. When administering IV diuretics, the nurse must be alert for

 a. side effects of weakness, vertigo, and postural hypotension.

 b. side effects of respiratory depression and cardiac toxicity.

 c. increased peripheral edema and pulmonary edema.

 d. hypertension, tinnitus, and jaundice.

26. When administering IV heparin infusions, the nurse must know that a safe adult dosage range is
    a. 5,000 to 15,000 U/24 hr.
    b. 20,000 to 40,000 U/24 hr.
    c. 40,000 to 60,000 U/24 hr.
    d. 60,000 to 80,000 U/24 hr.
27. When excessive anticoagulant effects occur, the antagonist for heparin is
    a. protamine sulfate.
    b. protamine zinc.
    c. platelet administration.
    d. thrombolytic agents.
28. Before administering IV histamine H-2 antagonists, the nurse should check
    a. the hematology profile.
    b. magnesium levels.
    c. baseline hepatic and renal studies.
    d. none of the above.
29. When preparing a parenteral dose of chlorpromazine, the nurse must be careful to avoid contact with the drug because it may cause
    a. headaches.
    b. yellow staining of the skin.
    c. a foul odor on the skin.
    d. skin irritation.
30. Streptokinase and urokinase promote the dissolution of a thrombus by
    a. inhibiting platelet aggregation.
    b. inhibiting the conversion of fibrinogen to fibrin.
    c. stimulating a fibrin-stabilizing factor.
    d. stimulating the conversion of plasminogen to plasmin.
31. The change that would be of least concern to the nurse when administering IV aminophylline is
    a. irregular cardiac rhythm.
    b. increased heart rate.
    c. increased urine output.
    d. increased restlessness.
32. The insulin preparation that can safely be given IV is
    a. regular insulin (crystalline zinc insulin).
    b. insulin zinc suspension (Lente).
    c. extended insulin zinc suspension (Ultralente).
    d. protamine zinc insulin suspension.
33. In the event of an anaphylactic reaction, the nurse should be prepared to administer the IV drug
    a. norepinephrine.
    b. hydrocortisone.
    c. Cromolyn.
    d. Betazole.
34. The drug that will inactivate carbenicillin when placed in the same container is
    a. chloramphenicol.
    b. clindamycin.
    c. gentamicin.
    d. penicillin G.
35. Creatinine clearance and BUN concentrations are important clinical guides to the toxicity and clearance of
    a. tetracycline.
    b. chloramphenicol.
    c. erythromycin.
    d. gentamicin.

36. The rate of administration of IV potassium chloride solutions should not exceed
    a. 10 mEq/hr.
    b. 20 mEq/hr.
    c. 30 mEq/hr.
    d. 40 mEq/hr.

CHAPTER 12: CENTRAL & PERIPHERALLY PLACED VASCULAR ACCESS DEVICES AND ADVANCED MEDICATION DELIVERY SYSTEMS

ADVANCED VASCULAR ACCESS

True/False

_____ 1. Any drug with an unusually high pH or osmolarity can cause severe venous irritation and subsequent chemical phlebitis.

_____ 2. The greater hemodilution of a central vessel precludes the vein irritation that occurs when hypertonic infusates are administered through peripheral veins.

_____ 3. The usual sites of insertion for CVCs are the subclavian vein and the internal and external jugulars, with access from the left side being preferable.

_____ 4. Superior vena cava (SVC) syndrome is not necessarily a contraindication to CVC placement.

_____ 5. A CVC needs to be positioned so that the tip terminates in the SVC or the right atrium.

_____ 6. The immediate complications associated with CVCs are usually related to problems involving insertion of the line, while long-term complications are often the result of inadequate catheter care or the patient's clinical situation.

_____ 7. The major preventable complication that can occur any time during therapy with a CVC, including the 24-hour period following removal, is infection.

_____ 8. The average adult lethal dose of air into the circulation is 70 to 150 ml or 5 to 15 ml/kg.

_____ 9. With cardiac tamponade, there is perforation of the pericardium that results in compression of the heart because of leakage of blood or infusate into the pericardial sac.

_____ 10. With pneumothorax there is perforation of the interpleural space with air accumulation in the mediastinum.

_____ 11. A patient complaint of a burning sensation or discomfort during infusions, as well as a gurgling sound in the ear, is indicative of CVC dislodgement or migration.

_____ 12. The Valsalva maneuver is the forced expiratory effort against a closed airway that is used to increase intrathoracic pressure, raise venous pressure, impede venous return to the right atrium, and slow the pulse rate.

_____ 13. Performing the Valsalva maneuver prevents air from entering the circulation and embolizing when a large vessel is cannulated or there is a breach in the IV line.

_____ 14. The CDC recommends that CVC dressings be changed every 72 hours, with antimicrobial ointment applied to the catheter exit site.

_____ 15. Prior to CVC insertion, the nurse should assist the patient to a 20-degree Trendelenburg position with a rolled towel between the shoulder blades.

_____ 16. Whenever a central line is disconnected for any reason, the pigtail extending from it must be clamped off with a hemostat.

Multiple Choice

17. One of the most important mechanisms used to maintain patency of a central line and prevent occlusion is
    a. irrigating or flushing.
    b. keeping the line heparinized at all times.
    c. maintaining the infusion running at a steady rate via an infusion pump.

18. When irrigating a CVC, the barrel capacity of the syringe must be no smaller than
    a. 1 cc.
    b. 3 cc.
    c. 5 cc.
    d. 10 cc.

19. When a central line is flushed, at least 10 ml of 0.9% NaCl should be used, instilling it with
    a. a slow, smooth push of irrigant.
    b. a rapid, forceful, and continual push of irrigant.
    c. a rapid succession of push-pause movements.
    d. a laminar flow.

20. If a needleless device is not employed, the correct gauge of a needle used to penetrate an injection cap should be within the range of
    a. 18 to 20 ga.
    b. 20 to 25 ga.
    c. 22 to 27 ga.
    d. 25 to 27 ga.

21. Intermittent catheter malfunction, difficulty drawing blood, and a positional IV, in conjunction with radiologic evidence of catheter compression, defines
    a. catheter malposition.
    b. catheter fracture.
    c. pinch-off sign.
    d. pinch-off syndrome.

22. Withdrawal or aspiration occlusion, which is not a true catheter occlusion, is caused by
    a. fibrin sheath formation.
    b. a fibrin tail extending from the catheter tip.
    c. the catheter tip being pressed up against the vein wall.
    d. all of the above.

23. When drawing blood samples from a CVC,
    a. the procedure should be done by laboratory phlebotomists.
    b. infusates containing glucose or electrolytes should be turned off 10 seconds prior to the blood draw.
    c. blood must not be left in the pigtail or cap following phlebotomy.
    d. all of the above.

24. Before using a declotting solution to clear a catheter occlusion, the nurse should try to
    a. vigorously irrigate the line.
    b. use the negative pressure POP method.
    c. use the stopcock method.
    d. force irrigant into the line.

25. The declotting agent of choice for the removal of blood clots from a central line is
    a. 0.1 N hydrochloric acid.
    b. 70% ethanol.
    c. sodium bicarbonate.
    d. tPa.

26. The declotting agent of choice for removal of lipid deposits from a central line is
    a. 0.1 N hydrochloric acid.
    b. 70% ethanol.
    c. sodium bicarbonate.
    d. urokinase.

27. When heparin-locking a Groshong® CVC, use
    a. heparin only.
    b. 0.9% NaCl only.
    c. normal saline followed by heparin.
    d. nothing. Groshong® catheters are closed systems.

28. If a CVC needs to be repaired (pigtail hub replacement, pigtail repair, or catheter stem repair), the nurse should
    a. use any universal repair kit.
    b. use a blunt-end needle and injection cap system.
    c. use the manufacturer-specific repair kit.
    d. call the physician, as nurses do not repair CVCs.

29. A tunneled CVC differs from a nontunneled CVC in that it
    a. is surgically inserted by a physician.
    b. has a Dacron® cuff around its circumference with a microbial barrier.
    c. has a Dacron® cuff near the subcutaneous exit that secures the device and provides a microbial barrier.
    d. is an antimicrobial-impregnated catheter.

30. The difference between a Broviac,® Hickman,® and Leonard® CVC is
    a. the size.
    b. their physical make-up.
    c. the infusates that may be delivered through each.
    d. that they are totally unrelated to each other.

31. The Groshong® catheter differs from other CVCs in that it
    a. has an open-ended tip with a three-position valve that stays open all the time.
    b. has a closed-end tip with a three-position pressure-sensitive valve that stays closed when not in use.
    c. has a chemical make-up that allows for minimal use of heparin for flushing.
    d. comes only in single-lumen styles.

32. In order for a nurse to insert a PICC
    a. he must have certification by his state and have additional employer training.
    b. he must be trained in a state-approved agency and show proficiency in insertion and maintenance.
    c. he must meet minimal educational requirements, have employer-granted certification, and demonstrate evidence of competency.
    d. he must be a registered nurse and meet minimum state-approved educational requirements.

33. The person who would not be a candidate for a PICC line is
    a. a construction worker.
    b. a swimming instructor or lifeguard.
    c. a nurse working in a dialysis unit.
    d. none of the above. All would be candidates.

34. The first vein of choice for a PICC line is the
    a. antecubital.
    b. basilic.
    c. cephalic.
    d. cubital.

35. The catheter tip position for a PICC line may be in
    a. the axillary or the subclavian vein.
    b. the axillary or the innominate vein.
    c. the subclavian vein or the SVC.
    d. the SVC.

36. The gloves worn by the nurse to insert a PICC should be
    a. sterile latex powdered.
    b. nonlatex powdered, that have been rinsed with sterile water or sterile NS.
    c. sterile latex or nonlatex powderless.
    d. any of the above.

37. The most frequent complication associated with PICCs is
    a. mechanical (sterile) phlebitis.
    b. infection.
    c. infusion pain.
    d. thrombosis.

38. For patients who use crutches to walk, the vein of choice for a PICC is the
    a. basilic.
    b. cephalic.
    c. axillary.
    d. none of the above. The patient is not a candidate for a PICC.

39. When flushing a PICC, the pulsatile, push-pause method should be employed, using sterile 0.9% NaCl in a syringe with a barrel capacity of
    a. 1 cc.
    b. 3 cc.
    c. 5 cc.
    d. 10 cc.

40. When changing a PICC dressing, the old dressing should be detached
    a. from the distal to the proximal edge.
    b. from the proximal to the distal edge.
    c. from the sides first, then top to bottom.
    d. any of the above.

41. Grade 4+ mechanical phlebitis would be assessed as
    a. erythema and swelling at the IV site, induration and a palpable venous cord <3 inches above the site.
    b. erythema and swelling at the IV site, induration and palpable venous cord >3 inches above the site.
    c. pain at the site, no erythema, swelling and induration at or around the site.
    d. severe pain and burning, redness, edema, and fever.

42. When removing a PICC, the most frequent cause of a *stuck* catheter is
    a. a catheter tear or rupture.
    b. phlebitis.
    c. thrombophlebitis.
    d. venospasm.

43. The intervention for removing a *stuck* PICC is to
    a. stretch the catheter and tape it to the arm for two to four hours, then remove it.
    b. pull gently on the catheter, stretching it, then tape the stretched portion to the arm for four to six hours, then remove it.
    c. leave it alone, apply gentle massage and/or moist heat to the area of the upper arm, and reattempt removal in 20 to 30 minutes after the vein relaxes.
    d. call the radiologist to remove it under fluoroscopy.

44. A midline catheter (MLC) is any percutaneously-inserted IV line that is placed
    a. between the antecubital fossa and the head of the clavicle with optimal tip location level with the axilla.
    b. with the tip in any location between the antecubital fossa and the subclavian vein.
    c. between the antecubital fossa and 3 to 5 cm distal to the axillary vein.
    d. between the antecubital fossa and 6 to 8 cm proximal to the innominate vein.

True/False

_____ 45. The difference between a subcutaneous vascular access port and any other CVC is that no portion of the device is placed on the external surface of the body.

_____ 46. For most implantable vascular ports (VAPs), only small-gauge hypodermic needles may be used to access the portal septum.

_____ 47. The best way to prevent the buildup of residual sludge in a VAP is through proper push-pause flushing techniques following the administration of infusates.

_____ 48. Teaching for patients who have VAPs includes reminding them not to rub or manipulate the skin over the port—a condition known as Twiddler's syndrome—to prevent internal catheter dislodgement.

_____ 49. The central venous pressure (CVP) is the force of venous blood ejected from the aorta.

_____ 50. The most accurate CVP readings are obtained when the CVC tip is positioned 3 to 4 cm superior to the Rt. atrial-SVC junction and the patient is sitting up.

_____ 51. Epidural administration consists of injecting medication directly into the epidural space for direct delivery to the tissues and vessels of the CNS.

_____ 52. With intrathecal administration, a drug is delivered into the cerebrospinal fluid.

_____ 53. When systemic intolerance and toxicity are a problem and higher concentrations of drug delivery are needed for some malignancies, the intraperitoneal route of administration is ideal.

Critical Thinking

54. Describe the correct way to explain to a patient how to perform the Valsalva maneuver, using terminology she can understand.

CHAPTER 13: INTRAVENOUS NUTRITIONAL SUPPORT

IV NUTRITIONAL SUPPORT

True/False

_____ 1. When stress or disease alters the ability to take in food or use energy sources, the body compensates by using its own stores of energy, resulting in a state of negative nitrogen balance.

_____ 2. Total parenteral nutrition (TPN) is indicated for patients who are malnourished or in danger of becoming malnourished and require IV nutritional support for periods of 7 to 10 days.

_____ 3. TPN products contain macronutrients including amino acids, dextrose, and fat emulsions.

_____ 4. Proteins supply 4 kcal/g and are more efficiently burned than carbohydrates.

_____ 5. High concentrations of dextrose are added to TPN products so that the amino acids can be retained by the body and utilized for protein synthesis.

_____ 6. The rapid infusion of hypertonic dextrose can result in fluid retention, hypoglycemia, and hyperosmolar coma.

_____ 7. The most concentrated source of energy in the body, oxidized to produce energy, are fats.

_____ 8. Lipids can be administered by peripheral or central venous access routes because they are isotonic.

_____ 9. The *breaking out* or *oiling out* of fat emulsions is normal and, once shaken up, they may be administered.

_____ 10. The rate of administration for lipid emulsions should not exceed 5 g/kg/day.

_____ 11. Total nutrient admixtures (TNAs) are used for relatively stable patients in whom it can be predicted that components of the admixture will not have to be altered within a 24-hour period.

_____ 12. Crystalline amino acid preparations are tolerated best by patients with liver diseases, such as cirrhosis or hepatitis.

_____ 13. Amino acid preparations for renal patients should contain only essential amino acids.

_____ 14. When TPN is initiated, it should be introduced at a rate of about 50 ml/hr, increasing the rate by 25-ml/hr increments until the desired rate is established.

_____ 15. If a TPN infusion flows faster or slower than its prescribed rate, it may be adjusted within no more than 20% of its original rate to compensate for any deviation in the infusion schedule.

_____ 16. Refeeding syndrome may be manifested as edema, hypernatremia, hypokalemia, hypomagnesemia, and hypophosphatemia.

_____ 17. Patients who are hypokalemic must always be assessed for hypomagnesemia as well, to avert cardiac problems.

_____ 18. Once the body has reestablished normal albumin and electrolyte balances, refeeding processes are reversed.

_____ 19. Peripheral parenteral nutrition (PPN) is indicated for patients who need a complete nutrient source, but who are not depleted.

_____ 20. PPN preparations usually contain 5% to 12% dextrose and may be administered through peripheral venous access.

CHAPTER 14: BLOOD & BLOOD PRODUCT ADMINISTRATION
BLOOD-BLOOD PRODUCTS
Fill in the Blank

1. The inherited glycoproteins or glycolipids located on the surface of the RBC membrane are known as _____.

2. The immunoglobulins that float freely in the plasma and are produced following exposure to foreign substances are know as _____.

3. The major cause of immediate fatal transfusion reactions is _____.

4. Blood collected from donors for transfusion to another individual, labeled *volunteer donor* is _____.

5. The safest type of blood transfusion to eliminate the risk of alloimmunization, immune-mediated transfusion reactions, and transmission of viral diseases is _____.

6. The blood component used to treat acute massive blood loss with hypotension, tachycardia, shortness of breath, pallor, and low hemoglobin and hematocrits is _____.

7. The transfusion of choice for patients with acute or chronic blood loss with tachycardia, shortness of breath, pallor, fatigue, and low Hgb/Hct is _____.

8. Under normal circumstances, in order for antibodies (agglutinins) to be produced, there must be exposure to red blood cell agglutinogens via _____ or _____.

9. The major immediate cause of fatal transfusion reactions, because of antibody formation against the missing A antigen, B antigen, or both is known as _____.

10. A universal donor is a person with blood type _____.

11. A universal recipient is a person with blood type _____.

True/False

_____ 12. Once the dose is determined, whole blood should be transfused as rapidly as the patient can tolerate, to stabilize the hemodynamic status.

_____ 13. Nothing, other than sterile 0.9% NaCl, may be added to blood.

_____ 14. The infusion time for one unit of packed RBC in the adult patient should not exceed six hours.

_____ 15. Irradiated blood products may pose a slight radiation risk to either the transfusionist or the recipient.

_____ 16. Patients with a history of febrile, nonhemolytic reactions may require leukocyte-poor platelets.

_____ 17. Granulocytes must be infused slowly, and the patient watched closely, as there is an increased incidence of febrile, nonhemolytic transfusion reactions when this product is administered.

_____ 18. Fresh frozen plasma is administered for volume expansion, and prophylactically with massive blood transfusion.

_____ 19. The expected outcomes following administration of colloid solutions are the acquisition and maintenance of adequate blood pressure and volume support.

_____ 20. A 20-gauge or smaller cannula should be used for adult transfusions.

_____ 21. It is usually not necessary to have a patient sign a consent form prior to a transfusion.

_____ 22. Whole blood can be stored under monitored refrigeration for up to two months.

_____ 23. Reactions from different causes can exhibit similar manifestations of a blood transfusion reaction.

_____ 24. Patients with a history of severe allergic reactions to plasma should not receive immune serum globulin.

_____ 25. An acute transfusion reaction can occur within five minutes of the start of a transfusion or as late as 48 hours after its discontinuation.

_____ 26. A delayed transfusion reaction may develop any time up to six months after the transfusion is administered.

Critical Thinking

_____ 27. What guidelines regarding vital signs and monitoring must the nurse follow when starting a blood transfusion?

_____ 28. What is an acute hemolytic transfusion reaction?

_____ 29. List the nursing interventions to be instituted for a transfusion reaction.

_____ 30. Why can hypocalcemia result from the rapid transfusion of stored blood?

Matching

Match the listed transfusion reaction with the described clinical manifestations.

_____ 31. anaphylactic

_____ 32. circulatory overload

_____ 33. mild allergic

_____ 34. acute hemolytic

_____ 35. febrile nonhemolytic

_____ 36. sepsis

a. chills, fever, low back pain, flushing, tachycardia, tachypnea, hypotension, vascular collapse, hemoglobinuria, hemoglobinemia, bleeding, acute renal failure, shock, cardiac arrest, death

b. sudden chills and rise in temperature one degree above baseline recording, anxiety, headache, flushing, muscle pain

c. flushing, itching, urticaria (hives)

d. anxiety, urticaria, wheezing, progressing to cyanosis, shock, and possible cardiac arrest

e. cough, dyspnea, pulmonary congestion with rales, headache, hypertension, tachycardia, distended neck veins

f. rapid onset of chills, high fever, vomiting, diarrhea, marked hypotension, and shock

CHAPTER 15: INTRAVENOUS INFUSION THERAPY FOR THE PEDIATRIC PATIENT

PEDIATRICS

True/False

_____ 1. Neonates generally have a higher relative body water content, requiring higher doses of very water-soluble drugs.

_____ 2. The seriousness of body water and fluid and electrolyte losses and gains is proportionate to the size of the child, with the larger child always at greater risk of imbalance.

_____ 3. In a premature infant, up to 85% of the body weight is water.

_____ 4. The percentage of body weight that is water varies according to the amount of body fat that is present; the more fat the child has, the smaller the amount of water in the body.

_____ 5. Fluid replacement in a child is essentially the same as for an adult.

_____ 6. In the unstressed infant, the basal metabolic rate is three times that of an adult.

_____ 7. The body surface area (BSA) of an infant or young child is proportionately greater than that of the older child or adult.

_____ 8. Because a child's kidneys are not able to concentrate urine as efficiently as those of an adult, more water is excreted with metabolic wastes.

_____ 9. When starting an IV on an infant, the nurse should instruct the mother not to feed the child immediately before the procedure.

_____ 10. When preparing to start an IV on a toddler, the nurse can expect little or no cooperation from the child and most likely will have to restrain him.

_____ 11. There is no point in explaining a proposed IV insertion to a preschooler; at this age, a child is totally unable to reason and understand cause and effect.

_____ 12. Before starting an IV on a school-age child, the nurse should consider allowing the child to look at and touch the equipment and ask questions about the proposed procedure.

_____ 13. The conditions that commonly result in dehydration and require IV replacement in a child are vomiting, diarrhea, fever, and tachypnea.

_____ 14. In a child with mild isotonic dehydration, there may be a weight loss of 5% or a fluid deficit of up to 50 ml/kg; with moderate isotonic dehydration, the weight loss is 10% with a fluid deficit of up to 100 mL/kg.

_____ 15. In a child with severe isotonic dehydration, there is usually a lack of response, the fontanels are sunken, there is a weight loss of 15% or more, and a potentially fatal situation exists.

_____ 16. There is more accuracy in calculating the severity of a child's dehydration by obtaining a serum potassium level, than by using subjective symptoms.

_____ 17. In a child with dehydration, signs of shock, and poor systemic perfusion, the nurse will most likely administer D_5W or $D_5\frac{1}{2}NS$ at 40 ml/kg.

_____ 18. In a child with isotonic or hypotonic dehydration, the goal is to replace one-half of the deficit in the first 8 hours, with the other half being replaced within the next 16 hours.

_____ 19. In a child with hypertonic dehydration, the goal is to replace the deficit over a 16- to 24-hour period.

_____ 20. The BSA method is less accurate than using weight in kilograms to calculate fluid maintenance needs for a child.

Multiple Choice

21. To prevent fluid overload and avoid unnecessary waste, a toddler's IV containers should contain no more than
    a. 50 ml.
    b. 100 ml.
    c. 250 ml.
    d. 500 ml.

22. An infant receiving IV fluids would have
    a. microdrip tubing connected to a 50-ml infusate container.
    b. a macrodrip tubing connected to a volume control cylinder.
    c. a microdrip volume control cylinder attached to a 250-ml infusate container.
    d. any tubing or container, as long as it is regulated with an EID.

23. The preferred vessel for administering IV fluids to a child is
    a. a peripheral vein.
    b. a scalp vein.
    c. a central vein.
    d. an intraosseous site.

24. The ONC of choice for a peripheral IV on a preschool child would be a
    a. 18 ga., $1\frac{1}{2}$ in.
    b. 20 ga., $1\frac{1}{4}$ in.
    c. 22 ga., 1 in.
    d. 24 ga., $\frac{3}{4}$ in.

25. The CVC most often used for small children is the
    a. Hickman.®
    b. Broviac.®
    c. Leonard.®
    d. Jelco.®

26. Intraosseous cannulation is recommended
    a. in emergency situations.
    b. for children who are six years of age or younger.
    c. when IV access is difficult.
    d. all of the above.

27. The most commonly used site for intraosseous access is the
    a. proximal humerus.
    b. distal humerus, 6 cm below the acromion process.
    c. anterior tibia, 1 to 3 cm below the tibial tuberosity.
    d. proximal posterior femur.

28. While rare, potential complications as a result of intraosseous infusions include
    a. cellulitis and skin necrosis.
    b. damage to the epiphyseal plate and tibial fractures.
    c. embolus from fat dislodgement within the bone marrow.
    d. all of the above.

29. When initiating home TPN for a child, the physician, nurse, and discharge planner must consider
    a. the clinical status of the patient.
    b. the parent's ability to perform or monitor the procedure.
    c. the family's understanding and ability to comply with infection control guidelines.
    d. all of the above.

CHAPTER 16: INTRAVENOUS INFUSION THERAPY FOR THE ELDERLY PATIENT
THE ELDERLY

Multiple Choice

1. *Elderly* is generally understood to mean people
   a. 50 years of age or older.
   b. 59 years of age or older.
   c. 62 years of age or older.
   d. 65 years of age or older.

2. The term *frail elderly* refers to people who are
   a. 70 or older.
   b. 75 or older.
   c. 85 or at high risk for health problems.
   d. terminally ill elderly.

3. The heart of the elderly person, as compared to a younger person,
   a. has less cardiac reserve with less flexible valves.
   b. has fewer pacemaker cells.
   c. does not respond to stress as quickly and, after stress is relieved, returns to normal more slowly.
   d. all of the above.

4. Indications of advanced age in the renal system include
   a. an increase in the weight and number of nephrons.
   b. diminished blood flow and glomerular filtration.
   c. increased renal adaptation to fluid overload.
   d. all of the above.

5. When initiating IV therapy, the nurse should consider changes in skin integrity in the elderly including
   a. loss of subcutaneous fat and decreased sweat glands.
   b. dry, fragile, thinning skin.
   c. decreased sensitivity to touch.
   d. all of the above.

6. Chronic dehydration in the elderly is usually associated with
   a. inadequate fluid intake, long-term diuretic use, and problems associated with getting and drinking fluids, often caused by altered mobility.
   b. loss of thirst sensation and disinterest in nutrition.
   c. illness.
   d. all of the above.

7. The major difference in drug absorption between younger and older adults is the decline in first-pass elimination of drugs with aging. The nurse should know that dosages in the elderly patient may need to be
   a. doubled to achieve the same effect.
   b. reduced to prevent excessive systemic levels.
   c. increased slightly to make up for diminished liver function.
   d. monitored for reduced clinical effectiveness.

8. The most common way to adjust drug therapy to compensate for physiologic changes in the older adult is to alter the
   a. dosage.
   b. route of administration.
   c. frequency of drug administration.
   d. duration of treatment.

9. The choices of IV sites for an elderly person
   a. are generally the same as for a younger adult.
   b. are far more limited than for the younger person.
   c. are much more difficult to access.
   d. are minimal.

10. When dilating a vein for venipuncture in an elderly person
    a. it may be better not to use a tourniquet; if a tourniquet is used, apply it loosely over the patient's sleeve.
    b. tap the vein vigorously to engorge it.
    c. use a great deal of friction when cleaning with alcohol to increase heat and dilate the vein.
    d. all of the above.

11. When performing venipuncture, the nurse should
    a. use the thumb of the nondominant hand to apply skin traction distal to the vein.
    b. use the third finger of the nondominant hand to stabilize the vein 2 to 3 inches above the venipuncture site to stabilize the vein and prevent it from rolling.
    c. not let the cannula hub abut the entry site, as the pressure could cause laceration of the skin or expansion of the cannulation site.
    d. all of the above.

12. When selecting an ONC for delivery of 75 ml/hr of a nonirritating infusate into a dorsal metacarpal vein of an elderly patient, the nurse should use a(n)
    a. 18 ga., 1½ in. cannula.
    b. 20 ga., 1½ in. cannula.
    c. 22 ga., 1 in. cannula.
    d. 24 ga., ¾ in. cannula.

13. When applying a dressing, the nurse should
    a. protect the skin by applying a skin polymer solution and a transparent semipermeable dressing.
    b. use minimal (and only hypoallergenic) tape or paper tape.
    c. stabilize the IV site to prevent tension on the catheter caused by the tubing.
    d. all of the above.

14. Frequent monitoring of the IV site is extremely important in the elderly person, because
    a. age-related neurologic changes can reduce tactile sensation, allowing infiltration or phlebitis to become severe before the patient notices any discomfort.
    b. old people always pull at their IVs.
    c. the veins of elderly people always rupture, causing infiltration.
    d. all of the above.

15. The potential for fluid volume overload is a major problem for an elderly person on IV therapy. The nurse can best safeguard the patient against this by
    a. using an EID and monitoring the IV hourly.
    b. using a small-bore cannula.
    c. using a volume control chamber and monitoring the IV.
    d. all of the above.

CHEMOTHERAPY

True/False

_____ 1. Cancer cells can arise anywhere in the body and fail to follow normal cell reproduction and growth patterns.

_____ 2. Most antineoplastic agents disrupt DNA synthesis.

_____ 3. Antineoplastic drugs are classified into one group of cell-cycle-specific agents.

_____ 4. Cancer treatment often involves combination chemotherapy in the attempt to destroy cells at different phases in the reproductive and growth cycle.

_____ 5. The safest method for antineoplastic drug preparation is to do it in a clean medication or utility room away from other people and supplies.

_____ 6. The G_1 phase of the cell cycle (postmiotic) is an active growth stage, preceding DNA synthesis, in which enzymes that are necessary for DNA synthesis are produced.

_____ 7. During the G_0 phase, the cell may enter a resting period in which all of the cell's activities occur except for those related to reproduction and growth.

_____ 8. During the S phase of the cell cycle, the alkylating agents are most effective.

_____ 9. During the M phase of the cell cycle, when the cell divides into two identical cells, the plant alkaloids are most effective.

_____ 10. The antineoplastic antibiotics are cell cycle nonspecific and bind with DNA to inhibit DNA and RNA synthesis.

_____ 11. The hormonal antineoplastic agents are cell cycle nonspecific and affect both resting and dividing cells, interfering with DNA replication.

_____ 12. Treatment with the nitrosureas acts to decrease growth fractions of cancer cells are usually palliative and not cytotoxic or curative.

_____ 13. All antineoplastic agents have toxic effects on the gastrointestinal system and cause severe nausea, vomiting, and stomatitis in the patient.

_____ 14. When preparing chemotherapy agents for administration to the patient, the nurse should wear powder-free, disposable surgical gloves.

_____ 15. Items contaminated with chemotherapeutic agents, such as needles, syringes, filters, tubings, and IV containers, must always be disposed of in plastic, puncture-proof, shatter-proof, closable hazardous waste containers.

_____ 16. Patient consent forms for chemotherapy must be signed only by patients in outpatient settings or in the home.

_____ 17. When initiating chemotherapy, patient/family teaching should include a discussion of the types of side effects the patient may be expected to experience and identify means of coping with these problems.

_____ 18. When teaching the patient about the side effect of alopecia, the nurse should tell him that his hair will probably never grow back.

_____ 19. Scheduling a patient's chemotherapy depends on two major factors: tumor growth patterns and the patient's recovery time.

_____ 20. A vesicant is an agent that causes blistering or tissue damage.

_____ 21. Administration of an irritant may result in itching, aching, a sensation of tightness, or phlebitis at the site of injection or along the vein track.

Multiple Choice

22. The most dangerous reaction to chemotherapy is
    a. nausea and vomiting.
    b. alopecia.
    c. malaise.
    d. myelosuppression.

23. The cells most commonly affected by the effects of chemotherapy are those of
    a. the bone marrow.
    b. the mucous membranes and GI tract.
    c. the hair follicles.
    d. all of the above.

24. Mood swings in the patient receiving chemotherapy are typically related to
    a. restlessness.
    b. nausea and vomiting.
    c. depression and fear of illness and dying.
    d. the side effects of the toxic drugs.

25. The nurse who administers chemotherapy must take precautions
    a. to prevent venous trauma and infiltration.
    b. to prevent nausea and vomiting.
    c. to determine the rate of drug administration.
    d. all of the above.

26. When administering Taxol to a patient, the nurse must know that
    a. it should never be diluted.
    b. it should not come into contact with Teflon® or plasticized PVC equipment.
    c. filters should never be used.
    d. all of the above.

27. When extravasation involves doxorubicin, mechlorethamine, or vinca plant alkaloids, protocols reported to be effective involve the administration of
    a. topical dimethyl sulfoxide.
    b. local steroid injections.
    c. sodium bicarbonate.
    d. any of the above. A definitive antidote has not been identified.

28. The best immediate treatment for the extravasation of doxorubicin is
    a. to apply ice to the site for 30 minutes to 12 hours.
    b. to discontinue the IV line and apply ice to the site for 30 minutes to 10 hours and intermittently for up to 7 days.
    c. to discontinue the IV, apply ice for 30 minutes, then infiltrate the tissue with phentolamine (Regitine).
    d. none of the above.

29. For extravasation of mechlorethamine, the immediate treatment of choice is usually
    a. IV and subcutaneous administration of an isotonic thiosulfate solution, followed by cold compresses to the site.
    b. subcutaneous administration of thiosulfate.
    c. ice compresses.
    d. to discontinue the IV and leave the site alone.

30. For extravasation of vinblastine, vincristine, or vindesine, the protocol is to
    a. discontinue the IV and apply warm compresses.
    b. discontinue the IV, infiltrate the extravasation with hyaluronidase dissolved in NaCl, and apply ice.
    c. discontinue the IV, infiltrate the extravasation with hyaluronidase dissolved in NaCl, and apply warm compresses.
    d. discontinue the IV, infiltrate the extravasation with prescribed steroids, and apply ice.

31. Which of the following laboratory results would be consistent with thrombocytopenia from chemotherapy?
    a. Low WBC count.
    b. Low platelet count.
    c. Low RBC count.
    d. High platelet count.

32. The nurse should continuously assess a patient receiving chemotherapy for bone marrow depression, which can cause
    a. fatigue and night sweats.
    b. weight loss and poor skin turgor.
    c. ecchymosis and weakness.
    d. decreased urine output and elevated serum creatinine levels.

33. A secondary metabolic effect from chemotherapy for malignancies such as leukemia is
    a. hyperuricemia.
    b. hyperthyroidism.
    c. hyperinsulinism.
    d. vasopressin release.

34. The point at which the blood counts drop to their lowest level is known as
    a. suppression.
    b. resistance.
    c. nadir.
    d. toxicity.

35. The nurse should take special precautions when handling the urine of patients receiving
    a. cyclophosphamide (Cytoxan).
    b. doxorubicin (Adriamycin).
    c. plicamycin (Mithracin).
    d. vincristine (Oncovin).

36. Although nausea is a side effect of many chemotherapeutic agents, it is usually most severe with the administration of
    a. carmustine (BCNU).
    b. cisplatin (Platinol).
    c. fluorouracil (5-FU).
    d. methotrexate (MTX).

37. When administering cyclophosphamide in combination with another chemotherapeutic agent, the cyclophosphamide should be given
    a. before the other drug.
    b. following the other drug.
    c. before or after the other drug is administered.
    d. mixed with the other drug in an isotonic preparation.

38. The chemotherapeutic agent that would be most harmful if it extravasated is
    a. doxorubicin (Adriamycin).
    b. fluorouracil (5-FU).
    c. methotrexate (MTX).
    d. 6-thioguanine.

39. Impaired renal function mainly reduces the elimination of
    a. methotrexate.
    b. 6-thioguanine.
    c. tamoxifen.
    d. vinblastine.

40. Unusual renal toxicity is associated with administration of
    a. cisplatin.
    b. doxorubicin.
    c. fluorouracil.
    d. prednisone.

41. Cardiotoxicity is induced by
    a. bleomycin.
    b. cisplatin.
    c. doxorubicin.
    d. vinblastine.

42. Pulmonary fibrosis may be caused by
    a. bleomycin.
    b. cisplatin.
    c. doxorubicin.
    d. vinblastine.

43. Because of its low bone marrow toxicity, the agent often used in combination with chemotherapy is
    a. cyclophosphamide.
    b. cytosine arabinoside.
    c. nitrogen mustard.
    d. vincristine.

44. Toxicity to the heart can result from excessive doses of
    a. cisplatin and bleomycin.
    b. daunorubicin and doxorubicin.
    c. methotrexate and 5-fluorouracil.
    d. vinblastine and vincristine.

Answers to Study Questions

Chapter 1: Introduction to Intravenous Infusion Therapy

The Nursing Process

1. g
2. c
3. h
4. a
5. j
6. b
7. e
8. i
9. d
10. f

General Concepts Regarding IV Therapy

1. d
2. False. See number 4.
3. True
4. True
5. False. The RN holds the first line of responsibility for IV therapy based on the dictates of the state in which she is licensed and on the employer's policies. The RN may delegate nursing tasks, but is responsible for appropriate delegation, must supervise the performance of delegates, and is held accountable for safe outcomes.
6.–8. Any of the following:
   - emergency access route for medications, fluids, and anesthetics
   - rapid systemic administration of a drug or fluid
   - multiple accesses to the circulation with one device
   - access route for an unconscious person or one unable to take oral medications
   - route of choice for products that cannot be absorbed by any other route
   - route of choice for products that are irritating to body tissues, such as chemotherapy drugs.

9.–11. Any of the following:
   - allergic reactions are immediate
   - potential for fatal reaction or overdose due to immediate absorption
   - skin barrier broken: potential for infection
   - transmission of HIV or hepatitis viruses

Chapter 2: Fluid and Electrolyte Fundamentals Related to Intravenous Infusion Therapy

Fundamental Concepts of Fluid and Electrolyte Balance

1. c	19. x	37. d
2. a	20. c	38. e
3. c	21. g	39. n
4. b	22. f	40. l
5. c	23. k	41. m
6. a	24. a	42. f
7. c	25. s	43. g
8. d	26. w	44. a
9. d	27. d	45. j
10. c	28. o	46. Sodium
11. c	29. j	47. Potassium
12. i	30. l	48. Chloride
13. m	31. u	49. sodium-potassium pump
14. n	32. b	50. Aldosterone
15. v	33. k	51. antidiuretic hormone (ADH)
16. z	34. c	52. b
17. r	35. h	53. c
18. b	36. i	54. a

Clinical Manifestations of Fluid and Electrolyte Imbalances

Potassium Imbalances

1. True	9. True	18. a
2. False. K leaves the cells.	10. True	19. b
3. True	11. True	20. b
4. True	12. True	21. a
5. False	13. True	22. a
6. True	14. True	23. a
7. False. Metabolic alkalosis promotes K movement to the ICF.	15. a	24. b
	16. b	25. a
8. True	17. a	26. b
		27. b

Sodium Imbalances

1. True	8. False	15. b
2. True	9. True	16. b
3. True	10. True	17. a
4. False	11. True	18. a
5. True	12. False	19. a
6. True	13. a	20. a
7. False	14. a	

Calcium Imbalances

1. False. Vitamin D is needed for calcium absorption.
2. False. The parathyroid glands regulate serum calcium levels.
3. True
4. True
5. True
6. a
7. a
8. b
9. a
10. a
11. a
12. a
13. b
14. b
15. b

Magnesium Imbalances

1. True
2. True
3. True
4. False. Magnesium contracts heart muscle.
5. True
6. b
7. b
8. a
9. a
10. b
11. b
12. a
13. a

Phosphorus Imbalances

1. True
2. True
3. False. Phosphorus is important for vitamin B utilization.
4. True. TPN is a phosphate-free or phosphate-poor solution. Also, if the TPN is administered too rapidly, (concentrated glucose and protein), the phosphorus shifts from the serum into the cells.
5. False. Phosphorus deficits can occur with excessive use of aluminum, calcium, and magnesium antacids.
6. a
7. b
8. b
9. a
10. b
11. a
12. a

Chloride Imbalances

1. True
2. True
3. True
4. False. Hypochloremic alkalosis.
5. True
6. True
7. b
8. a
9. a
10. b
11. a

Concepts of Acid-Base Balance

1. buffer system
2. bicarbonate-carbonic acid buffer system
3. phosphate buffer system
4. hemoglobin-oxyhemoglobin buffer system
5. protein buffer system
6. chloride shift
7. ion exchange regulatory mechanism
8. respiratory regulatory mechanism
9. renal regulatory mechanism for pH control
10. pH
11. $PaCO_2$
12. HCO_3 of the arterial blood gas (ABG)
13. base excess (BE) of the ABG
14. serum CO_2
15. pH
16. $PaCO_2$
17. pH
18. HCO_3
19. base excess (BE) of the ABG
20. serum CO_2

Clinical Manifestations and Treatment of Acid-Base Imbalances

1. b
2. d
3. c
4. a
5. d
6. a
7. c
8. d
9. b
10. b
11. d
12. a
13. True
14. True
15. True
16. False

Chapter 3: Legal Implications of Intravenous Infusion Therapy

Legal Considerations

1. True
2. True
3. False. Malpractice
4. False. Negligence

5. True
6. assault
7. battery
8. false imprisonment

9. abandonment
10. *respondeat superior* or the *captain of the ship doctrine*

Chapter 4: Infection Control and Safety Measures Related to Intravenous Infusion Therapy

Infection Control Principles

1. c
2. a
3. b
4. d

5. b
6. d
7. c
8. d

9. d
10. d
11. b
12. d

Chapter 5: Risks, Complications, and Adverse Reactions Associated with Intravenous Infusion Therapy

Complications of IV Therapy

1. h
2. c
3. d
4. e
5. f

6. b
7. g
8. i
9. a
10. c

11. c
12. b
13. b
14. d
15. d

Chapter 6: Intravenous Infusion Preparations

IV Infusion Preparations

1. a
2. b
3. c
4. a
5. b
6. c
7. a
8. b
9. b

10. a
11. c
12. c
13. a
14. c
15. b
16. a
17. c
18. a

19. c
20. a
21. c
22. c
23. a
24. c
25. b

Chapter 7: Patient Preparation and Site Selection for Peripheral Intravenous Infusion Therapy

Patient Preparation, Delivery and Care

1. d
2. c
3. d
4. c
5. c
6. c
7. d
8. a
9. c
10. b
11. b
12. b
13. d
14. a
15. a
16. b

17. a
18. d
19. c
20. a
21. d
22. True
23. False
24. False. The cannula size should allow for adequate blood flow.
25. False
26. True
27. True
28. True
29. False. Check for a blood return first and ensure patency with normal saline before medication is administered.

30. False. Ask the patient to state his name and check his identification band.
31. True
32. True
33. False. A needle may be used for only one stick.
34. False. The same nurse should try only two (or three) times at most.
35. False. Armboards should be used only when absolutely necessary.
36. True
37. False. Alcohol enhances bleeding. A gauze should be used.

Chapter 8: Equipment and Supplies Employed in the Preparation and Administration of Intravenous Infusion Therapy

IV Therapy Equipment and Supplies

1. False. A label should be affixed to the bag. A ballpoint pen could puncture the container and the ink of an indelible marker may leach into the plastic and contaminate the infusate.
2. False. The drop factor is the number of drops that equals 1 ml.

3. True
4. True
5. True
6. True
7. False. It is a TNC. The ONC is a flexible cannula that encases a steel needle or stylet.
8. False. A TSM dressing or gauze dressing may be used.

9. True
10. True
11. False. There is a lockout mechanism to prevent overdose.
12. False. The IV container should hang 36 inches above the site.
13. True
14. True

Chapter 9: Delivery, Care, Maintenance, and Discontinuation of Intravenous Infusion Therapy

1. d
2. b

3. a
4. a

5. d

Chapter 10: Mathematical Calculations for the Administration, Regulation, and Maintenance of Intravenous Infusion Therapy

Mathematical Calculations

1. 10 gtt/min.
2. 50 gtt/min.
3. 25 gtt/min.
4. 33 gtt/min.
5. a. 65 ml/dose
   b. 195 ml/24 hr
   c. 65 gtt/min
   d. 2 ml
   e. 48 ml
6. a. 20 ml/hr
   b. 5 gtt/min.
7. 2,240 hours (16 hours and 40 minutes from 0600 hours)
8. a. 0.5 ml/min.
   b. 30 ml/hr
   c. 5 gtt/min.
9. a. 240 ml/day
   b. 40 gtt/min.
   c. 1,760 ml/day
   d. 20 gtt/min.
   e. Set the regular IV of NS at 20 gtts/min. Every 8 hours, switch to the gentamycin IVPB at 40 gtt/min. for 30 minutes.
10. a. 60 gtt/ml
    b. 5 ml
    c. 25 ml
    d. 50 gtt/min
    e. one

Chapter 11: Pharmacological Principles Related to the Preparation and Administration of Intravenous Medications

Pharmacology

1. b
2. a
3. b
4. b
5. a
6. c
7. d
8. d
9. a
10. b
11. b
12. b
13. c
14. a
15. a
16. b
17. b
18. d
19. c
20. d
21. d
22. d
23. b
24. d
25. a
26. b
27. a
28. c
29. d
30. d
31. c
32. a
33. b
34. c
35. d
36. a

Chapter 12: Central and Peripherally Placed Vascular Access Devices and Advanced Medication Delivery Systems

Advanced Vascular Access

1. True
2. True
3. False. Access from the right is preferred.
4. False. SVC syndrome is a contraindication. In SVC syndrome there is partial occlusion of the SVC and interference of venous blood flow from the head and neck to the heart.
5. False. The tip should terminate in the SCV, within 3 to 4 cm for the right atrial-SVC junction.
6. True
7. False. Air embolism.
8. True
9. True
10. False. There is perforation of the visceral pleura with air accumulation in the pleural cavity.
11. True
12. True
13. True

14. False. Dressings are to be changed when they become damp, soiled, loose, or if inspection of the site or catheter change is necessary; ointment use is not recommended.
15. True
16. False. Never use a hemostat, as it may cut the line. Clamp it off with the attached slide clamp or with an atraumatic, nontoothed cannula clamp.
17. a
18. d
19. c
20. b
21. d
22. d
23. c
24. b
25. d
26. b
27. b
28. c
29. c
30. a
31. b
32. c
33. b
34. b
35. d
36. c
37. a
38. c
39. d
40. a
41. b
42. d
43. c
44. a
45. True
46. False. Only noncoring, nonbarbed needles are to be used.
47. True
48. True
49. False. The CVP is the force of venous blood return within the SVC-Rt. atrial junction.
50. False. The patient should be supine.
51. True
52. True
53. True
54. Tell the patient to take a deep breath, hold it, and bear down, as if pushing to have a bowel movement.

Chapter 13: Intravenous Nutritional Support

IV Nutritional Support

1. True
2. False. One to three weeks or longer.
3. True
4. False. Proteins are less efficiently burned.
5. True
6. False. It can result in diuresis, hyperglycemia, and hyperosmolar coma.
7. True
8. True
9. False. The infusate must be discarded.
10. False. The rate should not exceed 2.5 g/kg/day.
11. True
12. False. Patients with liver disease have low levels of branched chain amino acids and high levels of aromatic amino acids, making them intolerant of crystalline amino acid preparations.
13. True
14. True
15. False. It may be adjusted no more than 10%.
16. True
17. True
18. True
19. True
20. True

Chapter 14: Blood and Blood Product Administration

Blood-Blood Products

1. RBC antigens
2. antibodies
3. ABO incompatibility
4. homologous blood
5. autologous blood
6. whole blood
7. packed red blood cells
8. transfusion or pregnancy
9. ABO incompatibility
10. O
11. AB
12. True
13. True
14. False. It should not exceed 4 hours.
15. False
16. True
17. True
18. False. FFP is used to increase the level of clotting factors in patients with a demonstrated deficiency.
19. True
20. False. A 19-ga. or larger cannula should be used.
21. False
22. False. It may be stored for up to 35 days.

23. True
24. True
25. True
26. True
27. Vital signs taken and recorded: immediately prior to the start of the transfusion, at the start of the transfusion for three times at 5-minute intervals, at 30 minutes, and every 30 minutes until the transfusion is complete. The administration rate should not exceed 50 ml during the first 15 minutes and the nurse should stay with the patient during this time.
28. An acute hemolytic transfusion reaction is one in which hemolysis occurs when antibodies in the recipient's plasma attach to antigens on the donor's RBCs.

29.
   - Stop the transfusion immediately, but do not discontinue the IV line.
   - Connect new IV tubing to the cannula hub and KVO with 0.9% normal saline.
   - Stay with the patient.
   - Monitor vital signs.
   - Notify the physician.
   - Notify the lab to collect blood and urine samples specified by the blood services department.
   - Verify that the correct transfusion was given by using tags and numbers on the blood component containers and the patient's blood ID bracelet.
   - Send the blood bag, with its administration set and all attached labels, to the blood transfusion service.
   - Document all assessment data, nursing interventions, and patient responses in the medical record.
   - Fill out a transfusion reaction report.
30. Stored blood contains citrate, which binds with free calcium.
31. d
32. e
33. c
34. a
35. b
36. f

Chapter 15: Intravenous Infusion Therapy for the Pediatric Patient

Pediatrics

1. True
2. False. The smaller child is at greater risk.
3. True
4. True
5. False
6. True
7. True
8. True
9. True. The child may vomit and aspirate.
10. True
11. False
12. True
13. True
14. True
15. True
16. False. Serum sodium level.
17. False. Use NS or LR at 20 ml/kg until BP, capillary refill, pulses, and temperature of extremities improve.
18. True
19. False. Replacement is over 48 hours. A rapid administration will cause the serum sodium concentration to fall abruptly, causing rapid fluid shifts and potential neurologic complications.
20. False. BSA accounts for the patient's height and weight, thus making it a more accurate method of calculating fluid maintenance needs.
21. d
22. c
23. a
24. d
25. b
26. d
27. c
28. d
29. d

Chapter 16: Intravenous Infusion Therapy for the Elderly Patient

The Elderly

1. d
2. c
3. d
4. b
5. d
6. a
7. b
8. a
9. a
10. a
11. d
12. d
13. d
14. a
15. a

Chemotherapy

1. True
2. True
3. False. Antineoplastic agents are classified in two groups: cell-cycle-specific (CCS) and cell-cycle-nonspecific (CCNS)
4. True
5. False. Antineoplastic preparation should be done under a laminar air flow hood that has vertical ventilation to the outside to prevent exposure to harmful chemicals from aerosolization.
6. True
7. True
8. False. The antimetabolites are most effective during the S phase of the cell cycle.
9. True
10. True
11. False. This describes the alkylating agents.
12. False. This describes the hormonal agents.
13. False
14. True
15. True
16. False. Patient consent must always be obtained.
17. True
18. False. The hair will start to grow back about eight weeks after chemotherapy is completed, but it may be of a different color or texture.
19. True
20. True
21. True
22. d
23. d
24. c
25. a
26. b
27. d
28. b
29. a
30. c
31. b
32. c
33. a
34. c
35. a
36. b
37. c
38. a
39. a
40. a
41. c
42. a
43. d
44. b

Intravenous Infusion Therapy Nursing Skills Checklists

Skill 9-1 | Tourniquet Application

Name _____ Date _____ Instructor _____

ACTION TAKEN	COMPLETED SUCCESSFULLY	DID NOT COMPLETE	NOTES
1. Check the physician's order.			
2. Introduce yourself to the patient.			
3. Identify the patient by checking the wrist band against the doctor's order and asking the patient, if conscious, to state his/her name.			
4. Verify the allergy status of the patient.			
5. Explain the proposed procedure in terms the patient can understand.			
6. Carry out proper hand hygiene.			
7. Gather equipment.			
8. Provide for privacy.			
9. To correctly apply the tourniquet, hold one end in the dominant hand and the other end in the nondominant hand.			
10. Encircle the extremity 3 to 4 inches above the venipuncture site. Lay one length over the other, close to the skin, as if tying a knot. The end of the tubing in the nurse's dominant hand is not brought through completely (as it would be if tying a knot) but tucked under the other segment.			
11. Assess for a pulse distal to the application site.			
12. To remove the tourniquet, pull the end of the tucked portion.			

Skill 9-2 | Primary Infusion Setup

Name _____ Date _____ Instructor _____

ACTION TAKEN	COMPLETED SUCCESSFULLY	DID NOT COMPLETE	NOTES
1. Check the physician's order.			
2. Introduce yourself to the patient.			
3. Identify the patient by checking the wrist band against the doctor's order and asking the patient, if conscious, to state his/her name.			
4. Verify the allergy status of the patient.			
5. Explain the proposed procedure in terms the patient can understand.			
6. Carry out proper hand hygiene.			
7. Gather the ordered IV fluids, appropriate tubing, and a clean IV pole for set up in an uncontaminated area away from the patient's room. If a pole-mounted EID (electronic infusion device) is needed, check that it is in proper working order and that the batteries are charged.			
8. Check the IV fluid for type and amount, expiration date, clarity, and leaks in the bag or bottle. For plastic infusate containers, remove the outer tear-off wrap, following the manu-facturer's directions. (This will have been removed in the phar-macy if an admixture has been ordered.)			

Skill 9-2 | *(continued)*

Name _____ Date _____ Instructor _____

ACTION TAKEN	COMPLETED SUCCESSFULLY	DID NOT COMPLETE	NOTES
9. Check for the expiration date on the IV tubing container and open it. Ensure that the sterile cover is over the infusate spike and the distal end where the IV cannula connects are intact. (If the cannula end has a "breathable" attachment, it will not have a cover over it.) Once the set is removed from its package, keep it coiled and contained above waist level.			
10. Close the roller clamp on the administration set tubing (but not the slide clamps, if there are any).			
11. Hang the IV fluids that are in plastic bags on an IV pole. Place glass containers on a clean counter.			
12. To spike a plastic bag: a. Secure the neck of the bag with the thumb and index finger of the non-dominant hand and remove the sterile cover on the administration set port with the dominant hand. b. Remove the sterile cover from the tubing administration set spike. Do not touch the spike itself.			

(continues)

Skill 9-2 | (continued)

Name _____ Date _____ Instructor _____

ACTION TAKEN	COMPLETED SUCCESSFULLY	DID NOT COMPLETE	NOTES
c. To spike the bag, grasp the middle of the outside surface of the administration port, holding it vertically between the thumb and index and third finger of the non-dominant hand. Holding the finger-guard area below the spiked portion of the administration set, insert the spike into the administration port, using a straight, twisting motion.			
To spike a glass bottle... a. Be sure to use the appropriate administration set. A vented set must be used if there is no internal venting system in the bottle. b. With the bottle standing upright on a level surface, hold it in place with the nondominant hand and peel off the outer aluminum band from the top of the bottle with the dominant hand. c. Remove the rubber disk stopper, which seals the vacuum and sterile lid of the bottle where the administration port sits. If an admixture has been instilled, the aluminum cap and rubber stopper will already have been removed in the pharmacy and sealed with a tamperproof closure,			

Skill 9-2 | *(continued)*

Name _____ Date _____ Instructor _____

ACTION TAKEN	COMPLETED SUCCESSFULLY	DID NOT COMPLETE	NOTES
which must be torn off before spiking. Do not touch the top of the bottle where the administration port or vent outlet sits. If it is touched, the top must be thoroughly wiped with a 70% alcohol solution prior to spiking. d. Remove the sterile cap from the spike and push it into the port with a straight (not twisting) movement. e. Suspend the bottle on the IV pole by the aluminum bale at the bottom of the container.			
13. Squeeze the drip chamber to allow it to fill $^1/_3$ to $^1/_2$ full or to the level of the manufacturer's imprinted marking on the chamber.			
14. Remove the sterile cap from the distal end of the administration set. Make sure to maintain the sterility of the cap. Prime the administration tubing by holding the distal end of the administration set over (but not touching) a basin, paper towel, or sink. Slowly open the roller clamp to purge air from the set. As the fluid approaches the check valve or any injection ports, invert those sites and tap on them to remove any trapped air.			

(continues)

Skill 9-2 | *(continued)*

Name _____ Date _____ Instructor _____

ACTION TAKEN	COMPLETED SUCCESSFULLY	DID NOT COMPLETE	NOTES
15. Once the infusate reaches the distal end of the administration set and there are no visible air pockets, the tubing can be clamped, recapped (if appropriate), and hung over the top of the IV pole for transport to the patient's room.			
16. Connectors and add-on devices may be added before or after priming, depending on the manufacturer's guidelines. The priming volume is stated on the packaging.			
17. Label the infusate container and the administration set with date and time per institutional policy.			
18. Adjust the height of the infusate container to approximately 36 inches above the intended IV insertion site.			

Skill 9-3 | Preparing the Infusion Site

Name _____ Date _____ Instructor _____

ACTION TAKEN	COMPLETED SUCCESSFULLY	DID NOT COMPLETE	NOTES
1. Check the physician's order.			
2. Introduce yourself to the patient.			
3. Identify the patient by checking the wrist band against the doctor's order and asking the patient, if conscious, to state his/her name.			
4. Verify the allergy status of the patient.			
5. Explain the proposed procedure in terms the patient can understand.			
6. Carry out proper hand hygiene.			
7. Gather all necessary equipment.			
8. Choose the most appropriate vein.			
9. Assess for intact, non-bruised skin.			
10. If excessive hair is present, clip short with scissors.			
11. Assess the patient for allergies.			
12. Cleanse the site with 70% isopropyl alcohol. Using friction, begin at the intended cannulation site and work outward 2 to 3 inches, in a concentric circle, for 20 to 30 seconds. Do not backtrack over a previously cleaned area. Allow the alcohol to air-dry. Do not blow on or fan the skin and do not wipe the alcohol off the area.			

(continues)

Skill 9-3 | *(continued)*

Name _____ Date _____ Instructor _____

ACTION TAKEN	COMPLETED SUCCESSFULLY	DID NOT COMPLETE	NOTES
13. Using the same directional movement, cleanse the site thoroughly with 2% aqueous chlorhexidine gluconate, povidone-iodine, or tincture of iodine. If tincture of iodine is used, the site should be wiped gently with a sterile gauze.			
14. Proceed with venipuncture.			

Skill 9-4 | Starting an IV Over-the-Needle Catheter

Name _____ Date _____ Instructor _____

ACTION TAKEN	COMPLETED SUCCESSFULLY	DID NOT COMPLETE	NOTES
1. Check the physician's order.			
2. Introduce yourself to the patient.			
3. Identify the patient by checking the wrist band against the doctor's order and asking the patient, if conscious, to state his/her name.			
4. Verify the allergy status of the patient.			
5. Explain the proposed procedure in terms the patient can understand.			
6. Carry out proper hand hygiene.			
7. Set up all the necessary supplies on the bedside stand or overbed table in the order in which they will be used. Cut any tape that will be needed. Inspect the ONC to be sure that the needle bevel is sharp and smooth. Read the manu-facturer's directions regarding inspection and manipulation of the ONC.			
8. Provide privacy.			
9. Elevate the bed level.			
10. Place the patient in a Fowler's or semi-Fowler's position with extremity intended for can-nulation below the level of the patient's heart.			
11. Protect the patient's clothing and bed-ding with protective underpad or towel.			

(continues)

Skill 9-4 | *(continued)*

Name _____ Date _____ Instructor _____

ACTION TAKEN	COMPLETED SUCCESSFULLY	DID NOT COMPLETE	NOTES
12. Apply the tourniquet and identify the most appropriate vein for cannulation, preferably in the nondominant hand (Figure 9-19). a. Select a vein, using the most distal vein first. b. Avoid bony prominences. c. Use the nondominant hand. d. Avoid areas of rash or broken skin.			
13. Remove the tourniquet, leaving it under the extremity.			
14. If there is an excessive amount of hair at the venipuncture site, clip the hair at the site. Do not shave the area.			
15. Antiseptically prepare the site according to policy (Figure 9-20).			
16. Don gloves.			
17. Apply tourniquet to occlude venous flow.			
18. Palpate for and ensure presence of a pulse distal to the tourniquet.			
19. Remove the needle cover and tell the patient that the needle is going to enter the vein.			

Skill 9-4 | *(continued)*

Name _____ Date _____ Instructor _____

ACTION TAKEN	COMPLETED SUCCESSFULLY	DID NOT COMPLETE	NOTES
20. Anchor the vein below the intended insertion site with gentle skin traction. Using the thumb of the nondominant hand, pull the skin taut.			
21. Hold the ONC by the needle hub flash chamber, *not* the color-coded hub of the catheter unit, with the bevel up.			
22. Entry of the over-the-needle catheter can be either via a direct or indirect method. For the direct-entry method, position the needle over the vein with the needle in the bevel-up position and pointing in the direction of the blood flow. In this method, the needle passes through the skin, over and directly into the vein in one maneuver. For the indirect entry method, position the needle in the bevel-up position and alongside the vein, pointing in the direction of the blood flow. In this method, the needle enters the skin, is maneuvered alongside the vein, and then enters the vein.			
23. Use a 15-degree angle for insertion into superficial veins and a 25- to 30-degree angle for insertion into deeper veins.			

(continues)

Skill 9-4 | *(continued)*

Name _____ Date _____ Instructor _____

ACTION TAKEN	COMPLETED SUCCESSFULLY	DID NOT COMPLETE	NOTES
24. Observe for flash-back of blood in the flash chamber. *Note:* Upon entry into the tunica adventitia (outer-most) layer of the vein, the nurse may feel a slight "pop" (or sensation of release of pressure), depen-ding on the brand of catheter used. Some of the newer types, such as those made with Vialon®, provide such a sharp, smooth insertion that there is little or no charac-teristic "pop" upon vein access			
25. Once the over-the-needle catheter is in the vein, lower the needle until it is almost flush with the skin to avoid puncturing the opposite vein wall, then advance the needle and catheter unit so that the cath-eter tip is in the cen-ter of the vein lumen.			
26. Advance the catheter, using one of the following techniques: • Advance the whole unit—needle and catheter—into the vein, then retract the needle. • Stabilize the needle-flash chamber and gradually advance the catheter off the needle, threading it into the vein lumen, until the desired length has been inserted. If the catheter does not thread smoothly or blood flow ceases, remove the cath-			

Skill 9-4 | *(continued)*

Name _____ Date _____ Instructor _____

ACTION TAKEN	COMPLETED SUCCESSFULLY	DID NOT COMPLETE	NOTES
eter and needle together, apply pressure to the site, and attempt venipuncture in another site, using a new device. • To use the **hooding** method, hold the catheter unit stationary and advance the catheter off the needle no more than $1/4$ inch, *hooding* the tip of the needle inside the catheter. If preferred, pull the needle back no more than $1/4$ inch to achieve the same result. Grasp the color-coded catheter hub and advance the hooded needle or catheter as a unit into the vein. When it is in place, remove the needle. • To use the **floating** method, the needle and catheter are advanced about halfway into the vein (verified by flashback), at which point the tourniquet and needle are removed. The cannula hub is then attached to the infusion tubing, the flow control clamp is slowly opened, and the infusion is started. The catheter is then *floated* into the vein with the infusate. *Note:* For this method to work well, the skin and vein must remain anchored with one hand. If anchoring is not maintained, the catheter may meet resistance from			

Skill 9-4 | (continued)

Name _____ Date _____ Instructor _____

ACTION TAKEN	COMPLETED SUCCESSFULLY	DID NOT COMPLETE	NOTES
skin traction at the insertion site.			
27. Release the tourniquet. Do not touch the end of the catheter hub or the IV insertion site. A sterile 2 × 2-inch gauze pad may be placed under the catheter hub.			
28. Remove the needle and dispose of it in the sharps container.			
29. Connect the infusion tubing with a gentle push-and-twist motion.			
30. Place a strip of paper tape over the tubing.			
31. Open the flow clamp and observe the insertion site and vessel pathway as the infusate freely enters the vessel. Adjust the flow rate.			
32. Remove the strip of paper tape.Dress the site per agency policy.			
33. Remove gloves and carry out proper hand hygiene.			
34. Label the site at the side of the dressing with the date, time, IV device used, and your initials.			
35. Label the infusion container and all administration sets that are used.			
36. Return the bed to the lowest position, lower the head of the bed (if appropriate for the patient), and raise the bedrails.			

Skill 9-5 | Starting an IV: Insertion of a Winged Infusion Set

Name _____ Date _____ Instructor _____

ACTION TAKEN	COMPLETED SUCCESSFULLY	DID NOT COMPLETE	NOTES
1. Check the physician's order.			
2. Introduce yourself to the patient.			
3. Identify the patient by checking the wrist band against the doctor's order and asking the patient, if conscious, to state his/her name.			
4. Verify the allergy status of the patient.			
5. Explain the proposed procedure in terms the patient can understand.			
6. Carry out proper hand hygiene.			
7. Gather equipment.			
8. Provide for privacy.			
9. Assess for an appropriate vein in the nondominant hand/arm. A vein should be chosen at the most distal site, working upward in a proximal direction.			
10. Apply the tourniquet; this should be 2 to 3 inches above the intended venipuncture site for most patients.			
11. Cleanse the skin with alcohol starting at the insertion site and working outward in a circular motion. Once the site is cleansed, do not retouch the site, unless with a sterile gloved finger or a gloved finger that has been prepped with 70% isopropyl alcohol.			

(continues)

Skill 9-5 | *(continued)*

Name _____ Date _____ Instructor _____

ACTION TAKEN	COMPLETED SUCCESSFULLY	DID NOT COMPLETE	NOTES
12. Cleanse the skin with 2% aqueous chlorhexidine gluconate, povidone-iodine, or agency-approved iodophor if the patient is not allergic.			
13. Don gloves while the iodophor is drying.			
The following method works well for patients who have well-developed, elastic veins, with good venous pressure.			
14. Hold the skin below the insertion site taut.			
15. Pick up the winged needle, holding it by the plastic wings, bevel up.			
16. Insert the needle with the bevel up at a 20- to 30-degree angle.			
17. Assess for retrograde blood flow into the tubing of the set.			
18. Apply a strip of paper tape across the wings.			
19. Allow retrograde blood flow to purge the tubing of air, then connect the medication syringe and administration set tubing for the infusion, or apply a male-adapter plug as appropriate and instill a saline lock.			
20. Apply the appropriate dressing.			
21. Remove the tourniquet.			
22. Write (to the side of the dressing or on a piece of tape or labeling) the date, time, needle size (length and gauge), and your initials.			
23. Provide patient teaching.			

Skill 9-5 | *(continued)*

Name _____ Date _____ Instructor _____

ACTION TAKEN	COMPLETED SUCCESSFULLY	DID NOT COMPLETE	NOTES
24. Make the patient comfortable.			
25. Document the procedure in the medical record in the nurse's notes and appropriate infusion flow sheets. If medications are administered, document in the MAR.			
A variation in technique can be used when it is anticipated that backflow of blood into the winged set tubing will be sluggish.			
1. Attach a syringe containing 3 to 5 ml of normal saline to the winged infusion set and prime the tubing and the needle.			

Skill 9-6 | Adding Medication to an Infusion Container

Name _____ Date _____ Instructor _____

ACTION TAKEN	COMPLETED SUCCESSFULLY	DID NOT COMPLETE	NOTES
1. Check the physician's order.			
2. Introduce yourself to the patient.			
3. Identify the patient by checking the wrist band against the doctor's order and asking the patient, if conscious, to state his/her name.			
4. Verify the allergy status of the patient.			
5. Explain the proposed procedure in terms the patient can understand.			
6. Carry out proper hand hygiene.			
7. Gather equipment.			
8. Check the medication for the name, dosage, expiration date, appropriate appearance, and the integrity of the container.			
9. Draw up the medication dose as prescribed.			
10. Clamp the tubing on the infusate administration tubing.			
11. Remove the infusion container from the IV pole.			
12. Swab the injection port on the infusate container with the alcohol.			
13. Inject the medication into the injection port.			
14. Gently rock the infusion container back and forth.			
15. Hang the container on the IV pole.			
16. Discard the used syringe into the sharps container.			

Skill 9-6 | *(continued)*

Name _____ Date _____ Instructor _____

ACTION TAKEN	COMPLETED SUCCESSFULLY	DID NOT COMPLETE	NOTES
17. Open the clamp on the IV tubing and regulate the rate.			
18. Stay with the patient for five minutes.			
19. Affix a label to the infusate container to indicate the addition of the drug. The label should contain the following: a. Name of drug b. Dose of drug c. Date d. Time the drug was added e. Amount of infusate in container when drug was added. f. Expiration time g. Nurse's name			
20. Carry out proper hand hygiene.			
21. Document in the MAR.			

Skill 9-7 | IV Piggyback

Name _____ Date _____ Instructor _____

ACTION TAKEN	COMPLETED SUCCESSFULLY	DID NOT COMPLETE	NOTES
1. Check the physician's order.			
2. Introduce yourself to the patient.			
3. Identify the patient by checking the wrist band against the doctor's order and asking the patient, if conscious, to state his/her name.			
4. Verify the allergy status of the patient.			
5. Explain the proposed procedure in terms the patient can understand.			
6. Carry out proper hand hygiene.			
7. Provide privacy.			
8. Obtain the medication and verify that it is correct and compatible with the current infusate, and check the expiration date. If the medication is refrigerated, it should be removed from the refrigerator 20 to 30 minutes before administration. If the medication is stored at room temperature, it should be opened immediately before administration. Set up all the necessary supplies.			
9. Don gloves.			
10. Open the sterile container with the secondary medication administration set.			
11. Clamp the secondary medication administration set and spike the medication container without contaminating it.			

Skill 9-7 | *(continued)*

Name _____ Date _____ Instructor _____

ACTION TAKEN	COMPLETED SUCCESSFULLY	DID NOT COMPLETE	NOTES
12. Do not fill the drip chamber and do not prime the tubing in the conventional manner.			
13. Swab the injection port directly below the check valve on the primary tubing with alcohol.			
14. Attach the secondary tubing to the cleansed injection port with the appropriate needle or needleless adapter.			
15. Lower the secondary bag below the level of the port it is tethered into while the primary infusate is still running.			
16. Slowly open the clamp on the secondary administration set and let the infusate from the primary line purge the secondary tubing of air (via retrograde fluid flow). When the drip chamber is one-half to two-thirds full, close the roller clamp on the secondary set.			
17. Attach the hanger, included in the secondary set, and attach it to the primary infusate container (making the primary container hang lower than the secondary container).			
18. Open the roller clamp on the secondary tubing and infuse the piggybacked infusate at the prescribed rate. Do not close the clamp on the primary infusion.			

(continues)

Skill 9-7 | *(continued)*

Name _____ Date _____ Instructor _____

ACTION TAKEN	COMPLETED SUCCESSFULLY	DID NOT COMPLETE	NOTES
19. Tape or affix a manufactured coupling device to secure the connection between the primary and secondary line.			
20. Assess the patient's response.			
21. Document the procedure.			

Skill 9-8 | IV Drug Administration into an Existing Infusion Line

Name _____ Date _____ Instructor _____

ACTION TAKEN	COMPLETED SUCCESSFULLY	DID NOT COMPLETE	NOTES
1. Check the physician's order.			
2. Introduce yourself to the patient.			
3. Identify the patient by checking the wrist band against the doctor's order and asking the patient, if conscious, to state his/her name.			
4. Verify the allergy status of the patient.			
5. Explain the proposed procedure in terms the patient can understand.			
6. Carry out proper hand hygiene.			
7. Provide privacy.			
8. Elevate the bed level.			
9. Assess vital signs and LOC and record.			
10. Set up all the necessary supplies on the bedside stand or overbed table in the order in which they will be used.			
11. Ascertain that the medication to be injected is compatible with the existing infusion. (If it is not compatible, the injection must be preceeded and followed with normal saline [or manufacturer-provided diluent] while the tubing above the injection site is stopped of infusate flow either by pinching off or with the inherent slide clamp on the tubing set.)			

(continues)

Skill 9-8 | *(continued)*

Name _____ Date _____ Instructor _____

ACTION TAKEN	COMPLETED SUCCESSFULLY	DID NOT COMPLETE	NOTES
12. Don gloves.			
13. Swab the injection port nearest to the client with the alcohol.			
14. Insert the needle or needless adapter into the port.			
15. Stop the primary infusion by pinching the administration set tubing closed just behind the injection port (or, if the administration set has one, close the slide clamp).			
16. Inject the medication according to directions.			
17. Remove the syringe or needle and dispose of it properly in the sharps container.			
18. Check to be sure the infusion is running at the appropriate rate and adjust as required to maintain the schedule.			
19. Return bed to normal position.			

Skill 9-9 | Using a Peripheral Intermittent Infusion Device

Name _____ Date _____ Instructor _____

ACTION TAKEN	COMPLETED SUCCESSFULLY	DID NOT COMPLETE	NOTES
1. Check the physician's order.			
2. Introduce yourself to the patient.			
3. Identify the patient by checking the wrist band against the doctor's order and asking the patient, if conscious, to state his/her name.			
4. Verify the allergy status of the patient.			
5. Explain the proposed procedure in terms the patient can understand.			
6. Carry out proper hand hygiene.			
7. Provide privacy.			
8. Elevate the bed level.			
9. Set up all the necessary supplies on the bedside stand or overbed table in the order in which they will be used.			
10. Don gloves.			
11. Open the sterile container with the intermittent injection plug, remove the sterile cap, attach the syringe of normal saline, prime the plug, and leave the syringe attached.			
12. Stop the infusion.			
13. Loosen the existing infusion tubing, remove the tubing, remove the sterile cap (if present) on the Luer-Lok®, and insert the intermittent infusion plug, screwing it securely onto the cannula hub.			

(continues)

Skill 9-9 | *(continued)*

Name _____ Date _____ Instructor _____

ACTION TAKEN	COMPLETED SUCCESSFULLY	DID NOT COMPLETE	NOTES
14. Open the slide clamp on the set, aspirate, and slowly inject the saline. Stop injecting when the last 0.5 ml of saline remains and immediately close the slide clamp on the set.			
15. Dispose of the syringe in the sharps container.			
16. Properly dispose of the infusate and tubing.			
17. Remove gloves and carry out proper hand hygiene.			
18. Document the procedure.			

Skill 9-10 | Discontinuation of an IV

Name _____ Date _____ Instructor _____

ACTION TAKEN	COMPLETED SUCCESSFULLY	DID NOT COMPLETE	NOTES
1. Check the physician's order.			
2. Introduce yourself to the patient.			
3. Identify the patient by checking the wrist band against the doctor's order and asking the patient, if conscious, to state his/her name.			
4. Verify the allergy status of the patient.			
5. Explain the proposed procedure in terms the patient can understand.			
6. Carry out proper hand hygiene.			
7. Gather supplies.			
8. Provide privacy.			
9. Elevate the bed.			
10. Clamp infusion tubing and turn off electronic infusion device (if appropriate).			
11. Cut or tear off a few strips of tape.			
12. Don gloves.			
13. Remove all tape and loosen the skin from the edges of the dressing over the IV site very carefully, using the stretch method or alcohol (or adhesive remover) method. Be careful not to pull on the cannula.			
14. While stabilizing the cannula hub, remove the entire IV dressing, moving in the direction of the IV device, not away from it.			

(continues)

Skill 9-10 | *(continued)*

Name _____ Date _____ Instructor _____

ACTION TAKEN	COMPLETED SUCCESSFULLY	DID NOT COMPLETE	NOTES
15. Place a 2 x 2-inch sterile gauze (not alcohol) over the IV insertion site and apply gentle pressure while grasping the cannula hub and removing the catheter with one smooth movement.			
16. Place the catheter on the paper towel.			
17. Elevate the extremity and apply firm, gentle pressure to the IV site for 60 seconds, or until there is no bleeding.			
18. Assess the site and apply tape firmly over the gauze. If the patient is undergoing anticoagulation therapy or has a bleeding disorder, a larger pressure dressing may be needed.			
19. Examine the removed catheter.			
20. Dispose of the IV device in the sharps container.			
21. Return the bed to the lowest position and raise the bedrails.			
22. Recheck the IV site.			
23. Document the procedure.			

Skill 9-11 | Medication Administration by Bolus Delivery

Name _____ Date _____ Instructor _____

ACTION TAKEN	COMPLETED SUCCESSFULLY	DID NOT COMPLETE	NOTES
1. Check the physician's order.			
2. Introduce yourself to the patient.			
3. Identify the patient by checking the wrist band against the doctor's order and asking the patient, if conscious, to state his/her name.			
4. Verify the allergy status of the patient.			
5. Explain the proposed procedure in terms the patient can understand.			
6. Carry out proper hand hygiene.			
7. Draw the medication up in a syringe.			
8. Change the needle, attaching the smallest one that will deliver the ordered medication yet accommodate the patient's vein.			
9. Perform any preadministration nursing interventions, such as taking vital signs or performing neurologic or cardiovascular assessments.			
10. Cut or tear one 4-inch strip of tape and open the 2 × 2-inch gauze without contaminating it.			
11. Apply the tourniquet and engorge the vein.			

(continues)

Skill 9-11 | *(continued)*

Name _____ Date _____ Instructor _____

ACTION TAKEN	COMPLETED SUCCESSFULLY	DID NOT COMPLETE	NOTES
12. Prep the site using appropriate antiseptics. Work in a circular motion from the intended venipuncture site outward, extending to 2 inches. Do not backtrack. Allow the site to dry.			
13. Don gloves.			
14. Access the vein and pull back on the plunger to verify placement in the vein.			
15. Remove the tourniquet.			
16. Inject the medication.			
17. Place the 2 × 2-inch gauze over the injection site and remove the needle.			
18. Elevate the extremity until bleeding stops and apply tape over the gauze.			
19. Dispose of the syringe properly in the sharps container to prevent needle-stick injury and adhere to safety guidelines.			
20. Remove gloves and carry out proper hand hygiene.			
21. Stay with the patient and assess his response to the medication.			
22. Perform any postadministration nursing interventions associated with the medication.			

Skill 9-12 | Medication Administration by Bolus Using a Winged Administration Set

Name _____ Date _____ Instructor _____

ACTION TAKEN	COMPLETED SUCCESSFULLY	DID NOT COMPLETE	NOTES
1. Check the physician's order.			
2. Introduce yourself to the patient.			
3. Identify the patient by checking the wrist band against the doctor's order and asking the patient, if conscious, to state his/her name.			
4. Verify the allergy status of the patient.			
5. Explain the proposed procedure in terms the patient can understand.			
6. Carry out proper hand hygiene.			
7. Draw the medication up into a syringe and cap the needle.			
8. Draw up 2 to 3 ml of normal saline (0.9%) in each of two separate syringes and cap the needles.			
9. Attach a winged administration set with the smallest needle that will deliver the drug and be appropriate for the patient's vein to one of the syringes containing 0.9% saline and prime the tubing and needle on the set.			
10. Perform any preadministration nursing interventions, such as taking vital signs or performing neurologic or cardiovascular assessments.			

(continues)

Skill 9-12 | *(continued)*

Name _____ Date _____ Instructor _____

ACTION TAKEN	COMPLETED SUCCESSFULLY	DID NOT COMPLETE	NOTES
11. Cut or tear two 4-inch strips of tape and open the sterile 2 × 2-inch gauze without contaminating it.			
12. Apply the tourniquet to restrict venous blood flow and engorge the vein so venous access is facilitated.			
13. Prep the site using a circular motion extending 2 inches outward from the intended venipuncture site. Do not backtrack. Allow the site to dry.			
14. Don gloves.			
15. Remove the tourniquet to reestablish venous blood flow and facilitate IV medication delivery.			
16. Using the syringe attached to the 0.9% saline, insert the winged needle. Verify placement by retracting the plunger. If it's in the vein, flatten the administration set wings and place a strip of tape over them, securing the set to the patient's extremity. Slowly inject the 0.9% saline.			
17. Disconnect the empty syringe and attach the syringe containing the medication to the administration tubing.			
18. Inject the medication over the prescribed time.			

Skill 9-12 | *(continued)*

Name _____ Date _____ Instructor _____

ACTION TAKEN	COMPLETED SUCCESSFULLY	DID NOT COMPLETE	NOTES
19. When the medication has been administered, disconnect the empty syringe and attach the second syringe of 0.9% saline to the administration set tubing. Inject the normal saline.			
20. Remove the strip of tape and place the 2 × 2-inch gauze on the injection site and remove the needle.			
21. Elevate the extremity and apply pressure to the injection site until bleeding stops. Apply the clean strip of tape over the gauze.			
22. Dispose of the syringes and the winged administration set properly in the sharps container to prevent needlestick injury and adhere to safety guidelines.			
23. Remove gloves and carry out proper hand hygiene to prevent the spread of infection.			
24. Stay with the patient and assess his response to the medication.			
25. Perform any postadministration nursing interventions.			

Skill 12-1 | CVC Dressing Change and Site Care

Name _____ Date _____ Instructor _____

ACTION TAKEN	COMPLETED SUCCESSFULLY	DID NOT COMPLETE	NOTES
1. Check the physician's order.			
2. Introduce yourself to the patient.			
3. Identify the patient by checking the wrist band against the doctor's order and asking the patient, if conscious, to state his/her name.			
4. Verify the allergy status of the patient.			
5. Explain the proposed procedure in terms the patient can understand.			
6. Carry out proper hand hygiene.			
7. Provide privacy.			
8. Elevate the bed level.			
9. Secure all necessary supplies.			
10. Carry out proper hand hygiene.			
11. Nurse and patient don masks.			
12. Don clean, disposable gloves.			
13. Gently remove the soiled dressing, maneuvering the skin from the dressing, in the direction of (toward) the catheter insertion site, rather than from the insertion site outward. Use the stretch method if the dressing is a transparent semipermeable membrane dressing. Do not touch the catheter insertion site.			
14. Examine the dressing for purulent drainage or foul odor.			

Skill 12-1 | *(continued)*

Name _____ Date _____ Instructor _____

ACTION TAKEN	COMPLETED SUCCESSFULLY	DID NOT COMPLETE	NOTES
15. Remove disposable gloves and carry out proper hand hygiene.			
16. Examine the catheter site for abnormalities, such as the following: a. catheter malposition or slippage b. erythema c. dilated vessels d. drainage (Notify physician and obtain specimen for culture and sensitivity [C & S], per agency policy.) e. induration f. loose or absent sutures (Notify physician or appropriate personnel regarding resuturing, or obtain Steri-Strips, per agency policy.) g. tenderness			
17. Remove outer plastic wrap from the kit and tape it to the bedside.			
18. Aseptically open the supplies.			
19. Don sterile gloves.			
20. Clean the CVC site slowly, using friction and moving from the insertion site outward (including the catheter and catheter junction hub), in a concentric circle, to include the full area that will be covered by the final dressing. The sequence for cleaning is as follows: a. Clean, first with the alcohol swabsticks, removing all debris. Use each side of each			

Skill 12-1 | *(continued)*

Name _____ Date _____ Instructor _____

ACTION TAKEN	COMPLETED SUCCESSFULLY	DID NOT COMPLETE	NOTES
swab. Use all three swabsticks. Do not use organic solvents, such as acetone or ether. b. Allow the alcohol to dry completely. c. Clean with 2% aqueous chlorhex-idine gluconate or the iodophor, using all that are in the dressing kit. Use each side of the swabstick.			
21. Apply an agency-approved dressing. If a transparent semipermeable membrane (TSM) dressing is used, be sure it molds around the catheter and junction of the hub (and do not stretch it during application).			
22. Remove the gloves and discard. Dispose of all used materials.			
23. Secure the CVC pigtails to the skin above the dressing site.			
24. To the side of the dressing, place the label with the date, time, and nurse's initials.			
25. Carry out proper hand hygiene.			
26. Document in the nurse's notes all assessment data regarding the site and condition of the removed dressing, appropriate intervention data, and the evaluation of the patient's response to the procedure.			

Skill 12-2 | Flushing the CVC

Name _____ Date _____ _____ Instructor _____

ACTION TAKEN	COMPLETED SUCCESSFULLY	DID NOT COMPLETE	NOTES
1. Check the physician's order.			
2. Introduce yourself to the patient.			
3. Identify the patient by checking the wrist band against the doctor's order and asking the patient, if conscious, to state his/her name.			
4. Verify the allergy status of the patient.			
5. Explain the proposed procedure in terms the patient can understand.			
6. Carry out proper hand hygiene.			
7. Gather equipment. Have all necessary saline and heparin drawn up before beginning the procedure.			
8. Provide for privacy.			
9. Set up equipment.			
10. Put on gloves.			
11. Cleanse the central venous catheter cap with 70% isopropyl alcohol followed by povidone-iodine (or per agency policy). Allow each solution to air dry.			
12. Attach a syringe containing normal saline to the CVC.			
13. Instruct the patient to perform the Valsalva maneuver and open the CVC clamp.			
14. Flush the line with normal saline. Use the pulsatile, push-pause method. Clamp the line.			

(continues)

Skill 12-2 | *(continued)*

Name _____ Date _____ Instructor _____

ACTION TAKEN	COMPLETED SUCCESSFULLY	DID NOT COMPLETE	NOTES
15. Attach the syringe with the heparin.			
16. Instruct the patient to perform the Valsalva maneuver and open the CVC clamp. Flush the line with the heparin. Clamp the line while infusing the last 0.5 ml of solution.			
17. Document the procedure.			

Skill 12-3 | Changing Injection Caps on the CVC

Name _____ Date _____ Instructor _____

ACTION TAKEN	COMPLETED SUCCESSFULLY	DID NOT COMPLETE	NOTES
1. Check the physician's order.			
2. Verify the schedule.			
3. Introduce yourself to the patient.			
4. Identify the patient by checking the wrist band against the doctor's order and asking the patient, if conscious, to state his/her name.			
5. Verify the allergy status of the patient.			
6. Explain the proposed procedure in terms the patient can understand.			
7. Gather all necessary equipment.			
8. Carry out proper hand hygiene.			
9. Verify the schedule for injection cap replacement.			
10. Provide for privacy.			
11. Instruct the patient to position the head to the side opposite the CVC insertion site.			
12. Aseptically open the injection cap package.			
13. Prime the injection cap with normal saline per manufacturer's guidelines.			
14. Don gloves.			
15. Close the slide clamp on the catheter pigtail.			
16. Grasp the hub of the pigtail with the nondominant hand and the injection cap			

(continues)

Skill 12-3 | (continued)

Name _____ Date _____ Instructor _____

ACTION TAKEN	COMPLETED SUCCESSFULLY	DID NOT COMPLETE	NOTES
with the other. (For enhanced traction, use 2 × 2-inch gauze [optional] to hold the hub and injection cap.)			
17. Instruct the patient to perform the Valsalva maneuver and, as the breath is held, quickly twist off (counter-clockwise direction) and remove the used cap and connect the new cap. Be sure the Luer-Lok® is secure (clockwise twisting direction).			
18. Instruct the patient to resume her usual breathing pattern.			
19. Open the slide clamp.			
20. Prep the top of the injection cap (or remove the sterile cap from the needleless system, if applicable), first with the 70% isopropyl alcohol, then with the CHG or povidone-iodine (or agency-approved iodophor).			
21. Attach the 10-ml syringe containing the normal saline to the Luer-Lok® connection. Aspirate to confirm placement of the CVC. (There may not always be a blood return.) When aspirating, allow the blood to flow only a short distance into the pigtail. Do not aspirate blood back into the syringe.			

Skill 12-3 *(continued)*

Name _____ Date _____ Instructor _____

ACTION TAKEN	COMPLETED SUCCESSFULLY	DID NOT COMPLETE	NOTES
22. Inject 4.5 ml of NS with a continuous forward motion on the plunger, exerting the pulsatile flush movement on the plunger. If resistance is encountered while injecting, *do not exert pressure on the CVC by exerting force on the syringe plunger. No further attempts to flush should be made. NOTIFY THE PHYSICIAN.*			
23. Attach the 10-ml syringe containing the heparin solution to the Luer-Lok® connection. Inject the 2.5 ml of heparin solution (except for Groshong® CVCs), injecting only part of the last 0.5 ml, following the guidelines for needle and needleless systems.			
24. Change all other caps, if present, following the same guidelines.			
25. Discard the used injection cap and any syringes/needles used in the sharps container.			
26. Remove gloves.			
27. Carry out proper hand hygiene.			
28. Document the procedure.			

Skill 12-4 | Heparin-Locking the CVC

Name _____ Date _____ Instructor _____

ACTION TAKEN	COMPLETED SUCCESSFULLY	DID NOT COMPLETE	NOTES
1. Check the physician's order.			
2. Introduce yourself to the patient.			
3. Identify the patient by checking the wrist band against the doctor's order and asking the patient, if conscious, to state his/her name.			
4. Verify the allergy status of the patient.			
5. Explain the proposed procedure in terms the patient can understand.			
6. Gather all necessary equipment.			
7. Carry out proper hand hygiene.			
8. Provide privacy.			
9. Review the Valsalva maneuver with patient.			
10. Elevate the bed level.			
11. Carry out proper hand hygiene.			
12. Set up all the necessary supplies on the bedside stand or overbed table in the order in which they will be used.			
13. Assess the site.			
14. Don gloves.			
15. Swab the injection port with alcohol and let it air dry.			
16. Swab the injection port with the 2% CHG or iodophor; allow it to air dry.			

Skill 12-4 |(continued)

Name _____ Date _____ Instructor _____

ACTION TAKEN	COMPLETED SUCCESSFULLY	DID NOT COMPLETE	NOTES
17. Open the slide clamp and insert the syringe containing the normal saline, have the patient perform the Valsalva maneuver, unclamp the line, and aspirate.			
18. Instill the sterile normal saline, using the pulsatile, push-pause method of plunger movement, and close the slide clamp.			
19. Remove the syringe, maintaining positive pressure in the line, and clamp.			
20. Ask the patient to perform the Valsalva maneuver and unclamp the line.			
21. Instill the prescribed dose of medication, maintain positive pressure in the line, clamp the line, and remove the syringe.			
22. Prep the port as described in steps 12 and 13.			
23. Ask the patient to perform the Valsalva maneuver. Attach the syringe of normal saline, unclamp the line, and instill 3 ml of normal saline, maintaining positive pressure in the line. Clamp the line and remove the syringe.			
24. Prep the port, attach the syringe of heparin, and unclamp the line. Administer the heparin. Clamp, maintaining positive pressure in the line, and remove the syringe.			

(continues)

Skill 12-4 | *(continued)*

Name _____ Date _____ Instructor _____

ACTION TAKEN	COMPLETED SUCCESSFULLY	DID NOT COMPLETE	NOTES
25. Dispose of all used equipment and place used syringes in sharps container.			
26. Remove gloves and carry out proper hand hygiene.			
27. Lower the bed and raise the side rails.			
28. Document the procedure in the MAR. Report any problems encountered in the nurse's notes.			

Skill 12-5 | Drawing Blood from the CVC

Name _____ Date _____ Instructor _____

ACTION TAKEN	COMPLETED SUCCESSFULLY	DID NOT COMPLETE	NOTES
1. Check the physician's order.			
2. Check the orders for the lab work.			
3. Introduce yourself to the patient.			
4. Identify the patient by checking the wrist band against the doctor's order and asking the patient, if conscious, to state his/her name.			
5. Verify the allergy status of the patient.			
6. Explain the proposed procedure in terms the patient can understand.			
7. Carry out proper hand hygiene.			
8. Gather equipment. Have all necessary heparin and saline drawn up prior to beginning the procedure.			
9. Provide for privacy.			
10. Set up equipment.			
11. Put on gloves.			
12. If an infusion is running, and the patient has a single lumen CVC, do the following: a. Close the slide clamp on the pigtail.			

(continues)

Skill 12-5 | *(continued)*

Name _____ Date _____ Instructor _____

ACTION TAKEN	COMPLETED SUCCESSFULLY	DID NOT COMPLETE	NOTES
b. Instruct the patient to perform the Valsalva maneuver, then quickly disconnect the administration set tubing from the pigtail, cap the pigtail with the injection cap, and cap the distal end of the administration set with the sterile cap.			
13. For multilumen CVCs, use the proximal lumen to draw blood and turn off all electrolyte and glucose-containing infusates that are infusing into other lumens for one full minute.			
14. Prep the injection cap of the pigtail with the alcohol followed by the 2% CHG or iodophor.			
15. Attach a 10-ml saline-filled syringe. Open the slide clamp and ascertain placement and patency of the CVC, then vigorously flush with 10 ml of NS using the pulsatile, push-pause method. Clamp.			
16. Attach the vacuum container to the injection cap. Unclamp.			
17. Draw 5 to 10 ml of blood into the discard tube. (The first flow of fluid into the tube will be clear, as it is that which is in the pigtail.)			

Skill 12-5 *(continued)*

Name _____ Date _____ Instructor _____

ACTION TAKEN	COMPLETED SUCCESSFULLY	DID NOT COMPLETE	NOTES
18. Quickly insert and fill the required blood collection tube, then close the slide clamp on the pigtail and remove the vacuum container collecting device. Clamp.			
19. Prep the injection cap, open the slide clamp, and vigorously flush the line with at least 20 ml of NS to remove any residual blood. Clamp.			
20. Reconnect the infusion line and unclamp so the infusion may run (or unclamp, heparin-lock the pigtail, and then clamp).			
21. Label the blood tubes and deliver the sample to the laboratory as soon as the blood draw is complete and the integrity of the CVC is ensured.			
22. Dispose of used equipment and carry out proper hand hygiene.			
23. Document the procedure.			

Skill 12-6 | The POP Method

Name _____ Date _____ Instructor _____

ACTION TAKEN	COMPLETED SUCCESSFULLY	DID NOT COMPLETE	NOTES
1. Check the physician's order.			
2. Introduce yourself to the patient.			
3. Identify the patient by checking the wrist band against the doctor's order and asking the patient, if conscious, to state his/her name.			
4. Verify the allergy status of the patient.			
5. Explain the proposed procedure in terms the patient can understand.			
6. Gather all necessary equipment.			
7. Carry out proper hand hygiene.			
8. Follow the medical order or agency policy regarding clearing occluded CVCs.			
9. Gather equipment.			
10. Provide for privacy.			
11. Set up equipment.			
12. Put on gloves.			
13. Cleanse the central venous catheter cap with 70% isopropyl alcohol followed by 2% CHG or povidone-iodine. Allow each solution to air dry.			
14. Instruct the patient to perform the Valsalva maneuver, then open the CVC clamp.			

Skill 12-6 | *(continued)*

Name _____ Date _____ Instructor _____

ACTION TAKEN	COMPLETED SUCCESSFULLY	DID NOT COMPLETE	NOTES
15. Disconnect the catheter cap or IV infusion line (covering the tubing end with a sterile cap) and attach the 20-ml syringe containing the 5 ml of NS to the catheter hub. Tell the patient to breathe normally.			
16. Open the slide clamp.			
17. Pull back on the syringe plunger to the 15-ml mark and let go of the plunger. A popping sound results. Repeat the maneuver several times in rapid succession. (Follow the same procedure for the 3 French catheter, but pull back to the 10-ml mark on the syringe.)			
18. Ask the patient to perform the Valsalva maneuver.			
19. Remove the syringe and attach the syringe filled with the 20 ml of NS to the hub (or smaller syringe for smaller CVC). Tell the patient to breathe normally.			
20. Open the slide clamp.			
21. Attempt to flush. If no resistance is felt, flush vigorously, using the pulsatile, push-pause method.			
22. Close the slide clamp.			
23. Ask the patient to perform the Valsalva maneuver.			

(continues)

Skill 12-6 | *(continued)*

Name _____ Date _____ Instructor _____

ACTION TAKEN	COMPLETED SUCCESSFULLY	DID NOT COMPLETE	NOTES
24. Attach the sterile injection cap to the catheter hub and heparin-lock the catheter or attach the IV line to the catheter hub and regulate the infusion.			
25. Tell the patient to breathe normally.			
26. Document in the nurse's notes.			

Skill 12-7 | The Positive Pressure Method

Name _____ Date _____ Instructor _____

ACTION TAKEN	COMPLETED SUCCESSFULLY	DID NOT COMPLETE	NOTES
1. Check the physician's order.			
2. Introduce yourself to the patient.			
3. Identify the patient by checking the wrist band against the doctor's order and asking the patient, if conscious, to state his/her name.			
4. Verify the allergy status of the patient.			
5. Explain the proposed procedure in terms the patient can understand.			
6. Gather all necessary equipment.			
7. Carry out proper hand hygiene.			
8. Follow the medical order or agency policy regarding clearing occluded CVCs.			
9. Provide for privacy.			
10. Set up equipment.			
11. Put on gloves.			
12. Cleanse the central venous catheter cap with 70% isopropyl alcohol followed by 2% CHG or povidone-iodine. Allow each solution to air dry.			

(continues)

Skill 12-7 | *(continued)*

Name _____ Date _____ Instructor _____

ACTION TAKEN	COMPLETED SUCCESSFULLY	DID NOT COMPLETE	NOTES
13. If the CVC is connected to an infusion line, close the slide clamp, have the patient perform the Valsalva maneuver, disconnect the catheter cap or IV infusion line (covering the tubing end with a sterile cap), and attach the empty syringe to the CVC hub. Tell the patient to breathe normally.			
14. Open the slide clamp and attempt to aspirate. If successful, withdraw the clots/residue(s), close the slide clamp, detach the syringe, and proceed to the next step. If aspiration is unsuccessful, close the slide clamp. Have the patient perform the Valsalva maneuver, then detach the syringe and proceed to step # 13.			
15. Attach the syringe containing the 10 ml (or 20 ml) of NS and flush vigorously, using the pulsatile, push-pause method. Then, do one of the following: • Close the slide clamp, have the patient perform the Valsalva maneuver, attach the syringe with the heparin flush, have the patient breathe normally, open the slide clamp, heparin-lock the line, and close the slide clamp.			

Skill 12-7 | *(continued)*

Name _____ Date _____ Instructor _____

ACTION TAKEN	COMPLETED SUCCESSFULLY	DID NOT COMPLETE	NOTES
• Close the slide clamp, have the patient perform the Valsalva maneuver, connect the IV tubing to the CVC hub, have the patient breathe normally, unclamp, and regulate the infusion.			
16. Attach the syringe containing the thrombolytic agent (or other declotting agent) and have the patient breathe normally. Open the slide clamp.			
17. Open the slide clamp.			
18. Slowly and gently inject the declotting agent into the catheter, using a push-pull motion. Do not force the entire amount into the catheter if strong resistance is encountered.			
19. Leave the syringe attached to the catheter for 30 to 90 minutes (or per physician's order or agency policy) and do not attempt to aspirate during this period.			
20. Attempt to aspirate after the prescribed amount of time. If unsuccessful, repeat the procedure or notify the physician, depending on agency policy. If patency is restored, aspirate 5 ml to 10 ml of blood.			
21. Close the clamp.			

(continues)

Skill 12-7 *(continued)*

Name _____ Date _____ Instructor _____

ACTION TAKEN	COMPLETED SUCCESSFULLY	DID NOT COMPLETE	NOTES
22. Have the patient perform the Valsalva maneuver, attach the 20-ml NS-filled syringe, have the patient breathe normally, and open the clamp.			
23. Flush the line vigorously, using the pulsatile, push-pause method, then close the slide clamp.			
24. Attach the injection cap and heparin-lock the catheter or attach the IV line and regulate the infusion.			
25. Document the procedure.			

Skill 12-8 | The Stopcock-Negative Pressure Method

Name _____ Date _____ Instructor _____

ACTION TAKEN	COMPLETED SUCCESSFULLY	DID NOT COMPLETE	NOTES
1. Check the physician's order.			
2. Introduce yourself to the patient.			
3. Identify the patient by checking the wrist band against the doctor's order and asking the patient, if conscious, to state his/her name.			
4. Verify the allergy status of the patient.			
5. Explain the proposed procedure in terms the patient can understand.			
6. Gather all necessary equipment.			
7. Carry out proper hand hygiene.			
8. Follow the medical order or agency policy regarding clearing occluded CVCs.			
9. Provide for privacy.			
10. Set up equipment.			
11. Put on gloves.			
12. Cleanse the central venous catheter cap with 70% isopropyl alcohol followed by 2% CHG or povidone-iodine. Allow each solution to air dry.			
13. If the CVC is connected to an infusion line, close the slide clamp, have the patient perform the Valsalva maneuver, disconnect the catheter cap or IV infusion line (covering the tubing end with a sterile cap), and attach the			

(continues)

Skill 12-8 | *(continued)*

Name _____ Date _____ Instructor _____

ACTION TAKEN	COMPLETED SUCCESSFULLY	DID NOT COMPLETE	NOTES
empty syringe to the CVC hub. Tell the patient to breathe normally. Turn the three-way stopcock to the *off* position before it is attached to the CVC hub.			
14. Close the slide clamp, instruct the patient to perform the Valsalva maneuver, attach the closed stopcock to the CVC hub, and open the CVC clamp. Tell the patient to breathe normally.			
15. Cleanse one port of the stopcock with alcohol and 2% CHG or povidone-iodine (if sterility has been breached) and attach it to the empty 20-ml syringe.			
16. Cleanse the other port of the stopcock, as before (if sterility has been breached), and attach it to the 20-ml syringe containing the declotting agent.			
17. Turn off the stopcock to the syringe containing the declotting agent and open it to the empty 20-ml syringe.			
18. Open the slide clamp on the CVC.			
19. Gently aspirate the CVC until the plunger is pulled back to the 15-ml marking.			
20. With the plunger retracted to the 15-ml mark, turn off the stopcock to the plunger-aspirated syringe.			

Skill 12-8 *(continued)*

Name _____ Date _____ Instructor _____

ACTION TAKEN	COMPLETED SUCCESSFULLY	DID NOT COMPLETE	NOTES
21. Open the stopcock (*on* position) to the syringe containing the declotting agent.			
22. Turn the stopcock to the *off* position, leaving the declotting agent in the CVC lumen for the prescribed time (per manufacturer/ agency/physician recommendations).			
23. Open the stopcock and aspirate for a blood return. If blood is returned, aspirate a waste volume of 5 to 10 ml. Close the catheter clamp and proceed to the next step.			
24. Have the patient perform the Valsalva maneuver, remove the stopcock, and attach the 20-ml syringe containing the NS to the catheter hub. Tell the patient to breathe normally.			
25. Open the catheter slide clamp and vigorously flush the catheter, using the pulsatile, push-pause method. Close the slide clamp.			
26. Have the patient perform the Valsalva maneuver, then do one of the following: Open the slide clamp, and attach the heparin flush syringe. Have the patient breathe normally. Instill the heparin solution and close the clamp.			

(continues)

Skill 12-8 | *(continued)*

Name _____ Date _____ Instructor _____

ACTION TAKEN	COMPLETED SUCCESSFULLY	DID NOT COMPLETE	NOTES
After removing the syringe, connect the IV infusion line, open the slide clamp, and regulate the infusion.			
27. Document the procedure.			

Skill 12-9 | Removal of the CVC

Name _____ Date _____ Instructor _____

ACTION TAKEN	COMPLETED SUCCESSFULLY	DID NOT COMPLETE	NOTES
1. Check the physician's order.			
2. Introduce yourself to the patient.			
3. Identify the patient by checking the wrist band against the doctor's order and asking the patient, if conscious, to state his/her name.			
4. Verify the allergy status of the patient.			
5. Explain the proposed procedure in terms the patient can understand.			
6. Gather all necessary supplies.			
7. Carry out proper hand hygiene.			
8. Gather supplies.			
9. Provide privacy.			
10. Review the procedure for performing the Valsalva maneuver.			
11. Elevate the bed level.			
12. Position bed in Trendelenburg or flat position.			
13. Attach the plastic disposal bag to the side of the bed or overbed table or place the plastic sheeting in close proximity to the patient.			
14. Carry out proper hand hygiene.			
15. Clamp infusion tubing and turn off the electronic infusion device (if appropriate).			

(continues)

Skill 12-9 *(continued)*

Name _____ Date _____ Instructor _____

ACTION TAKEN	COMPLETED SUCCESSFULLY	DID NOT COMPLETE	NOTES
16. Close the slide clamp on the CVC.			
17. Apply disposable gloves.			
18. Remove the dressing, following the guidelines for dressing removal as described in *CVC Dressing Change and Site Care*.			
19. Inspect the dressing for purulent drainage or foul odor.			
20. Discard the dressing in the plastic bag or on the plastic sheeting.			
21. Remove gloves and carry out proper hand hygiene.			
22. Place 4 × 4-inch gauze, skin antiseptics, suture removal kit, and dressing materials in close proximity to the patient and open them, using aseptic technique.			
23. Don sterile gloves, leaving the inside (sterile portion) of the wrapper at the bedside.			
24. Inspect the site around the cannula insertion area.			
25. Cleanse the CVC insertion site and surrounding area, including the catheter and sutures, in a concentric circle, starting at the catheter exit site. Clean first with the alcohol, repeating as needed, to remove all debris. Use adhesive remover, if necessary, to eliminate			

Skill 12-9 *(continued)*

Name _____ Date _____ Instructor _____

ACTION TAKEN	COMPLETED SUCCESSFULLY	DID NOT COMPLETE	NOTES
any tape deposits. Follow with thorough cleansing with the 2% CHG or povidone-iodine and allow the area to air dry.			
26. Carefully clip and remove sutures, while securing the CVC.			
27. Place the 4 × 4-inch sterile gauze over the CVC exit site, holding in place with the nondominant hand. Instruct the patient to perform the Valsalva maneuver.			
28. As the patient performs the Valsalva maneuver, withdraw the CVC from the vein in one smooth, steady motion, continuing to hold the 4 × 4-inch gauze in place. Exert firm pressure over the exit site for one to five minutes after the catheter is out and discard the catheter on the sterile inner wrapper from the gloves. Instruct the patient to breathe normally. Continue to apply pressure until any bleeding stops.			
29. Apply the sterile air-occlusive dressing over the site and secure the edges so that air cannot enter.			
30. Leave the dressing in place for 24 to 72 hours.			
31. Examine the removed CVC and assess it for drainage, odor, integrity, and length. If there is any breach in the CVC structure,			

(continues)

Skill 12-9 | *(continued)*

Name _____ Date _____ Instructor _____

ACTION TAKEN	COMPLETED SUCCESSFULLY	DID NOT COMPLETE	NOTES
instruct the patient to maintain complete bed rest, save the catheter, and notify the physician immediately. If there is any drainage or foul smell, cut off the tip (2-3 inches) and place the tip portion of the CVC in a sterile specimen container for culture studies.			
32. Dispose of used equipment and carry out proper hand hygiene.			
33. Assess the dressing every 15 minutes for the first hour after removal, then hourly for the first 24 hours, post removal. The patient should maintain bedrest, as needed, until the exit site has epithelialized.			
34. Document the patient's response to CVC removal, the appearance of the site, dressing regimen, and the condition and length of the catheter as well as any associated interventions.			

Skill 12-10 | Insertion of the Peripherally Inserted Central Catheter

Name _____ Date _____ Instructor _____

ACTION TAKEN	COMPLETED SUCCESSFULLY	DID NOT COMPLETE	NOTES
1. Check the physician's order and institutional policy regarding insertion of a PICC.			
2. Introduce yourself to the patient.			
3. Identify the patient by checking the wrist band against the doctor's order and asking the patient, if conscious, to state his/her name.			
4. Verify the allergy status of the patient.			
5. Explain the proposed procedure in terms the patient can understand.			
6. Obtain patient consent for the procedure.			
7. Gather all necessary equipment.			
8. Carry out proper hand hygiene.			
9. Provide for privacy.			
10. Apply a tourniquet to the patient's arm and assess the arm for an appropriate insertion site. Remove the tourniquet.			
11. Measure the amount of line that will be needed according to agency policy and write that number down.			
12. Wash the patient's arm with soap and water 6 inches above and below the insertion site; dry thoroughly.			

(continues)

Skill 12-10 | *(continued)*

Name _____ Date _____ Instructor _____

ACTION TAKEN	COMPLETED SUCCESSFULLY	DID NOT COMPLETE	NOTES
13. Position the patient flat with the arm extended at a 90-degree angle.			
14. Carry out proper hand hygiene and open the PICC kit using sterile procedure. Any additional supplies should be dropped on the sterile field.			
15. Place the underdrape under the patient's arm and shoulder area.			
16. Don a mask, sterile gloves, and a sterile gown. Put a mask on the patient.			
17. Prepare three 10-ml syringes with normal saline.			
18. Remove the catheter from the tray and examine it; be sure the guidewire is straight.			
19. Prime the catheter with normal saline and place the sterile measuring tape alongside the catheter.			
20. For a closed-ended catheter, measure the distance from the tip of the catheter to where it will exit the body and mark it. For an open-ended catheter measure the distance from the exit site to where the tip of the catheter will lie in the vessel. Note this marking and allow for the distance of the catheter that will extend out of the arm. Retract the guidewire to where			

Skill 12-10 | *(continued)*

Name _____ Date _____ Instructor _____

ACTION TAKEN	COMPLETED SUCCESSFULLY	DID NOT COMPLETE	NOTES
the catheter tip will be cut, cut the tip straight across, advance the guidewire to within $1/8$–$1/4$ inch of the tip, bend the guidewire at a 90-degree angle at the external end of the device.			
21. Prime the catheter connector.			
22. Prep the insertion site first using three alcohol and then three 2% aqueous chlorhexidine gluconate or iodophor swabsticks. Work outward in a concentric circle. Allow each solution to completely dry before proceeding to the next step.			
23. Place sterile drapes around the insertion site.			
24. Apply the tourniquet; this should be above the elbow for most patients.			
25. Remove gloves used for preparation and apply second set of sterile gloves.			
26. Anesthetize the insertion site.			
27. Hold the skin below the insertion site taut.			
28. Perform the venipuncture holding the introducer needle at a 30-degree angle with the bevel up.			

(continues)

Skill 12-10 *(continued)*

Name _____ Date _____ Instructor _____

ACTION TAKEN	COMPLETED SUCCESSFULLY	DID NOT COMPLETE	NOTES
29. Look for a blood return in the flashback chamber and then slowly advance the introducer needle a fraction of an inch more so the sheath is in the vein.			
30. Remove the tourniquet.			
31. Maintain the stability of the introducer and advance it.			
32. Observe the pattern of blood flow.			
33. Remove the needle from the introducer, leaving the introducer in place.			
34. Thread the PICC into the vein through the introducer to the depth determined by previous measurements. Use a steady, moderate rate of passage.			
35. Hold pressure over the insertion site until bleeding stops.			
36. Cleanse the insertion site of all blood.			
37. Remove the guidewire by spreading the fingers of one hand over the length of the catheter outside the insertion site and gently pressing down while grasping the hub of the guidewire with the opposite hand and pulling it parallel to the skin with a slow, steady motion.			
38. Remove the introducer catheter from the PICC while applying pressure above the insertion site.			

Skill 12-10 | *(continued)*

Name _____ Date _____ Instructor _____

ACTION TAKEN	COMPLETED SUCCESSFULLY	DID NOT COMPLETE	NOTES
39. Cut the PICC so that approximately 10 cm are left extending from the insertion site.			
40. Insert the connector into the catheter and apply a suture wing.			
41. Using a 10-ml syringe of saline aspirate to confirm placement of the catheter tip, flush using the pulsatile, push-pause method.			
42. Apply an injection cap.			
43. Heparinize the injection cap.			
44. Place a 2 × 2-inch folded gauze over the insertion site and place a transparent dressing over that for the first 24 hours.			
45. Label the insertion site with date, time, length, and gauge of catheter and your initials.			
46. Remove gloves, gown, and mask and dispose of all materials in the proper waste receptacle.			
47. Carry out proper hand hygiene.			
48. Document the procedure.			
49. Catheter placement must be verified with a chest x-ray.			
50. Dressing should be changed in 24 hours. Assess for swelling, drainage, and tenderness. Assess for migration of the catheter by checking the length of the catheter.			

Skill 12-11 | PICC Dressing Change and Site Care

Name _____ Date _____ Instructor _____

ACTION TAKEN	COMPLETED SUCCESSFULLY	DID NOT COMPLETE	NOTES
1. Check the physician's order and institutional policy regarding a PICC dressing change.			
2. Introduce yourself to the patient.			
3. Identify the patient by checking the wrist band against the doctor's order and asking the patient, if conscious, to state his/her name.			
4. Verify the allergy status of the patient.			
5. Explain the proposed procedure, in terms the patient can understand.			
6. Gather all necessary equipment.			
7. Carry out proper hand hygiene.			
8. Provide for privacy.			
9. Put on the mask and assist the patient to put on a mask as well.			
10. Apply non-sterile gloves.			
11. Instruct the patient to turn her head in the opposite direction of the insertion site and not move until the procedure is over.			
12. Remove the old dressing using the stretch method, being careful not to dislodge the catheter. Note any abnormalities.			
13. Remove gloves and carry out proper hand hygiene.			

Skill 12-11 | *(continued)*

Name _____ Date _____ Instructor _____

ACTION TAKEN	COMPLETED SUCCESSFULLY	DID NOT COMPLETE	NOTES
14. Open central line dressing pack, apply sterile gloves.			
15. Pick up the sterile drape and drape the patient below the insertion site.			
16. Cleanse the site with each of three alcohol swabs. Cleansing should occur in a circular motion, starting at the center of the insertion site and spiraling outward. Allow the alcohol to dry between swabs.			
17. Cleanse the site with each of three 2% CHG or povidone-iodine swabs. Cleansing should occur in a circular motion, starting at the center of the insertion site and spiraling outward. Allow the area to air dry.			
18. Apply either a transparent semipermeable dressing or gauze dressing over the site with the insertion site in the center. If a gauze dressing is used, tape over all the gauze and edges.			
19. Note the date, time, the length of the catheter outside the insertion site, and the total length of catheter; then initial the dressing, being careful not to prevent visual inspection of the insertion site.			

(continues)

Skill 12-11 *(continued)*

Name _____ Date _____ Instructor _____

ACTION TAKEN	COMPLETED SUCCESSFULLY	DID NOT COMPLETE	NOTES
20. Dispose of used equipment and carry out proper hand hygiene.			
21. Document the procedure.			

Skill 12-12 | PICC Injection Cap Changes

Name _____ Date _____ Instructor _____

ACTION TAKEN	COMPLETED SUCCESSFULLY	DID NOT COMPLETE	NOTES
1. Check the physician's order and institutional policy regarding a PICC injection cap change.			
2. Check to be sure the cap needs to be changed.			
3. Introduce yourself to the patient.			
4. Identify the patient by checking the wrist band against the doctor's order and asking the patient, if conscious, to state his/her name.			
5. Verify the allergy status of the patient.			
6. Explain the proposed procedure in terms the patient can understand.			
7. Obtain patient consent for the procedure.			
8. Gather all necessary equipment.			
9. Carry out proper hand hygiene.			
10. Provide for privacy.			
11. Draw up 1 cc of normal saline in the syringe. Flush all air out of the injection cap.			
12. If the PICC cannot be clamped, place the patient in a supine position.			
13. Put on the gloves.			
14. Cleanse the connection site between the injection cap and the PICC thoroughly with the alcohol swab. Allow the site to air dry.			

(continues)

Skill 12-12 | (continued)

Name _____ Date _____ Instructor _____

ACTION TAKEN	COMPLETED SUCCESSFULLY	DID NOT COMPLETE	NOTES
15. Instruct the patient to turn her head away from the PICC during the procedure.			
16. If not contraindicated, clamp the PICC. If clamping is contraindicated, instruct the patient to perform the Valsalva maneuver.			
17. Remove the old injection cap by twisting the cap to the left.			
18. Add the new injection cap by twisting the cap to the right.			
19. Change all other caps, if present, following the same procedure.			
20. Dispose of all used equipment and carry out proper hand hygiene.			
21. Document the procedure.			

Skill 12-13 | Flushing the PICC

Name _____ Date _____ Instructor _____

ACTION TAKEN	COMPLETED SUCCESSFULLY	DID NOT COMPLETE	NOTES
1. Check the physician's order and institutional policy regarding PICC line flushes.			
2. Introduce yourself to the patient.			
3. Identify the patient by checking the wrist band against the doctor's order and asking the patient, if conscious, to state his/her name.			
4. Verify the allergy status of the patient.			
5. Explain the proposed procedure in terms the patient can understand.			
6. Gather all necessary equipment.			
7. Carry out proper hand hygiene.			
8. Provide for privacy.			
9. Set up equipment.			
10. Put on gloves.			
11. Cleanse the central venous catheter cap with 70% isopropyl alcohol followed by 2% CHG or povidone-iodine. Allow each solution to air dry.			
12. Attach syringe containing normal saline to PICC.			
13. Instruct the patient to perform the Valsalva maneuver and open the PICC clamp.			
14. Flush the line with normal saline. Use the pulsatile, push-pause method. Clamp the line.			

(continues)

Skill 12-13 | *(continued)*

Name _____ Date _____ Instructor _____

ACTION TAKEN	COMPLETED SUCCESSFULLY	DID NOT COMPLETE	NOTES
15. Attach the syringe with the heparin.			
16. Instruct the patient to perform the Valsalva maneuver and open the PICC clamp. Flush the line with the heparin. Clamp the line while infusing the last 0.5 ml of solution.			
17. Dispose of all used equipment and carry out proper hand hygiene.			
18. Document the procedure.			

Skill 12-14 | Drawing Blood from the PICC

Name _____ Date _____ Instructor _____

ACTION TAKEN	COMPLETED SUCCESSFULLY	DID NOT COMPLETE	NOTES
1. Check the physician's order and institutional policy regarding PICC line blood draws.			
2. Check the orders for the lab work.			
3. Introduce yourself to the patient.			
4. Identify the patient by checking the wrist band against the doctor's order and asking the patient, if conscious, to state his/her name.			
5. Verify the allergy status of the patient.			
6. Explain the proposed procedure in terms the patient can understand.			
7. Gather all necessary equipment.			
8. Carry out proper hand hygiene.			
9. Provide for privacy.			
10. Set up equipment.			
11. Put on gloves.			
12. If an infusion is running, close the slide clamp. It is necessary to turn off all electrolyte and glucose-containing infusates that are infusing into other lumens for one full minute prior to the blood draw.			

(continues)

Skill 12-14 | (continued)

Name _____ Date _____ Instructor _____

ACTION TAKEN	COMPLETED SUCCESSFULLY	DID NOT COMPLETE	NOTES
13. Instruct the patient to perform the Valsalva maneuver, and quickly disconnect the administration set tubing from the pigtail, cap the pigtail with the injection cap, and cap the distal end of the administration set with the sterile cap.			
14. Prep the injection cap of the pigtail with the alcohol followed by 2% CHG or iodophor.			
15. Attach a 10-ml saline-filled syringe. Open the slide clamp and ascertain placement and patency of the PICC, then vigorously flush with 10 ml of NS using the pulsatile, push-pause method. Clamp.			
16. Attach the vacuum container or the empty 10- or 20-ml syringe to the injection cap. Unclamp.			
17. Draw 5 to 10 ml of blood into the discard tube.			
18. Quickly insert and fill the required blood collection tube, then close the slide clamp on the pigtail and remove the vacuum container collecting device. Clamp.			

Skill 12-14 | *(continued)*

Name _____ Date _____ Instructor _____

ACTION TAKEN	COMPLETED SUCCESSFULLY	DID NOT COMPLETE	NOTES
19. Prep the injection cap, open the slide clamp, and vigorously flush the line with at least 20 ml of NS to remove any residual blood. Clamp.			
20. Reconnect the infusion line and unclamp so the infusion may run (or unclamp, heparin-lock the pigtail, and then clamp).			
21. Dispose of used equipment and carry out proper hand hygiene.			
22. Document the procedure.			
23. Deliver the sample to the laboratory as soon as the blood draw is complete and integrity of the PICC is ensured.			

Skill 12-15 | PICC Exchange

Name _____ Date _____ Instructor _____

ACTION TAKEN	COMPLETED SUCCESSFULLY	DID NOT COMPLETE	NOTES
1. Check the physician's order and institutional policy regarding PICC exchange.			
2. Introduce yourself to the patient.			
3. Identify the patient by checking the wrist band against the doctor's order and asking the patient, if conscious, to state his/her name.			
4. Verify the allergy status of the patient.			
5. Explain the proposed procedure, in terms the patient can understand.			
6. Obtain patient consent for the procedure.			
7. Gather all necessary equipment.			
8. Carry out proper hand hygiene.			
9. Provide privacy.			
10. Elevate the bed level.			
11. Secure all necessary supplies. The equipment and setup is the same as that for placing a new PICC, except for the use of an extra package of CHG or iodophor swabsticks.			
12. Place the patient comfortably in a semi-Fowler's position.			
13. Assess vital signs and level of consciousness and record.			
14. Remove the PICC dressing.			

Skill 12-15 | *(continued)*

Name _____ Date _____ Instructor _____

ACTION TAKEN	COMPLETED SUCCESSFULLY	DID NOT COMPLETE	NOTES
15. Following the procedure for inserting a new PICC, maintain a sterile field and drape the patient's arms appropriately.			
16. Don sterile gloves.			
17. Cover the end of the PICC with a sterile 4 × 4-inch gauze and remove the PICC from the insertion site to expose at least 5 inches of the line.			
18. Aseptically prepare the site, as for placement of a new PICC.			
19. Cleanse the existing PICC, using the additional CHG or iodophor swabsticks.			
20. Clamp the PICC 1 inch distal to its exit site from the body.			
21. Cut the PICC 3 inches distal to the clamp. Discard the removed portion of the PICC off the sterile field.			
22. Remove the introducer needle from the plastic introducer sheath.			
23. Thread the plastic introducer sheath over the end of the exposed PICC, advancing it up to the clamp.			
24. Fold the end of the PICC a short distance from the end of the introducer.			

(continues)

Skill 12-15 | *(continued)*

Name _____ Date _____ Instructor _____

ACTION TAKEN	COMPLETED SUCCESSFULLY	DID NOT COMPLETE	NOTES
25. While keeping the PICC doubled over, remove the clamp from its former position and place it between the introducer and the folded portion of the PICC.			
26. Advance the introducer sheath over the PICC up to its exit site on the arm.			
27. Apply normal saline around the PICC exit site and slowly advance the introducer into the site up to its hub.			
28. Gently pull down on the existing PICC.			
29. Pull the PICC out of the arm through the introducer. *Note:* Following removal there may or may not (more likely) be a retrograde flow of blood from the introducer. To stimulate a blood return, a tourniquet may be placed high on the upper arm.			
30. Introduce the new PICC into the introducer and advance it to its premeasured insertion length, following the usual insertion protocols.			
31. Withdraw the introducer sheath and retract it from the PICC.			

Skill 12-15 | *(continued)*

Name _____ Date _____ Instructor _____

ACTION TAKEN	COMPLETED SUCCESSFULLY	DID NOT COMPLETE	NOTES
32. Follow the same procedural guidelines for PICC placements, following advancement of the tip to its premeasured position.			
33. Lower bed to standard low position and raise rails.			
34. Remove personal protective equipment and dispose of used materials in appropriate waste containers.			
35. Carry out proper hand hygiene.			
36. Arrange for portable chest x-ray or transfer to radiology for x-ray.			
37. Document the procedure.			

Skill 12-16 | PICC Removal

Name _____ Date _____ Instructor _____

ACTION TAKEN	COMPLETED SUCCESSFULLY	DID NOT COMPLETE	NOTES
1. Check the physician's order and institutional policy regarding PICC removal.			
2. Introduce yourself to the patient.			
3. Identify the patient by checking the wrist band against the doctor's order and asking the patient, if conscious, to state his/her name.			
4. Verify the allergy status of the patient.			
5. Explain the proposed procedure, in terms the patient can understand.			
6. Obtain patient consent for the procedure.			
7. Gather all necessary equipment.			
8. Carry out proper hand hygiene.			
9. Provide privacy.			
10. Elevate the bed level.			
11. Secure all necessary supplies.			
12. Position the patient comfortably in a supine or semi-Fowler's position with arm extended at a 45- to 90-degree angle from the torso.			
13. Flush the PICC with normal saline.			
14. Don nonsterile gloves.			
15. Remove the dressing (and sutures, if present).			

Skill 12-16 *(continued)*

Name _____ Date _____ Instructor _____

ACTION TAKEN	COMPLETED SUCCESSFULLY	DID NOT COMPLETE	NOTES
16. If a culture is required, cleanse the PICC exit site.			
17. Gently grasp the catheter at its exit site from the skin.			
18. Remove the catheter, pulling it straight out while maintaining gentle, constant traction and regrasping the catheter every few centimeters.			
19. Measure the length of the removed catheter and compare it to the documented length that was inserted.			
20. Gently apply pressure with the 4 × 4-inch gauze.			
21. Fold the gauze over and apply a strip of tape or apply an adhesive bandage. Leave the dressing in place for 24 hours.			
22. Discard the catheter into the sharps container.			
23. Lower bed to standard low position and raise rails.			
24. Remove personal protective equipment and dispose of it in the appropriate container.			
25. Carry out proper hand hygiene.			
26. Document the procedure.			

Skill 12-17 | Preparation of the VAP Access Site

Name _____ Date _____ Instructor _____

ACTION TAKEN	COMPLETED SUCCESSFULLY	DID NOT COMPLETE	NOTES
1. Check the physician's order and institutional policy regarding VAP access.			
2. Introduce yourself to the patient.			
3. Identify the patient by checking the wrist band against the doctor's order and asking the patient, if conscious, to state his/her name.			
4. Verify the allergy status of the patient.			
5. Explain the proposed procedure, in terms the patient can understand.			
6. Obtain patient consent for the procedure.			
7. Gather all necessary equipment.			
8. Carry out proper hand hygiene.			
9. Provide privacy.			
10. Elevate the bed level.			
11. Secure all necessary supplies.			
12. Inspect the site.			
13. Wash insertion area with soap and rinse well with water and pat dry.			
14. Review the Valsalva maneuver with the patient.			
15. Assess vital signs and LOC and record.			
16. Set up the equipment in a sterile manner.			

Skill 12-17 | *(continued)*

Name _____ Date _____ Instructor _____

ACTION TAKEN	COMPLETED SUCCESSFULLY	DID NOT COMPLETE	NOTES
17. Expose the skin and palpate for the septum.			
18. Don gown, mask, and sterile gloves.			
19. Instruct the patient to turn her head away from the VAP site.			
20. Cleanse the septum site with each 70% isopropyl alcohol swab stick, starting at the intended puncture site and moving outward in a concentric circle 4 to 5 inches in diameter. Repeat for a total of three times. Allow the area to air dry.			
21. Repeat the above steps, using the 2% CHG or iodophor swabsticks and allow the area to air dry after the third application.			
22. Gently wipe off any residue of the iodophor at the needle insertion site.			

Skill 12-18 | Accessing and Deaccessing the VAP

Name _____ Date _____ Instructor _____

ACTION TAKEN	COMPLETED SUCCESSFULLY	DID NOT COMPLETE	NOTES
1. Check the physician's order and institutional policy regarding VAP access.			
2. Introduce yourself to the patient.			
3. Identify the patient by checking the wrist band against the doctor's order and asking the patient, if conscious, to state his/her name.			
4. Verify the allergy status of the patient.			
5. Explain the proposed procedure, in terms the patient can understand.			
6. Obtain patient consent for the procedure.			
7. Gather all necessary equipment.			
8. Carry out proper hand hygiene. Prepare the site as outlined in Skill 12-17, steps 9–22.			
Single Port Access			
23. Administer local anesthesia, if indicated, following agency protocols.			
24. Connect the needle with extension set to the 10-ml syringe filled with NS and clear the tubing of air, taking care not to contaminate the equipment, the site, or the nurse's gloved hands.			

Skill 12-18 | *(continued)*

Name _____ Date _____ Instructor _____

ACTION TAKEN	COMPLETED SUCCESSFULLY	DID NOT COMPLETE	NOTES
25. Locate the base of the port with the nondominant hand. Triangulate the port between the thumb and the first two fingers of the nondominant hand. Approximate the center of the port and aim for the center of these three fingers.			
26. Instruct the patient to perform the Valsalva maneuver.			
27. Insert the needle perpendicular to the port septum. Advance the needle through the skin and septum until reaching the bottom of the reservoir. Tell the patient to breathe normally.			
28. Aspirate for a blood return. Do not inject until placement is confirmed.			
29. Vigorously flush the line, using the push-pause, pulsatile method.			
30. Continue with procedure of administration of bolus injection, continuous/intermittent infusion, flushing, and heparin-locking, as indicated. Click here for a link to this skill.			
Dual Port Access Prepare the site as outlined in Skill 12-17, steps 9–22.			
23. Administer local anesthesia, if indicated, following agency protocols.			

(continues)

Skill 12-18 (continued)

Name _____ Date _____ Instructor _____

ACTION TAKEN	COMPLETED SUCCESSFULLY	DID NOT COMPLETE	NOTES
24. Connect the needle with extension set to the 10-ml syringe filled with NS and clear the tubing of air, taking care not to contaminate the equipment, the site, or the nurse's gloved hands.			
25. Palpate to locate the port septum to be accessed. i. Locate the base of the port with the nondominant hand. ii. Approximate the center of the dual port and place the index finger of the dominant hand to mark the spot. iii. Triangulate the right or left side of the dual port between the thumb and first two fingers of the dominant hand. Aim for the center point of these three fingers.			
27. Instruct the patient to perform the Valsalva maneuver.			
27. Insert the needle perpendicular to the port septum. Advance the needle through the skin and septum until reaching the bottom of the reservoir. Tell the patient to breathe normally.			
28. Aspirate for a blood return. Do not inject until placement is confirmed.			
29. Vigorously flush the line, using the push-pause, pulsatile method.			

Skill 12-18 | *(continued)*

Name _____ Date _____ Instructor _____

ACTION TAKEN	COMPLETED SUCCESSFULLY	DID NOT COMPLETE	NOTES
30. Each septum must be accessed separately and flushed with normal saline.			
31. Continue with procedure of administration of bolus injection, continuous/ intermittent infusion, flushing, and heparing-locking, as indicated.			
Deaccessing the VAP			
32. Stabilize the port with two fingers prior to withdrawal of the needle.			
33. Instruct the patient to perform the Valsalva maneuver.			
34. Slowly remove a noncoring needle while injecting the last 0.5 ml of infusate.			
35. Dispose of used equipment and carry out proper hand hygiene.			
36. Document the procedure.			

Skill 12-19 | Bolus Injection via the VAP

Name _____ Date _____ Instructor _____

ACTION TAKEN	COMPLETED SUCCESSFULLY	DID NOT COMPLETE	NOTES
1. Check the physician's order and institutional policy regarding VAP access.			
2 Introduce yourself to the patient.			
3. Identify the patient by checking the wrist band against the doctor's order and asking the patient, if conscious, to state his/her name.			
4. Verify the allergy status of the patient.			
5. Explain the proposed procedure, in terms the patient can understand.			
6. Gather all necessary equipment.			
7. Carry out proper hand hygiene.			
8. Provide privacy.			
9. Elevate the bed level.			
10. Secure all necessary supplies.			
11. Inspect the site.			
12. Wash insertion area with soap, rinse well with water, and pat dry.			
13. Review the Valsalva maneuver with the patient.			
14. Assess vital signs and LOC and record.			
15. Set up the equipment in a sterile manner.			
16. Expose the skin and palpate for the septum.			
17. Don gown, mask, and sterile gloves.			

Skill 12-19 | *(continued)*

Name _____ Date _____ Instructor _____

ACTION TAKEN	COMPLETED SUCCESSFULLY	DID NOT COMPLETE	NOTES
18. Instruct patient to turn her head away from the VAP site.			
19. Cleanse the septum site with each 70% isopropyl alcohol swab stick, starting at the intended puncture site and moving outward in a concentric circle 4 to 5 inches in diameter. Repeat for a total of three times. Allow the area to air dry.			
20. Repeat the preceding steps, using the 2% CHG or iodophor swabsticks, and allow the area to air dry after the third application.			
21. Gently wipe off any residue of the iodophor at the needle insertion site.			
22. Administer local anesthesia, if indicated, following agency protocols.			
23. Connect the appropriate needle with extension set to the 10-ml syringe filled with NS and prime the tubing and needle to displace any air, taking care not to contaminate the equipment, the site, or the your gloved hands.			
24. Triangulate the port between the thumb and the first two fingers of the nondominant hand. Aim for the center point of these three fingers.			
25. Instruct the patient to perform the Valsalva maneuver.			

(continues)

Skill 12-19 | *(continued)*

Name _____ Date _____ Instructor _____

ACTION TAKEN	COMPLETED SUCCESSFULLY	DID NOT COMPLETE	NOTES
26. Insert the needle perpendicular to the port septum. Advance the needle through the skin and septum until it reaches the bottom of the reservoir. Tell the patient to breathe normally.			
27. Aspirate for a blood return. Do not inject until placement is confirmed.			
28. Vigorously flush the line, using the push-pause, pulsatile method.			
29. Close the slide clamp on the extension tubing as the last 0.5 ml of NS is injected.			
30. Instruct the patient to perform the Valsalva maneuver.			
31. Disconnect the empty NS saline syringe and attach the 10-ml syringe containing the bolus medication.			
32. Instruct the patient to breathe normally.			
33. Open the slide clamp on the extension tubing.			
34. Administer the drug, according to directions, while examining the injection site.			
35. Clamp the extension set when the injection is complete.			
36. Instruct the patient to perform the Valsalva maneuver and remove the syringe.			

Skill 12-19 | *(continued)*

Name _____ Date _____ Instructor _____

ACTION TAKEN	COMPLETED SUCCESSFULLY	DID NOT COMPLETE	NOTES
37. Attach the 10-ml syringe containing the NS.			
38. Instruct the patient to breathe normally and open the slide clamp on the extension tubing.			
39. Flush the line vigorously, using the pulsatile, push-pause method. Clamp the line as the last 0.5 ml is instilled.			
40. Instruct the patient to perform the Valsalva maneuver and detach the empty NS syringe. If the VAP has a Groshong® tip, remove the needle at this time and do not flush with heparin.			
41. Attach the 10-ml syringe containing the heparin flush.			
42. Instruct the patient to breathe normally and open the slide clamp on the extension tubing.			
43. Heparin-lock the port, closing the slide clamp as the last 0.5 ml is injected.			
44. Stabilize the port with two fingers, instruct the patient to perform the Valsalva maneuver, and remove the needle. Instruct the patient to breathe normally.			
45. Return the bed to the low position and raise the siderails.			
46. Dispose of used equipment and carry out proper hand hygiene.			
47. Document the procedure.			

Skill 12-20 | Continuous Infusion into the VAP

Name _____ Date _____ Instructor _____

ACTION TAKEN	COMPLETED SUCCESSFULLY	DID NOT COMPLETE	NOTES
1. Check the physician's order.			
2. Introduce yourself to the patient.			
3. Identify the patient by checking the wrist band against the doctor's order and asking the patient, if conscious, to state his/her name.			
4 Verify the allergy status of the patient.			
5. Explain the proposed procedure, in terms the patient can understand.			
6. Gather all necessary equipment.			
7. Carry out proper hand hygiene.			
8. Provide privacy.			
9. Elevate the bed level.			
10. Secure all necessary supplies.			
11. Inspect the site.			
12. Wash insertion area with soap, rinse well with water, and pat dry.			
13. Review the Valsalva maneuver with the patient.			
14. Assess vital signs and LOC and record.			
15. Set up the equipment in a sterile manner.			
16. Expose the skin and palpate for the septum.			
17. Don gown, mask, and sterile gloves.			
18. Instruct the patient to turn her head away from the VAP site.			

Skill 12-20 | *(continued)*

Name _____ Date _____ Instructor _____

ACTION TAKEN	COMPLETED SUCCESSFULLY	DID NOT COMPLETE	NOTES
19. Cleanse the septum site with each 70% isopropyl alcohol swab stick, starting at the intended puncture site and moving outward in a concentric circle 4 to 5 inches in diameter. Repeat for a total of three times. Allow the area to air dry.			
20. Repeat the preceding steps, using the 2% CHG or iodophor swab sticks, and allow the area to air dry after the third application.			
21. Gently wipe off any residue of the iodophor at the needle insertion site.			
22. Administer local anesthesia, if indicated, following agency protocols.			
23. Connect the appropriate needle with extension set to the 10-ml syringe filled with NS and prime the tubing and needle to displace any air, taking care not to contaminate the equipment, the site, or your gloved hands.			
24. Triangulate the port between the thumb and the first two fingers of the nondominant hand. Aim for the center point of these three fingers.			
25. Instruct the patient to perform the Valsalva maneuver.			

(continues)

Skill 12-20 *(continued)*

Name _____ Date _____ Instructor _____

ACTION TAKEN	COMPLETED SUCCESSFULLY	DID NOT COMPLETE	NOTES
26. Insert the needle perpendicular to the port septum. Advance the needle through the skin and septum until it reaches the bottom of the reservoir. Tell the patient to breathe normally.			
27. Aspirate for a blood return. Do not inject until placement is confirmed.			
28. Vigorously flush the line, using the push-pause, pulsatile method.			
29. Close the slide clamp on the extension tubing as the last 0.5 ml of NS is injected.			
30. Place the 2 × 2-inch gauze (rolled up or folded in 4s) under the needle hub. Secure the needle and dressing in place with the transparent dressing.			
31. Open the slide clamp and vigorously flush the line using the pulsatile, push-pause method.			
32. Clamp the line, have the patient perform the Valsalva maneuver, and disconnect the syringe.			
33. Connect the fluid delivery system. Tell the patient to breathe normally.			
34. If an electronic infusion device is used, turn it on, open the slide clamp, and initiate the infusion.			

Skill 12-20 | *(continued)*

Name _____ Date _____ Instructor _____

ACTION TAKEN	COMPLETED SUCCESSFULLY	DID NOT COMPLETE	NOTES
35. Examine the site for signs of extravasation and initiate the appropriate interventions if needed.			
36. Tape all tubing connections with the paper tape.			
37. When the infusion is complete, turn off the electronic infusion device (EID), clamp the extension set, have the patient perform the Valsalva maneuver, and disconnect the IV line from the extension tubing of the needle.			
38. Connect the 20-ml syringe containing the NS, have the patient breathe normally, open the slide clamp and flush vigorously, as before.			
39. Heparin-lock the port (unless it has a Groshong® tip), closing the slide clamp as the last 0.5 ml is injected.			
40. Stabilize the port with two fingers, instruct the patient to perform the Valsalva maneuver, and remove the needle. Instruct the patient to breathe normally.			
41. Return the bed to the low position and raise the siderails.			
42. Dispose of used equipment and carry out proper hand hygiene.			
43. Document the procedure.			

Skill 12-21 | Blood Sampling from the VAP

Name _____ Date _____ Instructor _____

ACTION TAKEN	COMPLETED SUCCESSFULLY	DID NOT COMPLETE	NOTES
1. Check the physician's order.			
2. Check the orders for lab work.			
3. Introduce yourself to the patient.			
4. Identify the patient by checking the wrist band against the doctor's order and asking the patient, if conscious, to state his/her name.			
5. Verify the allergy status of the patient.			
6. Explain the proposed procedure, in terms the patient can understand.			
7. Gather all necessary equipment. Have all necessary heparin and saline drawn up prior to beginning the procedure.			
8. Carry out proper hand hygiene.			
9. Provide for privacy.			
10. Set up equipment.			
11. Put on gloves.			
12. Aseptically prepare the injection site (following the procedure for Accessing/ Deaccessing a VAP).			
13. Flush the extension tubing, stopcock, and needle, maintaining sterility.			
14. Insert the needle, aspirate for a blood return, and vigorously flush the port with 5 ml of NS.			

Skill 12-21 | *(continued)*

Name _____ Date _____ Instructor _____

ACTION TAKEN	COMPLETED SUCCESSFULLY	DID NOT COMPLETE	NOTES
15. Withdraw at least 5 ml of blood and discard the syringe into the sharps container.			
16. Aspirate the desired blood volume into the 20-ml syringe and transfer it to the appropriate blood sample tube (or use a Vacutainer® per the manufacturer's protocols).			
17. Flush the system vigorously with 20 ml of sterile NS, using the push-pause, pulsatile method.			
18. Heparin-lock the system (for ports with open-ended catheters).			
19. Label the blood tubes and deliver the sample to the laboratory as soon as the blood draw is complete and integrity of the VAP is ensured.			
20. Dispose of used equipment and carry out proper hand hygiene.			
21. Document the procedure.			

Skill 12-22 | Clearing a Blocked VAP

Name _____ Date _____ Instructor _____

ACTION TAKEN	COMPLETED SUCCESSFULLY	DID NOT COMPLETE	NOTES
1. Check the physician's order.			
2. Introduce yourself to the patient.			
3. Identify the patient by checking the wrist band against the doctor's order and asking the patient, if conscious, to state his/her name.			
4. Verify the allergy status of the patient.			
5. Explain the proposed procedure, in terms the patient can understand.			
6. Gather all necessary equipment.			
7. Carry out proper hand hygiene.			
8. Access the port.			
9. Using the 35-ml syringe, gently instill the declotting agent. Use a gentle pull-push action on the syringe to maximize mixing of the solution within the port and catheter.			
10. Leave the declotting agent in place for 15 minutes.			
11. Attempt to aspirate the declotting solution and the clot.			
12. Once the blockage has been cleared, vigorously flush the catheter with at least 10 ml of NS, using the pulsatile, push-pause method.			
13. Heparin-lock the port (for open-ended catheters).			

Skill 12-22 | *(continued)*

Name _____ Date _____ Instructor _____

ACTION TAKEN	COMPLETED SUCCESSFULLY	DID NOT COMPLETE	NOTES
Alternate (Two-Needle) Declotting Method An alternate method of declotting a VAP involves the use of two noncoring access needles. This method is especially useful when the blockage is in the port itself. It can be done by one nurse, but is more easily accomplished when done by two (with one maneuvering the syringe containing the declotting agent and the other pulling back on the empty syringe).			
1. Check the physician's order.			
2. Introduce yourself to the patient.			
3. Identify the patient by checking the wrist band against the doctor's order and asking the patient, if conscious, to state his/her name.			
4. Verify the allergy status of the patient.			
5. Explain the proposed procedure, in terms the patient can understand.			
6. Carry out proper hand hygiene.			
7. Connect the extension sets to each needle and syringe. Purge the air from the extension set and needle connected to the syringe containing the declotting agent.			

(continues)

Skill 12-22 | *(continued)*

Name _____ Date _____ Instructor _____

ACTION TAKEN	COMPLETED SUCCESSFULLY	DID NOT COMPLETE	NOTES
8. Access the port with both needles.			
9. Using the empty syringe, try the POP method to dislodge the clot. If this doesn't work, proceed to the next step.			
10. Gently instill a small volume of the declotting agent into the port, then pull back on the plunger of the empty syringe. Continue to gently push and pull until all the declotting agent has been instilled.			
11. Once the blockage has been cleared, vigorously flush the catheter with at least 10 ml of NS, using the pulsatile, push-pause method.			
12. Heparin-lock the port (for open-ended catheters). If the preceding methods do not remove the clot or obstruction, the blockage may be further down in the catheter. When this seems to be the problem, it is advisable to try the negative pressure method of declotting, using a stopcock. (See the procedure for Occluded CVCs.)			

Skill 12-23 | Accessing and Deaccessing the CathLink™ 20 Implanted Port

Name _____ Date _____ Instructor _____

ACTION TAKEN	COMPLETED SUCCESSFULLY	DID NOT COMPLETE	NOTES
1. Check the physician's order.			
2. Introduce yourself to the patient.			
3. Identify the patient by checking the wrist band against the doctor's order and asking the patient, if conscious, to state his/her name.			
4. Verify the allergy status of the patient. Assess for allergies, especially to iodine.			
5. Explain the proposed procedure, in terms the patient can understand.			
6. Gather all necessary equipment.			
7. Carry out proper hand hygiene.			
8. Provide privacy.			
9. Elevate the bed level.			
10. Secure all necessary supplies.			
11. Inspect the site.			
12. Wash the insertion area with soap, rinse well with water, and pat dry.			
13. Review the Valsalva maneuver with the patient.			
14. Assess vital signs and LOC and record.			
15. Set up the equipment in a sterile manner.			

(continues)

Skill 12-23 | *(continued)*

Name _____ Date _____ Instructor _____

ACTION TAKEN	COMPLETED SUCCESSFULLY	DID NOT COMPLETE	NOTES
16. Cleanse the septum site with each 70% isopropyl alcohol swab stick, starting at the intended puncture site and moving outward in a concentric circle 4 to 5 inches in diameter. Repeat for a total of three times. Allow the area to air dry.			
17. Repeat the preceding steps, using the 2% CHG or iodophor swab sticks, and allow the area to air dry after the third application.			
18. Attach a 10-ml syringe filled with sterile NS to the extension set. Expel air and close the clamp.			
19. Using a sterile gloved hand, locate the CathLink™ 20 implanted port and identify the funnel-shaped entrance by palpation.			
20. Stabilize the port by "holding" it between the thumb and forefinger of the nondominant hand.			
21. Aim for the funnel-shaped entrance (between two fingers) and insert the ONC into the port's funnel-shaped entrance until resistance is felt.			
22. Ask the patient to perform the Valsalva maneuver.			

Skill 12-23 | *(continued)*

Name _____ Date _____ Instructor _____

ACTION TAKEN	COMPLETED SUCCESSFULLY	DID NOT COMPLETE	NOTES
23. Using the thumb and forefinger of the dominant hand, advance the ONC completely into the port by grasping and advancing the catheter hub only, while simultaneously withdrawing the needle. (This can also be accomplished by advancing the ONC with one hand and withdrawing the needle with the other.) The IV catheter should be advanced a minimum of 1 cm.			
24. Place a gloved finger over the IV catheter hub until a secondary device can be attached.			
25. Immediately attach the syringe or extension set to the ONC and tell the patient to breathe normally.			
26. Dispose of the needle/stylet in the sharps container.			
27. Aspirate for a blood return.			
28. Flush with NS.			
29. Proceed with the infusion protocol.			
30. Following injection of medication/ infusion, the port is to be flushed with normal saline.			
31. Heparin-lock the port.			
32. To deaccess the port, stabilize the CathLink™ 20 with two fingers.			

(continues)

Skill 12-23 | *(continued)*

Name _____ Date _____ Instructor _____

ACTION TAKEN	COMPLETED SUCCESSFULLY	DID NOT COMPLETE	NOTES
33. Remove the ONC slowly while injecting the last 0.5 ml of infusate.			
34. Return the bed to the low position and raise the siderails.			
35. Dispose of used equipment and carry out proper hand hygiene.			
36. Document the procedure.			

Skill 14-1 | Transfusion of Blood Components

Name _____ Date _____ Instructor _____

ACTION TAKEN	COMPLETED SUCCESSFULLY	DID NOT COMPLETE	NOTES
1. Verify the prescriber's order.			
2. Verify informed consent. Assess the patient's understanding of the procedure, then describe the procedure, and provide the patient with the opportunity to ask questions and ventilate concerns. Ask if she has ever had any type of transfusion in the past (including cryoprecipitate, FFP, platelets, and RBCs). Assess for symptoms that may be misinterpreted for a reaction during the transfusion. If possible, although not absolutely contra-indicated, transfusion should be avoided in febrile (fever >38°C or 100.4°F) patients.			
3. Verify the patient's identity. If conscious, ask the patient to state her full name. She must have an identification band as well as a blood administration I.D. bracelet (put on by the blood administration service when a blood sample was drawn for type and crossmatching). Validate that the name and numbers on both I.D. bands correlate with those on the patient's chart and on the laboratory forms for pretransfusion testing of the blood.			

Skill 14-1 | *(continued)*

Name _____ Date _____ Instructor _____

ACTION TAKEN	COMPLETED SUCCESSFULLY	DID NOT COMPLETE	NOTES
4. If the patient is ambulatory, it is recommend that she go to the bathroom and empty her bladder. If bedridden, provide a bedpan (or urinal).			
5. Assemble all necessary equipment and start an infusion of 0.9% NaCl, if ordered, using the appropriate administration set, filter, and correct cannula size. *Never* piggyback blood into an existing IV line. Obtain an extra set of tubing and a container of 0.9% NaCl, (neither of which are opened, nor charged to the patient) and leave them at the bedside. Locate the availability of emergency drugs.			
6. Premedicate the patient with antihistamines, antipyretics, or diuretics, as ordered by the physician.			
7. Obtain the blood component from the transfusion service just prior to its administration. Unless an emergency exists, only one unit per patient is released at a time. Blood components, other than plasma derivatives (albumin and FFP), which are stored at room temperature, must be stored only in refrigerators (or freezers) that are strictly controlled and monitored (1–6°C or			

Skill 14-1 | *(continued)*

Name _____ Date _____ Instructor _____

ACTION TAKEN	COMPLETED SUCCESSFULLY	DID NOT COMPLETE	NOTES
33.8–42.8°F for refrigeration). *Never store any component in an unmonitored refrigerator.*			
8. Verification.			
9. Reassess the patient's condition and level of consciousness, ascertain vessel patency, take a full set of vital signs (temperature, pulse, respiration, and blood pressure), and document in the medical record. Abnormal vital signs require physician notification and documentation.			
10. Initiation of the transfusion. Carry out proper hand hygiene.			
11. Monitoring and maintenance.			
12. Discontinuation.			
13. Documentation.			

Skill 15-1 | Child with Acute Diarrhea

Name _____ Date _____ Instructor _____

ACTION TAKEN	COMPLETED SUCCESSFULLY	DID NOT COMPLETE	NOTES
1. Institute systematic assessment, head to toe approach, basing the assessment on clinical findings, lab values, and other monitoring systems (e.g., cardiorespiratory monitor, pulse oximeter).			
2. Keep the IV patent.			
3. Do not offer any food or fluids.			
4. Have oxygen and suction equipment at the bedside.			
5. Keep side rails up and the bed in low position.			

Glossary

Absolute Refractory Period The time period when the cell membrane is unable to react to any other stimulation because of changes occurring in the permeability of the membrane.

Absorption The process in which a drug or fluid moves from the site of administration into body fluids, which take it to the site of action (e.g., mouth [gastrointestinal system]—blood [circulatory system]—heart).

Accountability The state of being answerable for designated and accepted responsibilities.

Acid A substance that releases hydrogen ions when in solution; a hydrogen ion donor. *See also* **Nonvolatile (Fixed) Acid; Volatile Acid.**

Acid-Base Balance The balance between the acidity and alkalinity of body fluids.

Acidosis The accumulation of excess acids (hydrogen ions) or a deficiency of bicarbonate ions, dropping the plasma pH below 7.35. *See also* **Metabolic Acidosis; Respiratory Acidosis.**

Action Potential The rapid reversal and restoration of membrane potential polarity.

Activator Nonspecific substance that assists with an enzymatic reaction.

Active Transport The process whereby molecules are moved against either concentration, pressure, or electrical gradients utilizing cellular energy sources.

Activities of Daily Living (ADL) Activities that include bathing, feeding, dressing, and toileting.

Acute Normovolemic Hemodilution The preoperative removal of a client's blood via an arterial or venous catheter with the concurrent infusion of cell-free solutions to maintain normal volume.

Adaptation The process whereby the body adjusts to the ever-changing environment.

Adenosine Diphosphate (ADP) The molecule produced during muscle contraction that combines with inorganic phosphate to produce adenosine triphosphate (ATP).

Adenosine Triphosphate (ATP) The substance present in all cells that produces energy.

Administrative Law A rule made by an administrative agency or governing body to enforce statutory law.

Adverse Drug Reaction An unexpected or unintended effect of a drug; usually requires action such as discontinuing the drug, giving another drug, or decreasing the dosage.

Agent Any organism (bacteria, viruses, fungi, parasites, etc.) that is capable of eliciting a disease process.

Agglutination The clumping together of a solid antigen and a soluble antibody.

Agglutinin Antibody in the blood that attaches to an antigen and causes agglutination (clumping).

Agglutinogen The specific antigen that stimulates the recognition of an agglutinin.

Agonist A drug that fits to and interacts with the receptor site on a target cell to elicit a response.

Air Embolism The entry of air into the circulatory system during intravenous infusion therapy.

Alkalosis The reduction of acids (hydrogen ions) and the increase of bicarbonate ions, raising the plasma pH above 7.35. *See also* **Metabolic Alkalosis.**

Allele Form of a gene.

Allergen A substance that causes an immune response following sensitization.

Allergy An acquired abnormal immune response to an allergen.

Alligation The process of determining the proportion of components used in the preparation of an infusate of a specifically required strength not available commercially.

Alloantigen *See* **Isoantigen.**

Alloimmunization Lymphocytic response to specific antigens on the cell surfaces of transfused blood.

Alopecia Hair loss.

Amino Acid The building block of protein construction and the end product of protein digestion (hydrolysis).

Analgesic Agent used to relieve pain without altering consciousness.

Anaphylaxis Anaphylactic shock; a fatal allergic reaction that occurs because of the massive release of histamine.

Anesthetic An agent that produces loss of sensation, with or without loss of consciousness, and may be categorized as general, regional, or local.

Angina Pectoris Chest pain caused by myocardial ischemia; usually substernal pressure and pain that often radiates to the neck and jaw and down the left shoulder and arm; often mistaken for indigestion when pain is not severe.

Anion An ion with a negative charge.

Antagonism The combined effect of two agents (usually a fluid and/or medication) is less than the sum of each one acting alone.

Antagonist A drug that interacts with the target cell of a receptor site to inhibit or prevent the action of an agonist.

Antibiotic Destructive to life. Used to treat infectious diseases by inhibiting the growth of or destroying microorganisms.

Antibody An immunoglobulin (Ig) molecule that develops in response to an antigen that enters the system and combines with it.

Anticonvulsant Agent used to prevent or control seizure activity.

Antidiuretic Hormone A hormone produced in the hypothalamus and secreted by the posterior pituitary gland to act on the collecting tubules of the kidneys to promote water reabsorption; also called vasopressin.

Antiemetic An agent that prevents or arrests vomiting.

Antigen (immunogen) A molecular agent that is able to elicit an immune response by combining with an antibody.

Antigenic Determinant (epitope) The portion of an antigen to which an antibody attaches.

Anti-infective An agent that combats infection.

Antimicrobial Any natural or synthetic substance used to prevent the development of infection, kill existing microorganisms, or prevent their growth and development.

Antinauseant An agent that prevents the occurrence of nausea.

Antiseptic A product that can safely be applied to the skin or surface of mucous membranes to inhibit microbial growth or destroy organisms.

Anuria Loss of urinary output.

Arterial Laceration The inadvertent cut or puncture of an artery during CVC insertion.

Arteriole The smallest of the arteries.

Asepsis Absence of infectious organisms. *See also* **Medical Asepsis; Surgical Asepsis.**

Assault An intentional tort in which an individual threatens to do bodily harm to another.

Assessment First step of the nursing process, in which data is gathered.

Autoinfection Infection by resident flora. *See also* **Endogenous.**

Autologous Derived from the same person.

Autologous Blood Blood donated by an individual, in advance of its actual need, and stored for reinfusion at a later time.

Bacteremia Bacteria in the bloodstream.

Bactericidal Able to kill bacteria.

Bacteriostatic Tending to inhibit bacterial growth.

Band Immature neutrophil.

Baroreceptors Pressure-sensitive nerve endings located throughout the body in the aortic arch, blood vessels, atria of the heart, and carotid sinuses.

Basal Metabolic Rate Rate at which bodily waste products are metabolized.

Base A substance that accepts and combines with hydrogen ions; an alkali; hydrogen ion acceptor.

Battery An intentional tort involving the unlawful touching of another individual or his belongings without his consent.

Bioavailability The actual amount of a drug (as distinct from the amount administered) that enters the general circulation and is available for use.

Biotransformation The chemical alterations in pharmacologic activity that a drug undergoes once it enters the body, in order to be metabolized (syn: biodegradation).

Blood Salvage The collection and reinfusion of blood lost during the intraoperative and early (4-hour to 12-hour) postoperative period.

Blood Typing The tests run on a person's blood to determine blood type.

Brachial Plexus Injury Damage to the cervical and upper dorsal spin during CVC insertion.

Breach of Duty Failure to carry out the duty owed to another individual.

Buffer A substance that regulates acid–base balance.

Buffy Coat The thin layer between the RBCs and the plasma.

Capillaries The smallest blood vessels in the body.

Cardiac Tamponade Perforation of the pericardium by a CVC, resulting in compression of the heart.

Carrier An individual who harbors pathogens and transmits them to others without having the disease.

Carrier-Mediated Diffusion *See* **Facilitated Diffusion.**

Catabolism The phase of metabolism where complex substances are converted into simpler substances.

Catalyst An enzymatic activator.

Catheter Embolism Breakage of a portion of the CVC and entry into the circulatory system.

Catheter Malposition Position of the catheter outside the superior vena cava.

Cation An ion with a positive charge.

Causation Damage or harm that is caused by a breach of duty.

Causative Agent In the chain of infection, the organism capable of producing an infection.

Cellulitis The diffuse inflammation and infection of cellular and subcutaneous connective tissue.

Centrifuging The process by which whole, unclotted blood is placed in a tube in a centrifuge and spun at a high speed to separate the constituents.

Certification The granting, by a nongovernmental agency or private organization, of special recognition to one who has practiced and pursued an advanced role in a particular area.

Check Valve (back-check valve; one-way valve) A device that functions to prevent retrograde solution flow.

Chemotherapy The use of chemical agents to destroy malignant cells.

Child Life Specialist A professional (minimum of bachelor's degree) who, through medical play and dialogue, assists pediatric patients and their families to cope with the stressors of hospitalization.

Chloride Shift The diffusion of negatively charged bicarbonate ions out of the red blood cell and into the plasma, with the inward diffusion of chloride ions.

Chvostek's Sign Unilateral facial muscle contraction seen following tapping of the 7th cranial (facial) nerve anterior to the ear.

Chylothorax Lymph accumulation in the thoracic cavity due to laceration or perforation of the thoracic duct during CVC insertion.

Civil Law Private or common law regulating the rights of private individuals, as distinct from criminal law.

Clinical Pathway A case management tool that describes a sequence of events leading to desired outcomes for patient's with similar problems and treatment plans.

Colloid Glutinous substance whose particles, when submerged in a solvent, cannot form a true solution because the molecules, when thoroughly dispersed, do not dissolve, but remain suspended and uniformly distributed throughout the fluid.

Colloid Osmotic Pressure (oncotic pressure) The physical force created by colloids in suspension when crossing a semipermeable membrane.

Colonize The process whereby microorganisms take up residence in a host, making the host a carrier, which does not succumb to infection.

Combination Drug A brand-name drug made up of two generic drug products.

Communicable The ability to be passed from one person or object to another.

Communication All behavior in the presence of another; the dynamic interchange of self-expression, emotions, beliefs, information, and knowledge between individuals.

Community-Acquired Infection An infection that is picked up and present, or incubating, prior to admission to a health care facility.

Compartment Syndrome A condition in which nerves, vessels, or tendons are constricted within a space from the pressure of fluid or inflammation.

Competency A legal determination of an individual's capacity to make informed decisions.

Complete Protein One that contains all of the essential amino acids, such as that found in meat, milk, eggs, and cheese.

Concentration Gradient (concentration difference) A situation in which molecules become more populous in one area of a solution than in another.

Constant Portion The area on the end of each light and heavy chain of immune serum globulin that characterizes the properties of the antibody in terms of its ability to diffuse in tissues, adhere to certain substances, and pass through membranes. *See also* **Variable Portion.**

Constitutional Law Law addressing issues of governance that are the basis upon which the United States' government is built. The highest level of law directed at the powers and limitations of the federal government.

Contagious The ability of a disease to spread easily from one person to another.

Contamination The introduction of microorganisms or particulate matter into a normally sterile environment.

Cramp A strong, painful spasm.

Crime The act of violating a written law.

Criminal Law Law regulating actions that are harmful to society as a whole and prosecuted by state or local government.

Crossmatching The tests run to determine compatibility between the blood of a donor and recipient. *See also* **Major Crossmatching; Minor Crossmatching.**

Crystallization The ability to form crystals.

Crystalloid A substance that, when placed in solution, is capable of diffusing through membranes.

Crystalloid Osmotic Pressure The pressure created by the movement of dissolved ions.

Cubital Fossa The triangular area that lies anterior to and inferior to the elbow.

Database The written record of the objective and subjective information derived from the nursing assessment.

Deaminization The conversion to urea of any proteins not metabolized by the tissues.

Deep Vein Thrombosis (DVT) Inflammation of the larger, deeper veins of the extremities.

Defining Characteristics Observable cues related to a nursing diagnosis.

Definition A clear, accurate description that explains the meaning of a nursing diagnosis.

Dehydration Abnormal loss of body water. *See also* **Hypertonic Dehydration; Hypotonic Dehydration; Isotonic Dehydration.**

Denominator The bottom number in a fraction which indicates the total number of parts into which the whole is divided.

Depolarization   The reversal of membrane polarity during the production of an action potential.

Dermis (corium)   The true skin, composed of connective tissue, blood vessels, nerves, muscles, lymphatics, hair follicles, and sebaceous and sudoriferous glands.

Dimensional analysis   A logical, systematic approach to problem solving that does not require memorization of terms or formulas.

Disaccharide   A double sugar formed from two monosaccharide molecules; includes sucrose, lactose, and maltose.

Disease   Any combination of objective and subjective evidence that constitutes an abnormal health process in the human organism.

Displacement   The shift of the intravenous needle or catheter from its intended placement in the vein; inadvertent removal of the cannula from the vein.

Disseminated Intravascular Coagulation (DIC)   Diffuse pathologic coagulation process in which clotting mechanisms are used up and hemorrhage occurs.

Distribution   The process whereby a drug is transported to its intended site of action.

Drop Factor   The number of drops needed to deliver 1 ml of fluid.

Drug Action   The action of a therapeutic agent within the body and its physiologic alteration of existing bodily processes, which results in a therapeutic effect.

Drug Interaction   An adverse effect caused by the actions of two or more drugs.

Duty   Obligation owed to another individual.

Ecchymosis   Extravasation of blood into the interstitial spaces, resulting in skin discoloration; a black-and-blue mark.

Elder Abuse   Deliberate and willful act of a caregiver in inflicting injury.

Elderly   Individuals 65 years of age or older.

Elder Neglect   Failure to provide the necessities of life.

Elimination (drug)   Removal of a drug from the body.

Emboli   Plural of embolus.

Embolus   An aggregate of undissolved material carried in the blood. *See also* **Endogenous Embolus; Exogenous Embolus.**

Endocytosis   The process whereby the cell ingests particles that are too large to be taken in through passive or active transport systems.

Endogenous   That which originates within the body.

Endogenous Embolus   Embolus that arises from within the body and travels in the circulatory system.

Environment   The interacting group of conditions, surroundings, and influences in which a host and agent coexist.

Enzyme   A highly specialized molecule that coordinates and controls a cellular chemical reaction by serving as a specific activator (catalyst); the enzyme is not altered or diminished in the process.

Epidemiologic Triangle   The interaction of host, agent, and environment.

Epidemiology   The study of disease, its causes and determinants, its distribution within a population, and its control.

Epidermis   The outer layers of skin covering the body that is composed of epithelial cells and is devoid of blood vessels.

Epidural   The space surrounding the spinal cord.

Epitope (antigenic determinant)   The portion of an antigen to which an antibody attaches.

Erythema   Redness.

Evaluation   The fifth step of the nursing process where nursing care and the patient's goal achievement are measured.

Excitability (irritability)   The capability of nerves and muscles to make and transmit membrane potential changes.

Exocytosis   The process whereby molecules inside the cell that need to be transported out of the cell, but are too large to utilize passive or active transport processes, are removed by joining with the cell membrane, forming a vacuole, and exiting (in the reverse manner of pinocytosis).

Exogenous   That which originates outside the body.

Exogenous Embolus   Embolus that comes from outside the body and is introduced into the circulatory system.

Extension Set   A segment of IV tubing that is added to a primary administration line for the purpose of adding length.

Extracellular Fluid (ECF)   Fluid outside of the cells, comprising one-third (20%) of the body's total (60%) fluid; further divided into the intravascular, interstitial, and transcellular compartments.

Extracorporeal   Out of the body.

Extravasation   The leakage of material from a vessel into the surrounding tissue; the escape vesicant infusate from the vein into the surrounding tissue.

Facilitated Diffusion (carrier-mediated diffusion)   The process by which large polar lipid insoluble molecules cross the cell membrane by combining with carriers.

Factor   A number or quantity with a related measurement unit.

Fascia   The network of fibrous membranes that cover, bind, and support the muscular system.

Filter, IV   A porous medium through which impurities and particulate matter in an infusate pass for the purpose of separating and trapping them, thus preventing them from entering the patient's circulation during infusion therapy.

Filtration   The movement of fluid and diffusible particles through a membrane from an area of greater hydrostatic pressure to one of lesser pressure; the method of movement from the arterial capillary bed to the interstitial compartment. *See also* **Net Diffusion; Passive Diffusion; Net Filtration.**

Fistula Abnormal tubelike passage from a normal cavity or tube to a free surface or to another cavity or tube.

Five Rights of Medication Administration Right client, right medication, right dose, right route, and right time.

Floating A technique used to advance the IV catheter into the vein, whereby the catheter is inserted halfway into the vein and the tourniquet and needle are removed. The cannula hub is then attached to the infusion tubing and the control clamp on the tubing is slowly opened, floating the catheter into the vein with the infusate.

Flora Microbiologic organisms. *See also* **Resident Flora; Transient Flora.**

Fomites Inanimate objects that harbor microorganisms and serve as sources of contamination.

Foreseeability The aspect of an action or inaction implying the notion of cause and effect; the likelihood of a particular outcome.

Fowler's Position Semisitting with the head and torso elevated to a 40- to 60-degree angle. If the knees are flexed and supported with pillows, it is semi-Fowler's position.

Frail Elderly People over age 85 and at high risk for health problems.

Freeze-Drying *See* **Lyophilization.**

Freezing The process in which blood is frozen and all of the plasma and 99% of the WBCs are eliminated when thawing takes place and the nontransferable cryoprotectant is removed.

Fructose The sweetest of the monosaccharides; found in fruits, honey, sugar cane, and corn syrup.

Galactose A simple sugar formed, along with glucose, during the breakdown of lactose.

Genotype A combination of genes unique to each human being that determines the propensity for certain traits.

Geriatrics The branch of medicine concerned with medical problems of aging and diseases of the older person.

Germicide Agent capable of killing germs.

Gerontic Nursing Nursing care of the older person.

Gerontologic Nursing Application of scientific, logical practice to the nursing care of the older person.

Gerontology The scientific study of the process and problems of aging.

Glucose The most important monosaccharide in the body; the main source of cellular energy.

Glycogen Glucose that is stored in the body tissues and available when needed for metabolism.

Glyconeogenesis The formation of glycogen from body fat.

Harm *See* **Injury.**

Health Care Personnel Persons, including students and trainees, whose activities involve contact with patients or with blood or other body fluids from patients in a health care setting.

Hematogenous Spread The spread of pathogens through the blood or lymphatic systems.

Hematoma An accumulation of clotted blood in the tissue interstices.

Hemostasis The prevention of blood loss through the arrest of bleeding.

Hemothorax Blood accumulation in the pleural cavity due to vessel laceration or perforation during CVC insertion.

Histocompatibility The condition in which the tissue of the donor is compatible with that of the recipient.

Homans' Sign Calf pain with foot dorsiflexion.

Homeostasis The dynamic process that contributes to a state of internal constancy; the coordination of all bodily processes as well as the coordination of the human being as a dynamically integrated organism encompassing the biologic, physiologic, psychologic, sociocultural, and religious aspects of the person.

Homologous Having the same structure or genetic makeup.

Homologous Blood Blood collected from volunteer donors for transfer to other human beings.

Homotropic Pain in which the sensation of discomfort occurs at the point of injury.

Hooding A technique used to advance the IV catheter into the vein whereby the catheter is advanced $1/4$ inch off the needle, maintaining the tip of the needle inside the catheter, then the hub and needle as a unit is advanced into the vein and the needle is removed.

Host The living structure (person or animal) that provides the atmosphere in which organisms are able to live.

Humor Any fluid substance in the body.

Hydrogen Ion Acceptor Any substance that releases hydroxyl ions when placed in a solution; a base.

Hydrogen Ion Donor Any substance that releases hydrogen ions when placed in a solution; an acid.

Hydromediastinum Inadvertent puncture of the interpleural cavity during CVC insertion and infusion.

Hydrophilic Attracted to water.

Hydrophobic Repelled by water.

Hydrothorax Fluid accumulation in the thoracic cavity due to vessel laceration or perforation during CVC insertion.

Hydraulic Pressure The force of gravitational pressure that acts on hydrostatic pressure combined with the pumping pressure of the heart.

Hydrostatic Pressure The physical force of water as it pushes against a vessel wall or cellular membrane.

Hypercalcemia Abnormally elevated concentration of calcium in the blood.

Hypercapnia Abnormal increase of carbon dioxide in the blood.

Hyperchloremia An abnormal excess of chlorides in the blood.

Hyperkalemia An abnormally high concentration of potassium in the blood.

Hypermagnesemia Abnormally high concentration of magnesium in the blood.

Hypernatremia Abnormal excess of sodium in the blood.

Hyperosmolar A solution with an osmolality higher than that of plasma. *See* **Hypertonic.**

Hyperphosphatemia Abnormal excess of phosphorus in the blood.

Hypertonic (hyperosmolar) A solution with an osmolality higher than that of the plasma.

Hypertonic Dehydration Dehydration resulting from a greater loss of water than salt, producing increased sodium concentration and increased osmolality (hypernatremic dehydration).

Hypocalcemia Abnormally low concentration of calcium in the blood.

Hypochloremia An abnormal decrease in serum chloride.

Hypokalemia An abnormally low level of serum potassium.

Hypomagnesemia Abnormally low level of serum magnesium.

Hyponatremia Abnormal decrease in blood sodium levels.

Hypophosphatemia Abnormal deficiency of phosphorus in the blood.

Hyposmolar A solution with an osmolality lower than that of plasma. *See* **Hypotonic.**

Hypotonic (hyposmolar) A solution with an osmolality lower than that of plasma.

Hypotonic Dehydration Dehydration resulting from greater loss of salt than water, producing decreased sodium concentration and decreased osmolality (hyponatremic dehydration).

Idiosyncrasy An unusual or abnormal response to a medication or fluid.

Immune Response The ability of the immune system to recognize and respond to foreign invaders and prevent damage by neutralizing or eliminating them.

Immunity The state or condition in which an individual is protected from disease.

Immunogen (antigen) A molecular agent that is able to elicit an immune response by combining with an antibody.

Implementation (intervention) The fourth step of the nursing process in which the nurse puts the written plan of care into action.

Incompatibility The qualities of certain drugs and/or fluids that cause untoward effects when they are mixed.

Incomplete Protein One that does not contain all of the essential amino acids, such as vegetables and grains.

Indirect homologous donation Blood removed from a donor, stored under specific conditions, and then administered to a recipient at a later date.

Indurated Hardened.

Infarction Area of necrosis due to obstruction of blood flow.

Infection The process in which a host is invaded by microorganisms that are able to grow, reproduce, and cause injury, the result being disease. *See also* **Local Infection; Community-Acquired Infection; Nosocomial Infection; Systemic Infection.**

Infiltration The leakage of fluid out of the vein into the surrounding tissues; the escape of infusate (fluid, medication, or blood products) from the vein into the surrounding tissue.

Inflammation The body's normal immune response to any type of injury or invasion.

Inflammatory Pain that occurs as a result of the increased pressure that accompanies the inflammatory response.

Injury (harm) Physical damages (disability, disfigurement, pain, suffering, or wrongful death), emotional suffering, loss of reputation, or financial loss (past, present, or future).

Instrumental Activities of Daily Living Activities that include shopping, transportation, paying bills, and meal preparation.

Integumentary System The outer coverings that insulate and provide the first line of defense in protecting the body from microbial invasion and injury; composed of the epidermis and the dermis, including the hair and the nails.

Internal Environment The extracellular fluid that surrounds and bathes all body cells and communicates with the tissues, organs, and structures, which then make exchanges with the body's external surroundings.

Interstice Tissue space.

Interstitial Fluid (ISF) The fluid existing in the small spaces and gaps between body structures, cells, and tissues; where lymph forms.

Intima Inner lining of the vein wall.

Intracellular fluid (ICF) Fluid contained within the body cells, comprising two-thirds (40%) of the body's total (60%) fluid.

Intraosseous Within the medulla or marrow of the bone.

Intrathecal Into the cerebrospinal fluid.

Intravascular Within the vessels, arteries, veins, or capillaries.

Intravascular Fluid (IVF) The fluid found within the blood vessels of the body, containing serum (the water portion of blood) and serving as the vehicle for the transport and exchange of nutrients; plasma.

Ion An electrically charged molecule.

Ion Channel Submicroscopic passageway in the cell membrane matrix for the movement of charged organic ions.

Irrigate To gently flush a canal with fluid.

Irritability *See* **Excitability.**

Irritation Tenderness.

Ischemia Loss of blood supply to a part.

Isoantigen (alloantigen) A substance that can stimulate antibody production when introduced into members of the same species.

Isosmolar   A solution with the same osmolality as plasma. *See* **Isotonic.**

Isosmotic   Solutions with comparable molecular concentrations.

Isotonic (isosmolar)   A solution with the same osmolality of plasma.

Isotonic Dehydration   Dehydration resulting from a proportional loss of water and salt (isonatremic dehydration).

Judicial Law   The interpretation of statutes and regulations from which decisions are made; also called decisional or common law.

Label   Title that concisely names the nursing diagnosis.

Laminar Air Flow   Air that moves along parallel but separate flow paths into filters where contaminants are removed.

Learning   The taking in and processing of information, with a resultant change in behavior.

Legal Precedent   A court ruling that serves as basis for deciding future cases.

Leukopenia   Abnormal deficiency of leukocytes.

Liability   The state of being responsible for one's own actions.

Liable   Obligated or being responsible for (or to) something.

Lipid   A molecule that contains the elements carbon, hydrogen, and oxygen.

Litigation   The act or process of carrying on a lawsuit.

Local Infection   An infection in which microorganisms penetrate the tissues of a specific bodily area, then grow and exert their effect there.

Long-Term Goal   A goal that is reached over a relatively long period of time (weeks or months) or is ongoing.

Lymph   The interstitial fluid (ISF) that circulates within the lymphatic vessels, and is filtered in lymph nodes, containing proteins, salts, organic substances, and water.

Lyophilization (freeze-drying)   The process of rapidly freezing a product at an extremely low temperature and then dehydrating it in a high vacuum.

Lysosome   Intracellular digestive system containing hydrolytic enzymes that break down proteins and some carbohydrates for cellular use; digestive enzyme of the intracellular fluid.

Major Crossmatching   Mixing the donor's RBCs with the recipient's serum.

Malpractice   Negligence applied to professional behavior.

Manslaughter   Killing that is both unintentional and without malice.

Mediastinal Injury   Inadvertent puncture of the interpleural cavity during CVC insertion and infusion.

Medical Asepsis   The removal of pathogenic organisms; clean technique.

Medication Review   A process of matching each medication a patient is taking to a specific condition the client is known to have.

Membrane Potential   The state where the inside of the cell has a negative charge and the outside has a positive charge.

Microorganisms   All sources of life not perceptible to the naked eye, which include bacteria, fungi, molds, protozoa, viruses, yeasts, and other life forms.

Milliequivalent   The measurement of the concentration of electrolytes in a volume of solution.

Minor Crossmatching   Mixing the donor's serum and the recipient's blood.

Monosaccharide   A simple sugar, such as glucose, fructose, or galactose, that cannot be broken down to a simpler substance by hydrolysis.

Morbidity   Incidence of illness.

Mortality   Incidence of deaths.

Myocardial Infarction (MI)   Prolonged ischemia that causes irreversible damage to the myocardium.

Necrosis   Death of tissue.

Negligence   The unintentional tort that wrongs or harms another because of failure to act as any reasonable person would act; carelessness.

Net Diffusion   The movement that abolishes a concentration gradient and depends on membrane permeability, the difference in concentrations on each side of a membrane, the difference in electric potentials, and the difference in pressure across the membrane.

Net Filtration   The small amount of excess filtration in the interstitial compartment that is returned to the circulation by way of the lymphatics.

Neutralization   The process joining two opposing forces so that neither one dominates.

Noncarrier-mediated Transport   *See* **Passive Transport.**

Nonelectrolyte   Any solute present in the body fluid that is incapable of separating into particles when dispersed in fluid and does not carry an electrical charge.

Nonvolatile (Fixed) Acid   An acid that cannot be converted to vapors and eliminated in the lungs.

Nosocomial Infection   An infection that develops in a person during, or as a result of, a stay in a health care setting.

Nucleolus   A spherical body of granules within the nucleus where ribonucleoprotein is formed.

Numerator   The top number in a fraction which indicates the number of parts to be considered.

Nurse Practice Acts   Statutory laws that vary from state to state and define the parameters under which only those individuals who are qualified and licensed may practice nursing.

Nursing Diagnosis   The statement of an actual or potential patient health impairment that the nurse is able to identify and treat.

Nursing Process   The organized and systematized approach to nursing care with five steps: assessment, nursing diagnosis, planning, implementation, and evaluation.

Objective Data Information gathered through sensory input.

Obtunded A level of consciousness in which a patient has a limited response to his or her surroundings and is asleep, unless stimulated (auditory or tactile).

Oliguria Diminished urinary output.

Oncotic Pressure *See* **Colloid Osmotic Pressure.**

Onycholysis Loosening or detachment of the fingernail from the nail bed.

Osmolality The total number of solute particles in a unit weight of solvent.

Osmolarity (tonicity) The concentration of solute particles contained in a unit volume of solvent.

Osmosis The passage of water through a semipermeable membrane from an area of lower concentration of solutes to one of a higher concentration.

Osmotic Pressure The amount of hydrostatic pressure needed to draw a solvent across a membrane that develops as a result of a higher concentration of particles colliding with one another. *See also* **Colloid Osmotic Pressure; Crystalloid Osmotic Pressure; Oncotic Pressure.**

Osteomyelitis Infection of the bone marrow.

Oxidation The process in which oxygen combines with another substance.

Pain The sensatory and emotional experience associated with actual or potential tissue damage. It includes not only the perception of an uncomfortable stimulus but also the response to that perception (Source: International Association for the Study of Pain).

Paresthesia Sensation of numbness and/or tingling.

Passive (Simple) Diffusion The process whereby ions, water, and lipid-soluble molecules move randomly in all directions from an area of higher concentration to one of lower concentration through the pores in the matrix of a membrane.

Passive Transport (noncarrier-mediated transport) The movement of solutes through membranes without energy expenditure.

Pathogen A substance capable of producing disease.

Pathology The study of disease.

Patient-Controlled Analgesia (PCA) A drug administration system that allows the patient to self-administer and regulate delivery of medication for pain control on an as-needed basis.

Peau d'orange Skin surface that looks like orange peel (French).

Percent One part in one hundred.

Percutaneous Contact Penetration of the skin.

pH The potential of hydrogen; the chemical unit of measurement used to describe the degree of acidity or alkalinity of a substance.

Phagocytosis The process whereby the cell selectively ingests large particles of material such as bacteria, other cells, or particles of tissue degeneration.

Pharmacokinetics The study of drug action and drug metabolism.

Phlebitis Inflammation of a vein.

Phlebotomy The venipuncture and withdrawal of blood for autotransfusion or donor transfusion.

Phosphorylation The process of combining a phosphate with an organic compound.

Pinocytosis The endocytic process in which actual invagination of the cell membrane by the larger molecules occurs and channels are made that encapsulate to form vacuoles.

Planning Third step of the nursing process, in which the plan of care is formulated and goals are established.

Plasma Liquid portion of blood and lymph containing fibrinogen, which converts to fibrin in clot formation.

Pneumothorax Air accumulation in the pleural cavity due to perforation of the visceral pleura during CVC insertion.

Polar Molecule Molecule which is part negative, and part positive, making it neutral as a whole; soluble in water.

Polydipsia Excessive thirst.

Polymorphonuclear Cells with nuclei having several parts or lobes.

Polypharmacy The use of more than one medication for the same reason, no apparent reason, or as a treatment for a side effect of another medication.

Polysaccharide Large molecule, such as starch, glycogen, and cellulose, made up of numerous glucose molecules.

Polyuria Excessive urination.

Portal of Exit The site from which a microorganism leaves its reservoir.

Postinfusion Phlebitis Signs or symptoms of phlebitis that occur after an intravenous infusion or intermittent infusion device is discontinued.

Potential of Hydrogen *See* **pH.**

Potential Difference The difference, measured in voltage, between electrical charges on each side of a membrane.

Precipitation The suspension or crystallization of particles that occurs due to the mixing of incompatible solutions or adding solutes to incompatible solutions; results in the occlusion of an intravenous line.

Priming Volume The volume of infusate needed to replace the air in an IV adapter or connecting device.

Proportion Two equal ratios or an equation between them.

Protease An enzyme that breaks down protein.

Protein An organic compound composed of carbon, hydrogen, oxygen, and nitrogen molecules and usually phosphorus and sulfur; made up of molecular units called amino acids. *See also* **Complete Protein; Incomplete Protein.**

Protoplasm   The substance of the cell, composed of water, electrolytes, carbohydrates, lipids, and proteins.

Ratio   A quantitative relationship of one thing to another.

Reaction-Specific   The capability to act on certain substances or groups of closely related substances.

Reagin   A type of immunoglobulin E (IgE).

Reasonableness   The use of practical or sensible judgment; acting as any rational, prudent person would act in the same or similar situation, under the same or similar circumstances.

Red Flare   Area of redness around an IV site from the release of histamine and resulting vasodilation that occurs with a hypersensitivity reaction.

Related Factors   Patterned components that connect to the nursing diagnosis.

Relative Refractory Period   Time span toward the end of an action potential when potassium permeability increases and only an extremely strong stimulus can generate another action potential.

Repolarization   The reestablishment of the resting membrane potential.

Reservoir   The source of infection; the environment in which microorganisms are able to live and grow.

Resident Flora   Flora that reside in or on a person's body, are indigenous to that individual, and are not easily removed.

Resistance   The combination of internal and external barriers that prevent the invasion, reproduction, and impairment by invading pathogens (agents).

Resting Membrane Potential   The difference between the electrical charges on each side of a membrane when there is no cellular stimulation (negative on the inside; positive on the outside).

Risk-Benefit Analysis   Weighing the potential risks against the anticipated benefits of an action.

Risk Factor   Physiologic, psychologic, or genetic elements or environmental considerations that increase the individual, family, or communal potential for an unhealthful situation.

Salt   A chemical compound that results from the interaction of an acid and a base; it consists of the negative ion of an acid (other than hydroxyl) and the positive ion of a base (other than hydrogen).

Sebaceous   Containing, or pertaining to, sebum.

Semi-Fowler's Position   Semisitting position with the head and torso elevated at a 40- to 60-degree angle, with the knees flexed and supported by pillows.

Sensitization   The first exposure of the body to an allergen.

Sepsis   Pathologic state, usually with fever, that is the result of microorganisms and/or their toxic products in the bloodstream.

Serum   The water portion of the blood; plasma.

Short-Term Goal   A goal that is reached over a relatively short period of time (hours or days).

Side Effect   An interaction in which medication acts on one, intended, system, but also exerts an effect on another area.

Sign   Objective evidence of disease.

Slander   Verbal defamation of an individual between two parties in which a third party is witness to the defamation.

Sodium-Potassium Gates   Polypeptide ion channels in the cell membrane that selectively open and close according to membrane potentials.

Sodium-Potassium Pump   The active transport mechanism that acts to remove sodium from the cell and bring potassium into the cell.

Solute   Substance dissolved in a liquid (solvent).

Solution   Fluid composed of a solvent and dissolved solutes.

Solvent   Liquid that holds other substances (solutes) and acts to dissolve them.

Speed Shock   The systemic reaction to the rapid or excessive infusion of fluid or medication into the circulation.

Standard   Something established and used as the basis for comparison in evaluating the outcome of a performance.

Standard of Care   That which is used to determine the minimum acceptable level of nursing care within a practice setting.

State Board of Nursing   The regulatory body that oversees the practice of professional or practical (vocational) nursing within a state and enforces that state's nurse practice act.

Statute   A law enacted by a legislative body.

Steatorrhea   Fecal fat.

Stopcock   A valve that controls the directional flow of infusate through manual manipulation of a direction-regulating valve.

Subcutaneous   The area below the epidermis and dermis, made up of loose connective tissue and stored body fat; also called superficial fascia.

Subjective Data   Any information the nurse obtains from the patient regarding his or her condition.

Sudoriferous   Conveying sweat.

Superficial Thrombophlebitis   Inflammation of the subcutaneous vessels of the extremities.

Suppurative   To form pus.

Surfactant   An agent that lowers surface tension.

Surgical Asepsis   The removal of all microorganisms (pathogenic and nonpathogenic); sterile technique.

Susceptible   To have little resistance to an invading agent.

Symptom   Subjective evidence of disease.

Syncope   Fainting.

Synergism The combined effect of two or more agents (usually a medication and/or fluid) that is greater than the sum of each one acting alone.

Systemic Infection An infection in which microorganisms travel freely throughout the host's body and exert their virulence on several, or all, body systems.

Tachycardia Increased heart rate above normal.

Target Cell The cellular site of action where a drug exerts its effect.

Teaching The verbal, nonverbal, visual, or written act of transferring information from one person to another to impart knowledge and effect a desired change in behavior.

Therapeutic Communication The planned, goal-directed interchange between individuals that results in a desired, mutually agreeable outcome.

Threshold Potential The lowest amount of stimulation needed to change a membrane potential and reverse polarity.

Thrombophlebitis Inflammation of a blood vessel due to the development of a thrombus that obstructs or occludes the vessel.

Thrombosis Clot formation.

Thrombus Blood clot that obstructs or occludes a blood vessel.

Tort An intentional or unintentional wrong, injury, or damage to another person or his property, resulting from breach of duty, that can result in civil action.

Tourniquet An encircling device consisting of a segment of rubber tubing or a strip of Velcro® strapping that temporarily arrests blood flow from a distal vessel.

Transcellular Fluid (TSF) The fluid formed as a byproduct of cellular activity; smallest portion of the extracellular compartment.

Transient Flora Flora that are picked up, usually on the skin, and are removed fairly easily.

Transport Proteins Solute-specific carriers in the cell membrane that carry large polar (charged) lipid-insoluble materials into the cell.

Trousseau's Sign Carpal spasm following the inflation of a blood pressure cuff to the arm above systolic pressure for three minutes.

Tunica Adventitia The white fibrous connective tissue that makes up the outermost layer of the wall of an artery; also called the tunica externa.

Tunica Externa The white fibrous connective tissue that makes up the outermost layer of the wall of an artery; also called the tunica adventitia.

Tunica Intima A serous layer that forms the inner most wall of an artery; it is composed of endothelial cells, a subendothelial connective tissue layer, and a pliant inner lamina.

Tunica Media The yellow fibrous middle layer of an artery responsible for controlling the diameter of the artery; it is composed of smooth muscle and elastic fibers.

Universal Donor A person with blood type O, having no A or B antigens, who is able to donate blood for use by persons of any of the four blood types, as an emergency measure.

Universal Recipient A person with blood type AB, who has no plasma antibodies, and can receive all four blood types, as an emergency measure.

Vacuole Clear space, either fluid or air filled in the protoplasm.

Valence The electrical charge of an ion.

Variable Portion (immune serum globulin) The area on an antibody that gives it specificity in attaching to a particular antigen. *See also* **Constant Portion.**

Varices Twisted, dilated veins.

Vector A carrier that can transfer an agent between hosts.

Veins Blood vessels that return blood to the heart and lungs and transport waste products to excretory locations.

Venous Spasm The sudden involuntary movement or contraction of a vessel wall that occurs as a result of trauma or irritation.

Venous Stasis Inhibited or stagnated blood flow.

Venules The smallest of the veins; they are the first to receive blood containing carbon dioxide and waste products when it leaves the capillaries.

Vertigo Dizziness; the illusion of movement.

Vesicant An agent that irritates and causes blistering.

Vessel Collapse Retraction of the walls of a vein or artery.

Virulence The strength and ability of a microorganism to produce disease.

Volatile Acid An acid that can be vaporized, or evaporated and eliminated, through the lungs.

Washing The process in which 80% to 90% of the WBCs and almost all of the plasma are removed from the blood.

Reference List

Aitken, D. R., & Minton, J. P. (1984). The pinch-off sign: A warning of impending problems with permanent subclavian catheters. *American Journal of Surgery, 148,* 633–636.

Allen, K. (2000). How to remove a Huber needle without sticking yourself. *Nursing, 30*(10), 55–56.

Alvarado-Ramy, F., Alter, M.J., Bower, W., Henderson, D.K., Sohn, A.H., & Sinkowitz-Cochran, R.L. (2001). Management of occupational exposures to hepatitis C virus: Current practice and controversies. *Infection Control and Hospital Epidemiology, 22*(1), 53–55.

American Association of Blood Banks. (1990). *Technical manual* (10th ed.). Arlington, VA: Author.

American Heart Association. (2001). *Textbook of pediatric advanced life support*. Dallas, Texas: Author.

American Heart Association. (2002). *PALS Provider Manual.* Dallas, Texas: Author

American Nurses Association. (1980). *Nursing: A social policy statement*. Kansas City, MO: Author.

American Nurses Association. (1991). *Standards of clinical nursing practice*. Washington, DC: American Nurses Publishing.

American Nurses Association. (1995). *Nursing's social policy statement*. Washington, DC: American Nurses Publishing.

American Nurses Association. (2001). *Scope and standards of gerontological nursing practice* (2nd ed.). Washington, DC: American Nurses Publishing.

Association for Professionals in Infection Control and Epidemiology (2000). *APIC infection control and applied epidemiology: Principles and practices.* St. Louis, MO: Mosby.

Axton, S. E., & Hall, B. (1994). An innovative method of administering IV medications in children. *Pediatric Nursing, 20*(4), 341–344.

Banks, M. A. (1994). Home infusion of intravenous immunoglobulin. *Journal of Intravenous Nursing, 6,* 299–310.

Barber, Phil. (2002, September 27). Dirty Work: From hurried handwashing to faux fingernails, a disturbing rise in hospital-acquired infections prompts facilities to crack down. *Nurse Week: South Central Edition, 7*(19).

Beam, T. R., Goodman, E. I., Maki, D. G., Farr, B. M., & Mayhall, C. G. (1990). Preventing central venous catheter-related complications, a roundtable discussion. *Infections in Surgery, 10,* 1–13.

Behrman, R. E., Kliegman, R., & Jenson, H. B. (Eds.). (2001). *Nelson Textbook of Pediatrics* (16th ed.). Philadelphia: W. B. Saunders.

Bennett, J., & Brachman, P. S. (Eds.). (1998). *Hospital infections* (4th ed.). Philadelphia: Lippincott Williams & Wilkins.

Berger, T. G., James, W. D., & Odom, R. B. (2000). *Andrew's Diseases of the Skin* (9th ed.). Philadelphia: W. B. Saunders.

Bernard, G. R., Vincent, J.-L., Laterre, P.-F., LaRosa, S. P., Dhainaut, J.-F., Lopez-Rodriguez, A., et al., for The Recombinant Human Activated Protein C Worldwide Evaluation in Severe Sepsis (PROWESS) Study Group (2001, March 8). Efficacy and safety of recombinant human activated protein C for severe sepsis. *The New England Journal of Medicine.*

Brunner, L. S. (2001). *Lippincott manual of nursing practice* (7th ed.). Philadelphia: Lippincott Williams & Wilkins.

Burggraf, Virginia (2001). What the future holds for gerontology. *Nursing, 31*(1), 52.

California Department of Health Sciences. (2002, January 24). *SHARPS Injury Control Program*. Retrieved April 7, 2003, from http://www.dhs.ca.gov/ohb/sharps/default.htm

Carlson, R. D. (1992, January). Antiseptic-releasing catheter reduces infections: An interview with Dennis Maki, M.D. *Oncology Times, 14,* 1.

Carpenito, L. J. (2002). *Handbook of nursing diagnosis* (9th ed.). Philadelphia: Lippincott Williams & Wilkins.

Carrico, R.M. (2001). What to do if you're exposed to a bloodborne pathogen. *Home Healthcare Nurse, 19*(6), 362–368.

Carrieri, V. K., Lindsey, A. M., & West, E. M. (2003, March). *Pathophysiological phenomena in nursing: Human responses to illness* (3rd ed.). Philadelphia: W. B. Saunders.

Centers for Disease Control and Prevention (CDC). (1988). Update: Universal precautions for prevention and transmission of human immunodeficiency virus, hepatitis B virus, and other blood-borne pathogens in health care settings. *Morbidity and Mortality Weekly Report, 37*(24), 377–388.

Centers for Disease Control and Prevention (CDC). (1995a). A case-control study of HIV seroconversion in health care workers after percutaneous exposure to HIV-infected blood—France, United Kingdom, and United States, January 1988–August 1994. *Morbidity and Mortality Weekly Report, 44,* 929–933.

Centers for Disease Control and Prevention (CDC). (1995b). *HIV/AIDS Surveillance Report, 1,* 15.

Centers for Disease Control and Prevention (CDC). (1995c). Intravascular device-related infections prevention: Guideline availability notice. *Fed. Reg., Part II, 60*(187), 49978–50006.

Centers for Disease Control and Prevention (CDC). (1995d, September 22). Recommendations for preventing the spread of vancomycin resistance: Recommendations of the Hospital Infection Control Practices Advisory Committee (HICPAC). *Morbidity and Mortality Weekly Report, 44*(RR-12), 1–13. Retrieved April 7, 2003, from http://www.cdc.gov/mmwr/PDF/RR/RR4412.pdf

Centers for Disease Control and Prevention (CDC). (1996, June 7). Update: Provisional public health service recommendations for chemoprophylaxis after occupational exposure to HIV. *Morbidity and Mortality Weekly Report, 45*(22), 468–472. Retrieved April 7, 2003 from http://www.cdc.gov/mmwr/PDF/wk/mm4522.pdf

Centers for Disease Control and Prevention (CDC). (1997, December 26). Immunization of health-care workers: Recommendations of the Advisory Committee on Immunization Practices (ACIP) and the Hospital Infection Control Practices Advisory Committee (HICPAC). *Morbidity and Mortality Weekly Report, 46*(RR-18), 1–42. Retrieved April 7, 2003, from http://www.cdc.gov/epo/mmwr/preview/mmwrhtml/00050577.htm

Centers for Disease Control and Prevention (CDC). (1998a, May 15). *Appendix: First-Line Drugs for HIV Postexposure Prophylaxis (PEP).* Retrieved April 7, 2003 from http://www.cdc.gov/epo/mmwr/preview/mmwrhtml/00052801.htm

Centers for Disease Control and Prevention (CDC). (1998b). *Guideline for infection control in health care personnel, 1998.* Retrieved April 7, 2003 from http://www.cdc.gov/ncidod/hip/GUIDE/InfectControl98.pdf

Centers for Disease Control and Prevention (CDC). (1998c, May 15). *Public Health Service Guidelines for the Management of Health-Care Worker Exposures to HIV and Recommendations for Postexposure Prophylaxis.* Retrieved April 7, 2003 from http://www.cdc.gov/epo/mmwr/preview/mmwrhtml/00052722.htm

Centers for Disease Control and Prevention (CDC). (1998d, October 16). *Recommendations for Prevention and Control of Hepatitis C Virus (HCV) Infection and HCV-Related Chronic Disease.* Retrieved April 7, 2003 from http://www.cdc.gov/epo/mmwr/preview/mmwrhtml/00055154.htm

Centers for Disease Control and Prevention (CDC). (1998e). *Recommendations for prevention of infections in health care personnel.* Atlanta, GA: Centers for Disease Control and Prevention, The Hospital Infection Control Advisory Committee.

Centers for Disease Control and Prevention (CDC). (2001a). *Guideline for the Prevention of Intravascular Device-Related Infections.* Atlanta, GA: Author.

Centers for Disease Control and Prevention (CDC). (2001b). Recommendations for preventing transmission of infections among chronic hemodialysis patients. *Morbidity and Mortality Weekly Report 50*(RR-5), 1–43.

Centers for Disease Control and Prevention (CDC). (2001c, October 12). Deaths: Leading causes for 1999. *National Vital Stat Rep 49*(11):1–87. (DHHS Publication No.(PHS)2002 –1120 PRS 01-0594 (10/2001)). Retrieved April 7, 2003, from http://www.cdc.gov/nchs/data/nvsr/nvsr49/nvsr49_11.pdf

Centers for Disease Control and Prevention (CDC). (2001d). Updated U.S. public health service guidelines for the management of occupational exposures to HBV, HCV, and HIV and recommendations for postexposure prophylaxis. *Morbidity and Mortality Weekly Report 50*(RR-11):1–52. Retrieved April 7, 2003, from http://www.cdc.gov/mmwr/PDF/rr/rr5011.pdf

Centers for Disease Control and Prevention (CDC). (2002a, August 9). Guidelines for the prevention of intravascular catheter-related infections. *Morbidity and Mortality Weekly Report 51*(RR-10), 1–26.

Centers for Disease Control and Prevention (CDC). (2002b). Guidelines for the use of antiretroviral agents in HIV-infected adults and adolescents. *Morbidity and Mortality Weekly Report 51*(RR-7), 1–55.

Centers for Disease Control and Prevention (CDC). (2002c, October 25). Guidelines for hand hygiene in health-care settings: Recommendations of the Healthcare Infections Control Practices Advisory Committee and the HICPAC/SHEA/APIC/IDSA Hand Hygiene Task Force. *Morbidity and Mortality Weekly Report 51*(RR-16).

Centers for Disease Control and Prevention (CDC). (2003a). CDC prevention guidelines database. Retrieved April 7, 2003, from http://aepo-xdv-www.epo.cdc.gov/wonder/PrevGuid/PrevGuid.shtml

Centers for Disease Control and Prevention (CDC). (2003b). *Morbidity and Mortality Weekly Report (MMWR) home page.* Retrieved April 7, 2003, from http://www2.cdc.gov/mmwr/mmwr.html

Chaisson, R. E., Keruly, J. C., & Moore, R. D. (1995). Race, sex, drug use, and progression of human immunodeficiency virus disease. *New England Journal of Medicine, 333*(12), 751–756.

Chamberland, M. E. & Bell, D. M. (1992). HIV transmission from health care worker to patient. What is the risk? (Editorial). *Annals of Internal Medicine, 116,* 871–873.

Chamberland, M. E., Epstein, J., Dodd, R. Y., Persing, D., Will, R. G., DeMaria, A., Jr., et al. (1998). Blood safety. *Emerging Infectious Diseases, 4*(3).

Chiarello, L., Cardo, D.M., Panlilio, A.L., Alter, M.J., & Gerberding, J. (2001). Risks and prevention of blood-borne virus transmission from infected healthcare providers. *Seminars in Infection Control, 1*(1): 61–72.

Clinical. (2000). Giving up before surgery? *Nursing, 30*(7): 64.

Combating Infection (2001). Handwashing: First defense against infection. *Nursing, 31*(9): 20.

Combating Infection (2001). Handwashing: First defense against infection. *Nursing, 31*(10): 30.

Corbbett, J. V. (2000). *Laboratory tests & diagnostic procedures with nursing diagnoses* (5th ed.). Upper Saddle River, NJ: Prentice Hall.

Craven, R. F., & Hirnie, C. J. (2002). *Fundamentals of nursing: Human health & function* (4th ed.). Philadelphia: Lippincott Williams & Wilkins.

Crismon, C. (1992). Errors in subclavian administration of P.O. meds continue. *R.N. Update, 23*(3), 4.

Cunha, B. A. (2002). *Antibiotic Essentials.* Royal Oak, Michigan: Physicians' Press.

Curley, M. A. Q. & Moloney-Harmon, P. A. (2001). *Critical care nursing of infants and children* (2nd ed.). Philadelphia: Elsevier Health Sciences.

Daniels, J. M., & Smith, L. M. (1998). *Clinical calculations: A unified approach* (4th ed.). Albany, NY: Delmar Learning.

Decreases Seen in Leading Causes of Death. (2001, June 26). United Press International, on NewsMax.com.

DeCrosta, T. (1986a). Every patient is a target. Part I: The problem. *Nursing Life, 5,* 18–22.

DeCrosta, T. (1986b). Every patient is a target. Part II: Fighting the problem. *Nursing Life, 6,* 45–47.

DR Intravenous Therapy Consulting, Inc. (2003, February 15). *DR Intravenous Therapy Consulting home page.* Retrieved April 7, 2003, from www.drivt.com

Drinker, C. K., Drinker, K. R., & Lund, C. C. (1992). The circulation in the mammalian bone marrow. *American Journal of Physiology, 62*(1), 1–92.

Dudek, S. G. (2001). *Nutrition essentials for nursing practice* (4th ed.). Philadelphia: Lippincott Williams & Wilkins.

Ebersole, P., & Hess, P. (1998). *Toward healthy aging: Human needs and nursing response* (5th ed.). St. Louis, MO: Mosby.

Edlich, R. F., & Watkins, F. H. (1997). Glove powder—Facts and fiction. In *Surgical services management.* Denver, CO: Association of Operating Room Nurses.

Ehrlich, A. (2000). *Medical terminology for health professions* (4th ed.). Albany, NY: Delmar Learning.

Erbelding , E. J. (1999, May). Resistance testing: A primer for clinicians. *The Hopkins HIV Report, 11*(3), 1, 8, 9.

Ernst, J. (2001). Guide to needlestick prevention devices: Is your phlebotomy technique putting you at risk? *Home Healthcare Nurse, 19*(6): 345–347.

Estes, M. E. Z. (2002). Health assessment and physical examination (2nd ed.). Clifton Park, NY: Delmar Thomson Learning.

Evans, C. A., Kenny, P. J., & Rizzuto, C. (1993). Caring for the confused geriatric surgical patient. *Geriatric Nursing, 14*(5), 237–241.

Farber, T. M. (1991, September 29 – October 2). *ARROWgard ™ antiseptic surface—Toxicology review.* Paper presented at the 31st Interscience Conference on Antimicrobial Agents & Chemotherapeutic Agents.

Fitzpatrick, L. (2002). When to administer modified blood products. *Nursing, 32*(5): 36–42.

Fong, E., & Scott, A. (2004). *Body structures and functions* (10th ed.). Clifton Park, NY: Delmar Learning.

Fraser, D. (1993). Patient assessment: Infection in the elderly. *Journal of Gerontological Nursing, 19*(7), 5–11.

Friedman, G., Silva, E., & Vincent J.-L. (1998) Has the mortality of septic shock changed with time? *Crit Care Med., 26,* 2078–2086.

Friedman, M. M. (2001). The impact of the Needlestick Safety and Prevention Act on home care and hospice organizations. *Home Healthcare Nurse, 19*(6): 356–360.

Friend, T. (1997, January 22). Hospital's drug errors cost lives, drain resources. *USA Today,* p. D1.

Gahart, B. L. & Nazareno, A. R. (2003) *Intravenous Medications* (19th ed.). St. Louis, MO: Mosby.

Gaynes, R., Richards, C., Edwards, J., Emori, T. G., Horan, T., Alonso-Echanove, J., et al. (2001). Feeding back surveillance data to prevent hospital-acquired infections. *Emerging Infectious Diseases, 7*(2).

Gelb, L. (1991). *Food and Drug Administration medical alert.* Rockville, MD: U.S. Department of Health and Human Services.

Genentech. (2002). *Genentech products—disease education—central venous access devices.* Retrieved October 2, 2002 from www.gene.com/gene/products/education/cardiovascular/cvads.jsp

Gianino, S., Seltzer, R., & Eisenberg, P. (1996). The ABCs of TPN. *RN, 59*(2), 42–47.

Goodwin, D. (1992). Critical pathways in home health care. *Nursing Administration Quarterly, 22*(2), 35–40.

Gorbach, S. L., Mensa, J., & Gatell, J. M. (1999). *Pocket book of antimicrobial therapy & prevention.* Baltimore: Williams & Wilkins.

Guyton, A. C., & Hall, J. C. (1997). *Human physiology and mechanisms of disease* (6th ed.). Philadelphia: W. B. Saunders.

Guyton, A. C., & Hall, J.C. (2000). *Textbook of medical physiology* (10th ed.). Philadelphia: W. B. Saunders.

Hadaway, L. C. (2000a). IV rounds: Flushing to reduce central catheter occlusions. *Nursing, 30*(10), 74.

Hadaway, L. C. (2000b). IV rounds: Managing vascular access device occlusions, part 1. *Nursing, 30*(7), 29.

Hadaway, L. C. (2000c). IV rounds: Managing vascular access device occlusions, part 2. *Nursing, 30*(8), 14.

Hadaway, L. C. (2002). What you can do to decrease catheter-related infections. *Nursing, 32*(9), 46–48.

Haiduven, D. J., DeMaio, T. M., & Stevens, D. A. (1992). A five-year study of needlestick injuries: Significant reduction associated with communication, education, and convenient placement of sharps containers. *Infection Control and Hospital Epidemiology, 13*(5), 265–271.

Halderman, Francie. (2000). Selecting a vascular access device. *Nursing, 30*(11), 59–61.

Hall, J. K. (2002). *Law and Ethics for Clinicians.* Philadelphia: Jackhal.

Haney, Daniel Q. (2002, September 29). Alcohol gels speed hospital scrubbing. *Associated Press,* as reported in *The El Paso Times,* p. 7A.

Hawkins, D. A., Asboe, D., Barlow, K., Evans, B. (2001). Seroconversion to HIV-1 following a needlestick injury despite combination post-exposure prophylaxis. *Journal of Infection, 43*(1), 12–15.

Hazinski, M. F. (1992). *Nursing care of the critically ill child* (2nd ed.). St. Louis, MO: Mosby.

Henderson, D. K. (2001). HIV postexposure prophylaxis in the 21st century. *Emerging Infectious Diseases, 7*(2), 254–258.

Herbst, S. F. (1993). Accumulation of blood products and drug precipitates in VADs: A set-up for trouble. *Journal of Vascular Access Network, 3*(3), 9–13.

Hibberd, P. L. (1995). Patients, needles, and health care workers. *Journal of Intravenous Nursing, 18*(2), 65–76.

Hogstel, M. O. (2001). *Gerontology: Nursing Care of the Older Adult.* Clifton Park, NY: Delmar Learning.

Hospital Nursing Newsline. (2001). T-PA clears clogged catheters too. *Nursing, 31*(5), 32–38.

Hrouda, B. S. (2002). Warming up to IV infusion. *Nursing, 32*(3), 54–55.

Hunt, M. L. (1995). *Baxter training manual for intravenous admixture personnel* (5th ed.). Chicago: Precept Press.

Infusion Nurses Society. (2000). Infusion nursing standards of practice. *Journal of Intravenous Nursing* (Supplement). Note: This journal is now the *Journal of Infusion Nursing.*

INSERT Intravenous Access Network. (2003). *INSERT Intravenous Access Network home page.* Retrieved April 7, 2003, from www.ivteam.com

Institute of Medicine. (1999). *To err is human.* Washington: National Academy Press.

International Agency for Research on Cancer (IARC). (2000, February 28). *DEHP confirmed as non-carcinogenic: International Agency for Research on Cancer (IARC) reclassifies DEHP as non-carcinogenic to humans* [Press Release]. Brussels, Belgium: European Council for Plasticisers and Intermediates (ECPI). Retrieved April 7, 2003, from http://www.ecpi.org/pressrelease/current/index.asp

International Health Care Worker Safety Center, University of Virginia. (2001, April 18). *Safety devices.* Retrieved April 7, 2003, from http://www.people.virginia.edu/~epinet/products.html

Intravenous Nurses Society. (1998). Revised intravenous standards of practice. *Journal of Intravenous Nursing* (Supplement).

Intravenous therapy: The right stuff. (1994). Infection-control/Update 94. *Nursing, 24*(10), 54.

Iyer, P. W. (1991). Thirteen charting rules to keep you legally safe. *Nursing, 21*(6), 40–45.

Jackson, D. (1995). Latex allergy and anaphylaxis—What to do? *Journal of Intravenous Nursing, 18*(1), 33–52.

Jacobson, G. (1985). Handwashing, ring-wearing, and number of organisms. *Nursing Research, 34,* 186–187.

Jagger, J., and Perry, J. (2001a). Risky phlebotomy with a syringe. *Nursing, 31*(2), 73.

Jagger, J., and Perry, J. (2001b). Exposure prevention, point by point. *Nursing, 31*(6), 12–15.

Jagger, J., and Perry, J. (2001c). Beware of glass capillary tubes. *Nursing, 31*(11), 92.

Jagger, J., and Perry, J. (2002). Exposure safety: Realistic expectations for safety devices. *Nursing, 32*(3), 72.

Jagger, J., Hunt, E. H., Brand-Elnaggar, J., & Pearson, R. D. (1988). Rates of needlestick injury caused by various devices in a university hospital. *New England Journal of Medicine, 319*(5), 284–288.

James, L., & Hadaway, L. C. (1993). A retrospective look at tip location and complications of peripherally inserted central catheter lines. *Journal of Intravenous Nursing, 16*(2), 104–109.

Jezierski, M. (1997). Creating a latex-safe environment: Riddle Memorial Hospital's response to protect patients and employees. *Journal of Emergency Nursing, 23,* 191–198.

Johnson, M. (1998). *Working on a miracle.* New York: Bantam Doubleday Dell.

Joint Commission on Accreditation of Healthcare Organizations. (2002). *Comprehensive accreditation manual for hospitals: The official handbook.* Chicago: Author.

Kallenborn, J. C., Price, T. G., Carrico, R., & Davidson, A. B. (2001). Emergency department management of occupational exposures: Cost analysis of rapid HIV test. *Infection Control and Hospital Epidemiology, 22*(5), 289-293.

Kaunitz, K. K. (1996). Legal issues. In *APIC infection control and applied epidemiology: Principles and practice.* St. Louis, MO: Mosby.

Kee, J. L., & Paulanka, B. J. (2004). *Fluids and electrolytes with clinical applications: A programmed approach* (7th ed.). Clifton Park, NY: Delmar Learning.

Kelly, L. Y., & Joel, L. A. (1999). *Dimensions of professional nursing* (8th ed.). New York: McGraw-Hill.

Kenny, P. (1996). Managing HIV infection: How to bolster your patient's fragile health. *Nursing, 26*(8), 26–35.

Kite, P. (1999, October 30). Rapid Diagnosis of Central-Venous-Catheter-Related Bloodstream Infection without Catheter Removal. *Lancet.*

Kozier, B., Erb, G., & Olivieri, R. (1999). *Fundamentals of nursing: Concepts, process, and practice* (6th ed.). Redwood City, CA: Prentice Hall.

Larsen, E. A. (1988). APIC guidelines for infection control practice: Guideline for use of topical antimicrobial agents. *American Journal of Infection Control, 16*(6), 253–266.

Larson, E. L. (1996). Handwashing and skin preparation for invasive procedures. In *APIC infection control and applied epidemiology: Principles and practice.* St. Louis, MO: Mosby.

Lauer, G.M., & Walker, B.D. (2001). Hepatitis C virus infection. *New England Journal of Medcine, 345*(1), 41–52.

Lawson, M. (1991). Partial occlusion of indwelling central venous catheters. *Journal of Intravenous Nursing, 14*(3), 157–159.

Leddy, S., & Pepper, J. M. (1998). *Conceptual bases of professional nursing* (4th ed.). Philadelphia: Lippincott Williams & Wilkins.

LeMone, P. and Burke, K. M. (2000). *Medical-surgical nursing: Critical thinking in client care.* Upper Saddle River, NJ: Prentice Hall Health.

Lenox, A. C. (1990). IV therapy: Reducing the risk of infection. *Nursing, 20*(3), 60–61.

Levi, M, & ten Cate H. Disseminated intravascular coagulation. *New England Journal of Medcine, 341*(8), 586-592.

Linde-Zwirble W. T., Angus D. C., & Carcillo J. Age-specific incidence and outcome of sepsis in the US [abstract]. Critical Care Medicine, *27,* 3.

Lindley, C. M., & Deloatch, K. H. (1993). *Infusion technology manual: A self-instructional approach.* Bethesda, MD: American Society of Hospital Pharmacists.

Litjen, T., Hawk, III, J. C., Sterling, M. L. (2001, April 9). Preventing needlestick injuries in health care settings. *Archives of Internal Medicine, 161.*

Loftis, P. A., & Glover, T. L. (1993). *Decision-making in gerontologic nursing.* St. Louis, MO: Mosby.

Maki, D. G. (1989). Infection control and hospital epidemiology. *Infection Control and Hospital Epidemiology, 10*(6), 243–247.

Maki, D. G., & Ringer, M. (1987a). Evaluation of four dressing regimens for peripheral venous catheters, including gauze, a transparent dressing, and an iodophor-impregnated transparent dressing. *Journal of the American Medical Association, 258,* 2396–2403.

Maki, D. G., Botticelli, J. T., LeRoy, M. L., & Thielke, T. S. (1987b). Prospective study of replacing administration sets for intravenous therapy at 48-hour versus 72-hour intervals: 72 hours is safe and cost-effective. *Journal of the American Medical Association, 258*(13), 1777–1781.

Maki, D. G., Cobb, L., Garman, J. K., Shapiro, J. M., Ringer, M., & Helgerson, R. B. (1988). An attachable silver-impregnated cuff for prevention of infection with central venous catheters: A prospective randomized multicenter trial. *American Journal of Medicine, 85,* 307–314.

Maki, D. G., Ringer, M., & Alvarado, C. J. (1991). Prospective randomized trial of povidone-iodone, alcohol, and chlorhexidine for prevention of infection associated with central venous and arterial catheters. *Lancet, 338,* 339–343.

Maki, D. G., Wheeler, S. J., Stoltz, S. M., & Mermel, L. A. (1991, September 30 – October 2). Clinical trial of a novel antiseptic central venous catheter. In *Program and Abstracts of the 31st Interscience Conference in Antimicrobial Agents and Chemotherapy* (Abstract # 461, p. 176).

Malloy, J. (1991). Administering intraperitoneal chemotherapy: A new approach. *Nursing, 21,* 59–61.

Management of central venous catheter occlusions: The emerging role of alteplase. (1999, October). Littleton, CO: Postgraduate Institute for Medicine, sponsored by Genentech, Inc.

Masoorli, S. (1995). Know the pitfalls of IV therapy. *Nursing Service Risk Advisor, 95,* 2.

Masoorli, S. (1996). Home IV therapy comes of age. *RN,* *59*(10), 22–26.

Masoorli, S. (1997). Consult stat: Never assume anything when a patient's IV infiltrates. *Nursing, 60*(7), 65.

Masoorli, S. (1999). Iatrogenic injuries: Air embolism. *RN, 62*(11), 32–35.

Masoorli, S., & Angeles, T. (2002). Getting a line on central vascular access devices. *Nursing, 32*(4), 36–45.

Mawyer, D, & Perry, J. (2001). One nurse's fight. *RN, 64*(4), 59–60.

Mayhall, G. C. (Ed.). (1999). *Hospital epidemiology and infection control* (2nd ed.). Philadelphia: Lippincott Williams & Wilkins.

Mazur, S. (1997). *A different method of vein stimulation.* Presented at a PICC seminar sponsored by BARD Access Systems. (Available from BARD Access Systems, 5425 West Amelia Earhart Drive, Salt Lake City, UT 84116)

McCance, K. L. & Huether, S. E. (2001). *Pathophysiology: The biologic basis for disease in adults and children* (4th ed.). St. Louis, MO: Mosby.

McCloskey, J. C., & Bulechek, G. M. (Eds.). (2000). *Nursing interventions classification (NIC)* (3rd ed.). St. Louis, MO: Mosby.

McConnell, E. A. (1986). What the experts say: Air embolism in patients with central venous catheters. *Nursing Life, 2,* 47–49.

McCormick, R. D., Meisch, M. G., Ircink, F. G., & Maki, D. G. (1991). Epidemiology of hospital sharps injuries: A 14-year prospective study in the pre-AIDS and AIDS eras. *American Journal of Medicine, 91*(Supplement 3B).

McGovern, K. (1992). Ten golden rules for administering drugs safely. *Nursing, 22*(3), 49–56.

Mears, C. (1992). PICC and MLC lines: Options worth exploring. *Nursing, 22*(10), 52–55.

Medical Educational Services, Inc., & Kellett, P. B. (1996). *How to make your medical facility latex-safe.* Knoxville, TN: Medical Educational Services, Inc.

Merchant, R. C., Keshavarz, R. (2001). Human immunodeficiency virus postexposure prophylaxis for adolescents and children. *Pediatrics, 108*(2), E38.

Mermel, L. A. (2000, March 7). Prevention of intravascular catheter-related infectioins. *Annals of Internal Medicine, 132,* 391–402.

Mermel, L. A., Farr, B. M., Sherertz, R. J., Raad, I. I., O'Grady, N., Harris, J. S., & Craven, D. E. (2001, April). Guidelines for the management of intravascular catheter-related infections. *Infection Control and Hospital Epidemiology (Special Report), 22*(4).

Messner, R. L., & Pinkerman, M. L. (1992). Preventing peripheral IV infection. *Nursing, 22*(6), 34–41.

Metheny, N. M. (2000). *Fluid and electrolyte balance: Nursing considerations* (4th ed.). Philadelphia: Lippincott-Raven.

Millam, D. A. (1988). Managing complications of IV therapy. *Nursing, 18*(3), 34–42.

Millam, D. A. (1992). Starting IVs: How to develop your expertise. *Nursing, 22,* 33–48.

Millam, D. A., & Boutotte, J. (1993). Infection control update. *Nursing, 23*(10), 61–68.

Mirrop, M. (1992). *Intravenous catheterization: A guide to proper insertion techniques.* Tampa, FL: Critikon.

Moolenaar, R. L., Crutcher, J. M., San Joaquin, V. H., & Sewell, L. V. (2000). A prolonged outbreak of Pseudomonas aeruginosa in a neonatal intensive care unit: Did staff fingernails play a role in disease transmission? *Infection Control and Hospital Epidemiology, 21,* 80–85.

Moore, Kathleen. (1999). Consult Stat: AACN guidelines contain latest on PA catheter care. *RN, 62*(12), 71.

Moulton, P. J., Wray-Langevine, J., & Boyer, C. G. (1997). Implementing clinical pathways: One agency's experience. *Home Healthcare Nurse, 15*(5), 343–354.

Moureau, Nancy. (2001). Preventing complications with vascular access devices. *Nursing, 31*(7). 52–55.

Natanson, C., Esposito, C. J., Banks, S. M. (1998). The sirens' songs of confirmatory sepsis trials: Selection bias and sampling error. *Critical Care Medicine, 26,* 1927–1931.

National Alliance for Infusion Therapy. (1992). Home infusion fact sheet. *Journal of Nursing Administration, 22,* 8.

National Association for Home Care. (1999). *Basic statistics about home care.* Washington, DC: Author.

National Center for Chronic Disease Prevention and Health Promotion. (2002). *Healthy aging 2000.* Atlanta: Centers for Disease Control and Prevention.

National Center on Health Statistics. (2002). *Older Americans 2000: Key indicators of well-being.* Bethesda, MD: U. S. Department of Health and Human Services, National Institutes of Health.

National Institute for Occupational Safety and Health (NIOSH). (1997, June). *Preventing Allergic Reactions to Natural Rubber Latex in the Workplace* [DHHS (NIOSH) Publication No. 97-135]. Retrieved April 7, 2003, from http://www.cdc.gov/niosh/latexalt.html

National Institute for Occupational Safety and Health (NIOSH). (1998, January). *Selecting, Evaluating, and Using Sharps Disposal Containers* [DHHS (NIOSH) Publication No. 97-111]. Retrieved April 7, 2003, from http://www.cdc.gov/niosh/sharps1.html

Needlestick Safety and Prevention Act, Pub. L. No. 106-430 (2000). Retrieved April 7, 2003, from http://thomas.loc .gov/bss/d106/d106laws.html

Nightingale, F. (1992). *Notes on nursing: What it is and what it is not.* New York: Lippincott Williams & Wilkins.

North American Nursing Diagnosis Association (2001). *NANDA nursing diagnoses: Definitions and classification 1995–1996.* Philadelphia: Author.

A nurse with a mission: Lynda Arnold. (1996). *Advances in Exposure Prevention, 2*(2), 1, 10–11.

Nurses Service Organization. (1992). Q & As. *Nurses Service Organization Risk Advisor.* (Available from Nurses Service Organization, 159 E. County Line Road, Hatboro, PA 19040)

Occupational Safety & Health Administration (OSHA). (2001, November 27). *Enforcement procedures for the occupational exposure to blood borne pathogens, standard number: 1910.1030* [OSHA Instruction CPL 2-2.69]. Washington, D.C.: Author.

Occupational Safety & Health Administration (OSHA). (2002, August 26). *Safety and Health Topics: Latex Allergy.* Washington, D.C.: Author.

Occupational Safety and Health Administration (OSHA). (1999, February 22). *Glass capillary tubes: Joint safety advisory about potential risks.* Retrieved April 7, 2003, from http://www.osha.gov/pls/oshaweb/owadisp.show_document?p_table=INTERPRETATIONS&p_id=22695

Occupational Safety and Health Administration (OSHA). (2003, March 19). *Safety and health topics: Needlestick prevention.* Retrieved April 7, 2003, from http://www.osha-slc.gov/SLTC/needlestick/index.html

Opal, S. M. & Cohen, J. (1999). Clinical gram-positive sepsis: Does it fundamentally differ from gram-negative bacterial sepsis? *Critical Care Medicine, 27,* 1608–1616.

Otto, S. E. (1995). Advanced concepts in chemotherapy drug delivery. *Journal of Intravenous Nursing, 18*(4) 170–176.

Palmer, S., Giddens, J., & Palmer, D. (1996). *Infection control.* El Paso, TX: Skidmore-Roth Publishing, Inc.

Parry, M. F., Grant, B., Yukna, M., Adler-Klein, D., McLeod, G. X., Taddonio, R., Rosenstein, C. (2001). Candida Osteomyelitis and Diskitis after Spinal Surgery: An outbreak that Implicates Artificial Nail Use. *Clinical Infectious Diseases, 32*(3), 352–357.

Peck, K. R., & Altieri, M. (1988). Intraosseous infusions: An old technique with modern applications. *Pediatric Nursing, 14*(4), 296–298.

Pennsylvania Medical Society Center for Professional Drug Education. (2002, February 10). *Drug Alert! Streptase is not indicated for restoration of patency of intravenous catheters.* Retrieved April 7, 2003, from http://www.counterdetails.org/alert.html

Perry, J. (2001a). Attention All Nurses! *American Journal of Nursing, 101*(9), 24AA–24CC.

Perry, J. (2001b). The Bloodborne Pathogens Standard, 2001. *Nursing, 31*(6), 16.

Perry, J. (2001c). The Bloodborne Pathogens Standard, 2001: What's changed? *Nursing Management, 32*(6), 25–26.

Perry, J., Parker, G., & Jagger, J. (2001). Percutaneous injuries in home healthcare settings. *Home Healthcare Nurse, 19*(6), 342–344.

Perry, J. (2001d). The Bloodborne Pathogens Standard, 2001: What's changed. *Dimensions of Critical Care Nursing, 20*(5), 44–45.

Perry, J. (2001e). When home is where the risk is. *Home Healthcare Nurse, 19*(6), 338–341.

Petsonk, E. L. (1997). Nurses should take action to avoid occupational latex allergy. *Journal of Emergency Nursing, 23*(2), 91.

Phifer, T. J., Bridges, M., & Conrad, S. A. (1991). The residual central venous catheter track—An occult source of lethal air embolism: Case report. *Journal of Intravenous Nursing, 31,* 1558–1560.

Phipps, W. J., Long, B. C., Woods, N. W., & Cassmeyer, V. L. (2003). *Medical-surgical nursing: Concepts and clinical practice* (7th ed.). St. Louis, MO: Mosby.

Pickar, G. D. (1999). *Dosage calculations* (6th ed.). Albany, NY: Delmar.

Potts, N. (2002). Pediatric nursing: Caring for children and their families. Clifton Park, NY: Delmar Thomson Learning.

Pozzar, G. D. (2002). *Legal aspects of health care administration* (8th ed.). Gaithersburg, MD: Aspen.

Pugliese, G., Germanson, T. P., Bartley, J., Luca, J., Lamerato, L., & Cox, J. (2001). Evaluating sharps safety devices: Meeting OSHA's intent. *Infection Control & Hospital Epidemiology, 22*(7), 456–458.

Pugliese, G., & Salahuddin, M. (Eds.). (1999) Sharps injury prevention program: A step-by-sep guide. Chicago: American Hospital Association..

Rangel-Frausto, M. S., Pittet, D., & Costigan, M. (1995). The natural history of the systemic inflammatory response syndrome (SIRS): A prospective study. *Journal of the American Medical Association, 273,* 117–123.

Rathbun, J. (1996). A plague upon our houses. *Columns, The University of Washington Alumni Magazine, 16*(2), 14–17.

Reddy, Sumana. (1998, January 1). Latex allergy. *American Family Physician.*

Reiss, B. S., & Evans, M. E. (2002). *Pharmacological aspects of nursing care* (6th ed.). Albany, NY: Delmar.

Reiss, P. (1996). Battling the superbugs. *RN, 59*(3), 36–40.

Rhinehart, Emily. (2002). Infection control in home care. *Emerging Infectious Diseases, 7*(2).

Rice, J., & Skelley, E. G. (2001). *Medications and mathematics for the nurse* (9th ed.). Albany, NY: Delmar.

RN News Watch Clinical Highlights. (1999). Autologous blood donation isn't crucial anymore. *RN, 62*(4), 18–19.

Robertson, K. J. (1995). The role of the IV specialist in health care reform. *Journal of Intravenous Nursing, 18*(3), 130–144.

Sadovsky, R. (2000, August 15). Preventing Intravascular Catheter-Related Infections. *American Family Physician.*

Sandford, J. P., Gilbert, D. N., & Sande, M. A. (2002). *Guide to antimicrobial therapy* (32nd ed.). Dallas, TX: Antimicrobial Therapy, Inc.

Sands, K. E, Bates, D. W., & Lanken, P. N. (1997). Epidemiology of sepsis syndrome in 8 academic medical centers. *Journal of the American Medical Association, 278,* 234–240.

Sansivero, G. E. (1995). Why a PICC? What you need to know. *Nursing, 18*(3), 34–42.

Sapolsky, R. M. (1992). Stress and neuroendocrine changes during aging. *Generations, 16*(4), 35–38.

Scher, R. K. & Daniel, C.R. (1990). *Nails: therapy, diagnosis, surgery* (pp. 220–222). Philadelphia: W. B. Saunders.

Scott, B. D. (1996). *Techniques of regional anesthesia.* Norwalk, CT: Appleton & Lange/Mediglobe.

Spratto, G. R., & Woods, A. L. (2003). *PDR nurse's drug handbook.* Clifton Park, NY: Delmar Learning.

Springhouse Corporation. (2001a). *Clinical laboratory tests: Values & implications* (3rd ed.). Springhouse, PA: Author.

Springhouse Corporation. (2001b). *Professional guide to diseases* (7th ed.). Springhouse, PA: Author.

Springhouse Corporation. (2002). *Illustrated manual of nursing practice.* Springhouse, PA: Author.

St. Marie, B. (1994). *Management of cancer pain with epidural morphine independent study module.* St. Paul, MN: Sims Deltec, Inc. and Wyeth-Ayerst Laboratories.

Stedman's medical dictionary (27th ed.). (2000). Baltimore: Williams & Wilkins.

Stone, S. (1999). *Clinical gerontological nursing* (2nd ed.). Philadelphia: W. B. Saunders.

Swearingen, P. (2002). *Medical-surgical nursing diagnosis & interventions* (5th ed.). St. Louis, MO: Mosby.

Taber's Cyclopedic Medical Dictionary (19th ed.). (2001). Philadelphia: F.A. Davis Company.

Tappen, R. M., & Beckerman, A. (1993). A vulnerable population: Multiproblem older adults in acute care. *Journal of Gerontological Nursing, 19*(11), 38–42.

Thielen, J. B. (1996). Air emboli: A potentially lethal complication of central venous lines. *Focus on Critical Care, 17*(5), 374–383.

Thielen, J. B., & Nyquist, J. (1992). Subclavian catheter removal. *Journal of Intravenous Nursing, 14,* 114–118.

Townsend, Carolyn E. & Roth, R. (2002). *Nutrition & diet therapy* (8th ed). Clifton Park, NY: Delmar Learning.

Training for Development of Innovative Control Technologies (TDICT) Project. (n.d.) *Safety feature evaluation forms.* Retrieved April 7, 2003, from http://www.tdict.org/criteria.html

Ulrich, S. P., Canale, S. W., & Wendell, S. A. (2001). *Nursing care planning guides: A nursing diagnosis approach* (5th ed.). Philadelphia: W. B. Saunders.

U.S. Bureau of the Census. (2000, January 13). *Current population reports: Projections of the total resident population by 5 year age groups, race, and hispanic origin with special age categories: middle series, 1999 to 2000.* Washington, D.C.: Author.

U.S. Bureau of the Census (2002). *A profile of older americans: 2001.* Washington, D.C.: U.S. Administration on Aging.

U.S. Department of Health and Human Services (DHHS). (1990). *Transfusion therapy guidelines for nurses* [NIH Pub. No. 90-2668]. Bethesda, MD: National Institutes of Health.

U.S. Department of Health and Human Services (DHHS). (1991). *Transfusion alert: Use of autologous blood* [NIH Pub. No. 91-3038]. Bethesda, MD: National Institutes of Health.

U.S. Department of Health and Human Services (DHHS). (2001, January 18). *New needlestick rule: Occupational exposure to bloodborne pathogens; needlestick and other sharps injuries; final rule* [Federal Register# 66:5317-5325]. Atlanta, GA: Centers for Disease Control and Prevention.

U.S. Department of Veterans Affairs (VA). (2002, February 8). *Safety sharp device contracts.* Retrieved April 7, 2003, from http://www.va.gov/vasafety/page.cfm?pg=542

U.S. Food and Drug Administration (FDA). (1999a, January 25). *Important drug warning: Safety information regarding the use of Abbokinase (Urokinase).* Rockville, MD: Public Health Service.

U.S. Food and Drug Administration (FDA). (1999b, March 25). *Statement on latex allergies by Elizabeth D. Jacobson, Ph.D., Acting Director, Center for Devices and Radiological Health before the House Committee on Education and the Workforce, Subcommittee on Oversight and Investigations.* Rockville, MD: U.S. Department of Health and Human Services.

U.S. Food and Drug Administration (FDA). (2002a, February). *Keeping blood transfusions safe: FDA's Multi-layered protections for donated blood* [Publication No. FS 02-1]. Rockville, MD: U.S. Department of Health and Human Services.

U.S. Food and Drug Administration (FDA). (2002b, July 12). *Public Health Notification: PVC Devices Containing the Plasticizer DEHP.* Rockville, MD: U.S. Department of Health and Human Services.

U.S. Food and Drug Administration (FDA). (2003) *Safety alerts, public health advisories and notices from CDRH.* Retrieved April 7, 2003, from http://www.fda.gov/cdrh/safety.html

U.S. General Accounting Office. (2000, November 17). *Occupational safety: Selected cost and benefit implications of needlestick prevention devices for hospitals* [DCGAO-01-60R,: pp. 1–18]. Washington, DC: Author.

Veal, D. F., Altman, C. E., McKinnon, B. T., & Fillingim, O. (1995). Evaluation of flow rates for six disposable infusion devices. *American Journal of Health-System Pharmacists, 52,* 500–504.

Vervloet, M.G., Thijs, L. G., & Hack, C. E. (1998). Derangements of coagulation and fibrinolysis in critically ill patients with sepsis and septic shock. *Seminars in Thrombotic Hemostasis, 24,* 33–44.

Viall, C. D. (1990). Your complete guide to central venous catheters. *Nursing, 2,* 34–41.

Weinstein, Robert A. (1998, July-Sept,). Nosocomial Infection Update. *Emerging Infectious Diseases, 4*(3).

Wen-Tsung, L., Chih-Chien, A., & Mong-Ling C. (2002) A nursery outbreak of Staphylococcus aureus pyoderma originating from a nurse with paronychia. *Infection Control and Hospital Epidemiology, 23,* 153–155.

Wenzel, R. P., Rinsky, M. R., Ulevitch, R. J., et al. (1996). Current understanding of sepsis. *Clinical Infectious Diseases, 22,* 407–413.

Whaley, L. F., & Wong, D. L. (2001). *Nursing care of infants and children* (6th ed.). St. Louis, MO: Mosby.

Wheeler, A. P. & Bernard, G. R. (1999). Treating patients with severe sepsis. *New England Journal of Medicine, 340,* 207–214.

White, K. M. (1997). Understanding the hemodynamics of sepsis. In *Critical care choices 1997.* Bethlehem, PA: Springhouse Corp.

Whitehouse, M. J. (1992a). Nursing assessment of the elderly patient. *Journal of Intravenous Nursing, 15* (Supplement), S14–S17.

Whitehouse, M. J. (1992b). The physiology of aging. *Journal of Intravenous Nursing, 15* (Supplement), S7–S13.

Wilkes, G. M., Burke, M. B., & Ingwersen, K. (2002). *Oncology nursing drug handbook.* Boston: Jones and Bartlett Publishers, Inc..

Wilkinson, J. M. (2002). *Nursing diagnosis handbook with NIC interventions and NOC outcomes* (7th Ed.). Upper Saddle River, NJ: Prentice Hall.

Yamamoto, A. J., Solomon, J. A., Soulen, M. C., Tang, J., Parkinson, K., & Lin, R. (2002). Sutureless securement device reduces implications of peripherally inserted central venous catheters. *Journal of Vascular and Interventional Radiology, 13,* 77–81.

Zeni, F., Freeman, B., & Natanson, C. Anti-inflammatory therapies to treat sepsis and septic shock: A reassessment. *Critical Care Medicine, 25,* 1095–1100.

Zuger, A. (1995). When microbes can't be stopped. *Healthnews, 1*(4), 4.

Index

procarbazine, 273
progesterone, 283
prolactin, 281
proportions, mathematical calculations and, 247
proteases, 113
PROTECTIV IV catheter safety system, 178f
protein buffer system, 34
protein solutions, 137
proteins, 20, 24, 28, 137, 395, 396–397, 396f, 427
Proteus, 111
protoplasm, 19
proximal port, 299
Pseudomonas, 66, 70, 74, 111, 296
psychodynamics in elderly and geriatric patients, 490
psychological preparation of patient, 150–153, 152f
psychosocial needs of pediatric patients and, 468–469
pulmonary artery monitoring, 383–384, 385f
pulmonary circulation, 147f, 488
pulmonary edema, 35, 39
pulmonary embolism, 35, 116, 116f
pulsatile flushing (push-pause) technique, 309
pumps, for EIDs, 188
pus, 102
push, IV push (*See also* bolus injections), 230, 237

quinolones, 270

random donor platelets, 421–422
ratio and proportions, 247
reactions to blood transfusions, 436–441
reaction-specific enzymes, 19
reagins, 113
reasonableness doctrine, in malpractice, 51
red blood cells, 414–416, 419–420
red flare, 114
refeeding syndrome, 409
refractory period, 30
refusal by patient for procedure, 160
registered nurse (RN), 3–4
regulating infusions, 253
regulation of fluids and electrolytes, 30–32
regulations, 3–4
related factors, 5
related to (RT), 6
relative refractory period, 30
releasing factor (RF), 280
removal and discontinuation routines, 325–328
renal disease, 36, 39, 43
renal failure, 41, 44, 45
renal formulas, nutritional support and, 402

renal system, 31
  elderly and geriatric patients and, 488–489
  pediatric patients and, 455–456
RenAmine, 137
repolarization, 30
reporting, 56, 226
reporting errors, 56
Resectisol, 131
reservoir of infection, 68
resident flora, infection control and, 67
resistance, of host to disease, 69
resistant organisms, 67–68, 77, 78, 268–269
respiration, 31
respiratory acidosis (carbonic acid excess), 34–35, 36f
respiratory agents, 285
respiratory alkalosis (carbonic acid deficit), 35, 36f
respiratory system, 32
respiratory crisis in pediatric patients, 463
respiratory rate in pediatric patients and, 466
resting membrane potential, 29
restraints, pediatric patients and, 473
retrograde leakage, 356
retrograde medication administration technique, 477, 477f
Rh factor (Factor D), 415–416
Rh immune globulin, 430
rifampin, 271
right to refuse treatment, 9
Ringer's lactate (*See* lactated Ringer's)
Ringer's solution, 128
risk-benefit analysis, 496
risk factors, 5
risks, complications, adverse reactions, 92–120
  anaphylaxis and, 113–114
  catheter and needle displacement in, 99
  cellulitis and, 108–109
  contamination and infection in, 110
  elderly and geriatric patients and, 493–494
  embolism in, 114–118
  extravasation and, 96–99, 100f
  hematoma in, 106–107
  hypersensitivity reactioin in, 113–115
  infiltration and, 96–99
  local problems and complications in, 94–110
  medication and fluid interaction in, 112–113
  nerve, tendon, ligament, limb damage in, 109–110
  occlusion and loss of patency in, 232–236
  occlusion and loss of patency in, 99–102

  pain and irritation in, 94–96
  pediatric patients and, 475–476
  phlebitis in, 102–105
  sepsis in, 110–112, 112f
  speed shock and, 118–119
  systemic complications in, 95, 110–119
  thrombosis and thrombophlebitis in, 105–106, 105f
  venous spasm and, 107–108
  vessel collapse and, 108
rounding off, mathematical calculations and, 251
route of medication, 54–55

safety (*See also* infection control and safety), 63–89, 153
safety of blood supply, 432
salicylate poisoning, 35, 36
saline locks, 102, 368
Salmonella, 463
salts, 18, 33, 39
scalp access, pediatric patients and, 473, 473f
sclerosis, 194, 201
scoop technique, 87
score card for pediatric patients, 469–470
sebaceous glands, 145
secondary administration sets, 170, 170f
secondary medication administration piggybacking, 229–230
securing site with dressing and tape, 223–225
sedatives, 280–283
seizure disorders, 43
Seldinger technique, PICCs, 351
selenium, 400, 409
semi-Fowler's position, 154, 156f
semirigid plastic containers, 165–166, 166f
sense organs, elderly and geriatric patients and, 489–490
sensitization, 113
sepsis, 10–11, 66, 77, 110–112, 112f, 294, 296, 439
septicemia, 501–502, 503
serotonin, 283
Serratia, 111
serum, 123
serum ammonia elevation, 407
serum globulins, 427–430
serum sodium level, pediatric patients and, recovery rate in, 460
serum urea elevation, 407
setup for IV therapy, 204–205
Shigella, 463
shock, 36, 118–119
short term goals, 6
shunt, 155f, 194
side effects of drugs, 112–113, 265, 286, 495
SideKick positive pressure drug delivery system, 190f